1

Mathematics, Physics, and Engineering in Medicine

GH-Method: Math-Physical Medicine

VOLUME ONE

Mathematics, Physics, and Engineering in Medicine

GH-Method: Math-Physical Medicine

VOLUME ONE

By Gerald C. Hsu

For additional information, please visit: www.eclairemd.com

978-1-7332583-1-9

Mathematics, Physics, and Engineering in Medicine
GH-Method: Math-Physical Medicine
Volume One
Gerald C. Hsu

978-1-7332583-1-9

First Edition June 2021
Printed in the United States of America

Website: www.eclairemd.com

Cover and Interior Design: Epicenter Creative

Introduction:

Diagnosed with Type II diabetes at the height of his career as a Silicon Valley CEO, Gerald Hsu spent the next decade relying on prescribed medication to control his condition. Unfortunately, his health continued to deteriorate.

From 1991 to 2006, he suffered five cardiac episodes due to severe stress from work and an unhealthy lifestyle. By 2010, having been on three diabetes medications for 15 years, he was further diagnosed with several severe complications. This included obesity, chronic kidney damage, diabetic neuropathy, foot ulcer, bladder infections, retinopathy, and hypothyroidism.

Refusing to succumb to a life of insulin injections and dialysis treatments, Gerald took it upon himself to study and research chronic diseases and food nutrition. Since 2010, he has studied and performed medical research every day, averaging twelve to fourteen hours a day. Thus far, he has spent nearly 30,000 hours on the study of internal medicine.

Utilizing the software system he developed to identify, assess, treat, and monitor his diabetes, Gerald was able to reverse much of the damage done to his health and reduce the dosages of his medications until he ceased taking them completely by December 2015, five years after taking personal responsibility for his health.

Throughout his seventeen-year academic career, he has studied seven disciplines, including mathematics, computer science, mechanical engineering, structural engineering, bioengineering, ocean engineering, and business (finance and marketing) at seven universities. He spent nine additional years studying abnormal psychology and behavioral science on his own and established four psychotherapy centers that specialized in the care of hundreds of abused and traumatized children and women from 2002 to 2010.

Having spent more than half his life studying and learning ten different academic disciplines, Gerald had a unique perspective on how to approach medical research despite his lack of formal training in biology and chemistry. He relied on his knowledge and experience with mathematics, physics, computer science, statistics, engineering, quantum mechanics, theory of elasticity, energy theory, signal processing, wave theory, optical physics, big data analytics, machine learning, and artificial intelligence to conduct his medical research work.

He named his engineering and mathematics-based quantitative approach "math-physical medicine" to distinguish it from traditional "biochemical medicine." His main focus is on precision and preventive medicine using various medical prediction tools he developed with his Silicon Valley high-tech experience. He believes that the more accurate prediction a patient has, the better control that patient will have over their health. This has proven to be the case for Gerald.

Thus far, he has written four hundred thirty-four papers and published over four hundred of them in over one-hundred medical and science journals. Prior to the COVID-19 pandemic, he attended over sixty-five international medical conferences and delivered one hundred twenty oral presentations.

In the past six months, four international journals (including three Medical journals and one Science & Engineering journal) published four special editions which exclusively featured twenty to twenty-five of his papers. This book is the assembled volume of published papers in those four journals.

After eleven years thus far of continuous efforts, Gerald has saved his own life. Now, his new goal is to share his knowledge so he can help his family, other patients like himself, and medical professionals.

Gerald does not have a medical degree, nor a professional medical license to practice medicine. He has not received financial assistance from any organization and has relied solely on his own financial resources to conduct his research. He has no connection or alliance with any medical institution, industrial sponsor, or governmental agency.

Gerald holds a Master of Engineering degree from the Massachusetts Institute of Technology. He also holds an honorary PhD in applied mathematics.

Acknowledgements:

Foremost, I would like to express my deep appreciation to my former professors: Professor James Andrews at the University of Iowa, who helped develop my foundation in basic engineering and computer science, and Professor Norman Jones at the Massachusetts Institute of Technology, who taught me the right work attitude combined with useful and excellent research methodologies to solve tough scientific problems.

I owe a deep debt of gratitude to my father, a western medicine-trained MD, for passing along his wisdom to me and exposing me to the medical world; and to my mother, a retired nurse, for raising me to be persistent and to have strong willpower in life.

Last, but not the least, I would like to acknowledge and thank my beloved wife, Li Li, who is the best partner anyone could have. Her tireless love, encouragement, and support for everything I have done in my life has made all the difference. Thank you, Li Li, for sticking by me through twenty-eight years of my entrepreneurship struggles, and eleven years of my obsessive medical research.

Table of Contents

Preface

An introduction of the author's medical research history and methodologies from 2010 to 2021

Introduction

From 2010 to 2021, the author utilized his previously learned knowledge from seven academic disciplines to develop various medical research methodologies, models, and techniques in order to analyze and present results of multiple health issues related to chronic diseases.

This article is organized into 5 parts:
  1. Background
  2. Stage 1 (2010-2013): Self-study of endocrinology and software development
  3. Stage 2 (2014-2017): Metabolism and glucose control of type 2 diabetes
  4. Stage 3 (2018-2021): Diabetes induced complications and other chronic diseases
  5. Epilogue

Part 1:
Background

The author spent seventeen years studying seven disciplines across seven colleges. These seven disciplines include: applied mathematics, computer science, mechanical engineering, biomechanics, ocean engineering, structural engineering, and business (finance & marketing).

In addition, he self-studied electronics engineering for twelve years during his professional career in artificial intelligence (AI) based auto-design of various semiconductor chips.

From 1976 to 2002, the author alternated between working as an engineer or starting new ventures as an entrepreneur. During this time, he worked in seven major industries which include: aerospace & defense, naval battle ships and weapon systems, nuclear power, earthquake engineering, computer hardware, computer software, and semiconductors. Most of his professional experiences related to real applications of industrial projects, computer science products (both hardware and software), and artificial intelligence (AI) applications. He also invented a portable computer, a smart printer, a three-dimensional computer-aided design software for architecture and mechanical design, scientific development of software robotics, and medical AI prediction systems. Throughout his early professional career, he conducted research and development tasks daily, but did not publish any academic papers since college.

After selling his successful and publicly traded semiconductor company in mid-2002, he spent seven more years studying abnormal psychology and an additional two years studying behavioral psychology. Throughout this nine-year period, he read sixty-eight psychology textbooks and over five hundred clinical reports on psychotherapy along with several published psychology papers. He went on to establish five psychotherapy centers to treat over two hundred traumatized women and children. During 2002-2010, he gained practical knowledge through his day-to-day involvement with the psychotherapy centers. In 1994, he attempted his 8th venture and later built it into the leading AI-based semiconductor chip design tool company in the world. This new venture catapulted him into the position of highest paid CEO among 15,000 CEOs in Silicon Valley between 1999 to 2002. Through his continuous hard work and dedication over twenty-six years, he accumulated his wealth and success in the high-tech industry.

However, this business fortune did not contribute to his overall wellbeing. On the contrary, it was detrimental to his health. He suffered five cardiac episodes between 1994 and 2006. At that time, he believed the heart attacks were a result of work-related stress only. However, he eventually came to realize it was from a combination of intense stress and neglect of his diabetic condition.

In 2010, his Albumin-to-Creatinine Ratio (ACR) reached 116 (maximum normal range is 30). Also, his weight was at 220 pounds (99.8 kilograms), his Body Mass Index (BMI) was 32.5, his A1C was above 10 percent, and his average glucose was at ~380 mg/dL. He suffered from hypertension, hyperlipidemia (triglycerides at 1161 mg/dL), cardiac episodes, bladder infections, foot ulcers, diabetic fungal infections, and hypothyroidism. Three separate medical doctors advised him that he would most likely need to begin kidney dialysis treatment soon if his condition didn't improve. At the time, he was sixty-three years old and had been taking the maximum dosages of three diabetes medications for the past decade. The three doctors also informed him that he was likely to die within three to five years. This life-threatening message, combined with the threat of painful kidney dialysis treatments, was the final wakeup call.

In August 2010, he moved from Silicon Valley to Las Vegas to escape his daily stress associated with the fast-paced Bay Area high-tech lifestyle. By October 2010, he closed all his remaining business operations and activities and decided to focus on saving his life. *He made a vow to himself that he would figure out what went wrong with his health and how to fix it through his own medical study and research.*

The three diabetes medications he took for the past decade had not improved his diabetes condition and various related complications. Through his study and research, he found that these medications only dealt with his symptoms and not the root causes of his condition. Therefore, his diabetic symptoms continued to go up and down based on his lack of a consistent healthy lifestyle. Through much trial and error, he was able to slowly taper off his medications over a four-year period. By December 2015, he was able to cease taking all prescribed medications. He has since successfully managed his diabetic condition solely through lifestyle management (diet, exercise, sleep, and stress management). As of October of 2021, his A1C is at 5.8 percent, estimated average glucose (eAG) is 106 mg/dL, weight is 168 pounds (76.2 kilograms), and BMI is 24.8. There are no more presented signs of diabetic complications, except for a diabetic fungal infection.

This is the short version of his story on how *he had no choice but to rely on his own efforts to save his life!*

In the author's personal view, there is a hierarchy structure of sciences. At the bottom, or foundation, is mathematics. Mathematics presents clear problems and exact answers. Applied mathematics (above mathematics) has three branches consisting of physics, computer science, and statistics. Further up this hierarchy (above physics) is applied physics which has three branches consisting of engineering, biology, and chemistry. Above biology and chemistry are medicine and pharmacology. Finally, psychology sits above medicine and pharmacology. The higher position in this science hierarchy, the more applicable it is at addressing practical problems. However, it also moves further away from the foundation of mathematics. Therefore, it's ability to solve tough problems in the real world can become somewhat limited and difficult.

Another personal view from the author is that there is an abundance of intelligent and capable predecessors (i.e. innovators, scholars, scientists) who have already discovered or invented so many amazing and useful facts, concepts, theories, equations, and models. The author feels there is no need to reinvent the wheel and instead should apply existing theories, equations, models, and inventions (using mathematics and physics as bases) in order to save research time and effort, and develop new breakthroughs in the process. Under this logic, the author's developed GH-Method: math-physical medicine is not an invention, it is merely another application using the most fundamental branches of mathematics and physics to apply them within medical research.

Part 2:
Stage 1 (2010-2013): self-study & software development

From the fortune the author made through his high-tech venture successes, it became a habit for him to "buy" rather than to "make" something he needed. From 2010-2011, he used his own funds to hire eighty-two medical doctors in China and six part-time doctors in the US to assist him on his medical research project. By November 2011, he realized he had not achieved his goal of learning more about diabetes and its complications. He spent most of his time and effort managing other people's work instead of expanding his own knowledge sphere.

By the end of 2011, he decided to start over and do everything himself, without the aid of hired medical researchers. The main purpose of his research was to further expand his knowledge base in order to save his own life. During the past twelve years of dedicated medical research work, he finally figured out how to turn himself from an engineer and a businessman into a medical research scientist.

However, his "do-it-yourself" approach had one major drawback. It took him much longer and with much more effort to read all the medical papers and textbooks in order to figure out the hidden inter-connectivity between different internal organs and diseases.

Initially, he decided to focus on studying endocrinological diseases and food nutrition. At first, he couldn't fully understand the medical terminology in the textbooks and papers he read. He only understood parts of introductions and conclusions and didn't understand the sections on methods and results. Sometimes he would reread papers ten or more times in order to truly understand their methods and conclusions. Through his stubborn and tenacious approach to conquering all challenges, he was finally able to comprehend the readings. Thus far, he has skimmed or read through 50-80 medical textbooks and ~2,000 published medical papers.

The central pathway of his self-study and research is from lifestyle through metabolism to chronic diseases and then into their induced complications, such as heart, brain, kidney, eyes, nerves, etc. Recently, he also expanded his self-learning scope from metabolism through immunity to infectious diseases, as well as into areas such as cancers and dementia (which are metabolic disorder related diseases). His focus has always been on prevention and control of diseases, not medical interventions or treatments, because he does not have a medical license.

From 2002 to 2010, he developed a "software robot" product. One of his previous dreams was to develop an AI-based software architecture which can automatically generate the needed software codes using Java language based on user defined and described system requirements via a common interface language of English. By 2009, he completed the design and code development of this software robot's prototype which was ready for commercialization. However, in 2010, he became very sick and had to give up on this product. When he started his self-learning of internal medicine in 2011, he decided to develop a dedicated medical research software tool utilizing his ready-made software robot as its architecture base. Since 2011, the development and enhancement of his medical software tool, "eclaireMD Chronic", has been ongoing and will continue into the foreseeable future. He continues to add and strengthen the software while collecting his own and a few other patients' real-life data of medical conditions and lifestyle details for analyses. Thus far, he has collected ~3 million data regarding his own health conditions and lifestyle details along with an additional ~6 million cleaned and reorganized food nutrition data transferred from the United States Department of Agriculture (USDA).

The "big data analytics" approach is extremely practical and useful for his medical research project. Almost ~90% of existing medical papers he has read uses the statistics approach. Unfortunately, statistics has its fair share of shortcomings and is sometimes mathematically debatable (depending on certain situations and constraints). The author has also used some statistics tools, such as regression models and probabilities, to conduct some of his medical research projects. A well-organized and cleaned database can indeed provide many different and useful views of a problem from different angles. For example, a person can depict a fruit cake using equations, formulas, or languages to describe the starchy outer shell with white creamy surface color, various fruits inside, and chocolate as the topping. However, the big data analytics approach is like using a knife to cut this fruit cake in any desirable angle. Each different cutting angle can reveal different views of this same fruit cake; therefore, they can offer additional information about the inside views of this cake. If we compare this cake analogy to a human body, we can see its power and applicability on dealing with human health and medical issues.

Artificial intelligence is just another add-on tool to collect all stored knowledge and previous experiences to provide an accurate prediction of the future. This AI approach is extremely useful for the tasks of a simulation or prediction.

Since 2010, the author has spent between 30,000 to 40,000 hours during the past ~12 years to study and research nutrition, lifestyles, diseases, and health. In total, including his previous nine years of psychology study, he has already spent ~21 years on the general subject of "health and happiness." This twenty-one year investment has no relation to his younger self's desire of chasing power, fame, and money. Now, he strives for the two fundamental elements of any person's life - health and happiness.

Part 3
Stage 2 (2014-2017): Metabolism and Glucoses
GH-Method: math-physical medicine
Since the author has never studied biology or chemistry, he cannot apply his knowledge and tools to these two disciplines to study medicine in a traditional way. He must rely on his learned theories and concepts from mathematics, physics, modeling techniques, and engineering to observe different biophysical phenomena (a result of biological structure and its internal chemical interactions) before collecting, organizing, and analyzing collected data in order to derive accurate analysis results or useful predictions. After data analysis, he will then establish some accurate mathematical models and derive adequate equations in order to predict their future behaviors, outcomes or outputs correctly. During this data process and data analysis, knowledge of computer science applications, including both big data analytics and artificial intelligence, are heavily utilized. That was the process he previously used to design space shuttle, naval battle ships, nuclear power plants, computer devices, software robots, and semiconductor design tools. In December 2017, he attended the International Diabetes Federation annual conference in Abu Dhabi and made his first presentation on his unique medical research approach, which he would later name the GH-Method: math-physical medicine (MPM).

Metabolism Index Model

The author spent the entire year of 2014 to develop his metabolism model. Metabolism is dealing with energy inputs and outputs of the body. At first, he was inspired by the topology concept of mathematics. He observed that the human body with its various internal organs are very similar to the mathematical concept of a topological subject because its fundamental characteristics are retained and unchanged even under various types and degrees of deformation. If there is no partial rupture of an organ or a total break-down of certain biomedical systems inside a body (poor lifestyle practices and bad habits may damage or deform the organs and the total system of a body), then the basic characteristics of a body and its organs remain the same. Even if the subjects' or body's biomarker values are altered and is still within its allowed limitations, the human body's life and organ functions are savable because the body's original characteristics and functions are preserved.

Secondly, he applied the finite element method of engineering that he studied at MIT in 1973 to build up his metabolism model. He subdivided human health and energy into ten different but interrelated categories and a total of nearly five hundred detailed elements. These ten categories are four basic medical conditions (weight, glucose, blood pressure, and blood lipid) and six lifestyle details (food and meals, water consumption, exercise, sleep, stress, and daily routines). Each category contains a different number of elements. For example, stress has over forty elements, sleep has over ten elements, and daily life routines and habits have over fifty elements. The category of food and meals is the most complex category, which contains several hundred elements. This metabolism is not a "big data" problem but rather a "big relationship" problem. This is because the total possible relationships among those ten categories is a large number. In theory, there are ~3.629 million possible relationships (=10!), like having 3.629 million rubber bands encircling ten nails on a piece of a wooden board. At first, we nail in those ten category nails at thirty-six degrees each, centered around the origin of the circle. When we start to change the location of these nails by either moving toward the inside or toward the outside of the circle which is similar to moving the glucose value outward (higher glucose) or inward (lower glucose), it creates stress (expansion or contraction) inside of these rubber bands. He further defines the total metabolism as the summation of all those stresses inside of those 3.629 million rubber bands. Of course, this is a difficult problem to be solved if we want to identify an exact answer. Therefore, he came up with an approximation model using geometric algebra operations to calculate his desired Metabolism Index (MI) value. The final equation derived for calculating this approximated MI value has been written on paper, totaling fourteen pages.

Glucose and HbA1C predictions:

From 2015 to 2018, he developed the following 4 math-physical models (using prediction equations, not relying solely on statistical tools):

1. Weight prediction model (2015)
2. Postprandial Plasma Glucose (PPG) prediction models (2015)
3. Fasting Plasma Glucose (FPG) prediction model (2016)
4. HbA1C prediction models (2016)

The above four prediction models achieved a linear accuracy between 95 percent to 99.9 percent. In addition, he was able to figure out the major influential factors and their contribution margins for these four biomarkers. For example, FPG has five contributing factors and PPG has nineteen contributing factors.

Optical Physics, Big Data & AI:

The most complicated category of the MI model is food and diet which possesses the biggest portion of his collected data. Furthermore, the link between PPG and carbohydrate and sugar (carbs/sugar) intake amounts is the toughest to deduce. He has tried the PPG prediction method using a popular concept in the nutrition field, glycemic index (GI) and glycemic load (GL), but the derived results based on GI were unsatisfactory. GL involves quantity of food which is troublesome to collect on a daily basis. In 2015, he thought that the different ingredients, especially carbs/sugar amounts, were the reflection of the different internal molecular structure of plants or meats, and that different molecular structures would result in different optical waves (further turning into a different color of food material). The amplitude, frequency, and wavelength of those optical waves (color of food material) could indicate the type of ingredient and the portion amount. Therefore, by applying optical physics principles and optical wave theory, he explored their internal linkages through software programming. A standard iPhone camera can take a meal's photo with 20 megapixels in one picture, or 20 million optical pixels. Each light pixel is represented by a unique combination of 8 alpha-numerical digits. Each meal's photo using an iPhone camera would capture 160 million digits, which could be utilized to calculate the intake amount of carbs/sugar within each meal. By utilizing his developed PPG prediction model, he could obtain the predicted PPG value instantly. The iPhone's computer processing unit (CPU) is fully capable of processing these 160 million digits within a few seconds. Using this optical physics approach, along with big data analytics and developed AI algorithms, it yielded an extremely high prediction accuracy of greater than 99.5 percent on his Predicted PPG values. This calculated prediction accuracy is based on a total of 7,568 food photos (7,128 daily meals with 440 snacks/fruits) during the past six and a half years.

Input versus output (root cause vs. symptom):

When the author was an engineering student, his professor told the students that they should always try to locate or identify the inter-connection or inter-relationship between the input (root causes of disease or external forces on a structure) and output (symptom of disease or structural deformation). In early 2015, the author struggled for almost one year trying to identify the real reason behind his elevated FPG. At first, he analyzed his FPG data (metabolism output or symptom of disease) against lifestyle inputs, such as food, exercise, sleep, and stress, but could not find any connections. On March 17, 2016, he woke up at 3AM from a dream and realized that he must not be constrained by his previous learning from engineering schools, and instead should think out-of-the-box about this elevated FPG problem. He then started to compare his FPG against his other biomarkers (metabolism outputs). He analyzed the relationship between FPG against PPG, blood pressure, and lipid without any success. By 7:00 in the morning, he finally found that his body weight and his FPG (both belong to the outputs of a body) had an extremely high correlation coefficient of over 90 percent. It turns out that his elevated FPG of 17 mg/dL was caused by his elevated weight of six pounds from March 2014 to March 2015. He had over-eaten fatty nuts and seeds (both food quantity and food quality, lifestyle input elements m9a and m9b), therefore his body weight gradually increased from 175 to 181 pounds, which then further elevated his FPG (medical conditions output m2) by 17 mg/dL from 118 md/dL to 135 mg/dL. This medical example explains that we can examine one symptom against another symptom in order to identify some hidden connections.

In 2021, he read an article on cancer which had some difficulties identifying the direct linkage of symptoms between diabetes and cancers. However, the author started to compare their root causes and identified that around 60 to 70 percent of root causes for both diabetes and cancers are identical. After all, cancers are just another type of metabolic disorder and chronic disease. But cancers have rather unique "environmental" root causes, such as poison, pollution, radiation, and hormone treatments, while diabetes do not have those environmental causes.

Part 4:
Stage 3 (2018-2021): Diabetes induced complications and other chronic diseases

Data Presentation of Segmentation and Contribution Analyses

Every biomarker's data range can be segmented using "from-to" time ranges or "high, medium, low" amplitude ranges, such as the ADA diabetes guidelines of time-below-range (TBR) <70 mg/dL, time-in-range (TIR) 70-180 mg/dL, and time-above-range (TAR) >180 mg/dL. After segmenting a dataset into different ranges, we can then calculate each segment's contribution percentage of certain biomarkers, such as glucose.

For presentation of certain analysis results, we can combine two contributing factors with one resulting biomarker performance into one graphic diagram, such as plotting carbs/sugar and exercise with glucose together in one graphic diagram. The author developed a three-dimensional (3D) diagram, but with a presentation model of "2.5-dimension" diagram, to demonstrate this type of multiple relationships. For example, the x-axis is the carbs/sugar intake amount from 0 to 50 grams, the y-axis is the post-meal walking steps from 0 to 5000 steps, and the third dimension (glucose) on the z-axis is shown as a skewed radio wave starting from the origin at the lower-left corner (the lowest glucose) and moving toward the upper-right corner (the highest glucose) on the x-y two-dimensional (2D) plane. That is why he calls it a two-and-half dimension diagram which represents 3D information together. He uses this presentation model for many of his diabetes and psychology papers given that one input usually involves at least two critical inputs.

Candlestick Model vs. Density Model

The author was the CEO of a publicly traded semiconductor company from 1995 to 2002. Not only is he a finance specialist and businessman, but he is also familiar with various mathematical financial models used for stock trading. In nature, both stock price and glucose values are waveforms which fluctuate continuously due to different driving forces. In early 2019, he borrowed the concept of the *candlestick model (aka K-line model) used on Wall Street* and reprogrammed it into a presentation model for glucose fluctuations in his diabetes papers. For example, using a continuous glucose monitoring (CGM) sensor device, he can collect 96 glucose values per day every fifteen minutes and 288 glucose values per day every five minutes. He then selects five key glucose values per day: *opening* glucose, maximum *high* glucose, minimum low glucose, *average* glucose, and *closing* glucose. The 4 glucose values, without the minimum low glucose value, constitute an *"OHAC model" with a triangular shape*, for an approximate PPG diagram within a three-hour time frame after the first bite of a meal.

However, this Candlestick model and OHAC model only deals with a few key data points per day. Therefore, he has further developed a more completed *"Density*

Model" which includes all the collected data within a selected time frame, not daily averaged data. The selected time frame can be any period but having a longer time span is recommended. Not only is the Density Model useful for glucose analysis, but it can also be used for analyzing food, exercise, blood pressure, heart rate, and other disease biomarkers. This model covers a complete spectrum of his collected data, where its graphic representation of final results is quite similar to a normal distribution or Gaussian distribution curve. Therefore, the concepts of mean and standard deviation can also be applied. Incidentally, the density model can be linked with other tools, such as segmentation analysis or contribution analysis.

From Wave Theory to Energy Theory via Fast Fourier Transform

All biomarkers can be represented by different waveforms as long as they have sufficient data. All waves have three basic characteristics: amplitude, frequency, and wavelength. In a general practice, many biomarker performances are expressed in a time domain initially with the horizontal x-axis as the time scale with the vertical y-axis as the biomarker wave's amplitude scale. We can then use Fast Fourier Transform (FFT) to convert the time domain data or curve into a frequency domain data or curve. In the frequency domain diagram, the horizontal x-axis becomes the frequency scale while the vertical y-axis becomes the original time-domain wave's associated energy scale. Once the glucose wave in the time domain is transformed into the frequency domain, we can then have a clear idea of how much the associated energy of glucose is corresponding to a certain glucose occurrence frequency. After we have the associated energy information, it will be simpler for us to determine how much damage occurs on the internal organs by the associated glucose energies. For example, hypoglycemia (<70 mg/dL) or hyperglycemia (>180 mg/dL) usually occur in the lower frequency range because these two serious conditions should not appear too often unless the patient has severe diabetes. For severe diabetic patients, their lower-frequency numbers would be higher than non-severe diabetic patients. This is how the frequency-domain analysis links with segmentation and contribution analyses along with utilizing time domain to frequency domain transform technique. Therefore, by using frequency domain analyses, we can estimate the risk probability of developing certain induced complications from chronic diseases, such as heart attacks, stroke, kidney failure, diabetic retinopathy, neuropathy, etc.

Linear Elastic Glucose Theory

The author studied mechanical engineering undergraduate courses at the University of Iowa. In the course of strength of materials taught by Professor James Andrews, he learned the basic stress-strain relationship via Young's modulus. He then applied this basic engineering concept to his developed PPG prediction model that involves FPG serving as the baseline of PPG in his ongoing medical research work. By introducing and including 3 GH-Modulus, he can then build a simple, easy, yet accurate predicted PPG model. He defined GH.f Modulus using FPG as the calculated baseline for PPG, GH.p Modulus for converting carbs/sugar intake amount into energy influx to raise the PPG value, and GH.w modulus for converting exercise amount into energy burnout to reduce the PPG value. The three GH-Modulus are dependent on the patient's overall health condition and individual diabetes severity within different timeframes. This situation is similar to Young's modules being dependent on different materials, such as diamond, steel, copper, concrete, etc. The following equation is his developed linear elastic glucose theory (LEGT) model:

Predicted PPG
= FPG*GH.f + carbs/sugar*GH.p + walking k-steps*GH.w

This developed LEGT model has been proven that it can achieve >95% of PPG prediction accuracy.

Regretfully, he did not keep personal data of medical conditions and lifestyle details prior to 2012 when his HbA1C was above 10%, eAG was around 380 mg/dL, BMI over 30, along with suffering from 5 cardiac episodes, kidney problems, and more. In conjunction with the missing data, he is not a licensed medical doctor and does not have access to other patients' records. Moreover, there are very few patients who have strong will power, stubborn persistence, adequate knowledge and experience on data collection, organization, cleaning, along with preparation to be capable for useful data processing and analysis. Otherwise, the author can apply a "nonlinear plastic" model which he learned from Professor Norman Jones at MIT to develop a "nonlinear plastic glucose theory" (NPGT) which can be extremely beneficial for saving patients with severe diabetic conditions. Nevertheless, the LEGT should be sufficient to provide a useful tool for the purpose of prevention and control for most type 2 diabetes (T2D) conditions. This situation is similar to the engineering elasticity theory, which is suitable for most engineering situations, while plasticity theory is valuable for certain special, extreme, or severe circumstances, such as structural impact, structural fracture, or structural failure. In the medical field, the plasticity situation is similar to the damaged pancreatic beta cells.

Glycemic Variability (GV) and Statistics
Using a mean value of glucoses, such as average glucose or HbA1C value, it can reveal certain useful information about the diabetes conditions. However, it definitely misses the description of glucose excursion, i.e., glucose fluctuations (GF) which provides significant data. There are various ways to present GF or excursion detailing the glucose impact on different internal organs. This glucose excursion or glycemic variability (GV) deals with glucose wave theory from a distinct approach, specifically belonging to the scope of "Statistics". The ADA published "TxR" guidelines of time-in-range (TIR%) with 70-180 mg/dL for normal glucose range, time-above-range (TAR%) with >180 mg/dL for hyperglycemia, and time-below-range (TBR%) with <70 mg/dL for hypoglycemia (insulin shock) are located somewhere between the average glucose and glucose excursion picture. As a result, the ADA's TxR model can be considered as a "pseudo" analysis tool. There are also other GV statistical methods available such as standard deviation (SD), coefficient of variation (CV), adjusted M-value, mean amplitude of glycemic excursions (MEGA), continuous overall net glycemic action (CONGA), mean of daily differences (MODD), etc. In some of the author's papers, he applied simpler and easier "GF" model which is the daily maximum glucose minus daily minimum glucose. Using this simpler GF term which covers a "wider" range than SD and combined with the mean value of glucose, such as

HbA1C; it can offer additional information than the present diabetes clinical practice of relying on HbA1C only. Furthermore, GF provides a quick and rough picture of a patient's overall health along with the risk in developing various complications from diabetes. In addition, the author has also applied certain statistics regression models (such as linear, nonlinear, single variables, multiple variables) to develop regression predicted biomarker values.

Continuous Glucose Monitoring (GCM) Sensor Device Collected Data

The author has utilized the Libre lifestyle CGM sensor device on his upper arm since May 5, 2018 and has changed it every fourteen days. Furthermore, he installed a Bluetooth device on top of the CGM device in order to automatically transmit sensor glucose data to his developed app software EclaireMD Chronic. These glucose values are organized in two datasets. The first dataset contains 96 glucoses per day every fifteen minutes and the second dataset contains 288 glucoses per day every five minutes. As of October 24, 2021, he has already collected a total of 348,288 sensor glucose data which include 87,072 from 15-minutes and 261,216 from five-minutes. This data collection process utilizes both computer hardware and software.

By using the five-minute sensor glucose (average 113.78 mg/dL) and fifteen-minute sensor glucose (average 113.23 mg/dL) during a period from February 18, 2021 to October 25, 2021, it has a small difference of 0.55 mg/dL or 0.49%; therefore, a denser data collection done at every 5 minutes does not provide more accurate results. As a result, the author continued with the fifteen-minute sensor glucose model for his research work, since it is a sensible and reliable time duration for measuring blood glucose changes. Luckily, a glucose wave has significant changes every ten to fifteen minutes, unlike seismic waves changing every second.

With such a big database available, the research techniques mentioned above, such as candlestick K-line, GV, and glucose excursion, can assist him with his efforts in his medical research work using CGM sensor device collected glucoses.

Big Data Analytics:

Since January 2012, the author has collected his glucose via the traditional finger-prick method four times a day, once in the early morning when he wakes up, and two hours after the first bite of every meal. After applying the CGM sensor device on May 8, 2018, for the purpose of data consistency with the doctor's recommended testing for diabetes patients, he has used the CGM data at 120-minutes moment after first bite of meal as his finger PPG value in his Chronic software. Over the past three and a half years (907 days) of CGM usage period, he still continues with the finger pricking method as the calibration data for his CGM sensor data. This is due to the CGM data being usually higher in the first two to three days of installation and then becoming lower for the last two to three days. Therefore, only the Libre CGM sensor data collected from the middle range of eight to ten days for the fourteen-day lifespan is more reliable. However, the two extreme ends of the first two to three days and the last two to three days, he always uses the finger-pricking glucose data to serve as a calibration tool. Furthermore, he has modified his software to accept the calibrated data only as the stored glucose values. In summary, thus far, his collected finger glucoses have reached 14,328 data over the past ten years (3,582 days) and 348,288 over the last three and a half years (907 days). The raw data includes 362,616 with additional 18,140 processed data of average (mean), maximum, minimum, open, close, SD, glucose fluctuation (GF=max-min), FG/eAG, PPG/eAG, FPG/PPG, CV, MAGE, CONGA, MODD, finger A1C, sensor A1C from 15-minutes, sensor A1C from 5-minutes, combined sensor A1C, A1C with GF, and the ADA's A1C. In the category of glucose alone, there are 380,756 data stored in his database. With other glucose related items, the total glucose data size has around 500,000 data points.

The category of Food Nutrition related data is another big data set. Since May 1, 2015, he kept a record of his food information which comprises of 7,528 meal photos (on his iPhone), carbohydrates amount, sugar amount, post-meal walking steps, corresponding PPG, twelve food material categories, 238 consumed food materials, 6,719 eaten food items, 238 different food glycemic index, AI predicted PPG (using optical physics), Natural Intelligence or NI predicted PPG (using his eyes and brain to estimate PPG), 7,528 food portion % (food quantity), bowel movement amount (for weight prediction and gastrointestinal health). In addition, he has a rough estimate of his food related data size which has reached to over 500,000 data points.

Finally, the Metabolism Index (MI) contains all ten categories and nearly 500 elements to summarize his health condition and be used for risk assessment of developing into various complications affecting the heart, brain, kidney, eyes, foot, skin, and nervous system. These direct input data for around 500 elements for 3,582 days contain 1,791,000 data points.
There are other miscellaneous data with a total size between 200,000 to 300,000 data points.

By combining his glucose, diet, metabolism and miscellaneous data sets together, his collected and stored total data size has reached around 3 million data on his iPhone, which is backed up on his cloud storage. This database does not take account of the purchased, cleaned, and transferred of over six million publicly-available food nutritional data from the USDA for his optical physics and AI application of PPG prediction.

Various HbA1C Formulas
Using certain linear regression analysis methods and his collected HbA1C data from 43 "near-quarterly" lab-tested results (mainly from one single lab to avoid data integrity issues), he has developed several predicted HbA1C formulas as shown below:

(1) Finger A1C
= finger eAG /16.7
(2) Sensor A1C
= sensor eAG /18.7
(3) Combined A1C
= 0.4*finger A1C + 0.6*sensor A1C
(4) A1C with glucose fluctuation
= (0.3*sensor eAG + 0.7*sensor GF) / 16.25

(5) ADA defined A1C
= (finger eAG or sensor eAG +46.7) / 28.7

Without using the ADA defined formula, his average predicted HbA1C result utilizing the four predicted A1C formulas would match almost perfectly with the average forty-two lab-tested HbA1C result along with high correlation coefficients (67% - 70%) between his predicted A1C curve and lab-tested A1C curve. The lower correlation is due to insufficient lab-tested A1C data.

It should be mentioned that based on glucose density distribution and segmentation & contribution analyses, his finger PPG occupies 75 percent of A1C and finger FPG occupies 25 percent of A1C. On the other hand, the CGM sensor PPG occupies 38 percent of A1C, sensor FPG occupies 29 percent of A1C, sensor between-meals and pre-bed glucoses occupy 33 percent of A1C.

Excerpt from the "Metabolical" book written by Lustig, Robert H. MD, HarperWave, Harper Collins Publisher, New York, 2021 and some of his related research work:

"The following 8 intra-cellular or sub-cellular pathological processes (or pathways) are the basic causes of chronic diseases which are not mutually exclusive. Each interacts with the others, and so they tend to cluster together.

These 8 processes are:
1. *Glycation*
   The carbohydrates (fructose, i.e., sugar, or glucose) and an amino acid (e.g., proteins) are related for glycation. *(The author: Sugar has connection).*
2. *Oxidative stress*
   If there are more oxygen redials than antioxidants, it causes cellular dysfunction and cell death. The color of real food is an indication that these plants contain antioxidants we can't make on our own. *(The author: Consuming real food helps oxidative stress).*
3. *Mitochondrial dysfunction*
   Chronic disease is mitochondrial. The single best stimulus to make more and fresh mitochondrial is "exercise." Your mitochondrial can't overturn a bad diet. (The author: Both diet and exercise are important).
4. *Insulin resistance*
   Insulin lowers the blood glucose. Its main job is to store energy for a rainy day. Two organs need insulin to function, liver and adipose tissues. *(The author: Even the brain needs insulin).* Insulin resistance is the central problem in metabolic syndrome. Processed food is by far the biggest player. *(The author: Eating real food, not processed food makes a huge difference on insulin resistance).*

5. ***Cell membrane integrity & fluidity***
   Cell membranes are composed of a lipid belayer. There are 7 different types of fats in your diet, and all can impact your cell membranes in different ways. Saturated fatty acids could reduce the cells'overall fluidity. Unsaturated fats are better than saturated fats. *(The author: Excessive fat from food is bad for health)*.

6. ***Inflammation***
   Foreign invaders (e.g., viruses and bacteria) can damage cells directly. We need an inflammatory response, unfortunately there are 4 downsides. There are connections between metabolism and inflammation. *(The author: Metabolism and immunity are two sides of the same coin and immunity defends inflammation)*. Chronic diseases have four inter-connected problems, nutrition, metabolism, inflammation, immunity. Screw up one and you screw up the other three. *(The author: Nutrition helps metabolism and immunity)*.

7. ***Epigenetics, not genetic***
   The metabolic syndrome studies say only 15% is genetic, the rest is environmental. (The author: The term of environmental includes lifestyles). But environment can change gene as well through a phenomenon called epigenetics. Altered nutrition, such as processed food, appears to be a primary driver of altered epigenetics. *(The author: Avoid consuming any processed food)*.

8. ***Cell autophage***
   Clearing biological waste products is a process known as autophage, and it plays a key role in healthy aging, especially in the brain. All organs do better with autophage, which is an essential process that maintain healthy cells by removing damaged proteins and malfunctioning organelles, especially mitochondria. *(The author: Mitochondria is an organelle containing enzymes responsible for producing energy)*. Old mitochondria make a lot of oxygen radicals. Autophage is under various nutritional controls. Intermittent fasting lowers insulin and raises ketones, both of which promote autophage. *(The author: He has been conducting intermittent fasting since November 8, 2020)*.

All of these 8 pathologies are directly related to food and nutrition. In order to maintain excellent health and avoid metabolic disorder syndrome, we must consume real food with good nutrition. ***Processed food must be avoided since it causes the most damage to the body and our metabolism system.***

The key to fending off chronic diseases is to keep the eight intra-cellular pathological pathways running correctly.

Drugs and nutraceuticals don't work for metabolic syndrome. All of the eight pathologies are driven by and are responsive to specific components of real food, because real food gets where it needs to inside the cell. Processed food poisons the eight pathways instead.

Food is related to all of the eight pathologies. However, exercise is only related to 5 pathologies, i.e., mitochondrial dysfunction, insulin resistance, inflammation, epigenetics, and cell autophage. Exercise has no relationships with glycation, oidative stress, cell membrane integrity & fluidity.

The author has conducted various Segmentation and Correlation analyses of glucoses which is one of the key methods of diabetes research. For example, FPG is highly related to body weight and body weight is controlled by food portion (quantity) mainly with exercise, sleep, stress as secondary contributors. In addition, he has also identified that FPG in the early morning is also highly correlated to body temperature in the early morning. PPG's nineteen contribution factors are largely due to diet (~60 percent) and exercise as the secondary factor (~40 percent) if he ignores other third-tier factors. Therefore, the ratio of food (60 percent) versus exercise (40 percent) is 1.5 (=60/40) while food contributes into 8 intra-cellular or sub-cellular pathological processes (or pathways) and exercise contributes only 5 pathways with a ratio of food versus exercise of 1.6 (=8/5).

These research results have linked his results using GH-Method: math-physical medicine approach almost exactly with the Dr. Robert H. Ludwig's book-mentioned biomedical pathological approach.

Quantum Mechanics & Perturbation Theory:

In 2020, the author compared the human body (inner space) to the universe (outer space). All of the different but interconnected internal organs and diseases are similar to the planets existing in outer space which are mutually influenced (for example, the ocean tide waves on earth are influenced by moon). Therefore, he started to apply certain quantum mechanics concepts and equations to his internal organ study, especially to diabetic-related diseases. At first, he transformed his glucose data from time domain into frequency domain via Fast Fourier Transform (FFT). Second, he modified Albert Einstein's famous theory of relativity equation of $E=m*(c**2)$ into his desired glucose energy equation of $E=n*(a**2)$. Einstein's m is mass and c is the speed of light. The author's glucose energy equation's *n is the frequency number and a is the glucose amplitude of Y-axis value in the time domain. As energy is proportional to the square of a wave's amplitude;* therefore, the glucose associated energy is directly proportional to the square of glucose amplitude times its corresponding frequency number. After calculating the glucose energy *using the equation of $E=n*(a**2)$, we can then estimate the glucose induced damages to the internal organs*.

The perturbation theory is another application from quantum mechanics which has already been proven to be one of the best approximation techniques. The author applies the first-order, second-order, and third-order interpolation perturbation equations in order to obtain his "perturbed PPG." This is another form of predicted PPG using one measured sample PPG waveforms and one selected *perturbation factor*, such as carbs/sugar intake amount, which is the "*Slope*." The "measured PPG" waveform is used as his reference or baseline waveform.

The following polynomial function is the **perturbation equation:**

$$A = f(x)$$
$$= A0 + (A1*x) + (A2*x**2)+(A3*x**3) + ... + (An*x**n)$$

Where A is the perturbed glucose, A i is the measured glucose, and x is the perturbation factor based on a chosen carbs/sugar intake amount.

The first-order interpolation perturbation equation can also be expressed in the following simplified format for risk probability studies:

A i = A1 + (A2-A1)(slope 1)*

Where:
A1 = original risk A at time 1
A2 = advanced risk A at time 2
(A2-A1) = (Risk A at Time 2 - Risk A at Time 1)

The perturbation factor or **Slope** is an arbitrarily selected parameter that controls the size of the perturbation. The author has chosen a "slope" for his perturbed glucose as follows:

Slope
= (Selected value - Low-bound value) / (High-bound value - Low-bound value)

By applying the perturbation theory from quantum mechanics, for certain biomarkers, he was able to reach **~95 percent accuracy using the first-order equation, ~97 percent accuracy using the second-order equation, and ~99 percent accuracy using the third-order equation.** The perturbed glucoses can be used as another predicted glucoses with extremely high accuracy.

Metabolic Disorder Induced Complications and Longevity

1. *Risk probability of having complications*

   Since his metabolism model contains four basic biomarkers and six major lifestyles; therefore, it can serve as the foundation of his risk model for many chronic disease complications with certain selected and emphasized factors based on previous medical research findings. For example, the CVD/CHD (heart) and stroke are mainly resulted from macro-vessel (artery) complications. As a result, he added an amplified contribution factor by blood pressure for the artery rupture scenario and blood lipids for artery blockage situation. The neuropathy, retinopathy, and chronic kidney problems contain amplified contribution factor by blood pressure for micro-vessels leakage scenario. Furthermore, triglycerides provide an amplified contribution factor for diabetic retinopathy. Albumin creatinine ratio (ACR), protein in urine, contributes to chronic kidney disease (CKD), but ACR also has a strong relationship with blood pressure, thyroid stimulating hormone

(TSH), and triglycerides (blood lipids).

2. *Longevity*

In December 2019, he developed a mathematical equation using MI values as the base to estimate a patient's expected life span by comparing the calculated health age against biological age. This health age formula is expressed as follows:

Effective Health Age
*= Real Biological Age ***
(1+((MI-0.735)/0.735)/AF)

Where AF (amplification factor) = 2

He has written a few papers regarding longevity and published them in several geriatric journals.

Neuro-science study on glucose and self-repair of pancreatic beta cells

The glucose production is controlled by our brain. Once we wake up and light enters our retina or when food arrives in our stomach, this process turns into a neuro-message to be sent to the brain. After receiving these transmitting messages, the brain then makes a decision and provides feedback. It informs the liver to produce or release glucose and for the pancreas to produce or release insulin to regulate glucose. These observed phenomena explain why the 10+ mg/dL glucose increase between the moment we wake up and the first bite of breakfast, with increasing PPG amount between the first-bite moment of meal and 15-20 minutes after the first bite.

The author has conducted an experiment of eating over four-hundred specific meals over the past two years. The increased PPG at 60-minutes after the first bite are 30-40 mg/dL for solid egg meals and ~10 mg/dL for liquid egg meals. These 20-30 mg/dL PPG difference between two different food preparation methods can be interpreted using a neuro-scientific viewpoint. At the first-bite of meals, the stomach sends two messages immediately to the brain that include the food arrival and the specific physical state of the food entry. Therefore, liquid foods can trick our brain to treat them as if we were drinking water. This neuro-scientific interpretation can explain these observed PPG differences. *Based on his various research projects, he has tried to apply both eating liquid foods (~200 experiments) and maintaining intermittent fasting practice (~300 experiments) to control his glucose excursion. This practice has contributed to his lower average glucose during 2020-2021.*

By analyzing and observing detailed glucose behaviors over the past seven years, including FPG improvements without food and exercise, PPG improvement with reduced amounts of carbs/sugar and increased post-meal walking steps, the author has drawn a bold conclusion regarding his pancreatic health. *His pancreatic beta cells have been self-repaired at an annual rate of 2.8 percent to 4.5 percent; therefore, over the past seven years, his insulin conditions, including either insulin secretion or insulin resistance or both, have been improved approximately 20 percent to 30*

percent (assuming an annual improvement rate of ~3 to 4 percent).
Other diabetic complications or metabolic disorder induced diseases

Utilizing his developed GH-Method: math-physical medicine approach, he has studied many diseases, including neuropathy (e.g. foot ulcers), retinopathy, immunity, diabetic constipation, diabetic fungal infection, cancers prevention, dementia (Alzheimer's disease) prevention, and even psychological issues (diabetes patient's behavior, border-line personality disorder, patients' behavior during the COVID-19 quarantine period, MD suicides, etc.).

Part 5:
Epilogue:

Since the author's presentation at the International Diabetes Federation (IDF) annual conference in 2017, along with being recognized by several diabetes research organizations and medical research scientists, he has continued writing medical papers and working on several book publications. To date, he has written 564 medical papers and published over 500 papers in various journals, including 20 percent of them in journals of physics, science, and engineering (his original learned disciplines). His published papers and conference presentations include over 100 non-endocrinology conferences or journals, such as Cancer, Dementia, Alzheimer's, Central Nervous System, Neurology, Infectious Diseases, Oncology, Pharmacology, Toxicology, Pediatrician, Antibiotics, Vaccine, Biomedicine, Stem Cell, System Biology, Liver and Pancreatic diseases, Nephrology and Urology. Over one hundred non-endocrinology conferences and journals have expressed interested his presentations and/or reading his papers regarding his research method, the GH-Method: math-physical medicine research methodology.

His mission is to help diabetics worldwide through the existing medical community or by directly outreach. The author has found that publications appear to be a more effective way than conferences to reach a broader spectrum of medical professionals and patients. Since late 2020, he has also began publishing his books which consist of his medical papers. Through Amazon's highly effective publishing and distribution channels, his books can reach both medical professionals and patients worldwide. The core reason of doing so is to prevent diabetics from suffering from complications similar to himself, therefore, the author felt compelled to spread his lifestyle management message of preventive medicine and his 12-years medical research results to whomever wishes to save their own lives or their patients' lives.

The author believes that everyone deserves to have the basic human rights of health, happiness, and freedom. That is why *he has spent twenty-one years continuously conducting his study and research on both psychology and internal medicine. The author considers this as his mission in the next chapter of his life, and ultimately, his life's calling.*

Applying the first-order interpolation perturbation method to establish predicted PPG waveforms based on carbs/sugar intake amounts using GH-Method: math-physical medicine (No. 154)

By: Gerald C. Hsu
eclaireMD Foundation, USA
12/27-28/2019 Taipei

Introduction:

In this paper, the author presents his numerical techniques of applying the first-order interpolation perturbation method to establish and predict a new postprandial plasma glucose (PPG) waveform based on the "perturbation factor" of carbs/sugar intake amount. This is part of his GH-Method: math-physical medicine research methodology. He also uses two previously measured PPG datasets (waveforms) of high-carbohydrates breakfasts to validate this numerical methodology.

Methods:

The exact solution of many nonlinear problems encountered in the biomedical field cannot be achieved analytically for most situations. Normally, a given complex function can get certain approximated solutions via a class of simpler operations. Most of the general complex problems can be expressed by the following polynomial function of nth degree:

$$P(x) = a_0 + a_1x + a_2x^2 + ... +$$

This nth degree polynomial function could be solved by approximating the values outside the available data table with the help of the calculating points that correspond to the approximate locations within the proximity of the available data table. This approach could be achieved via function approximation simplification and interpolation perturbation methods.

First, in many cases, this nth degree polynomial function could be further simplified via truncating off the higher order terms to achieve the following first-order polynomial function:

$$Y = f(X) = A0 + A1*X$$

Second, the above first-order polynomial function's approximate solution could be obtained via a specific "interpolation or extrapolation" method.

Interpolation is implemented within the range covered by data of both the PPG due to high-carbs amount ("high glucose") and PPG due to low-carbs amount ("low glucose"). The interpolation method replaces Y (glucose level) with an easily calculated function, usually a polynomial and a simple straight line. In short, the interpolation method, also known as the intermediate value, is a scientific term that could be defined as arriving at an unknown intermediate values (e.g. glucose level Y mg/dL) of a function by using known values (e.g., carbs amount X grams). For the complex problem of glucose variation study, this simplified equation can be expressed in the following format of ***Equation 1***:

New Glucose Y mg/dL at new X carbs gram
= function of carbs amount, i.e. f(X)
= Y1 + slope * (Y2 - Y1)

Where:
slope = (new X - low carbs) / (high carbs - low carbs)
Y1 = low glucose
Y2 = high glucose

The above-described steps of the calculation (Equation 1) have utilized an applied mathematics methodology of "first-order interpolation perturbation method" which have been frequently used in quantum mechanics, fluid dynamics, and solid mechanics.

Results:

The author has selected a period of 601 days (5/5/2018 - 12/26/2019) as the time window of his segmented PPG pattern analysis associated with two separate meal groups. The first one has 240 breakfasts with either an egg or McDonald's breakfast, including egg, sausage, hash brown or muffin occasionally, and the other has 228 breakfasts at McDonald's restaurant exclusively.

A summarized data table of breakfast PPG analysis is listed below with the format of (averaged carbs/sugar grams; averaged post-meal walking steps; averaged finger PPG; averaged sensor PPG):

Egg: (7.5g; 4700 steps; 114.7 mg/dL; 136.72 mg/dL)
McDonald's: (10.0g; 4616 steps; 117.7 mg/dL; 137.68 mg/dL)

The major difference between these two breakfast groups is the first perturbation factor of carbs/sugar intake amount, 7.5 grams for Egg vs. McDonald's and 10.0 grams for McDonald's exclusively. Post-breakfast walking steps and PPG values for both cases are comparable.

He was then able to construct two separated PPG waveforms (curves) between 0-minute and 180-minutes, for high-carbs input and low-carbs input. The data table and waveforms are shown in Figure 1.

Finally, he used these two breakfast cases (7.5 g and 10g) as known values (X1, X2, Y1, Y2) to construct two new approximate waveforms associated 7.5 g and 10g, respectively using interpolation perturbation methods (Equation 1).

Figures 2 depicts two data tables of these two-interpolation perturbation calculated results. Figure 3 shows the comparison between measured waveform versus perturbed waveform for 7.5g case and 10g case, respectively.

It is clear that the PPG waveform comparison between perturbed PPG and measured PPG offer a high correlation coefficients, i.e. high similarity of curves, of 76% and 86%. The perturbed PPG peaks are at 94% and 96% of measured PPG peaks, while the perturbed average PPG value is at 96% of measured average PPG value. Although these two perturbed breakfast PPG values are only approximated values, both of them still have ~ 95% degree of accuracy.

Conclusion:

Glucose variance is an extremely complex biochemical and biophysical phenomenon. In addition, glucose testing using finger piercing is both troublesome and painful. Most diabetes patients do not like to measure their glucose constantly.

The authors paper numbers *153-2019 and 154-2019* describe his application of perturbation theory to develop a 3-hour approximate PPG waveform based on one single input data, the carbs/sugar intake amount, with high accuracy.

Based on this technique and his developed artificial intelligence glucometer's estimated carbs/sugar intake amount (via optical physics), a diabetes patient can predict and control his PPG in a much easier way.

After a diabetes patient measures and establishes two separate initial waveforms with low-carb meal and high-carb meal respectively, we can then apply this interpolated perturbation method to predict and plot out this patient's 3-hour PPG waveform (curve) prior to eating. Even though these approximated PPG values sacrifice some degree of prediction accuracy, this prediction method is fast, easy, painless, and at no cost to diabetes patients to control their glucose levels.

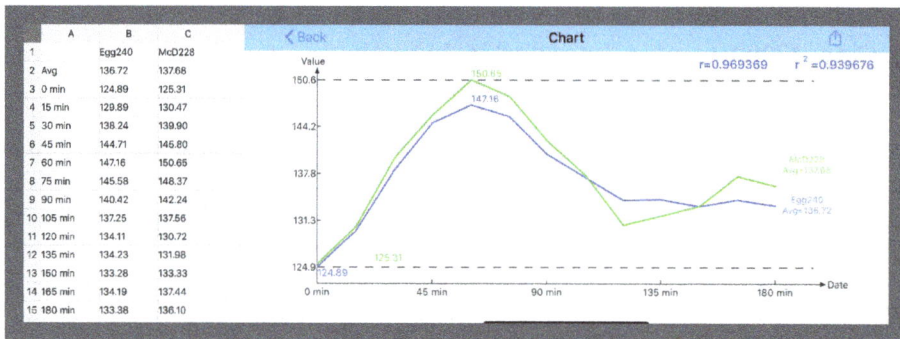

A	B	C
1	Egg240	McD228
2 Avg	136.72	137.68
3 0 min	124.89	125.31
4 15 min	129.89	130.47
5 30 min	138.24	139.90
6 45 min	144.71	145.80
7 60 min	147.16	150.65
8 75 min	145.58	148.37
9 90 min	140.42	142.24
10 105 min	137.25	137.56
11 120 min	134.11	130.72
12 135 min	134.23	131.98
13 150 min	133.28	133.33
14 165 min	134.19	137.44
15 180 min	133.38	136.10

Figure 1: Low-carbs PPG and High-carb glucose

Egg plus McDonald Carbs = 7.5 g			McDonald Carbs = 10 g		
1	EggReal	EggPert	1	McdReal	McdPert
2 Avg	136.72	130.80	2 Avg	137.68	132.75
3 0 min	124.89	128.42	3 0 min	125.31	128.72
4 15 min	129.89	131.14	4 15 min	130.47	131.72
5 30 min	138.24	136.07	5 30 min	139.90	137.16
6 45 min	144.71	139.40	6 45 min	145.80	141.12
7 60 min	147.16	139.44	7 60 min	150.65	141.53
8 75 min	145.58	135.89	8 75 min	148.37	138.35
9 90 min	140.42	131.93	9 90 min	142.24	134.50
10 105 min	137.25	128.20	10 105 min	137.56	131.04
11 120 min	134.11	125.84	11 120 min	130.72	128.59
12 135 min	134.23	125.45	12 135 min	131.98	128.10
13 150 min	133.28	125.65	13 150 min	133.33	127.95
14 165 min	134.19	126.62	14 165 min	137.44	128.77
15 180 min	133.38	126.41	15 180 min	136.10	128.20

Figure 2 : Interpolation perturbation method to generate two datasets for both egg breakfast and McDonal breakfast

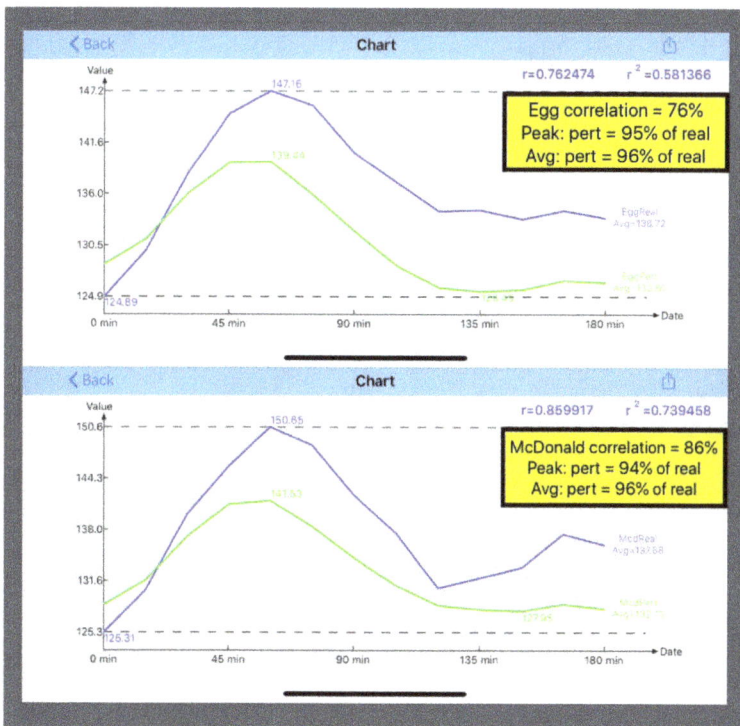

Figure 3: Comparison between perturbed and measured PPG for both egg and McDonal breakfasts

Effective health age resulting from metabolic condition changes and lifestyle maintenance program (No. 223)

By: Gerald C. Hsu
eclaireMD Foundation, USA
12/31/2019 - 1/1/2020 Taipei
1/12/3020 - 1/14/2020 Taipei

Introduction:

In this paper, the author reviewed his past 8-years data from 2012 through 2019 and focused on both of his metabolic conditions and health lifestyle details. He then developed an "Effective Health Age" model by using the GH-Method: math-physical medicine approach in comparison with the "Real Biological Age".

Method:

He defined the "Effective Health Age" based on the evaluation of his multiple medical examination reports and his ~2 million data of his lifestyle, metabolism, and diseases over an 8-year period. This is different from the "Real Biological Age" or "Chronological Age" defined as the actual amount of time a person has been alive.

As shown in Figure 1, approximately 2.1 million people died in 2017 from multiple causes of death in the United States. Among them, almost 79% (~1.7 million deaths) were related to metabolic conditions, whether directly or indirectly. It should be noted that in 2018, the total death figure reached more than 2.8 million people with ~2.2 million deaths related to metabolic conditions and diseases.

In 2014, the author developed a mathematical metabolic model, including 4-categories of diseases (body outputs) and 6-categories of lifestyle details (body inputs). He started to collect his data of weight and glucose beginning on 1/1/2012 and other lifestyle data from 2013-2014. Thus far, he has collected nearly 2 million data regarding his body health and lifestyle details. He further assembled those 10-categories (with a total of ~500 detailed elements) and combined them into two new biomedical terms: the metabolism index (MI), which is a combined daily score to show the body health situation, and general health status unit (GHSU), which is the 90-days moving averaged number to show the health trend.

Figures 2 and 3 demonstrate the above-mentioned details of his metabolic diseases and conditions during the past 8-years (2012 - 2019).

He has also identified a "break-even line" at 0.735 (73.5%) to separate his metabolic conditions between the healthy state (below 0.735) and unhealthy state (above 0.735).

He further developed a simple equation to calculate his effective health age as follows:

Effective Health Age
*= Real Biological Age ***
(1+((MI-0.735)/0.735)/2)

He then utilized his annualized MI data to calculate his effective health age in order to compare against his real biological age.

Results:

As shown in Figure 4, both of his MI and GHSU were >73.5% during 2012-2014 (unhealthy) and <73.5% during 2014-2019 (healthy). During 2014, his overall health condition improved significantly. It should be noted that his MI and GHSU during the years 2018 and 2019 were increased slightly due to his heavy travel schedule of attending more than 60 medical conferences worldwide. As a result, his risk probability of having a heart attack or stroke also increased by approximately 2% to 3%.

Figure 5 depicts the comparison between his real biological age and effective health age. Of course, the real biological age increases annually, while the effective health age was higher than his real biological age during 2012-2014 and lower than his real biological age during 2015-2019. These changes are results of improvements on his bad metabolic conditions and poor lifestyle habits. These factors were significantly improved during 2015 and then maintained through 2019. Figure 5 also shows the two age differences between effective health age and real biological age. The age difference has changed from +8 years in 2012 to -7 years in 2019 (here, + is getting worse and - is getting better).

An interesting fact from the past decade is that three of his physicians indicated his age was about 10 years older after reviewing his medical examination reports when he was 63 years old. However, the same physicians told him during 2016-2019 that he was about 10 younger when he reached ~70 years old. This range of +10 years to -10 years was an *empirical* judgement based on their many years of clinical experiences from seeing hundreds of patients. However, the author used a *scientific* approach which is based on physical phenomena observations, big data analytics, and mathematical derivations to draw a conclusion of the range of +8 to -7 years. Nevertheless, these two guesstimated age ranges are actually quite comparable.

The life expectancy of an American male is 78.69 years (2016 data). If the author continues his metabolic conditions improvement, chronic disease control, as well as his existing lifestyle maintenance program, he may stand a good chance to extend his life for an additional eight years to reach to a real biological age of 87 (79 plus 8).

Conclusions:

This simple numerical calculation based on big data analytics and sophisticated mathematical metabolic model has depicted a possible way to extend our life expectancy via an effective metabolic condition improvement and lifestyle maintenance program. This practical method has been applied and proven effectively in his own diabetes conditions control.

The author hopes that this method can also be applied in the field of geriatrics, longevity, or other forms of chronic diseases control. For example, if a particular patient is able to collect sufficient data regarding his particular chronic disease conditions, he can then replace those input data of M1 through M4 with his own disease data, and utilizes similar lifestyle model of M5 through M10. In this way, he can then guesstimate his own effective health age and life expectancy under his own disease conditions.

Life is precious and health is important. A long and healthy life is the dream for everyone. This article provides a logical and practical way of achieving longevity.

2017 Death Cause	Sub-Category	Metabolism related
Heart	647,457	647,457
Cancer	599,108	599,108
Accidents	169,936	
Respiratory	160,201	
Stroke	146,383	146,383
Alzheimer's	121,404	121,404
Diabetes	83,564	83,564
Pneumonia	55,672	
Kidney	50,633	50,633
Suicide	47,173	
Total	2,081,531	1,648,549
Percentage	100%	79%

Figure 1: US leading death causes

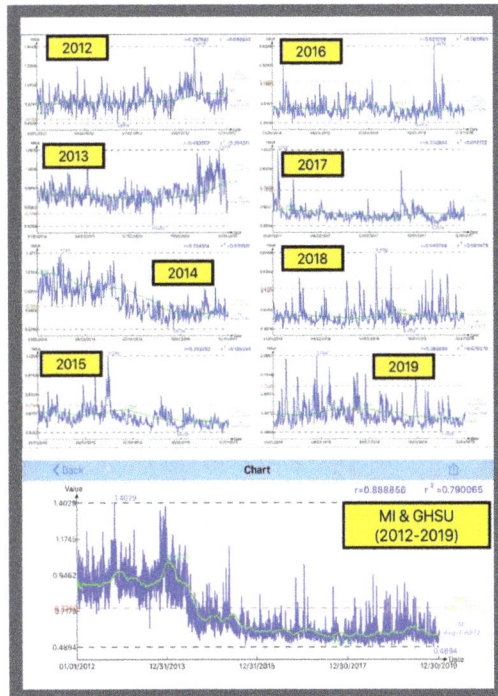

Figure 2: Metabolism model of inputs and outputs

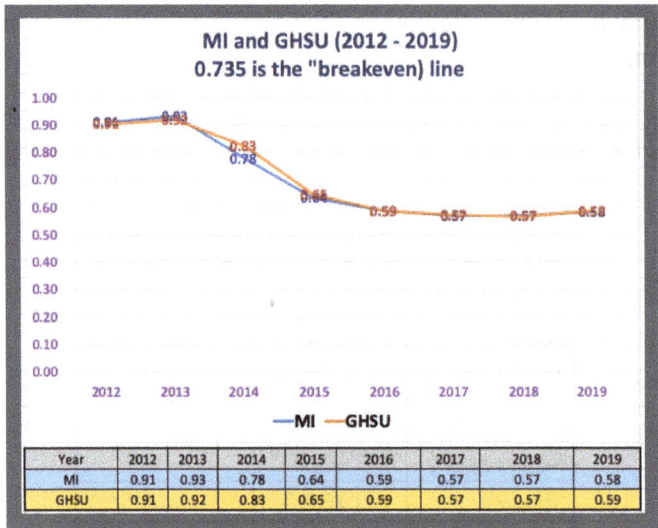

Figure 3: MI & GHSU (2012-2019)

Year	2012	2013	2014	2015	2016	2017	2018	2019
MI	0.91	0.93	0.78	0.64	0.59	0.57	0.57	0.58
GHSU	0.91	0.92	0.83	0.65	0.59	0.57	0.57	0.59

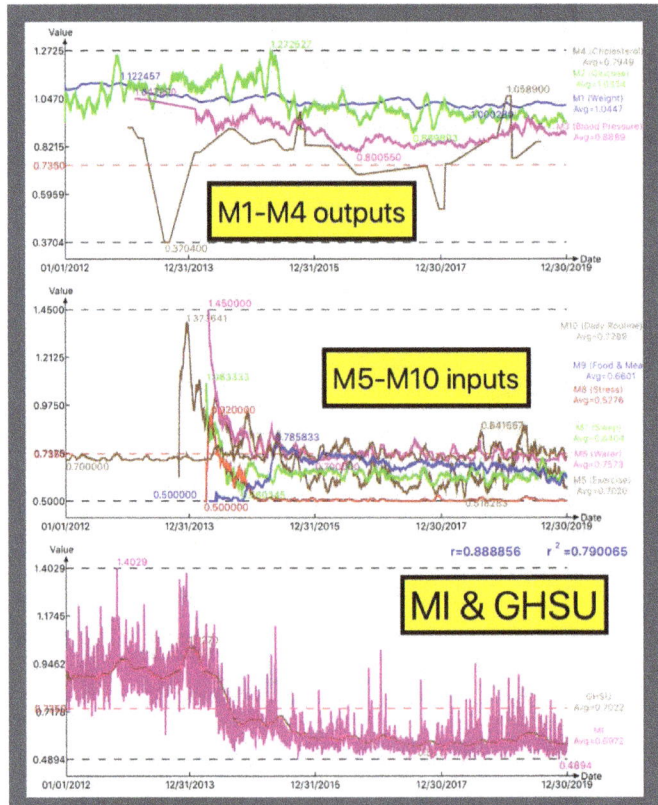

Figure 4: Annualized MI & GHSU

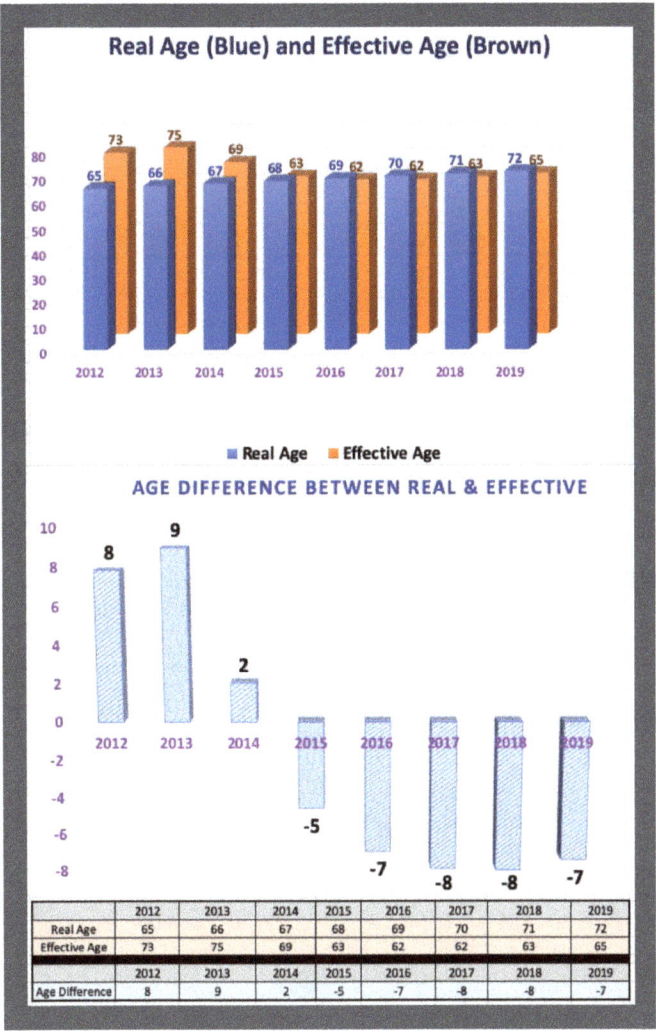

Real Age (Blue) and Effective Age (Brown)

AGE DIFFERENCE BETWEEN REAL & EFFECTIVE

	2012	2013	2014	2015	2016	2017	2018	2019
Real Age	65	66	67	68	69	70	71	72
Effective Age	73	75	69	63	62	62	63	65

	2012	2013	2014	2015	2016	2017	2018	2019
Age Difference	8	9	2	-5	-7	-8	-8	-7

Figure 5: Differences between Real & Effective Ages

Diabetic Retinopathy study via metabolism improvements and chronic diseases medical conditions control of HbA1C, SBP, and Triglycerides (using GH-Method: math-physical medicine) (No.247)

Gerald C. Hsu
eclaireMD Foundation, USA
4/16-21/2020

Introduction:

The author used his own medical data to investigate the impact on his diabetic retinopathy condition and its risk probability percentage or hazard ratio (HR) over a period of 7-years.

Methods:

The author suffered from type 2 diabetes (T2D) since 1996. By year 2010, he experienced cardiovascular disease, renal complications, bladder infection, foot ulcer, thyroid disorder, and vision problems. In July of 2010, three of his physicians warned him that he would have three to five remaining years to live. Therefore, he decided to study and research diabetes and its complications in order to save his own life. For the past 10 years, he has spent 30,000 hours on endocrinology with a specialty in diabetes and food nutrition.

The following timetable illustrates the focused area of each stage:

- 2000-2013 - Self-study diabetes and food nutrition, developing a data collection and analysis software

- 2014 - Develop a mathematical model of metabolism, using engineering modeling and advanced mathematics ·

- 2015 - Weight & FPG prediction models, using neuroscience

- 2016 - PPG & HbA1C prediction models, using optical physics, artificial intelligence (AI), and neuroscience

- 2017 - CVD and Stroke research, using segmentation analysis and pattern analysis

- 2018 - Complications due to micro-vascular research, for example, renal, bladder, and foot

- 2019 - CGM glucose big data analysis, using wave theory, energy theory, frequency domain analysis, quantum mechanics, and AI

- 2020 - Geriatrics, Longevity, Diabetic Retinopathy, Diabetic Hypothyroidism, linkage between Metabolism and Immunity

To date, he has collected ~2 million data regarding his medical conditions and lifestyle details. He has written 246 medical papers and made ~120 presentations at ~70 international medical conferences.

Under the leadership of American Diabetes Association (ADA), a group of 14 authors quoted 137 references to publish a long editorial article, "Perspectives in Diabetes: Diabetic Retinopathy, Seeing Beyond Glucose-Induced Microvascular Disease" (Reference 1).

Here is an excerpt:

The diabetic retinopathy remains the leading cause of vision impairment and blindness. The risk of developing vision loss from diabetes is predicted to double over the next three decades.

The fundamental functions of retina are to capture photons, convert the photochemical energy into electric energy, integrate the resulting action potentials, and transmit them to the occipital lobe of the brain, where they are deciphered and interpreted into recognizable images. Although the retina is easily visible, it is, ironically, the only major tissue affected by diabetes that cannot be biopsied in human.

*Established **neurobiological** principles can inform us how diabetes impairs vision, **and metabolism knowledge may lead to new treatments**. Retina physiology may underlie its vulnerability to diabetes. The combination of high metabolic demand and minimal vascular supply may limit the inner retina's ability to adapt to the metabolic stress of diabetes. The pathogenesis of diabetic retinopathy includes glucose-mediated micro vascular damage. Although micro vascular changes are undeniably integral to retinopathy, **the retina is actually a vascularized neural tissue, not a network of blood vessels. Diabetic retinopathy involves more than elevated glucose and micro vascular lesions.** Plenty of evidences for **neural retinal involvement in diabetic retinopathy** have already been presented.*

*To the best of our knowledge, there is no evidence that a primary, selective defect in vascular cells is sufficient to cause diabetic retinopathy. Clearly, **it is essential to treat both the vascular and neural elements of the retina to preserve vision.***

*Excess glucose (elevated **HbA1C**) is the primary culprit in the development and progression of diabetic retinopathy. However, disordered lipid (especially **triglycerides**) and protein metabolism are also linked to the central biochemical abnormality in all forms of impaired insulin action.*

In reference 2, a paper titled "Risk factors associated with progression to referable retinopathy" was written and presented by J. J. Smith, D. M. Wright, P. Scanlon, & N. Lois:

*This study was conducted in a dynamic cohort of 2,770 type 2 diabetes patients, recruited between April 2005 and July 2013 (~8 years) in Ireland. In this diabetic retinopathy paper, the authors demonstrated that Higher current values of **HbA1C, systolic blood pressure (SBP), and triglycerides were associated with increased risk of referral diabetic retinopathy.***

Based on learnings from these excerpts, the author conducted a study on his own diabetic retinopathy development and progression for the past 7-years (2013-2019). He has collected and further calculated the following data categories associated with his own medical conditions:

Weight: 2 body weight, BMI
Glucose: 1 FPG, 3 PPG, 1 daily A1C
Blood Pressure: SBP, DBP, pulse
Lipid: Triglycerides, HDL, LDL

The data for the top three categories were collected (weight, glucose, and BP) or calculated (i.e. HbA1C, BMI and predicted glucoses) on a daily basis. However, his lipid results were obtained from 22 hospital lab-tests with an averaged testing period of every four months.

Initially, he listed his lab-tested Triglycerides data, and then extracted data from both measured HbA1C and SBP from his stored database to match the actual dates of his lab-test for triglycerides (a total of 22 dates). In summary, 38,385 data of these 2,555 days (7-years) were used in this study.

Next, he selected the following medical conditions as his baseline conditions (i.e. "normal conditions") for his risk probability analysis.

Triglycerides: 150 mg/dL
SBP: 120
HbA1C: 6.0%

Finally, he applied a linear regression analysis model with 7 different cases to conduct his numerical analysis.

In addition, he also applied Cox proportional-hazards regression model to conduct one more set of calculation. The Cox Hazard Model can be expressed as follows:

$$h(t) =$$
$$h0(t) * exp(b1x1+b2x2+...+bnxn)$$

where h(t) is the expected hazard at time t, h0(t) is the baseline hazard and represents the hazard when all of the predictors (or independent variables) x1, x2 ... xn are equal to zero. Notice that the predicted hazard (i.e., h(t)), or the rate of suffering the event of interest in the next instant, is the product of the baseline hazard (h0(t)) and the exponential function of the linear combination of the predictors. Thus, the predictors have a multiplicative or proportional effect on the predicted hazard.

Results:

Figure 1 shows his records of Triglyceride, SBP, and HbA1C, where his SBP curve is expressed with 90-days moving average data.

After he matches the dates of both HbA1C and SBP with the actual lab-test dates of Triglycerides, he then normalized those daily medical values by using baseline or normal conditions. These original data and normalized results are shown in Figure 2.

Since, from external references, the author could not find the contribution margins (i.e. weighting factors) related to these three primary factors of diabetic retinopathy study (i.e. A1C, SBP, and Triglycerides), he then decided to conduct a sensitivity analysis by using a range of possible weighting factors. Figures 3, 4, 5, and 6 reflect the operational results and his 7 different cases of weighting factors.

Here is the list of these 7 different weighting factors:

Case 1: Trig 33%, SBP 33%, A1C 33% (even distribution at 33% each)
Case 2: Trig 30%, SBP 30%, A1C 40% (A1C is slightly heavier, 40%)
Case 3: Trig 60%, SBP 20%, A1C 20% (Trig is the heaviest, 60%)
Case 4: Trig 20%, SBP 60%, A1C 20% (SBP is the heaviest, 60%)
Case 5: Trig 20%, SBP 20%, A1C 60% (A1C is the heaviest, 60%)
Case 6: Trig 20%, SBP 30%, A1C 50% (A1C is heavier, 50%)
Case 7: Trig 30%, SBP 36%, A1C 34% (using Ref. 2's HR findings as a clue or source)

Figure 6 is a simplified Bart chart of risk probability % of these 7-cases.

From Figures 3, 4, 5, 6 and 7, we can observe the following conclusive phenomena:

(1) Upper bound: Both Case 5 (A1C 60%) and Case 6 (A1C 50%) have the highest risk probability % (106%-108%).
(2) Middle Ground: All of Case 7 (Ireland HR case), Case 1 (even distribution of 33% each), and Case 2 (A1C 40%) are within a range of moderate risk probability % (100-102%) .
(3) Lower Bound: Both Case 3 (Trig 60%) and Case 4 (SBP 60%) have the lowest risk probability % (94-98%).

Based on the author's medical data and personal feelings of his diabetic retinopathy conditions at different progression stages, the upper bound curves (Case 5 and Case 6) seem to be closely matched with the situation of his real conditions. On the opposite, the lower bound (Case 3 and Case 4) seem to be further apart from his real conditions.

Although lacking of available medical test data, but in general, he feels his overall diabetic retinopathy progression slowing down during the past 7 years. This feeling matched with the trend of this set of curves.

Although both blood pressure and lipids share their responsibility of damaging retina, but based on this specific study, it seems that HbA1C plays a major role of his diabetic retinopathy conditions and developments.

In summary, he applied both linear regression analysis and Cox proportional-hazard model to calculate his "relative" risk probability % and his hazard ratio (HR) using 0.366 as its baseline. The comparison of these two approaches can be seen in Figure 7. Although the absolute values are slightly different on certain test dates, but these two curves have an extremely high correlation coefficient (99.991%). These slight numerical differences are a result from HR Model utilizing exponential operation of the risk % value. The most important thing is that both of them demonstrate the relative risk probability % and relative hazard ratio (HR) of an upper bound Case 6 with a very high correlation.

Conclusion:

From this diabetic retinopathy sensitivity regression analysis results, it appears that diabetes, in particular HbA1C, plays a more dominating role as the murderer, while both hypertension (SBP) and hyperlipidemia (Triglycerides) play supporting roles as the accomplices. It is no wonder that the medical community calls it *diabetic* retinopathy! Nevertheless, the combination of these three chronic diseases may definitely cause severe damage to the retina. Furthermore, as stated in Reference 1, the diabetic retinopathy is not only a metabolic microvascular blood vessel issue, but also a serious neuroscience problem. The author strongly agrees with this viewpoint. In his recent research work of glucose, he has also identified the amounts for both fasting and postprandial glucoses' production and timing are controlled by our brain and neuro-system. He has already proved that diabetes itself is also closely related to our brain and nervous system.

As pointed out in Reference 1, this particular study may shed light on using an approach to strengthen metabolic conditions, combination of HbA1C, SBP, and triglycerides, to improve existing conditions of diabetic retinopathy in the patient.

References:

1. David A. Antonetti, Alistair J. Barber, Sarah K. Bronson1, Willard M. Freeman, Thomas W. Gardner, Leonard S. Jefferson, Mark Kester, Scot R. Kimball1, J. Kyle Krady, Kathryn F. LaNoue, Christopher C. Norbury, Patrick G. Quinn, Lakshman Sandirasegarane, Ian A. Simpson. (2006). Perspectives in Diabetes: Diabetic Retinopathy, Seeing Beyond Glucose-Induced Microvascular Disease. Diabetes. 55:2401–2411, 2006.
   doi.org/10.2337/db05-1635

2. J. J. Smith D. M. Wright P. Scanlon N. Lois. (2020). Risk factors associated with progression to referable retinopathy: a type 2 diabetes mellitus cohort study in the Republic of Ireland. Presented partially at the annual meeting of the Association for Research in Vision and Ophthalmology (ARVO), Vancouver, Canada, 28 April to 2 May 2019. doi.org/10.1111/dme.14278

3. Hsu, Gerald C. (2018). Using Math-Physical Medicine and Artificial Intelligence Technology to Manage Lifestyle and Control Metabolic Conditions of T2D. *International Journal of Diabetes & Its Complications,* 2(3),1-7. Retrieved from http://cmepub.com/pdfs/using-mathphysical-medicine-and-artificial-intelligence-technology-to-manage-lifestyle-and-control-metabolic-conditions-of-t2d-412.pdf

4. Hsu, Gerald C. (2018). A Clinic Case of Using Math-Physical Medicine to Study the Probability of Having a Heart Attack or Stroke Based on Combination of Metabolic Conditions, Lifestyle, and Metabolism Index. *Journal of Clinical Review & Case Reports*, 3(5), 1-2. Retrieved from https://www.opastonline.com/wp-content/uploads/2018/07/a-clinic-case-of-using-math-physical-medicine-to-study-the-probability-of-having-a-heart-attack-or-stroke-based-on-combination-of-metabolic-conditions-lifestyle-and-metabolism-index-jcrc-2018.pdf

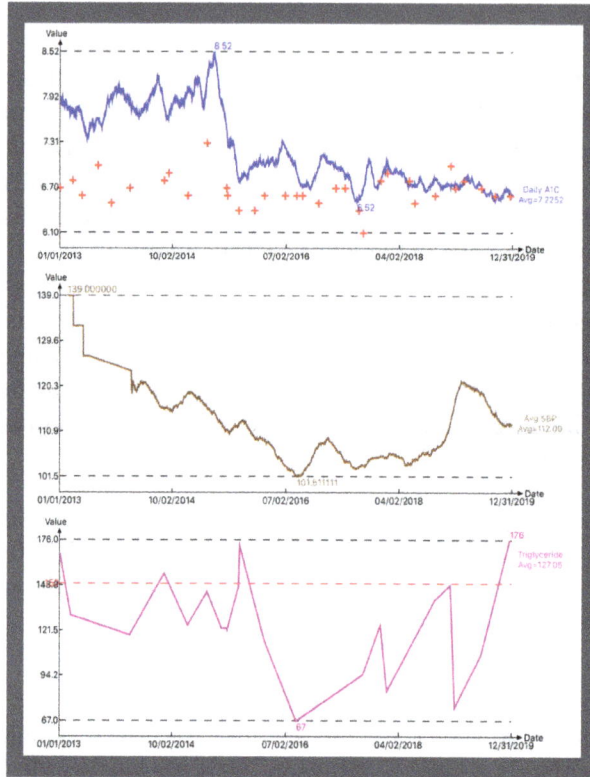

Figure 1: HbA1C, SBP, Triglycerides during 2013 - 2019

Original Data				Standard %	150	120	6.0
Date	Trig.	SBP	HbA1C	Date	Trig.	SBP	HbA1C
1/4/13	168	139	7.83	1/4/13	1.12	1.16	1.31
3/8/13	131	139	7.74	3/8/13	0.87	1.16	1.29
2/5/14	119	124	7.86	2/5/14	0.79	1.03	1.31
8/20/14	156	116	7.77	8/20/14	1.04	0.97	1.30
12/30/14	125	119	8.02	12/30/14	0.83	0.99	1.34
4/16/15	145	116	8.20	4/16/15	0.97	0.97	1.37
7/6/15	123	112	7.85	7/6/15	0.82	0.93	1.31
8/4/15	123	111	7.39	8/4/15	0.82	0.93	1.23
10/9/15	148	112	6.79	10/9/15	0.99	0.93	1.13
10/15/15	173	113	6.78	10/15/15	1.15	0.94	1.13
3/4/16	116	109	6.98	3/4/16	0.77	0.91	1.16
9/1/16	67	102	6.91	9/1/16	0.45	0.85	1.15
9/12/17	95	104	6.81	9/12/17	0.63	0.87	1.14
12/20/17	125	106	6.89	12/20/17	0.83	0.88	1.15
1/26/18	85	105	7.01	1/26/18	0.57	0.88	1.17
10/22/18	140	107	6.84	10/22/18	0.93	0.89	1.14
1/18/19	149	113	6.74	1/18/19	0.99	0.94	1.12
2/12/19	75	117	6.77	2/12/19	0.50	0.98	1.13
7/11/19	107	109	6.72	7/11/19	0.71	0.91	1.12
12/20/19	176	113	6.64	12/20/19	1.17	0.94	1.11
Avarage	**127**	**114.3**	**7.23**	**Avarage**	**0.85**	**0.95**	**1.20**

Figure 2: Original data and normalized value of HbA1C, SBP, Triglycerides of selected dates during 2013 - 2019

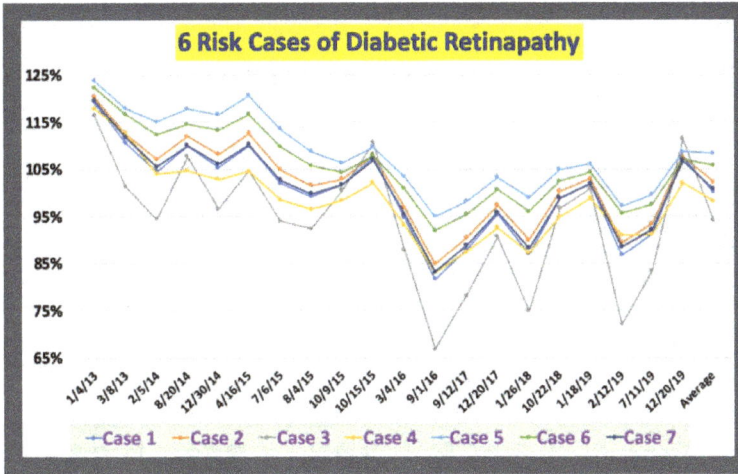

Figure 3: Time series Line Chart of diabetic retinopathy risk probability % of 7 cases

Risk Case	Case 1	Case 2	Case 3	Case 4	Case 5	Case 6	Case 7
1/4/13	119%	121%	116%	118%	124%	122%	120%
3/8/13	111%	113%	101%	113%	118%	117%	112%
2/5/14	105%	107%	94%	104%	115%	112%	106%
8/20/14	110%	112%	108%	105%	118%	115%	110%
12/30/14	105%	108%	97%	103%	117%	113%	106%
4/16/15	110%	113%	105%	105%	121%	117%	110%
7/6/15	102%	105%	94%	99%	114%	110%	103%
8/4/15	99%	102%	92%	97%	109%	106%	100%
10/9/15	102%	103%	101%	98%	106%	104%	102%
10/15/15	107%	108%	111%	102%	110%	108%	107%
3/4/16	95%	97%	88%	93%	103%	101%	95%
9/1/16	82%	85%	67%	83%	95%	92%	83%
9/12/17	88%	90%	78%	87%	98%	95%	89%
12/20/17	95%	97%	91%	93%	103%	101%	96%
1/26/18	87%	90%	75%	87%	99%	96%	88%
10/22/18	99%	100%	97%	95%	105%	102%	99%
1/18/19	102%	103%	101%	99%	106%	104%	102%
2/12/19	87%	89%	72%	91%	97%	96%	88%
7/11/19	91%	93%	83%	91%	100%	98%	92%
12/20/19	107%	108%	111%	102%	109%	107%	107%
Average	100%	102%	94%	98%	108%	106%	101%

Figure 4: Data Table of Diabetic Retinopathy risk probability % of 7 cases

Risk Case	Risk %	Trig.	SBP	A1C
Case 1	100%	33%	33%	33%
Case 2	102%	30%	30%	40%
Case 3	94%	60%	20%	20%
Case 4	98%	20%	60%	20%
Case 5	108%	20%	20%	60%
Case 6	106%	20%	30%	50%
Case 7	101%	30%	36%	34%
Case 7	HR	1.10	1.29	1.22

Figure 5: Table of contribution weighting factors and risk probability % of 7 cases

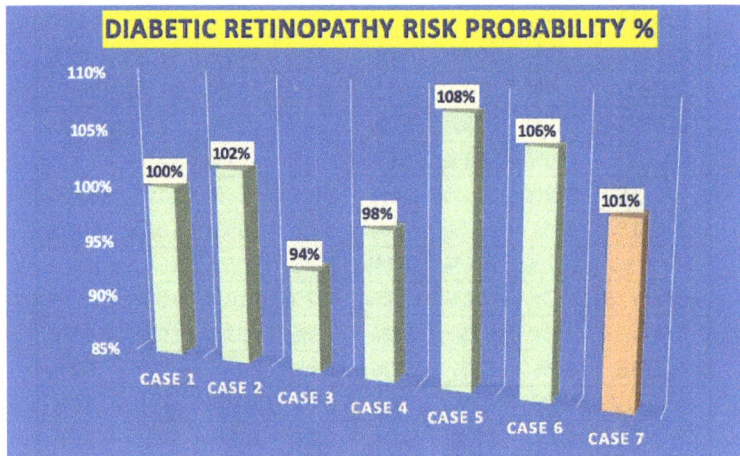

Figure 6: Bar Chart of diabetic retinopathy risk probability % of 7 cases

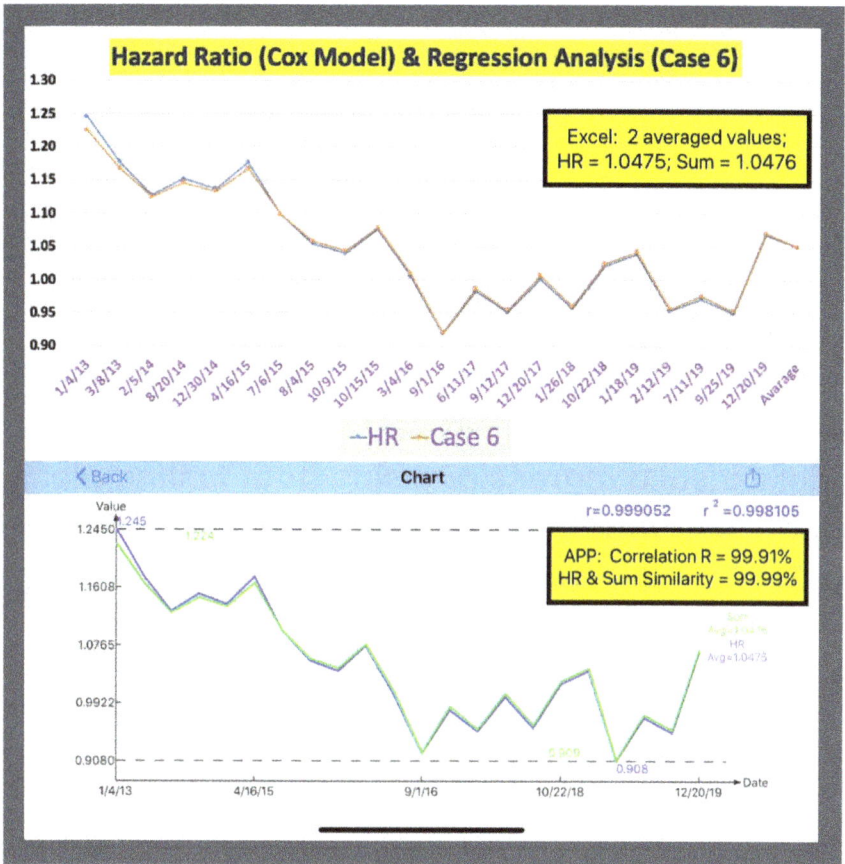

Figure 7: Comparison of Case 6 between weighted risk probability (Sum) % and HR Model results

A summary report on self-repair of the pancreatic beta cells insulin regression using both fasting plasma glucose, postprandial plasma glucose and HbA1C data using GH-Method: math-physical medicine (No. 252)

By: Gerald C. Hsu
eclaireMD Foundation, USA
5/2-3/2020 Stanford

Introduction:

In this paper, the author describes his hypothesis on the "self-recovery" of partial insulin regeneration capacity of the pancreatic beta cells from a type 2 diabetes (T2D) patient (himself). By using the collected big data of postprandial plasma glucose (PPG) of both Finger piercing PPG and Synthesized PPG via Sensor PPG pattern, fasting plasma glucose (FPG of Finger piercing), and HbA1C for six years from 1/1/2014 to 12/31/2019.

Methods:

Background

The author has had T2D for 25 years and took various diabetes medications to control his elevated glucose levels starting in 1998. For the last 20 years, he has suffered from many complications from his diabetes, including five cardiac episodes, foot ulcer, bladder infection, renal complications, diabetic retinopathy, and hypothyroidism; however, he did not have a stroke.

In 2013, he started different stages to reduce the dosages from his three prescribed diabetes medications. On 12/8/2015, he finally ceased his last one, the classic metformin HCL. For more than four years, his body has been free of any medications.

Since then, he has completely relied on a stringent lifestyle management program to control his diabetes conditions. As a result, his HbA1C has been reduced from 10% in 2010, while taking medications, to an average of 6.63% during 2016-2019 without any medication or use of insulin injection (Figure 1).

Thus far, he has kept ~2 million data of his own medical conditions and lifestyle details. He has also developed a sophisticated computer software by using big data analytics, artificial intelligence, physics concepts and principles, mathematics equations and formulas, as well as some engineering modeling techniques to analyze, process, manage his massive health data, and even predict future development of certain important biomedical variables, such as HbA1C.

To summarize prominent findings from the glucose data analysis based on his own observations for the past 4 to 6 years, he has noticed two "opposite" phenomena. The first observation, his peak PPG value around 60-minutes after the first bite of his meal, occasionally reaches to 200-300 mg/dL when he does not follow his stringent diet and exercise guidelines. This explicitly shows the true status and severity of his existing T2D conditions in terms of insulin resistance or lack of insulin production supply. The second observation, from checking his massive data since 2014, his natural health state of pancreatic beta cells seems to be on a "slow" self-recovery path, even though its recovery rate might be on a small scale.

Other research:

Recently, he read an article online, *"Diabetes: Can we teach the body to heal itself?"* on *Medical News Today*, which was published on January 8, 2019.

Here is an excerpt:

"A new study by researchers from the University of Bergen in Norway, Maria Cohut, Ph.D. and Luiza Ghoul, suggests that, with just a small "push," we may be able to train the body to start producing adequate levels of insulin once more, on its own. The researchers were able, for the first time, to uncover some of the key mechanisms that allow cells to "switch" identity, looking specifically at pancreatic alpha- and beta-cells in a mouse model. They found that alpha-cells respond to complex signals they receive from neighboring cells in the context of beta-cell loss. **Approximately 2 percent of alpha-cells can thus "reprogram" themselves and start producing insulin.** *By using a compound able to influence cell signaling in the pancreas, the researchers could boost the number of insulin-making cells by 5 percent.*

The author's research methodology is a "math-physical medicine" approach, rather than a "biochemical medicine" approach as used in the article above. Furthermore, he uses his own body, instead of a "mouse model" cited in Norway's lab test.

Methodology:

Math-physical medicine approach has three key steps of research methodology. For the first step, it starts with observing physical phenomena of some prominent biomedical characteristics from collected data. All of the biological and chemical work including their actions and chain reactions in the human body and organs would show or expose some sort of physical phenomena in terms of exterior appearances, because both biology and chemistry are applied physics. In the second step, he then forms a hypothesis from these specific physical observations based on physics theories or concepts. The third step, if possible, he utilizes existing mathematical equations (along with their given constraints) or derives his own mathematical equations and constraints based on both original physics concept and engineering models (engineering is applied physics and physics is applied mathematics), in order to verify or prove his hypothesis. Finally, once his hypothesis is proven by using his collected data, he can then apply these mathematical prediction equations to recreate future outcomes or reproduce the final results based on future input data. It should be noted that computer science techniques, such as artificial intelligence and big data analytics, are only served as convenient and useful "tools" for his simulation model work and massive data processing.

This research work:

This project started in July of 2019 and lasted through May of 2020. During this 10-month period, he has already written 10 medical papers (No. 103, 108, 112, 133, 138, 139, 241, 242, 243, 244) regarding the subject of beta cells. In those referenced papers, he has described his suspicion and hypothesis regarding the probability of his pancreatic beta cells' "self-recovery". He will try to summarize his efforts on how he determined his annualized self-recovery rate of his damaged pancreatic beta cells due to either insufficient insulin production and/or insulin resistance.

Results:

(A) Baseline PPG: Lower-Bound

Applying signal processing technique of wave theory from electronics and earth science, the author was able to successfully decompose his PPG waveform into 19 sub-waves of carbs/sugar intake (39%) and post-meal walking exercise (41%) plus other 17 secondary factors and "left-over" or remaining insulin's biological functionality (a total of ~20%). He developed a linear equation for a newly termed "Baseline PPG" which is further defined as follows:

Baseline PPG =
Measured PPG + PPG Adjustment

Where PPG Adjustment =
(diet *B - walking/1000 * C)
B and C are different multipliers

We can observe from Figure 2 that both increased PPG amount by food intake and decreased PPG amount by walking steps are almost equal and cancel each other for both periods (6/1/2015-5/3/2020 and 1/1/2017-5/3/2020). However, the PPG moving average curves still have noticeable variances due to some of remaining secondary factors, and mostly the "left-over" insulin functionalities of the pancreatic beta cells.

He then calculated these Baseline PPG values using the above equation and segregated the Baseline PPG data into annualized average Baseline PPG datasets for the 6-year period between 2014 and 2019 (Figure 3). Finally, he computed the baseline PPG's change rate (%) of each year as well as the average change rates of these 6 years. *For this lower-bound case of Baseline PPG, the annualized change rate is 1.5%.*

(B) Segment turning points PPG: Medium

During the period of ~5 years (June of 2015 through April of 2020), there are 7 "turning-points" PPG values (i.e. peaks or bottoms of a wave). By connecting these turning-points and then calculating the decline rate of each segment, he was able to get the overall average dropping rate (see Figure 4). If we include the first PPG peak of 141 mg/dL, then the overall average declining rate is 3.8%; and if we exclude the first peak, then the overall average declining rate is 2.3%. *For this medium case of Segment Turning-point PPG, the annualized change rate is 2.3%. The author choose this conservative rate of 2.3% in order to remove the perturbation caused by the first peak data).*

(C) Synthesized PPG via OHCA Model: Upper-bound

The author has applied his created OHCA (Open, High, Close, and Average) Model of the CGM Sensor PPG data during 5/5/2018 to 4/5/2020 to build a hypothetical synthesized sensor PPG model for the pre-CGM period of 1/1/2014 - 5/4/2018 (see Figure 5). Since the average sensor PPG value is about 18% higher than Finger PPG value, this is the reason he created "synthesized PPG" value, which would serve as an upper bound of his research results. Following the same calculation scheme, we get a higher bound of PPG change rate result. This effect is due to the observation of

CGM sensor monitoring the entire 3-hour time span of a PPG wave, while Finger PPG measuring around 2-hours after the first bite of food, usually catching a much lower PPG value. *For this upper-bound case of Synthesized PPG via OHCA Model, the annualized change rate is 3.5% (see Figure 6).*

(D) Combined average PPG

When we add the above three PPG models change rates we then get *the combined average PPG change rate of 2.3% per year.*

(E) FPG

By applying the signal processing technique similar to the PPG case, we can identify the most significant contribution factor of FPG is the body weight in the morning (> 90% of influence). The remaining 4 other secondary factors and "left-over" or "remaining" insulin functionalities contribute only ~10% or less. As shown in Figure 7, the correlation between the annualized body weight vs. annualized FPG is as high as 93%. The author notices that for the past 6 years, his weight dropped moderately from 177 lbs. in 2014 down to 173 lbs. (- 2.3%) in 2019. However, his FPG decreased more noticeably from 128 mg/dL down to 113 mg/dL (- 11.7%). This observation is another indirect proof that his pancreatic beta cells have been self-repairing over the past 6 years. *For this FPG case, the FPG change rate is 2.3% per year.*

Currently, we can see that both of his combined average PPG change rate and FPG change rate are at 2.3% per year (see Figure 8).

(F) HbA1C

He developed a mathematical model to predict his HbA1C level on daily basis. He utilized his past 4-moth glucoses data, including both FPG and PPG, and then assigned different weighting factors for each month input data. Combining with some other assumptions and adjustments, this daily HbA1C model becomes a "nonlinear" mathematical model which he named as the "N-2 model" inside of his computer software program. Due to this difficulty, it is not easy to decompose his HbA1C wave similar to his PPG wave using signal processing technique. *For this HbA1C case, the HbA1C change rate is 2.9% per year (see Figure 9), which is higher than 2.3% for both FPG and PPG cases.*

Conclusion:

The author has spent 10-months to research the self-recovery of his pancreatic beta cells via different entry-points and various methods. He has written a total of 10 medical articles regarding this specific subject (see References). Finally, after summarizing all of his past findings at different research stages, he has confirmed that, via his continuous and stringent lifestyle management efforts, he has seen a self-recovery rate of 2.3% to 2.9% per year. This percentage range is actually quite close to the cited Norwegian Lab's mouse result of ~2% conversion rate from alpha cells into beta cells to produce insulin.

Although this is only a moderate improvement, it is still promising. If his self-recovery rate is 2.3% to 2.9%, then for the past 6 to 7 years, his beta cells insulin functionalities have been repaired by 13% to 20%. This solid evidence of "glucose improvement" for nearly 7-years is a non-arguable fact. Most medical professionals stated that diabetes is an "irreversible" or "non-curable" disease. At least, the author has now proven that not only has he stopped the "deterioration" of his T2D conditions, but he may have "reversed" his damaged pancreatic beta cells. Hopefully, by sharing his lifestyle program, research methods, and positive results, other T2D patients can also be encouraged to achieve similar positive results on their battles against diabetes.

References:

Hsu, Gerald C., eclaireMD Foundation, USA

1. Using GH-Method: math-physical medicine methodology and four clinical cases to study type 2 diabetes patients' liver and pancreas baseline conditions

2. Changes in relative health state of pancreas beta cells over eleven years using GH-Method: math-physical medicine

3. Changes in relative health state of pancreas beta cells over eleven years using GH-Method: math-physical medicine

4. Probable partial recovery of pancreatic beta cells insulin regeneration using annualized fasting plasma glucose (GH-Method: math-physical medicine)

5. Probable partial self-recovery of pancreatic beta cells using calculations of annualized fasting plasma glucose (GH-Method: math-physical medicine)

6. Guesstimate probable partial self-recovery of pancreatic beta cells using calculations of annualized glucose data using GH-Method: math-physical medicine

7. Using signal processing techniques to decompose PPG waveform and investigate the regeneration of pancreatic beta cells insulin production (GH-Method: math-physical medicine)

8. Probable self-recovery of pancreatic beta cells insulin regeneration using annualized PPG, postprandial plasma glucose (GH-Method: math-physical medicine)

9. (Probable partial self-recovery of pancreatic beta cells using various glucose data (GH-Method: math-physical medicine)

10. Using GH-Method: math-physical medicine approach and various glucose data to investigate the health state of a type 2 diabetes patient's pancreatic β- cells

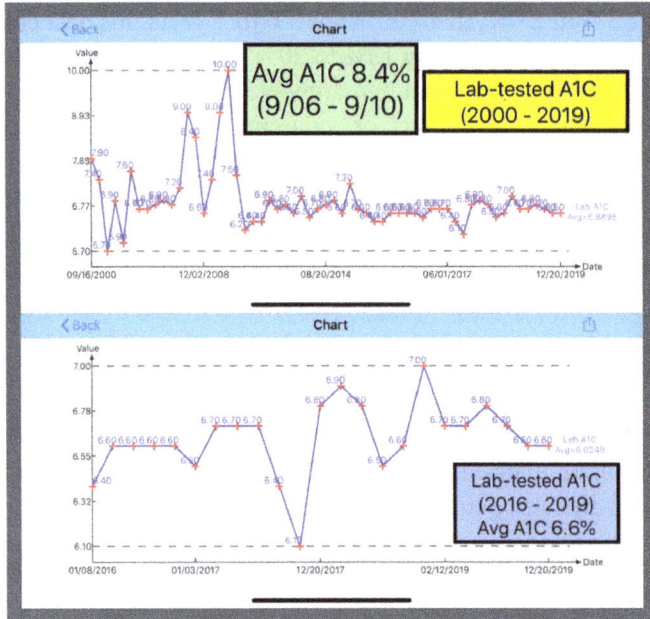

Figure 1: HbA1C results

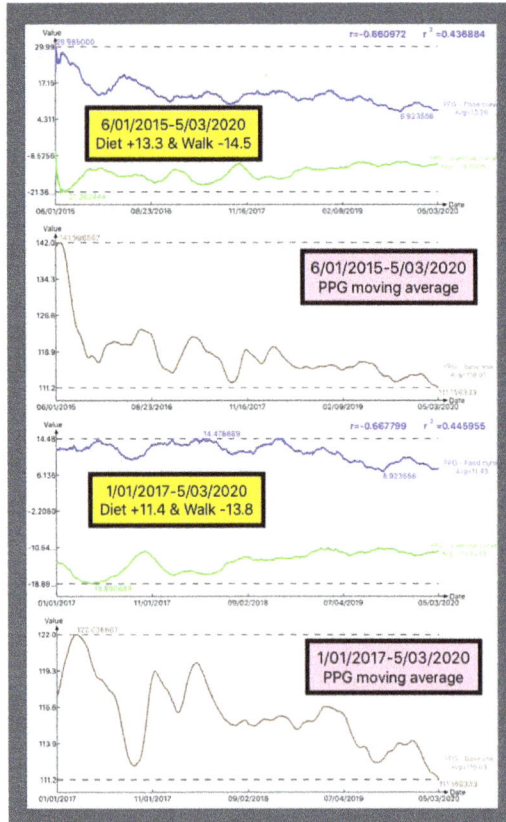

Figure 2: PPG with food and exercise

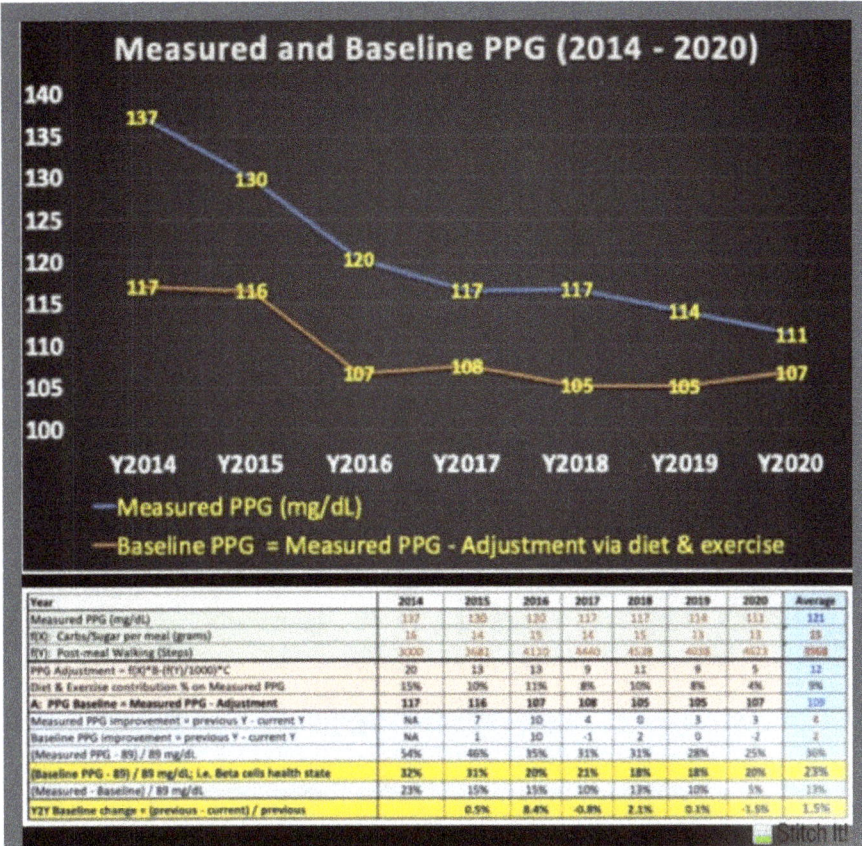

Figure 3: Baseline PPG (minus adjustments) improvements (lower-bound)

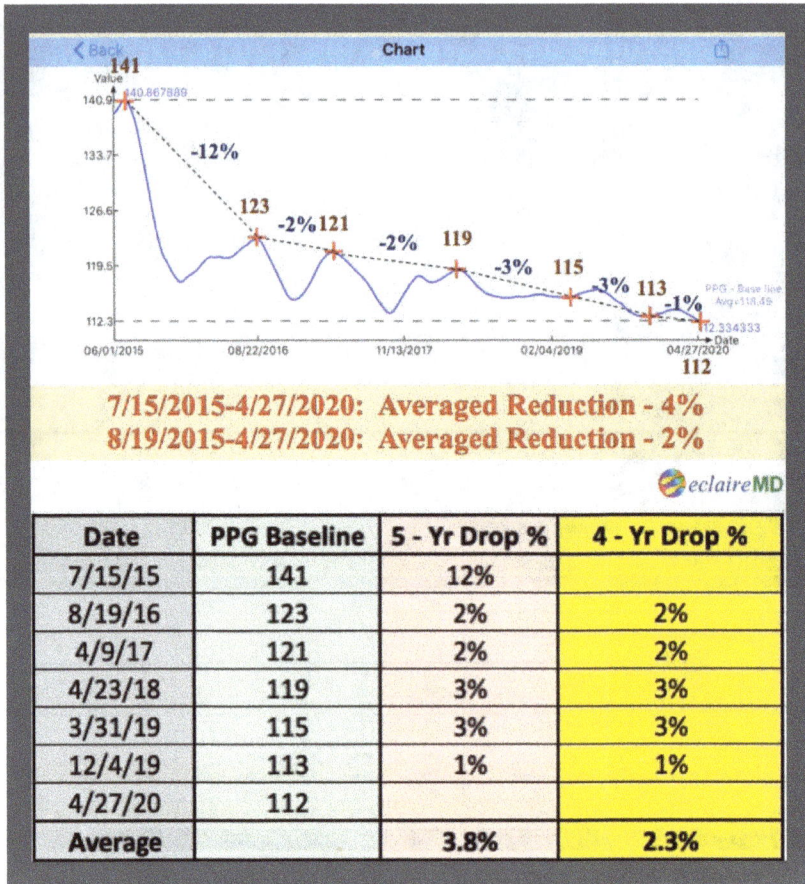

Date	PPG Baseline	5 - Yr Drop %	4 - Yr Drop %
7/15/15	141	12%	
8/19/16	123	2%	2%
4/9/17	121	2%	2%
4/23/18	119	3%	3%
3/31/19	115	3%	3%
12/4/19	113	1%	1%
4/27/20	112		
Average		3.8%	2.3%

Figure 4: Segment turning-points PPG improvements (medium)

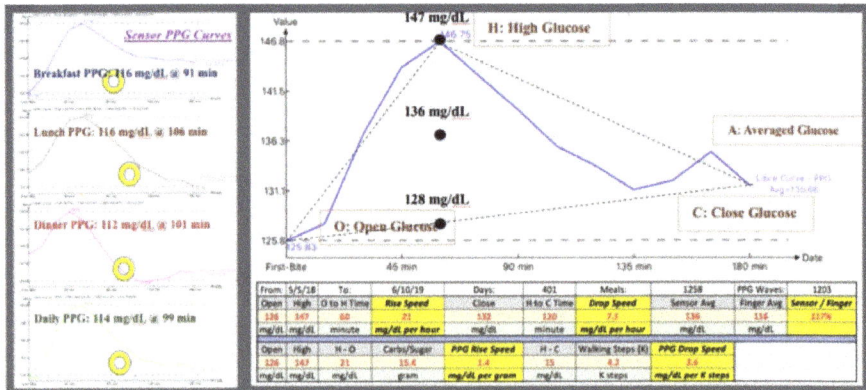

Figure 5: OHCA Model to extend CGM Sensor PPG to Finger PPG

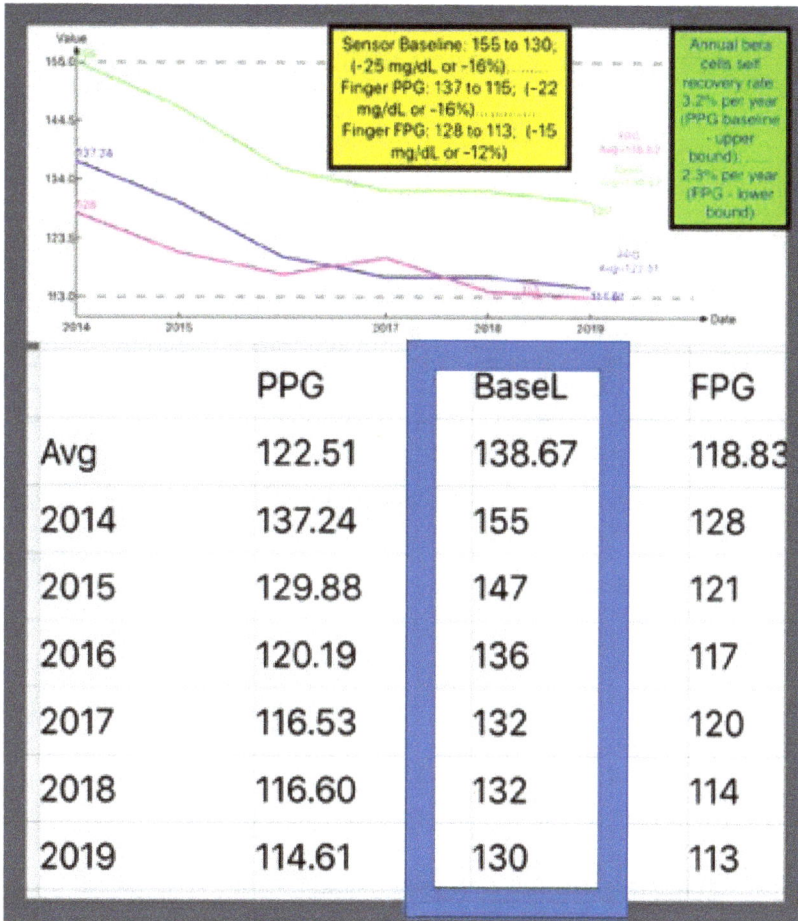

	PPG	BaseL	FPG
Avg	122.51	138.67	118.83
2014	137.24	155	128
2015	129.88	147	121
2016	120.19	136	117
2017	116.53	132	120
2018	116.60	132	114
2019	114.61	130	113

Figure 6: Synthesized PPG improvements (upper bound)

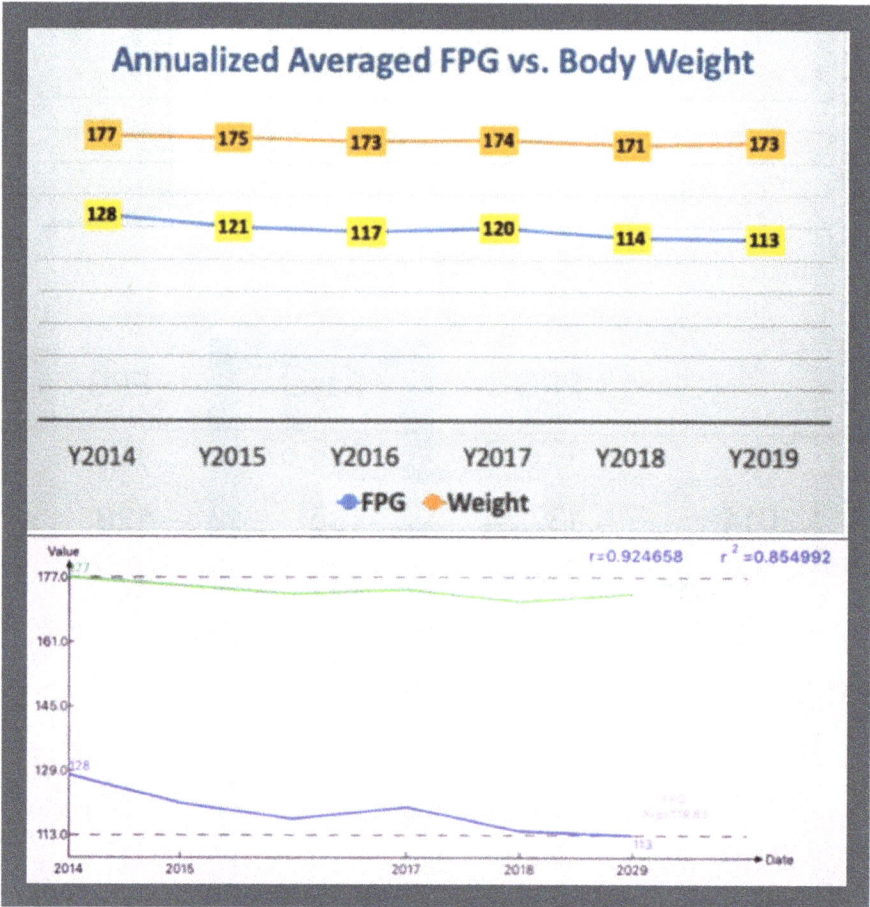

Figure 7: Finger FPG improvements

Entry Point of Analysis	Repaire Rate
PPG: Baseline (Measured - Adjustments)	1.5%
PPG: Segment Peaks	2.3%
PPG: Synthesized via OHCA Sensor Model	3.2%
PPG: Average of above 3	2.3%
FPG: Correlated with Weight	2.3%

Pancreatic Beta Cells are "self-recovering" at a rate of 2.3% per year

Figure 8: Summary Table of pancreatic beta cells "self-recovery" rate of 2.3% (PPG & FPG)

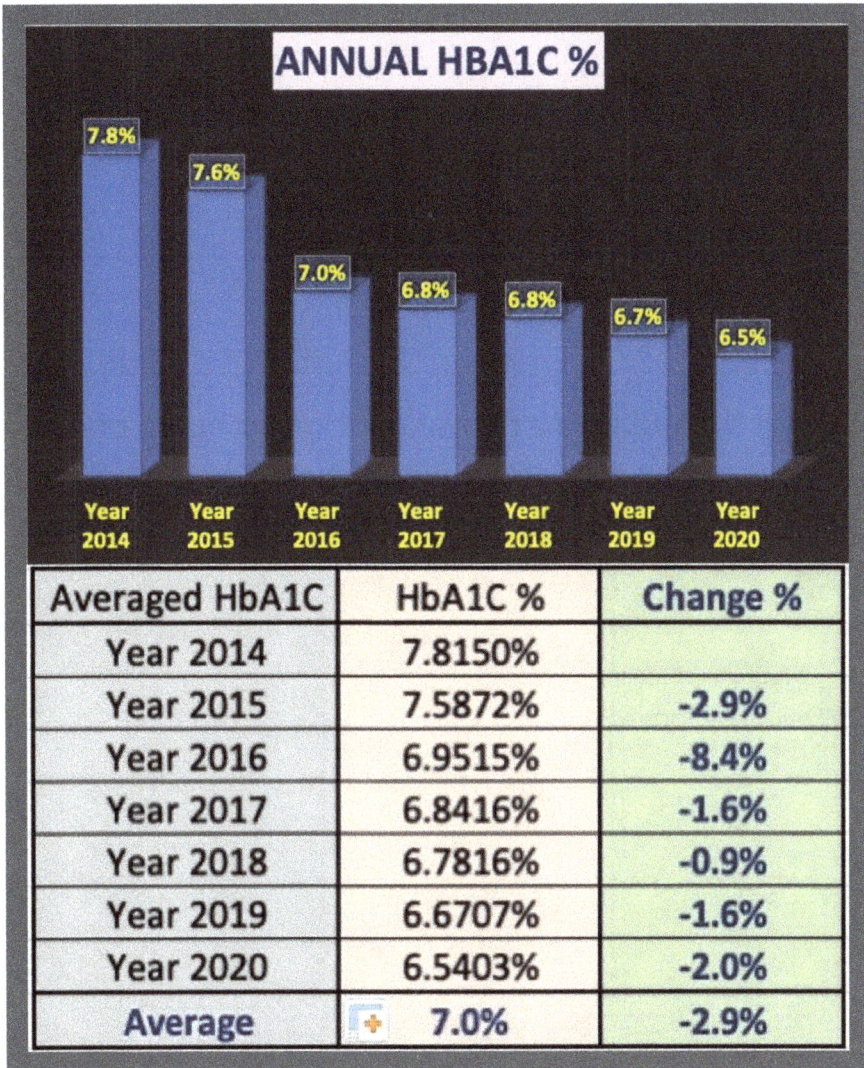

ANNUAL HBA1C %

Averaged HbA1C	HbA1C %	Change %
Year 2014	7.8150%	
Year 2015	7.5872%	-2.9%
Year 2016	6.9515%	-8.4%
Year 2017	6.8416%	-1.6%
Year 2018	6.7816%	-0.9%
Year 2019	6.6707%	-1.6%
Year 2020	6.5403%	-2.0%
Average	7.0%	-2.9%

Figure 9: Pancreatic beta cells "self-recovery" rate of 2.9% (HbA1C)

How to reverse chronic disease induced heart conditions using a simple and effective "cookbook of quantitative formulas" using GH-Method: math-physical medicine (No. 256)

Gerald C. Hsu
eclaireMD Foundation, USA
5/7-9/2020

Introduction:

The author uses GH-Method: math-physical medicine (MPM) approach to investigate his risk probability (Risk) of having a cardiovascular disease (CVD) or stroke. Here, the word of CVD implies the most common type of heart diseases. It is also called coronary artery disease (CAD), or coronary heart disease (CHD). All of these situations relate to plaque buildups to block the blood flow in arteries due to high glucose and high lipid, or rupture of arteries caused by high glucose and high blood pressure. Based on the research findings of his CVD and stroke risks investigation (Reference 1), this article specifically addresses how he "reversed" his chronic diseases induced heart conditions in a quantitative manner, via a stringent lifestyle management program without drugs or surgeries. The word "reverse" used in this context is to change the direction of his heart condition's progression in order to prevent the condition from worsening.

Methods:

Background:

The author is a 73-year-old male who has a history of three severe chronic diseases for over 25 years. He experienced five cardiac episodes, without having a stroke, from 1994 through 2008. During that period, he thought the cause of his cardiac episodes were outcomes from his stressful business life. In mid-2010, he was diagnosed with an acute renal problem with an albumin-to-creatinine ratio (ACR) level of 116 mg/g (30 -300 mg/g refers to albumin excretion above the normal range) and would eventually require dialysis treatment. At that time, he also consulted with three independent physicians and received similar warnings that he would die within 3 to 5 years if he did not reverse his overall poor health conditions. This kidney episode was his final "wake up call". Therefore, he launched his own efforts of study and research internal medicine, especially endocrinology. Since 2010, he spent 30,000 hours to focus on research of diabetes and its various complications, especially heart and kidney. Now, he has extended his research into diabetic retinopathy and hyperthyroidism.

During 2010-2013, he self-studied diabetes and food nutrition via reading many textbooks and medical publications. In 2012, he developed a customized computer software to collect vital data of his own health conditions. By 2014, he further developed a complex mathematical model of metabolism and also started his stringent lifestyle management program. As a result, his overall health conditions have been noticeably improving since 2014. In the same year, he decided to gradually reduce the dosage of his three different diabetes medications. By December 8th of 2015, he completely stopped taking all kinds of diabetes medications. Within 2015-2016, he also created four mathematical prediction models for body weight, fasting plasma glucose (FPG), postprandial plasma glucose (PPG), and HbA1C values, and achieved accuracy rates above 97%. Due to his high-tech background, he also applied optical physics and artificial intelligence to develop an iPhone APP to estimate the carbs/sugar amount contained inside of his food from meal photo, and then predicted his finger-piercing PPG level at two hours after first bite of his meal. During the entire post-medication period of 12/8/2015 through 5/5/2020, his lab-tested HbA1C averaged value is around 6.6% which decreased from his peak value of 10% in 2010.

Glucose:

Arteries in our body carry glucose (nutrition) and oxygen via blood flow to our heart and other organs which then provide energy (i.e. metabolism) for living our life. This situation is remarkably similar to the tubes that transmit gasoline and air to the engine and other parts of the car which provide energy to move the car.

In his various research subjects of diabetes and complications, including heart (CVD, CAD, CHD), stroke, kidney, bladder, nervous system, foot, eyes, and thyroid, he has identified high glucose (diabetes) as the "principal criminal" while high blood pressure (hypertension) and high lipid (hyperlipidemia) are "accessory criminals" that work together to cause various diabetes complications. Glucose contributes somewhere near 40% to 60% weight of the total influences.

There are many contributing factors to high glucose in spite of two biological factors which are pancreatic beta cells damage and being overweight (obesity). In total, there are 24 influential factors, such as food, exercise, weather temperature, sleep, stress, etc. Among those many influential factors, the most prominent two are carbs/sugar intake (39%) and post-meal exercise (41%). Exercise not only reduces inflammation in our body organs but also highly effective to bring down our glucose level quickly. The "post-meal" exercise impacts PPG even more obviously. Although some human psychological behaviors, including love to eat and lazy on exercise, are quite common for most people, diet control is indeed far more complicated than exercising in terms of scope of knowledge, variety of choices, and degree of difficulty.

Once diet and exercise are in place, most likely, glucose and HbA1C will be under well control. Now, let us expand the glucose control to combine with the management of both blood pressure (reduce salt consumption, avoid stress, exercise) and lipid (avoid fat, reduce cholesterol consumption, exercise), your blood system (both artery and micro-vessels) will then be in a healthy state. This will definitely reduce our risks of having artery problems, such as CVD & stroke; and micro-vessel & nerves problems, such as renal failure, bladder infection, foot ulcer, diabetic retinopathy, and erectile dysfunction, and so forth.

Nutrition:
The author has been practicing the following listed rules in terms of his diet nutrition control:

(1) In general, 90% of his meals are plant-based diets and 10% are animal-based diets. Among all of those popular diets on consumer market, the Mediterranean Diet is his choice of diet, not Atkins diet or Paleo diet.

(2) He maintains a well-balanced nutrition diet which includes carbohydrates and sugar coming from vegetables mainly. Due to diabetes sensitivity to sugar, he eats

only limited quantity and carefully selected fruits, such as berries. Besides, he prefers high quality proteins from fish, chicken, egg white, cheese, and tofu. He cooks his meal with olive oil mainly, uses flaxseed oil for salad at least 1.4 gram per day since it contains high omega 3. He eats small amount of seeds and nuts every day, frequently eats reasonable amount of whole grains, legumes, soy products and also makes sure that his daily supplies of multiple vitamins are met.

(3) He avoids eating white rice; white flour-based food, e.g. bread, noodle, or cake; potatoes, vegetable roots; or any refined food with high carbohydrates or sugar in it. Occasionally he eats small amount of brown rice, oatmeal or whole wheat toast.

(4) He avoids any high-fat animal-based red meat, such as beef, pork, or lamb. He only eats fish and limited amount of shell fishes. He does not like to eat chicken, but chicken (without skin and fat) is a good protein source.

(5) He tries to eat "whole food" which is defined as food that naturally produced from farm and have not been processed or refined by any machine in any factory and are free from any chemical additives or artificial substances.

(6) In summary, he mainly eats lots of vegetables, plant-based diet with low sugar, low fat, low refined-carbs, low animal proteins, high plant-based protein, high in good fat (omega-3 fatty acids).

Results:

The above section of "Methods" are mainly described in a qualitative manner, however, this section of "Results" will be described in a quantitative manner. All of these results are measured and analyzed from data collected during the period of 12/8/2015 through 5/5/2020, the so called his "post- medications period".

Weight Control (Figure 2):
He maintains an **82% of his normal food portion** as guidelines of his regular meal amount. In this way, he could maintain his **BMI around 25** and his weight would bounce between 170 lbs. to 176 lbs. (77.2 kg to 80 kg) with an averaged weight of 173 lbs (78.6 kg). As a reference, he weighed 220 lbs. (100 kg) in 2000 and weighted 198 lbs. (90 kg) in 2010.

FPG Control (Figure 2):
FPG would drop between 1.5 mg/dL and 3.6 mg/dL for each pound of weight reduction. The daily FPG variance range also depends on some other factors, such as sleep condition, stress, cold weather temperature, etc. During this period of research data, the variance range of his FPG is bouncing between 93 mg/dL and 140 mg/dL with an averaged FPG of 116 mg/dL.

PPG Control (Figure3)
PPG would increase 1.8 mg/dL for each gram of carb/sugar intake. During this period, his averaged carbs/sugar intake was 14.48 grams and his averaged PPG increased by 26.1 mg/dL.

PPG would decrease 5.0 mg/dL for each 1,000 steps of post-meal walking. During this period, his averaged post-meal walking was 4,285 steps and his averaged PPG decreased by 21.4 mg/dL.

FPG would decrease 0.3 mg/dL for every degree Fahrenheit weather temperature decrease, while PPG would increase 0.9 mg/dL for every degree Fahrenheit weather temperature increase. During this period, the weather temperatures varies between 58 degree to 87 degree with an average temperature of 72.4 degree. During this period, most of the time, he moved around according to weather change, except for trips to attend various medical conferences. As a result, his PPG increased amount from weather temperature influence is +3.4 mg/dL.

The author utilized signal processing technique to decompose seven waveforms of secondary influential factors and then combined with waves of both carbs/sugar and post-meal walking to obtain a predicted finger PPG at 117.6 mg/dL (Figure 8). This gives a prediction accuracy of 99.2% in comparison with the actual measured finger PPG at 116.7 mg/dL.

HbA1C control (Figure 4):
FPG occupies ~25% of influential weight on HbA1C formation while PPG occupies ~75% of influential weight on HbA1C formation. During this period, his averaged FPG was 116.4 mg/dL while his averaged PPG was 116.7 mg/dL. They are amazingly close to each other. This is not coincidence, but rather due to his diligence and persistence on implementing his lifestyle management program. As a result, his mathematically predicted daily HbA1C value was 6.8% (97% prediction accuracy) while his 23 collected lab-tested HbA1C averaged value was 6.6%.

Blood Pressure, Lipid (Figure 5):
His **averaged SBP/DBP/Heart Rate was 109/66/56. His averaged Triglycerides/ LDL/HDL was 108/109/47**. All of these values are normal and healthy.

Metabolism Index (MI Figure 5):
His **averaged MI was 0.58** which is extreme healthy (below the break-even line of 0.735, see Reference 1). By implementing and following his stringent lifestyle management program, he could completely control his Type 2 Diabetes conditions. As an associated consequence, his hypertension (high blood pressure) and hyperlipidemia (high lipid) conditions were also well under-controlled since those three areas are inter-related (Reference 2).

CVD Risk Assessment (Figure 6):
In 2017, he developed a sophisticated and complex mathematical model to calculate his risk probability of having a chronic diseases induced CVD or stroke. This model includes personal & genetic data, such as age, gender, race, family medical history, personal health history, BMI (weight & height), waistline, bad habits (smoking, alcohol drinking, illicit drugs), probability of blockage and rupture of blood vessels due to different medical conditions (mainly chronic diseases), and lifestyle details. Here is his annualized risks probability **based on MI** of having a CVD or stroke (see Figure 3):

Y2000: 85% (weight 220 lbs., BMI 32.5, waistline 44 inches)
Y2010: 82% (weight 198 lbs., BMI 29.2, glucose 280 mg/dL)
Y2012: 82% (glucose 128 mg/dL)
Y2013: 84% (glucose 133 mg/dL)
Y2014: 71% (developed metabolism model, glucose 135 mg/dL)
Y2015: 60% (weight & FPG control, glucose 129 mg/dL)
Y2016: 55% (PPG control & stopped medication, glucose 119 mg/dL)
Y2017: 54% (BMI 25, glucose 117 mg/dL)
Y2018: 53% (heavy traveling, glucose 116 mg/dL)
Y2019: 55% (heavy traveling, glucose 114mg/dL)
Y2020 : 51% (weight 171 lbs., BMI 25, waistline 32.5 in, glucose 112 mg/dL)

It should be noted here that the risk probability percentages are expressed on a "relative" scale, not on an "absolute" scale.

Due to his heavy traveling schedules of attending more than 60 medical conferences during 2018-2019, his risks of having a CVD or stroke were in the range of 53%-55%; however, during this recent stabilized self-quarantined life in 2020 (since 1/19/2020) has actually helped him to bring his risk down to 51%.

It is quite obvious that his chronic diseases induced CVD risks and annual averaged glucoses have an extremely high correlation of 83% (Figure 7). As he mentioned earlier, through his research results of the past 5-years, he has already detected that glucose is the "principal criminal" plus the help from both blood pressure and lipids as the "accessory criminals" in terms of chronic diseases induced CVD. Not only his overall health conditions have been greatly improved which can be seen from his regular medical examination reports, but also his "reversed" heart conditions can also be observed from his past medical examination reports.

Conclusion:

Lifestyle change and its continuous management provide better results than medications and/or surgeries. Stents and angioplasties are indeed limited in their functionality. Of course, medications and surgeries can also save patient's lives; however, they can coexist with a lifestyle management program. It should be further noted that about 5% of the total patients account for up to 80% of the total healthcare costs with the number one expense case being for heart disease.

This article describes the author's cookbook of reversing his CVD conditions via lifestyle management. His CVD risk probability research results for the past 10-years and his lifestyle management related "cookbook of qualitative guidelines and quantitative formulas" from his past 4.5 years work have provided a detailed explanations of his proven ways to reverse his heart conditions. Human organs are amazing. They have their own memories and strengths to repair themselves if properly taken care of.

References:

1. Hsu, Gerald C., eclaireMD Foundation, USA. No.255: "Using mathematical model of metabolism to estimate the risk probability of having a cardiovascular diseases or stroke during 2010-2019 (GH-Method: math-physical medicine)

2. Hsu, Gerald C., eclaireMD Foundation, USA. No.43 "Using GH-Method: math-physical medicine to investigate the triangular dual-correlations among weight, glucose, blood pressure with a Comparison of 2 Clinic Cases"

3. Hsu, Gerald C., eclaireMD Foundation, USA. No.13: "Using GH-Method: math-physical medicine and signal processing techniques to predict PPG"

	Biomedical Variable	Conversion Formula
From:	Food Portion	82%
To:	Weight	173 lbs
From:	Weight	1 lb
To:	FPG	1.5 - 3.6 mg/dL
From:	Carbs/Sugar	1 gram
To:	PPG	+ 1.8 mg/dL
From:	Walking	1,000 steps
To:	PPG	- 5.0 mg/dL
From:	Temperature	- 1 degree F
To:	FPG	- 0.3 mg/dL
From:	Temperature	+ 1 degree F
To:	PPG	+ 0.9 mg/dL
From:	FPG & PPG	25% FPG + 75% PPG
To:	HbA1C	/ 17.1931

Figure 1: Table of Conversion formulas

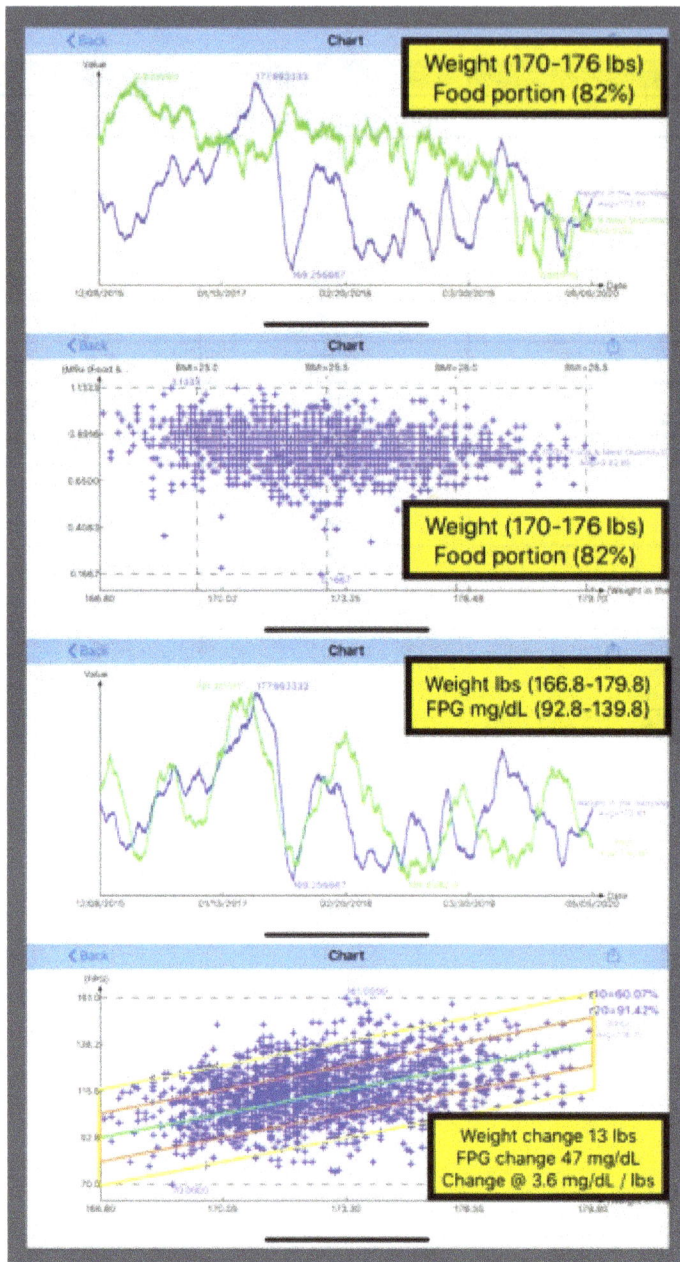

Figure 2:   Weight and FPG

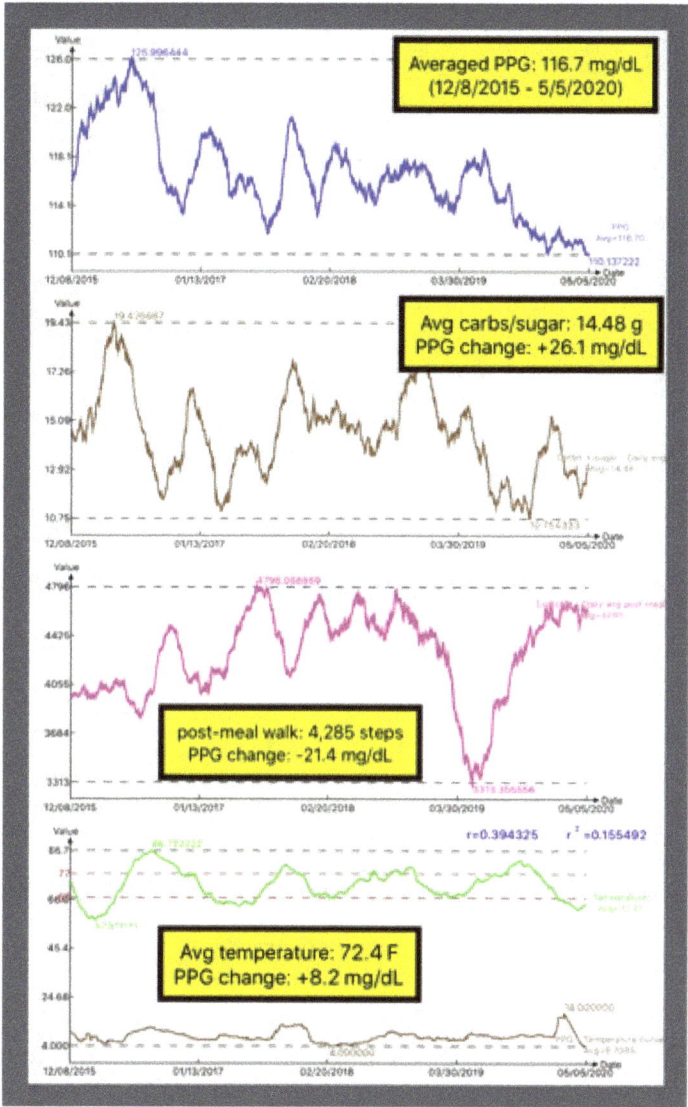

Figure 3: PPG and carbs/sugar, post-meal walking, & temperature

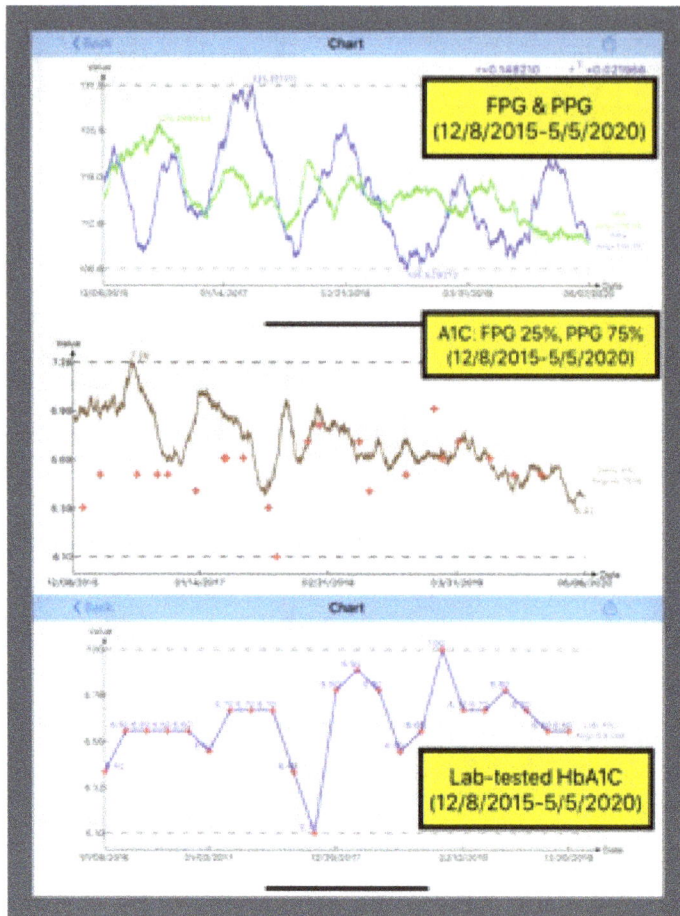

Figure 4: FPG, PPG, and HbA1C

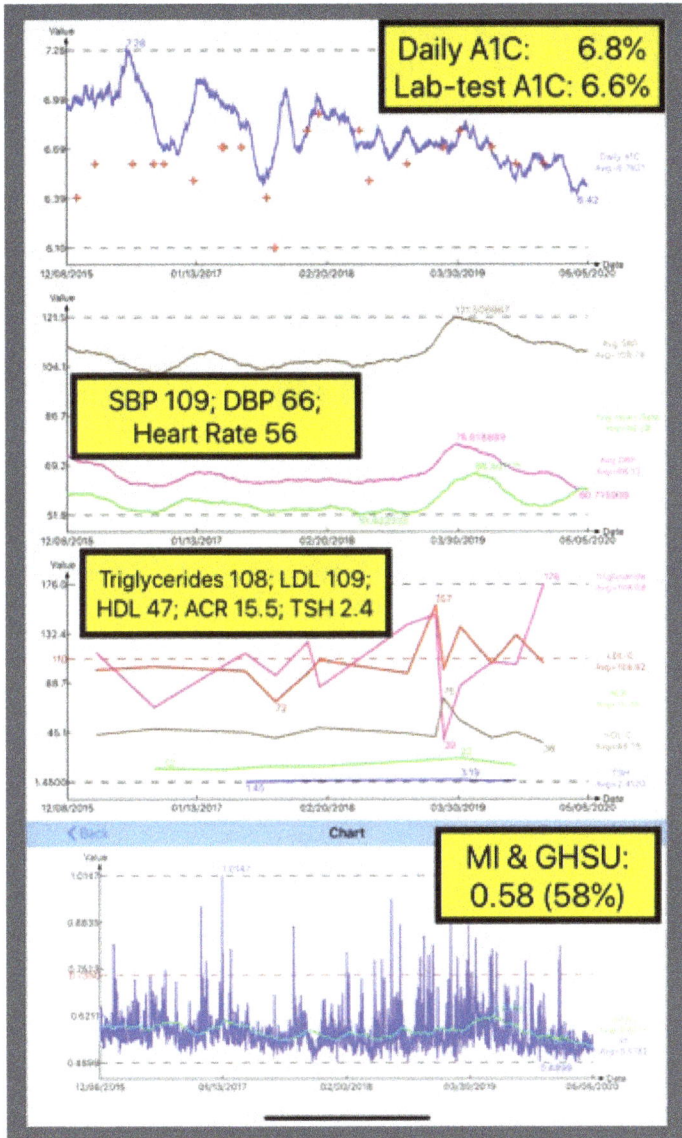

Figure 5: HbA1C, BP, Lipid, MI

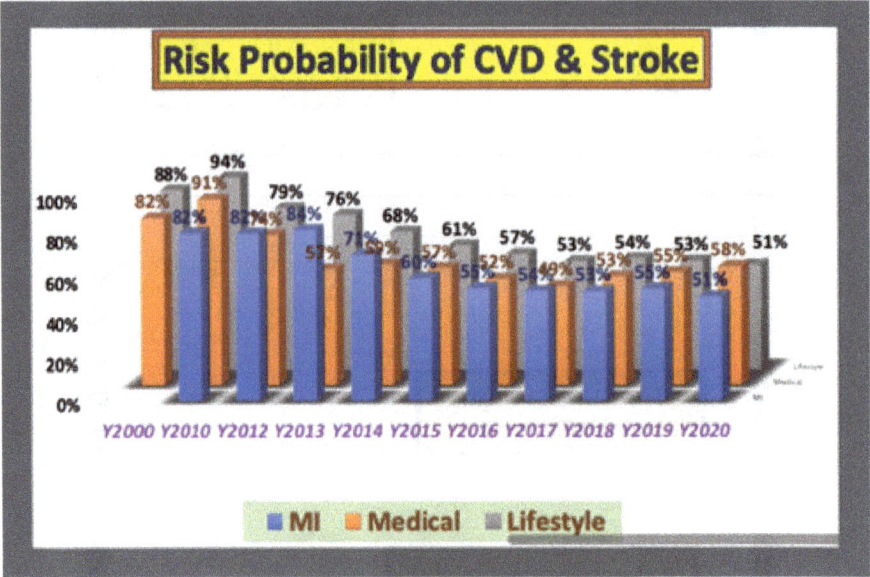

Figure 6: CVD Risk (2010-2020)

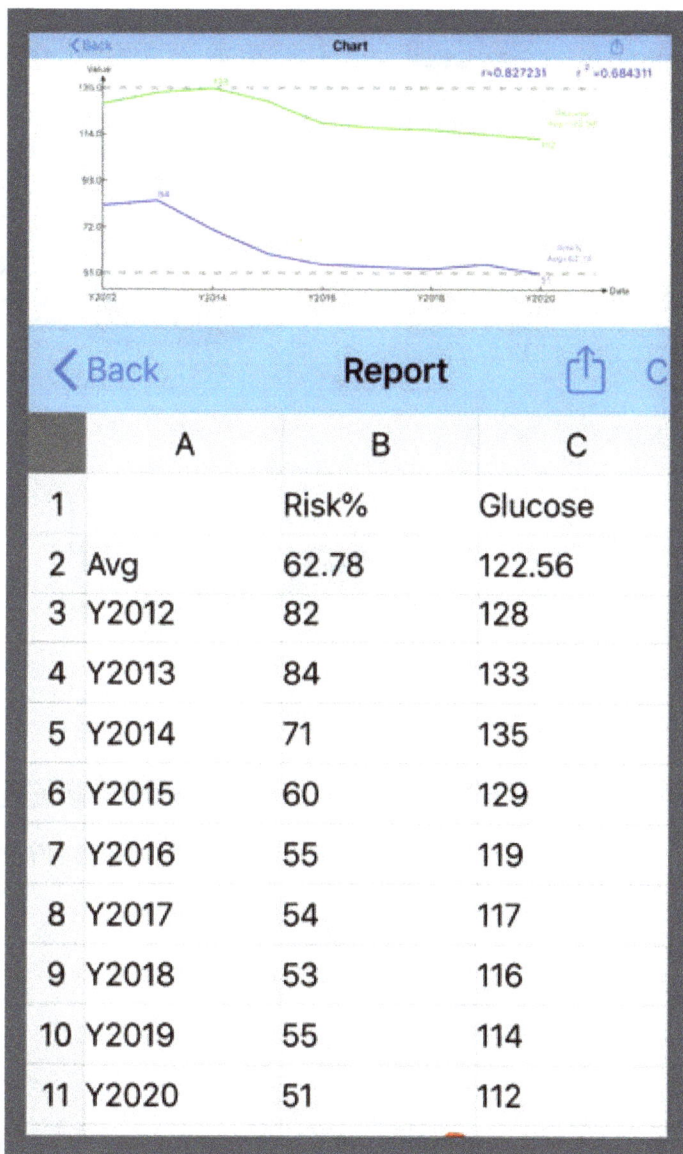

	A	B	C
1		Risk%	Glucose
2	Avg	62.78	122.56
3	Y2012	82	128
4	Y2013	84	133
5	Y2014	71	135
6	Y2015	60	129
7	Y2016	55	119
8	Y2017	54	117
9	Y2018	53	116
10	Y2019	55	114
11	Y2020	51	112

Figure 7: CVD Risks and Glucoses

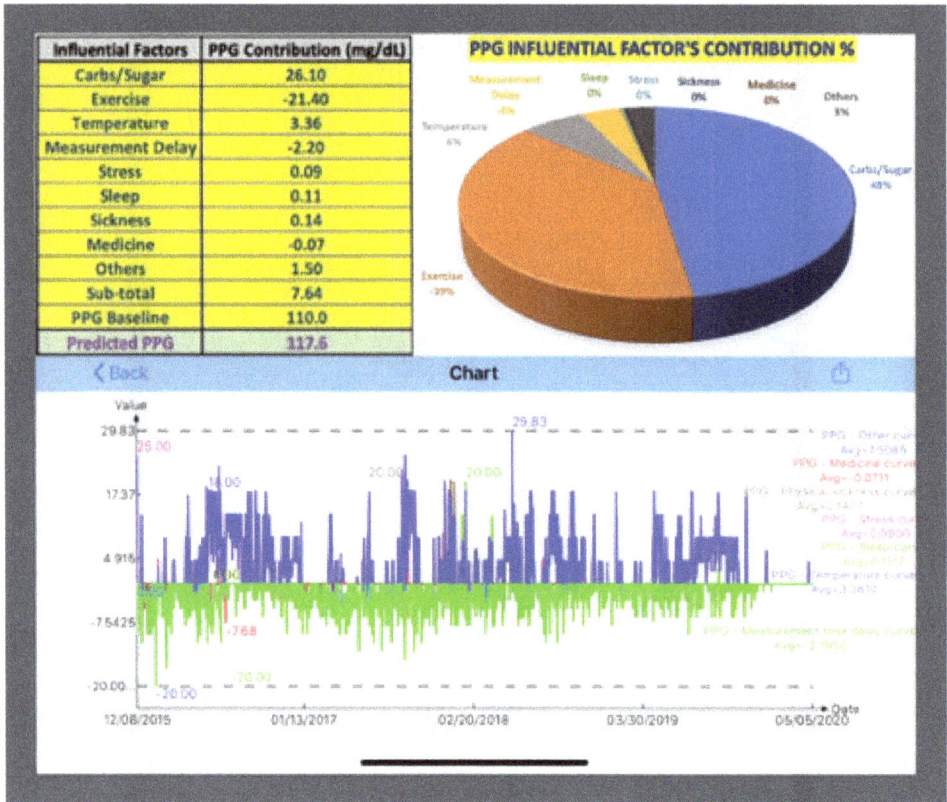

Influential Factors	PPG Contribution (mg/dL)
Carbs/Sugar	26.10
Exercise	-21.40
Temperature	3.36
Measurement Delay	-2.20
Stress	0.09
Sleep	0.11
Sickness	0.14
Medicine	-0.07
Others	1.50
Sub-total	7.64
PPG Baseline	110.0
Predicted PPG	117.6

Figure 8: Secondary influential factors of predicted finger PPG via signal processing

Relationship between metabolism and risk of cardiovascular disease and stroke, risk of chronic kidney disease, and probability of pancreatic beta cells self-recovery using GH-Method: Math-Physical Medicine (259)

By: Gerald C. Hsu
eclaireMD Foundation, USA
5/12-13/2020

Introduction:

The author uses GH-Method: math-physical medicine (MPM) approach to investigate his risk probability on metabolic disorder induced cardiovascular disease (CVD), stroke, or chronic kidney disease (CKD), as well as probability of pancreatic beta cells self-recovery. He addresses the damages caused by metabolic disorders affecting arteries and micro-vessels in terms of blockage, rupture, or leakage along with the probability assessment of pancreatic beta cells self-recovery. Furthermore, he uses mathematical correlations to distinguish the weighted impact by metabolism on heart, brain, kidney, and pancreas.

Methods:

In 2014, the author applied topology concept, finite-element engineering technique, and nonlinear algebra operations to develop a mathematical metabolism model which contains ten categories, including four basic output categories such as weight, glucose, BP, and other lab-tested data (lipid, ACR, and TSH), and six basic input categories such as food, water drinking, exercise, sleep, stress, routine life patterns and safety measures, with approximately 500 detailed elements.

He further defined a new parameter, metabolism index (MI), as the combined score of the above 10 metabolism categories and 500 elements. He also defined another term, General Heath Status Unit (GHSU), as the 90-days moving average value of MI for indicating the trend of metabolism. This MI value is continuously and dynamically calculated whenever the patient has encountered some condition changes and their relevant data were collected regarding his medical conditions and lifestyle details. He has identified a mathematical normalized "break-even line" at 0.735 (73.5%) to separate his metabolism conditions between healthy (below 0.735) and unhealthy (above 0.735).

He started to collect his above-mentioned personal detailed data on 1/1/2012. Thus far, he has collected and stored ~2 million data of his own body health and personal lifestyle.

Through his developed four prediction models of weight and glucose (FPG, PPG, and HbA1C), he has successfully reduced his glucose level from 280 mg/dL (A1C 10%) in 2010 to 113 mg/dL (A1C 6.4%) in 2020. It should be noted that, for the period of 2016-2020, he did not take any diabetes drugs or insulin injections.

In 2017-2018, he developed two similar but rather different mathematical models to calculate risk probability of having a CVD/Stroke and CKD, respectively.

In 2019-2020, he further conducted a special research on probability and improvement rate of his pancreatic beta cells self-recovery situation.

At first, he built a baseline model, including genetic factors such as steady state and unchangeable conditions (race, gender, family history, and personal medical history), semi-permanent factors such as weight and waistline, and bad habits such as hard to change conditions (smoking, alcohol drinking, and illicit drugs).

Next, he developed a risk probability calculation model for estimating the following three scenarios:

(1) For CVD & Stroke: blood flow blockage of arteries due to diabetes and hyperlipidemia; and blood vessel rupture of arteries due to diabetes and hypertension.

(2) For CKD: leakage from micro-blood vessels due to diabetes and hypertension.

(3) For Pancreatic beta cells: this is a quite different subject since it involves hormone production capability and capacity, mainly insulin which are not the same as his research work on heart/brain and kidney complications. CVD and CKD dealt with physically observed phenomena, such as blood vessel's structural damage or weakening by high glucose or artery rupture by high blood pressure. He finally found a way to cut into the problem of " beta cells insulin" through "glucose" phenomena. Beta cells structure with insulin production is a kind of "black box" problem which is rather difficult for him at the beginning since he is a professionally trained mathematician, physicist, and engineer, and lack of academic training in biology and chemistry.

Finally, he applied his collected several hundred thousand data of medical conditions regarding four basic chronic diseases and more than 1 million data of lifestyle details, from the past eight and one-half years (2012-2020), to calculate their combined contribution to cause following situations related to CVD, Stroke, CKD, and pancreatic beta cells:

(1) blockage and rupture of arteries in heart or brain, including situations of CVD, CAD, CHD due to diabetes, hypertension, and hyperlipidemia. We already know that more than 50% of heart diseases or stroke patients also have different chronic diseases due to their metabolic disorders.

(2) kidney complications, including glucose, blood pressure, kidney, glomeruli, bladder, urinary tract, etc.

We already know that two main causes of chronic kidney disease are diabetes and hypertension, which are responsible for up to two-thirds of the CKD cases.

(3) elevated glucose were caused by insufficient insulin production or insulin resistance of damaged pancreatic beta cells. Once he removed the element of medications out from the equation, he started to notice the changes of fasting plasma glucose (FPG) are directly related to the health state of pancreas since both diet and exercise play no rules in FPG formation. He then further investigated changes due to both postprandial plasma glucose (PPG) and HbA1C in order to figure out the possible changes and ranges of both functionality (i.e. insulin resistance) and production amount (i.e. insufficient insulin) of pancreatic beta cells.

For CVD and CKD, his calculation results are further divided into the following three groups:

(A) Medical conditions (individual M1 through M4: i.e. weight, glucose, blood pressure, lipid, and ACR).

(B) Lifestyle details (individual M5 through M10).

(C) MI scores (a combined score of M1 through M10).

With these mathematical risk probability assessment models, he can obtain three separate percentages of risk probability (i.e. medical-based, lifestyle-based, and MI-based, but these three results are quite close to each other) to offer a range of the risk prediction of having cardiovascular diseases, stroke, or chronic kidney diseases resulted from metabolic disorders, unhealthy lifestyles, and their combined impact on the human body.

For self-recovery of pancreatic beta cells, he examined annual change rate of FPG, PPG, and HbA1C, (its outcome, "glucose" only). However, there is a data reliability issue associated with existing medical testing and measurement community, including finger-piercing glucose devices, continuous glucose monitoring (GM) sensor devices, and lab-tested HbA1C devices and process. Sometimes, their output data's deviation could be in the range of 25% or more. Therefore, the author decided to derive the following three sets of simple formulas for his "Beta-cells %" calculation which are used in his calculation table (Figure 5).

(1) Averaged glucose = (FPG + PPG) / 2
(2) Averaged HbA1C = (Lab A1C + math A1C) / 2
(3) Beta cell % = (Averaged glucose + (Averaged HbA1C * 17.1931)) / 4; where 17.1931 is the glucose conversion factor he has used in his mathematical daily predicted HbA1C value. The reason of "dividing by 4" is for a purpose of better viewing for his data or curve that it would give a final number within the general data range of other three datasets. After all, all of these data or curves are "relative", not "absolute", and for serving the porpoise of investigating their relative relationship.

Regarding these four prominent influential biomarkers, i.e. MI %, CVD risk %, CKD risk %, and Beta cells %, he further calculated three pairs of correlation coefficients using time-series method. Due to the small data volume in this study using "annualized" averaged data, he cannot apply the powerful spatial analysis method. Spatial analysis method can provide an accurate and clear picture of data relationship pattern and moving trend; however, it also requires a bigger size of collected data than time-series method in order to conduct its analysis.

During the past 8+ years, all of his measurements of weight, glucose and blood pressure were performed using home-based devices. However, to obtain his tested data of HbA1C, albumin, creatinine, and albumin-creatinine ratio (ACR), these were done in a laboratory or hospital.

Finally, it should be noted here that the risk probability percentages and pancreatic beta cells self-recovery rate are expressed on a "relative" scale, not on an "absolute" scale.

Results:

Figure 1 demonstrates the author's overall metabolic conditions, including both MI and GHSU for the past eight and one-half years (1/1/2012 - 5/10/2020), along with the detailed descriptions of MI category's measurement standards. Both his MI and GHSU were >73.5% during 2012-2014 (unhealthy) and <73.5% during 2014-2020 (healthy). In 2014, his health greatly improved due to his knowledge gained from development of metabolism model and his discipline on implementing the lifestyle management program.

Figures 2 shows his risk probability % of having a CVD or stroke (heart or brain). It is obvious that his CVD risk % is decreasing from 82% in 2012 gradually down to 51% in 2020 with a linear decreasing speed of 4.3% per year. The year of 2014 is the turning point.

Figures 3 depicts his risk probability % of having a CKD (kidney). His CKD risk % is decreasing from 69% in 2012 gradually down to 35% in 2018 through 2020 with a linear decreasing speed of 5.8% per year. The year of 2013 as the turning point.

Figure 4 depicts a table which lists all of numerical values of MI %, CVD risk %, CKD risk %, and Beta cells %.

Figure 5 shows the calculation table of beta cells % from both glucose and HbA1C.

Furthermore, in Figure 6, three additional interesting discoveries are observed:

(A) The correlation between MI % and CVD % is 99.9% while the correlation between MI % and CKD % is 78.2%. Both correlations are quite high (greater than 50%) which indicates that metabolism conditions indeed causing the risk probabilities of having both heart/brain and kidney complications.
(B) He further delves into the question of why there is a gap between these two correlation coefficients. It is obvious that the 99.9% of the damage on the heart and brain's arteries is **21.7% higher** than the 78.2% of the damage on the kidney's micro-vessels. This difference probably indicates a closer and stronger relationship between MI and CVD than MI and CKD. In order to provide more confirmation regarding this hypnoses, more clinical data analyses will be needed.
(C) The correlation between MI % and beta cells % is 95.1%, but the actual difference between the beta cell value of 65 in 2012 and 56 in 2020 is only 13.85% over 8.5 years. This difference provides 1.6% reduction rate per year which is close to his prior findings of possible self-recovery rate of pancreatic beta cells around 2.3% per year. The small difference of 0.7% is due to many simplification steps used in beta cells % formation in this paper with its main objectives being "trend" and "relationship".
In Figure 7, we can see the combined four curves of these different cases.

Conclusions:

These annualized big data analytics using four different sophisticated mathematical models for MI, CVD, CKD, and Pancreatic beta cells have demonstrated the close relationships between metabolism and two major chronic disease induced complications, CVD/Stroke (heart/brain) and CKD (kidney), as well as the beta cells self-recovery rate. By using the GH-Method: MPM math-physical medicine approach (mathematics, physics, engineering modeling, and computer science), it can certainly attain similar conclusions without lengthy and expensive biochemical experiments performed in a laboratory.

References:

1. Hsu, Gerald C., eclaireMD Foundation, USA, No.225

2. "Health improvements using Metabolism Indexes of four different time periods (2012-2019)"

3. Hsu, Gerald C., eclaireMD Foundation, USA, No.256 "How to reverse chronic disease induced heart conditions using a simple and effective "cookbook of quantitative formulas" (GH-Method: math-physical medicine)"

4. Hsu, Gerald C., eclaireMD Foundation, USA, No.257 "Risk Probability of having chronic kidney disease over the past ten years using GH-Method: Math-Physical Medicine"

5. Hsu, Gerald C., eclaireMD Foundation, USA, No.115 "Using GH-Method: math-physical medicine to investigate the risk probability of metabolic disorders induced cardiovascular diseases or stroke"

6. Hsu, Gerald C., eclaireMD Foundation, USA, No.252, "A summary report on partial regeneration of the pancreatic beta cells insulin regression using both FPG, PPG, and HbA1C data (GH-Method: math-physical medicine)"

7. Hsu, Gerald C., eclaireMD Foundation, USA, No.258, "Relationship between metabolism and probability risks of having cardiovascular diseases or renal complications using GH-Method: Math-Physical Medicine"

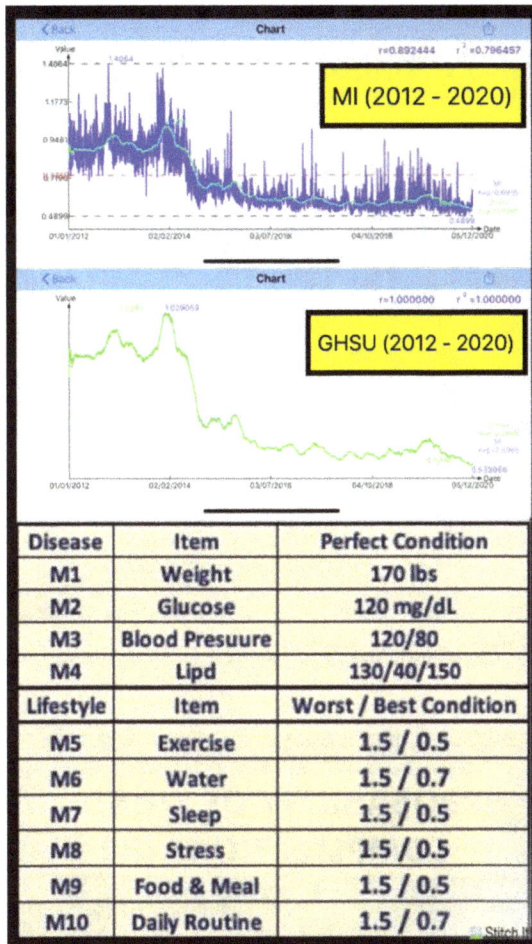

Disease	Item	Perfect Condition
M1	Weight	170 lbs
M2	Glucose	120 mg/dL
M3	Blood Presuure	120/80
M4	Lipd	130/40/150
Lifestyle	Item	Worst / Best Condition
M5	Exercise	1.5 / 0.5
M6	Water	1.5 / 0.7
M7	Sleep	1.5 / 0.5
M8	Stress	1.5 / 0.5
M9	Food & Meal	1.5 / 0.5
M10	Daily Routine	1.5 / 0.7

Figure 1: Metabolism Index (2012-2020) & measurement standards (M1-M10)

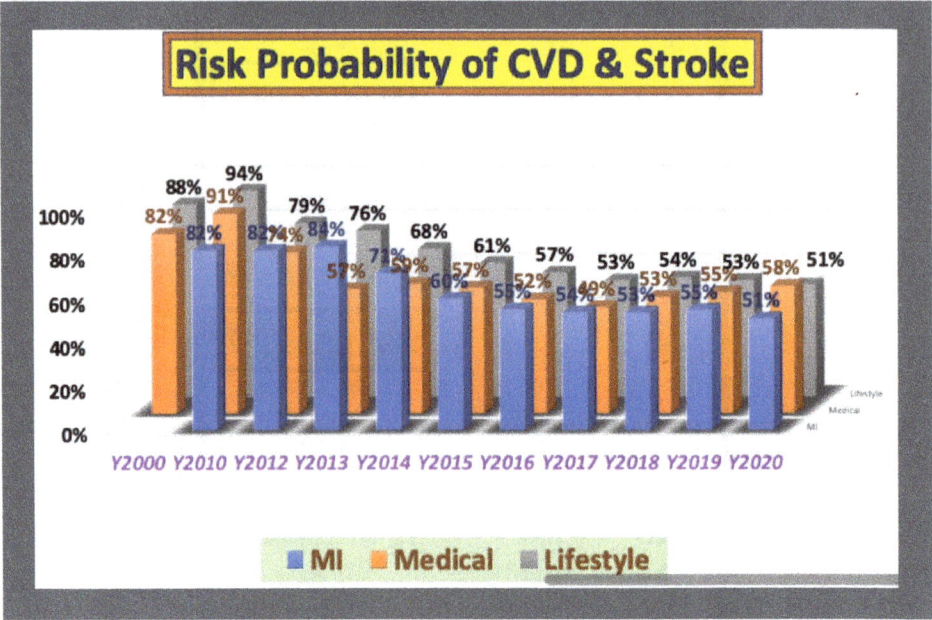

Figure 2: Probability Risk % of having a CVD or Stroke (2012-2020)

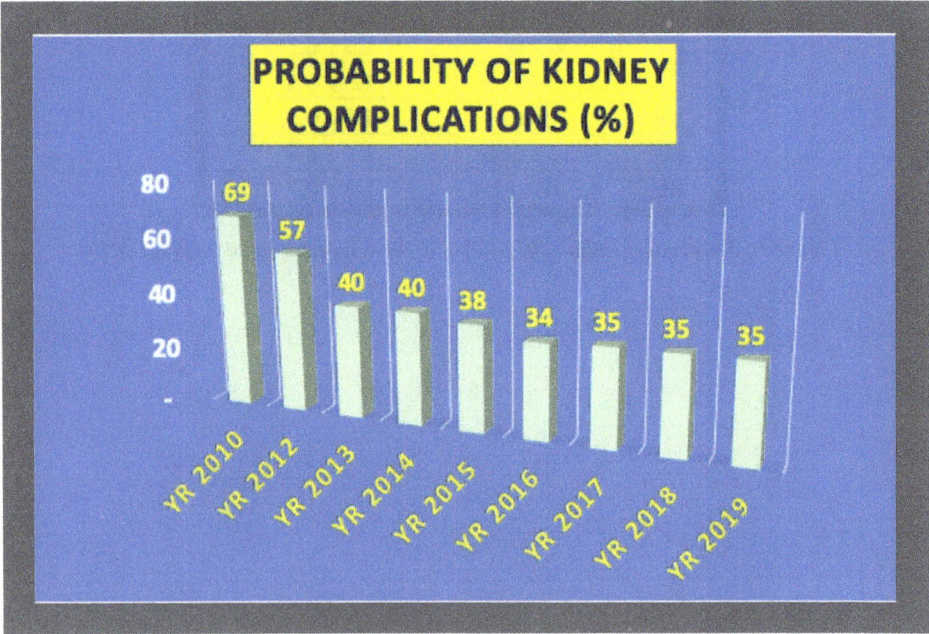

Figure 3: Probability Risk % of having a CKD (2012-2020)

Year	MI %	CVD risk %	CKD risk %	Beta cells %
Y2012	91	82	57	65
Y2013	94	84	40	65
Y2014	78	71	40	64
Y2015	64	60	38	61
Y2016	59	55	34	59
Y2017	57	54	35	58
Y2018	57	53	35	58
Y2019	58	55	35	57
Y2020	54	51	33	56

Figure 4: Table of MI %, CVD Risk %, CKD Risk %, & Beta cells (2012-2020)

Year	Beta cells %	Lab A1C	Daily A1C	Avg A1C	FPG	PPG	Avg Glucose
Y2012	65	6.9	7.37	7.1	139	128	136
Y2013	65	6.9	7.70	7.3	135	133	135
Y2014	64	6.8	7.82	7.3	128	137	130
Y2015	61	6.6	7.59	7.1	121	130	123
Y2016	59	6.6	6.95	6.8	117	120	118
Y2017	58	6.5	6.84	6.7	120	117	119
Y2018	58	6.8	6.78	6.8	114	117	115
Y2019	57	6.7	6.67	6.7	113	115	114
Y2020	56	6.5	6.54	6.5	112	111	112

Figure 5: Calculation Table of Beta cells from both Averaged Glucose and Averaged HbA1C

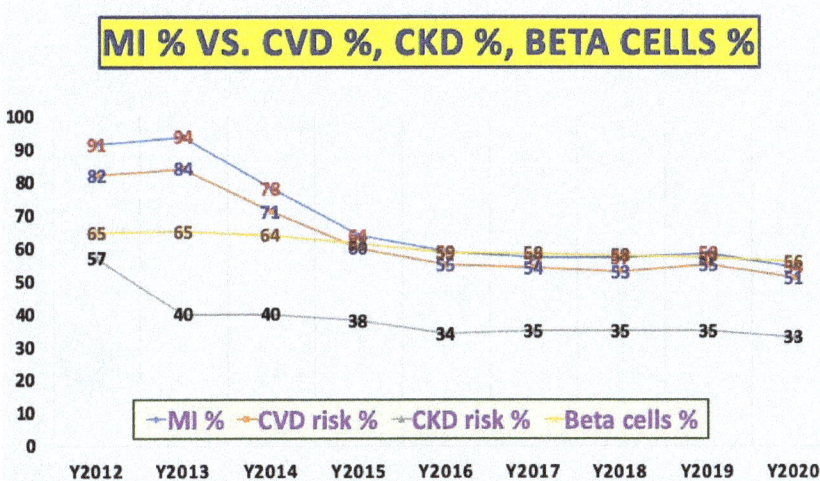

Figure 6: Correlation of MI % vs. CVD %, MI % vs. CKD %, and MI % vs. Beta cells (2012-2020)

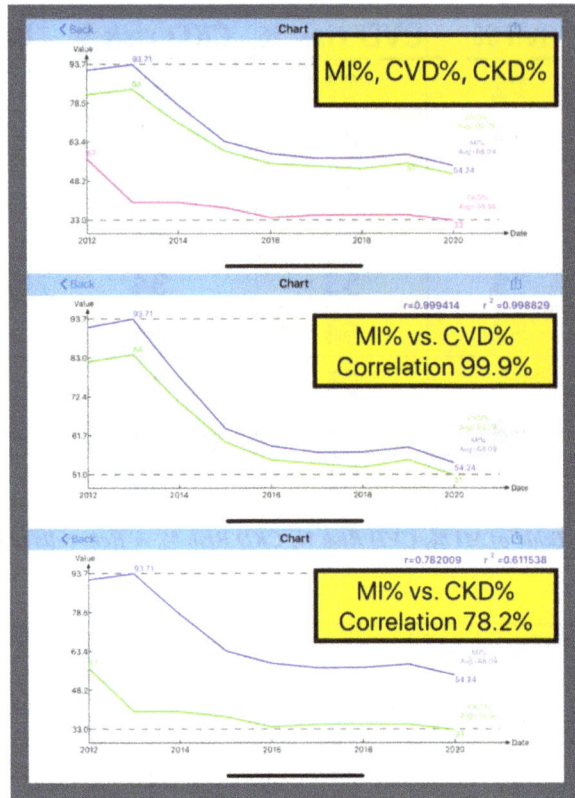

Figure 7: Four curves of MI %, CVD Risk %, CKD Risk %, Beta cells (2012-2020)

Comparison study of postprandial plasma glucose characteristics from candlestick model using GH-Method: Math-Physical Medicine (No. 261)

Gerald C. Hsu
eclaireMD Foundation, USA
5/20-21/2020

Introduction:

This paper describes the author's investigation results of his glucose behaviors based on a continuous glucose monitoring (CGM) sensor collecting postprandial plasma glucose (PPG) data from breakfast, lunch, and dinner using a candlestick charting techniques from Wall Street and his developed GH-Method: Math-Physical Medicine approach.

Method:

A Japanese merchant, who traded in the rice market in Osaka, Japan, started the candlestick charting around 1850. An American fellow, Steve Nison, brought the candlestick model concept and method to the Western world in 1991. These techniques are largely used in today's stock market to predict the stock price trend.

On 4/17/2018, the author had an idea to study glucose behavior by using the candlestick chart (aka "K-Line") and subsequently developed a customized software to analyze his big data of glucose. The analogies between fluctuations of stock price and glucose value are described as follows:

1. Stock prices are closely related to the psychology of the buyers and sellers, which is similar to the glucoses related to a patient body's biochemical interactions and behavior psychology.

2. Stock price wave of a public traded company is dependent upon its product line, internal management, marketing efforts, and public events and perception. This is remarkably similar to the PPG wave of a diabetes patient being dependent on his/her complex food & diet, exercise pattern and amount, weather temperature, and pancreatic beta cell insulin function. From a trained mathematician's eyes, both waves are just two mathematical representations.

3. When there are more buyers than sellers, the price goes up, which is similar to the glucose value rising when carbs/sugar intake increases (more buyers) or lack of exercise (less sellers).

4. When there are more sellers than buyers, price goes down, which is similar to the glucose value decreasing when carbs/sugar intake decreases (less buyers) or exercise increases (more sellers).

During his period of using CGM sensor to collect his glucoses data (5/5/2018 - 5/19/2020), he has compiled a total of 56,730 data via a sensor placed on his upper left arm with an average of 76.25 measurements per day approximately every 15 minutes. His standard PPG wave covers a period of 180 minutes, or 3-hours from the first bite of his meal. Each PPG waveform contains the following five key characteristic data:

1. "Open" value as his PPG at first-bite, 0 minute
2. "Close" value as PPG at 180 minutes
3. "Minimum" value as the lowest PPG "Maximum" value as the highest PPG
4. "Average" glucose - average value of 12 recorded PPG data per meal over 3-hours

Based on his 2,232 meal candlestick bars, glucose patterns and moving trends can be observed and analyzed through further mathematical and statistical operations. Finally, he interpreted these operational results with his acquired knowledge of biomedical phenomena of his body in order to discover some hidden medical truth or potential health dangers.

Since the stock market is much more lucrative than the medical research field, it attracts more talented mathematicians and engineers to work in the highly rewarded financial industry. They even call themselves, "Finance Engineers". On the contrary, most financial rewards in the medical community are distributed to pharmaceutical companies, healthcare institutions, and clinical medical doctors. From the author's personal observation, a large amount of medical research scientists are self-motivated through their interests and dedication, which are mostly associated with either universities or research institutions. They are rarely rewarded financially. The author is a professionally trained mathematician, physicist, engineer, and computer scientist. He accidentally wandered into the medical research field due to his strong motivation of saving his own life after suffering many diabetes complications, such as five cardiovascular episodes (CVD), chronic kidney disease complications (CKD) and faced the possibility of death. As a result, he thought about how to import his learned candlestick techniques, when he was the CEO of a public traded corporation, and how to apply them to his medical research activities. This allowed him to learn and gain from other intellectuals' knowledge and professional experiences.

Results:

Figure 1 shows the normal time-series analysis results of the finger-piercing tested PPG, CGM sensor collected PPG, meal's carbs/sugar intake amount in grams, and post-meal walking steps for the period from 5/5/2918 to 5/19/2020.

Figure 2 depicts three candlestick models for breakfast, lunch, and dinner during the same period. It is rather difficult to identify useful and significant characteristics from these candlestick charts directly without further pattern analysis. This situation is similar to analyzing a publicly listed company's stock performance via its candlestick charts without detailed analysis of its product lines, internal management, marketing programs, and market perception.

We can extract more PPG associated values from the candlestick charts of three meals regarding five key values of opening, maximum, minimum, closing, and average; then, put them into one consolidated table as shown in Figure 3. It is obvious that the lunch data is higher than both the breakfast and dinner data. In this table, his carbs/sugar intake amount and post-meal walking steps are also listed. The average PPG values from both finger and sensor are only listed here as a reference purpose. It is important to mention that the author normally eats a simple breakfast with high-quality protein and small amount of carbohydrates (average PPG 135 mg/dL and maximum PPG 160 mg/dL) and a very light dinner due to weigh control purpose (average PPG 129 mg/dL and maximum PPG of 153 mg/dL). Both post-breakfast and post-dinner walking amounts are within the range of 4,400 to 4,500 steps. His heaviest meal is his lunch which contains a higher carbs/sugar intake amount from a plant-based diet (17g for lunch in comparison with 12g for breakfast and 16g for dinner) and the lowest post-lunch exercise level (4,150 walking steps) due to hot weather temperature around noon time. These are the reasons of his high lunch results with the highest average PPG (139 mg/dL) and the highest maximum PPG (166 mg/dL). This section also describes the closed relationship between lifestyle and metabolism. Figure 4 uses both bar chart and point chart to further graphically demonstrate the same data from Figure 3.

Similar to the study of a publicly traded company's stock performance via its stock candlestick charts, we must study and understand why its stock price is trending upward, in what speed, and how high it reaches to; why is the stock price trending downward, in what speed, and how low it reaches to; and what is the average price for that day. When we connect their daily candlesticks together into a complete waveform, we can then investigate the wave's past performance and future trend to predict the wave moving direction and its future performance.

We can apply the same concept and method to analyze the glucose waveforms since, in nature, both waves of the stock price and blood sugar are two similar waves with the identical mathematical form. Based on this fundamental understanding, the author further calculated 10 more different values derived from these five key candlestick characters, i.e., open, max, average, min, and close. These 10 different items are listed in the table and by the line chart in Figure 5. Due to the complexity of each "key character difference" and their secondary significance, he will not put these detailed findings and their meanings in this article.

In Figure 6, he would like to point out one interesting observation of the overall pattern behaviors of these 10 different characteristics of the three meals PPG. The breakfast is similar but has differences from lunch (R=84%) and from dinner (R = 79%), where R is the correlation coefficient. However, lunch and dinner are highly correlated with each other (R = 98%). This phenomenon is similar to the stock price situation of three hypothetical publicly listed companies with different names of breakfast, lunch, and dinner. Two company performances, lunch and dinner, are quite similar companies with similar product lines and belong to the same market. The lunch values are higher than dinner values probably due to some differences of their product quality (such as carbs/sugar amount). However, the breakfast pattern is quite different from both lunch and dinner which is similar to a third company with a vastly diverse product line to serve a different market.

Finally, in Figure 7, it illustrates his TIR analysis demonstration based on the American Diabetes Association's new guideline regarding TAR (> 180 mg/dL), TIR (70 - 180 mg/dL), and TAR (< 70 mg/dL). His TIR percentages are in the range of 91% to 96% which means his T2D conditions control has been highly effective during this reporting period. His TAR percentages are in the low range of 4.3% to 8.6% (lunch) which means his chances of having hyperglycemia damage is quite low. His TBR percentages are in the smallest range of 0.01% to 0.27% which means his chance of having insulin shock is near zero. It should be emphasized that the author has ceased taking any diabetes medication since 12/8/2015. Therefore, all of the above discovered biomedical phenomena are under "medicine-free" conditions.

Conclusion:

This paper further demonstrated the power of using both the candlestick model and GH-Method: Math-Physical Medicine approach to observe and analyze the PPG phenomena. The methodology of observation for the physical phenomena, derivation of mathematical equations, utilization of various computational tools, and finally combined with the discovery of biomedical interpretations have been proven repeatedly in the author's previous 260 medical papers.

References:

1. Hsu, Gerald C., eclaireMD Foundation, USA: No.76 "Using Candlestick Charting Techniques to Investigate Glucose Behaviors (GH-Method: Math-Physical Medicine)".

2. Hsu, Gerald C., eclaireMD Foundation, USA: No.238 "The influences of medication on diabetes control using TIR analysis (GH-Method: Math-physical medicine)".

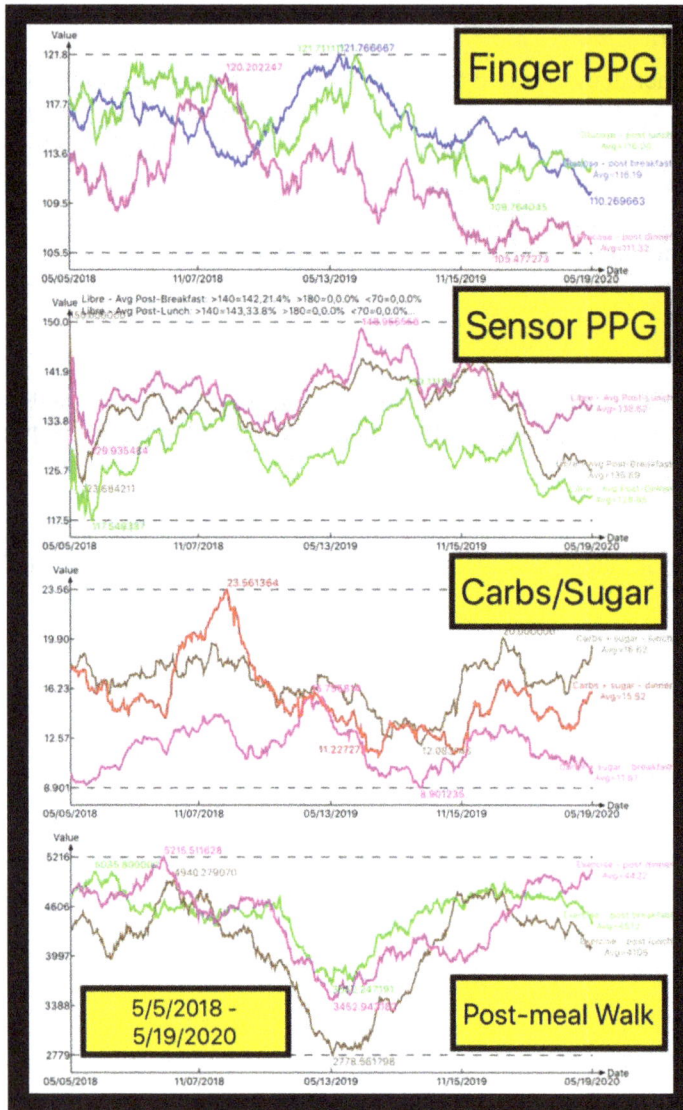

Figure 1: PPG (Finger & Sensor) and Carbs/sugar Walking

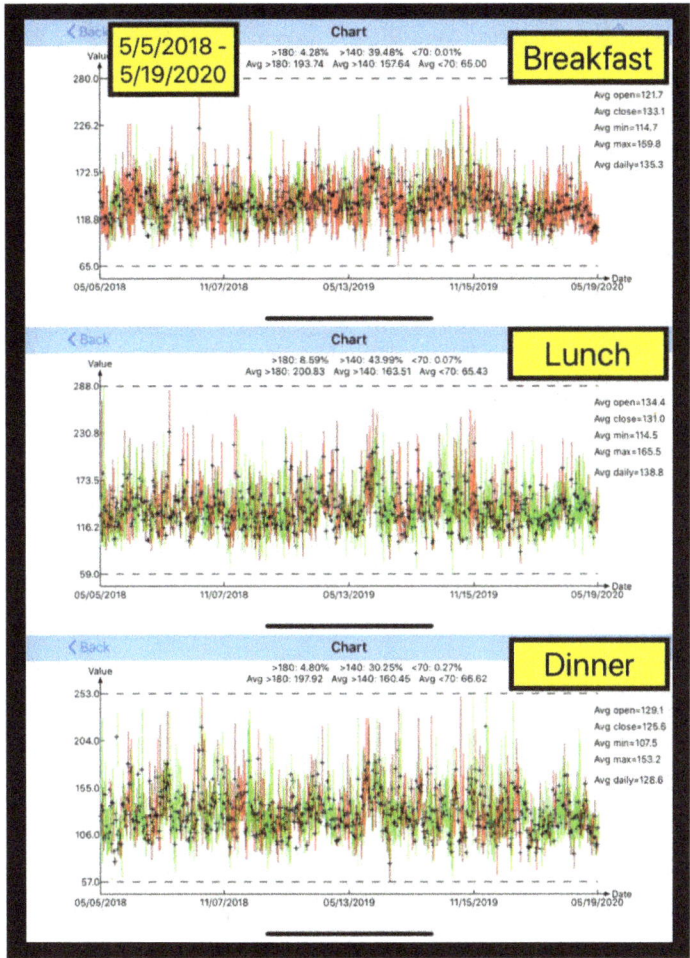

Figure 2: Candlestick charts of 3 meals and Post-meal

Candlestick	Breakfast	Lunch	Dinner
Max	160	166	153
Close	133	131	126
Average	135	139	129
Open	122	134	129
Min	115	115	108

Candlestick	Breakfast	Lunch	Dinner
Carbs/Sugar (g)	12	17	16
Walking (steps)	4512	4105	4422
Finger avg PPG	116	116	111
Sensoe avg PPG	136	139	129

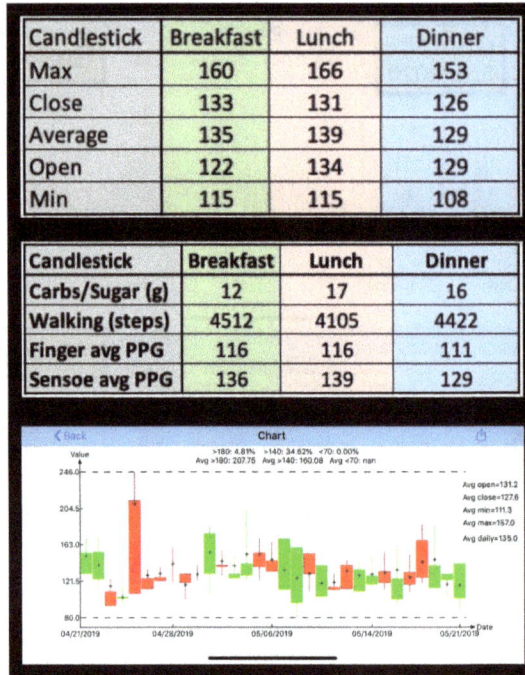

Figure 3: Data Table of 5 key PPG characteristics, carbs/sugar, walking, and magnified view of Candlestick

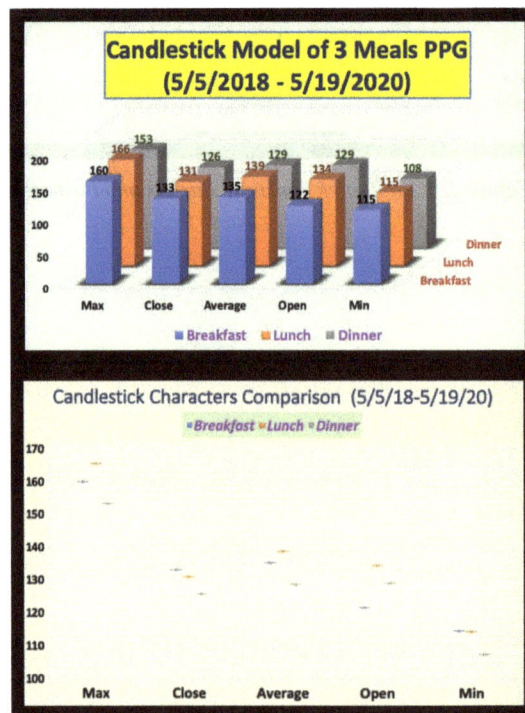

Figure 4: Bar and Point charts of 5 key PPG waveform characteristics

Candlestick	Breakfast	Lunch	Dinner
Max	160	166	153
Close	133	131	126
Average	135	139	129
Open	122	134	129
Min	115	115	108

Candlestick	Breakfast	Lunch	Dinner
Max - Min	45	51	46
Max - Open	38	31	24
Max - Close	27	35	28
Max - Avg	25	27	25
Avg - Open	14	4	-1
Avg - Close	2	8	3
Avg - Min	21	24	21
Close - Open	11	-3	-4
Close - Min	18	17	18
Open- Min	7	20	22

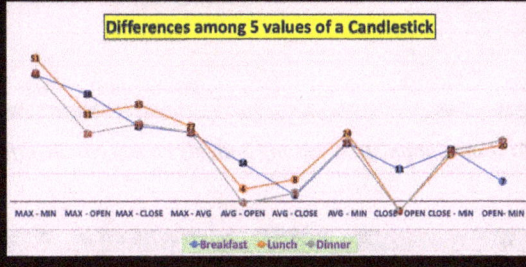

Figure 5: 10 differences among 5 key characteristics of 3 meal PPG

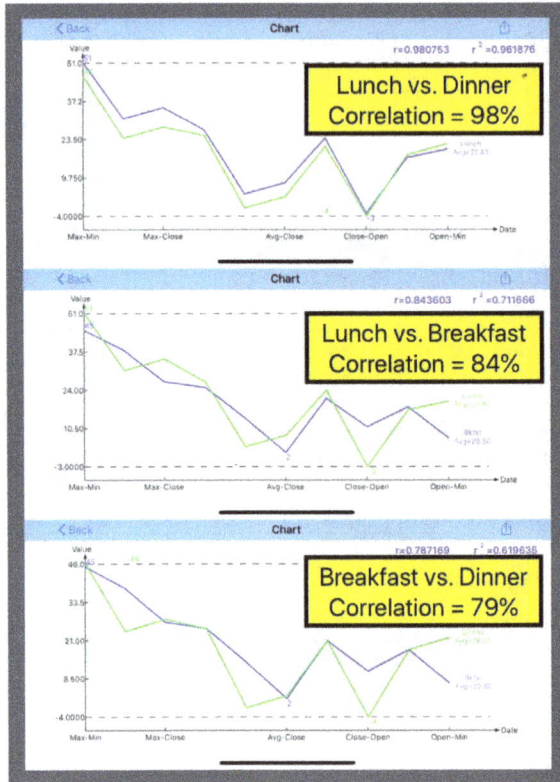

Figure 6: Correlation study among 3 meals characteristic differences

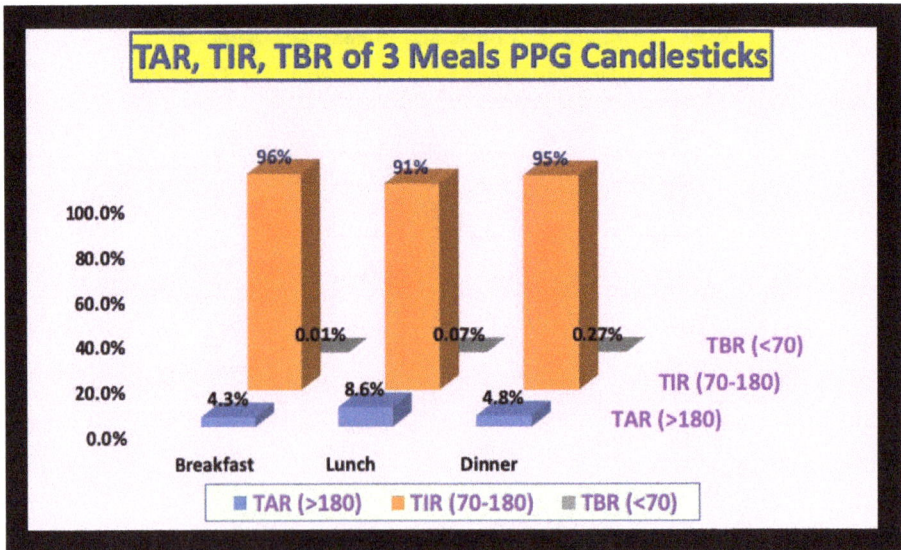

Figure 7: TAR, TIR, TBR study of Candlestick PPG of 3 meals

Medical research of PPG characteristics using candlestick model from Wall Street using GH-Method: Math-Physical Medicine (No. 261a)

Gerald C. Hsu
eclaireMD Foundation, USA
5/20-21/2020
6/15/2020

Introduction:

This paper describes the author's investigation results for his glucose behaviors based on a continuous glucose monitoring (CGM) sensor collecting postprandial plasma glucose (PPG) data from breakfast, lunch, and dinner, using a candlestick charting techniques from Wall Street and his developed GH-Method: Math-Physical Medicine approach.

Method:

A Japanese merchant, who traded in the rice market in Osaka, Japan, started the candlestick charting around 1850. An American fellow, Steve Nison, brought the candlestick model concept and method to the Western world in 1991. These techniques are largely used in today's stock market to predict the stock price trend.

On 4/17/2018, the author had an idea to study glucose behavior by using the candlestick chart also known as the "K-Line" and subsequently developed a customized software to analyze his big data of glucose. The analogies between fluctuations of stock price and glucose value are described as follows:

(1) Stock prices are closely related to the psychology of the buyers and sellers, which is similar to the glucoses related to a patient body's biochemical interactions and behavior psychology.
(2) The stock price wave of a public traded company is dependent upon its product line, internal management, marketing efforts, and public events and perception. This is remarkably similar to the PPG wave of a diabetes patient being dependent on his/her complex food & diet (buying stock), exercise pattern and amount (selling stock), weather temperature (buying stock), and pancreatic beta cell insulin function (SEC regulations). From a trained mathematician's eyes, both waves are just two similar mathematical representations.
(3) When there are more buyers than sellers, the price goes up, which is similar to the glucose value rising when carbs/sugar intake increases (more buyers) or lack of exercise (less sellers).
(4) When there are more sellers than buyers, price goes down, which is similar to the glucose value decreasing when carbs/sugar intake decreases (less buyers) or exercise increases (more sellers).

During his period of using CGM sensor to collect his glucoses data, from 5/5/2018 to 5/19/2020, he has compiled a total of 56,730 data via a CGM sensor placed on his upper left arm with an average of 76.25 measurements per day approximately every 15 minutes. His standard PPG wave covers a period of 180 minutes, or 3-hours from the first bite of his meal. Each PPG waveform contains the following five key characteristic data:

1. "Open" value as his PPG at first-bite, 0 minute
2. "Close" value as PPG at 180 minutes
3. "Minimum" value as the lowest PPG
4. "Maximum" value as the highest PPG
5. "Average" glucose - average value of 12 recorded PPG data per meal over 3-hours

Based on his 2,232 meal candlestick bars, glucose patterns and moving trends can be observed and analyzed through further mathematical and statistical operations. Finally, he interpreted these operational results with his acquired knowledge of biomedical phenomena of his body in order to discover some hidden medical truth (Figures 3 through 7) or potential health dangers via time-in-range or TIR analysis (Figure 8).

Since the stock market is much more lucrative than the medical research field, it attracts more talented mathematicians and engineers to work in the highly rewarded financial industry. They even call themselves, "Finance Engineers". On the contrary, most financial rewards in the medical community are distributed to pharmaceutical companies, healthcare institutions, and clinical medical doctors. From the author's personal observation, a large amount of medical research scientists are self-motivated through their interests and dedication, which are mostly associated with either universities or research institutions. They are rarely rewarded financially.

The author is a professionally trained mathematician, physicist, engineer, computer scientist, and a successful entrepreneur. He accidentally wandered into the medical research field due to his strong motivation of saving his own life after suffering many diabetes complications, such as five cardiovascular episodes (CVD), chronic kidney disease (CKD) complications, and faced the possibility of death. As a result, he thought about how to import his learned physics principles and mathematical analysis methods from his academic educations and professional experiences, as well as his accumulated knowledge regarding stock price and other financial analyses techniques, such as the Candlestick model, from his position as the CEO of a public traded corporation, and apply them to his medical research activities. This allowed him to learn and benefit from the financial world intellectuals based on their knowledge and professional experiences.

Results:

Figure 1 shows the normal time-series analysis results of the finger-piercing tested PPG, CGM sensor collected PPG, meal's carbs/sugar intake amount in grams, and post-meal walking steps for the period from 5/5/2918 to 5/19/2020.

Figure 2 depicts three candlestick models for breakfast, lunch, and dinner, respectively during the same period. It is rather difficult to identify useful and significant characteristics from these candlestick charts directly without further pattern analysis. This situation is similar to analyzing a publicly listed company's stock performance via its candlestick charts without detailed analysis of its product lines, internal management, marketing programs, and market perception.

We can extract more PPG associated values from the candlestick charts of three meals regarding five key values of opening, maximum, minimum, closing, and average. Next, put them into one consolidated table, which also includes a "blow-up view" of different types of candlestick bars as shown in Figure 3.

It is obvious that the lunch data is higher than both the breakfast and dinner data. In this table, his carbs/sugar intake amount and post-meal walking steps are also listed.

The average PPG values from both finger and sensor are only listed here as a reference purpose. It is important to mention that the author normally eats a simple breakfast with high-quality protein and small amount of carbohydrates (average PPG 135 mg/dL and maximum PPG 160 mg/dL) and a very light dinner due to weigh control purpose (average PPG 129 mg/dL and maximum PPG of 153 mg/dL). Both post-breakfast and post-dinner walking amounts are within the range of 4,400 to 4,500 steps. His heaviest meal is his lunch which contains a higher carbs/sugar intake amount from a plant-based diet (17g for lunch in comparison with 12g for breakfast and 16g for dinner) and the lowest post-lunch exercise level (4,150 walking steps) due to hot weather temperature around noon time. These are the reasons of his high lunch results with the highest average PPG of 139 mg/dL and the highest maximum PPG of 166 mg/dL. The data in this section also describe the tight relationship between lifestyle and metabolism.

Figure 4 displays the candlestick bars for breakfast, lunch, dinner respectively, using each meal's 5 key values.

Figure 5 uses graphic presentations of both bar chart and point chart to clearly demonstrate the same data as shown in Figure 3.

Similar to the study of a publicly traded company's stock performance via its stock candlestick charts, we must study and understand why its stock price is trending upward, in what speed, and how high it reaches to; why is the stock price trending downward, in what speed, and how low it reaches to; and what is the average price for that trading day. When we connect their daily candlesticks together into a complete waveform, we can then investigate the wave's past performance and future trend to predict the wave moving direction and its future performance. We can also analyze the reasons of sudden significant changes of glucose candlesticks similar to COVID-19 did on Wall Street trading candlesticks.

We can apply the same concept and similar method to analyze the glucose waveforms since, in nature, both waves of the stock price and blood sugar are two similar waves with the identical mathematical form. Based on this fundamental understanding, the author further calculated 10 more different values which are derived from these five key candlestick characters, i.e. open, max, average, min, and close. These 10 different values are listed in the table and shown by the line chart in Figure 6. Due to the complexity of each "key character difference" and their secondary significance, he will not put these detailed findings and their meanings in this article.

Through Figure 7, one particular correlation behavior of the meal overall patterns from their 10 different characteristics (Figure 5) can be observed. The breakfast is similar but has differences from lunch (R=84%) and from dinner (R = 79%), where R is the correlation coefficient. However, lunch and dinner are highly correlated with each other (R = 98%). This phenomenon is similar to the stock price situation of three hypothetical publicly listed companies with different names of breakfast, lunch, and dinner. Two company performances, lunch and dinner, are quite similar companies with similar product lines and belong to the same market. The lunch values are higher than dinner values probably due to some differences existed in their product quality (such as carbs/sugar amount). However, the breakfast pattern is quite different from both lunch and dinner which is similar to a third company with a vastly diverse product line to serve a different market. Indeed, the author's breakfast nutritional ingredients are vastly different from his lunches and dinners.

Finally, in Figure 8, it illustrates his TIR analysis demonstration based on the American Diabetes Association's new guideline regarding TAR (> 180 mg/dL), TIR (70 - 180 mg/dL), and TAR (< 70 mg/dL). His TIR percentages are in the range of 91% to 96% which means his T2D conditions control has been highly effective during this reporting period. His TAR percentages are in the low range of 4.3% to 8.6% (lunch) which means his chances of having hyperglycemia damage is quite low. His TBR percentages are in the smallest range of 0.01% to 0.27% which means his chance of having insulin shock is near zero. It should be emphasized that the author has ceased taking any diabetes medication since 12/8/2015. Therefore, all of the above discovered biomedical phenomena are under "medicine-free" conditions. This Figure 7 has graphically summarized his overall diabetes safety analysis.

Conclusion:

This paper has further demonstrated the power of using both the Wall Street candlestick model and GH-Method: Math-Physical Medicine approach to observe and analyze the PPG phenomena. The methodology of observation for the physical phenomena, derivation of mathematical equations, utilization of various computational tools, and finally combined with the discovery of biomedical interpretations have been proven repeatedly in the author's previous 260 medical papers.

References:

1. Hsu, Gerald C., eclaireMD Foundation, USA. May 2019. No. 76: "Using Candlestick Charting Techniques to Investigate Glucose Behaviors via GH-Method: Math-Physical Medicine."

2. Hsu, Gerald C., eclaireMD Foundation, USA. May 2020. No. 238: "The influences of medication on diabetes control using TIR analysis via GH-Method: Math-physical medicine."

3. "Candlestick Chart Basics." *RJO Futures*, RJ O'Brien, rjofutures.rjobrien.com/ learning-center/technical-analysis/candlestick-chart-basics.

4. Cattlin, Becca. "16 Candlestick Patterns Every Trader Should Know | IG US." *IG*, www.ig.com/us/trading-strategies/16-candlestick-patterns-every-trader-should-know-180615.

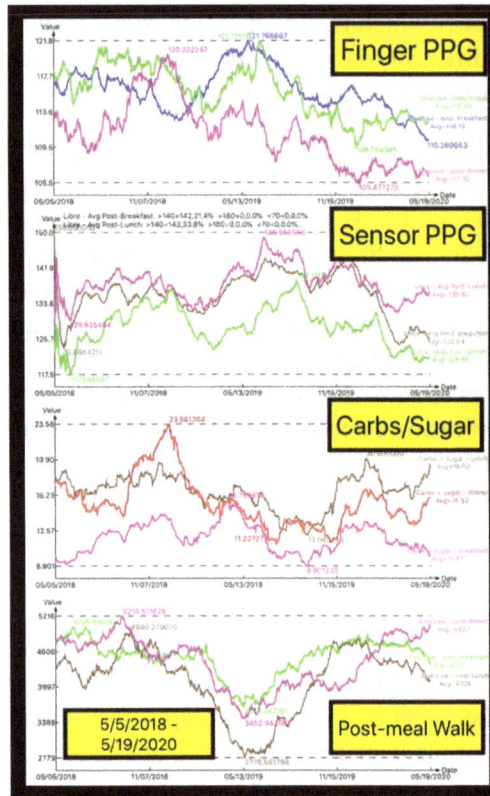

Figure 1: PPG (Finger & Sensor), Carbs/sugar, and Post-meal Walking

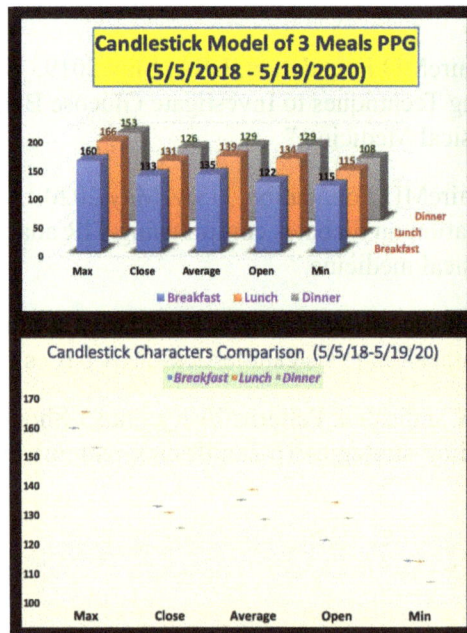

Figure 2: Candlestick charts of 3 meals

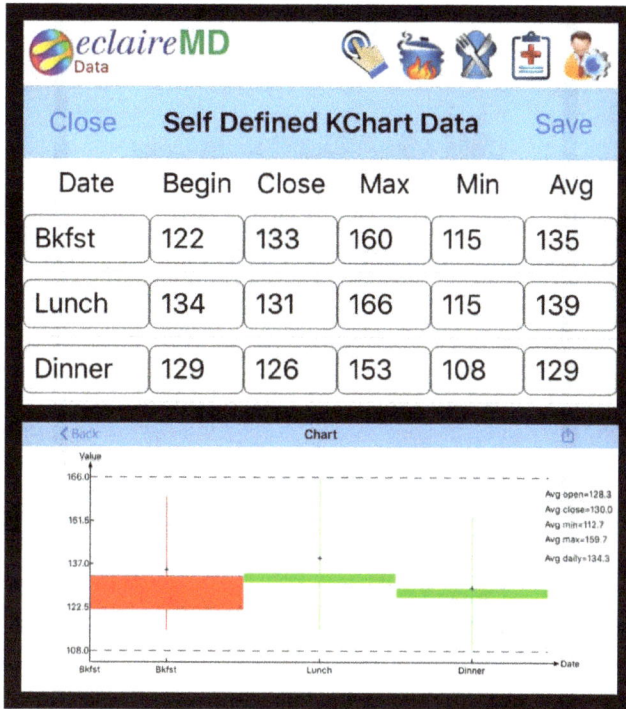

Figure 3: Data Table of 5 key PPG characters, carbs/sugar, walking, and a blowup view of Candlestick

Candlestick	Breakfast	Lunch	Dinner
Max	160	166	153
Close	133	131	126
Average	135	139	129
Open	122	134	129
Min	115	115	108

Candlestick	Breakfast	Lunch	Dinner
Carbs/Sugar (g)	12	17	16
Walking (steps)	4512	4105	4422
Finger avg PPG	116	116	111
Sensoe avg PPG	136	139	129

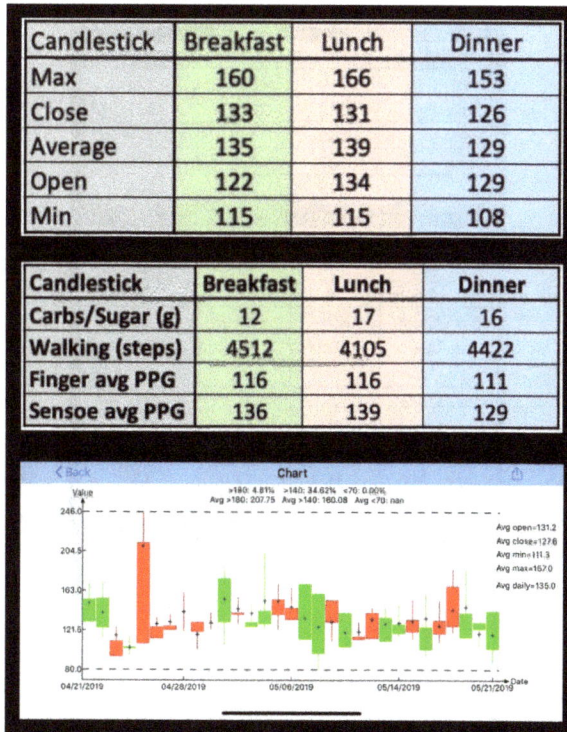

Figure 4: Candlestick bars of breakfast, lunch, and dinner

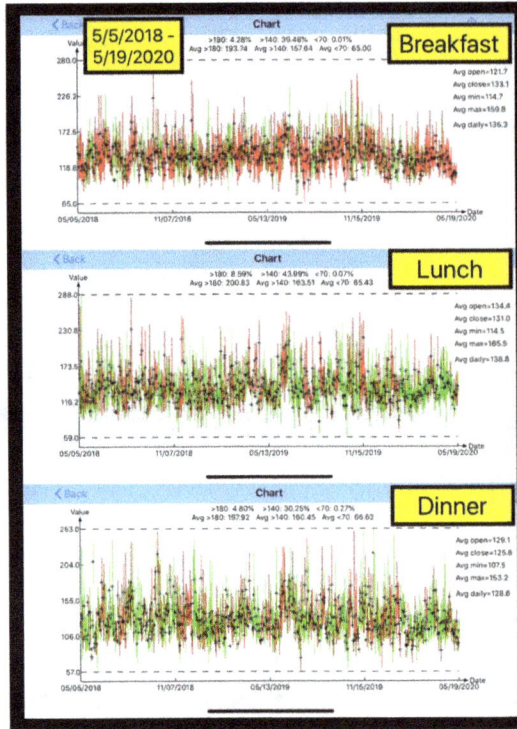

Figure 5: Bar and Point charts of 5 key PPG waveform characteristics

Candlestick	Breakfast	Lunch	Dinner
Max	160	166	153
Close	133	131	126
Average	135	139	129
Open	122	134	129
Min	115	115	108

Candlestick	Breakfast	Lunch	Dinner
Max - Min	45	51	46
Max - Open	38	31	24
Max - Close	27	35	28
Max - Avg	25	27	25
Avg - Open	14	4	-1
Avg - Close	2	8	3
Avg - Min	21	24	21
Close - Open	11	-3	-4
Close - Min	18	17	18
Open- Min	7	20	22

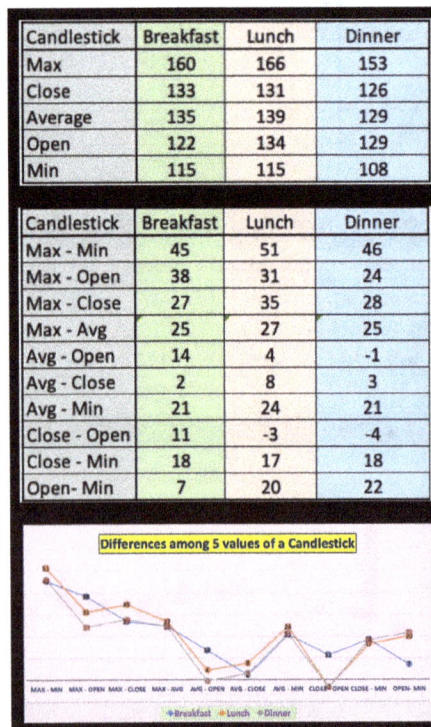

Figure 6: 10 differences among 5 key characters of 3 meal PPG

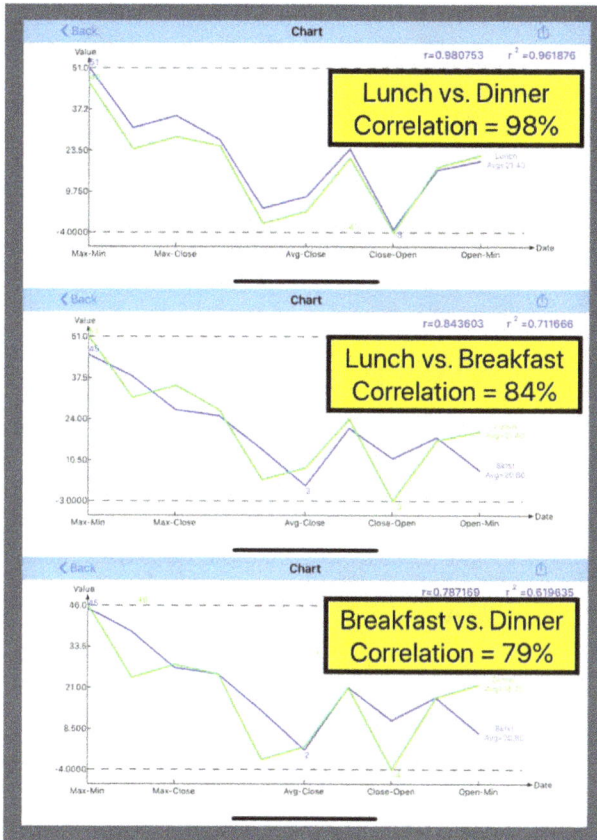

Figure 7: Correlation study among 3 meal character differences

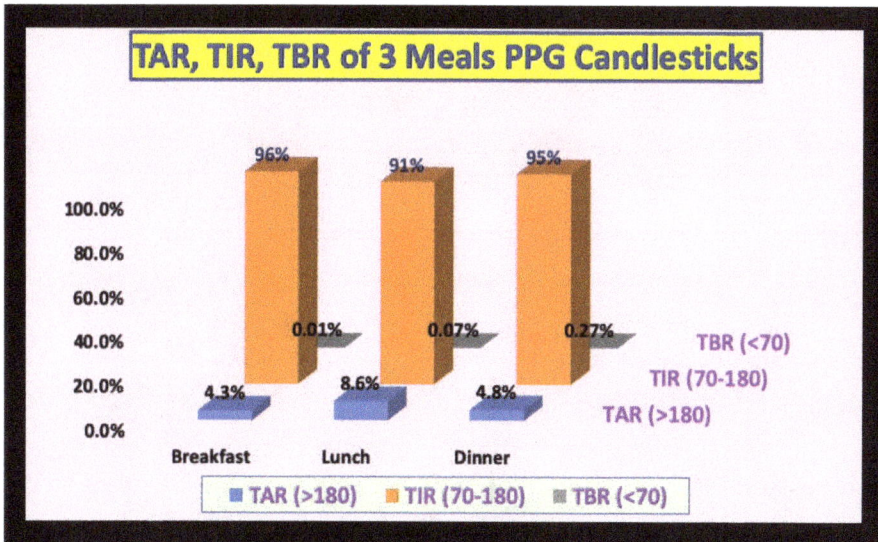

Figure 8: TAR, TIR, TBR safety study of Candlesticks of 3 meals

Different glucose levels produced by coffee versus decaffeinated coffee using GH-Method: Math-physical medicine (No. 277)

By: Gerald C. Hsu
eclaireMD Foundation, USA
6/15-16/2020

Introduction:

In this research note, the author describes his preliminary findings of two different glucose levels produced by "coffee-only" meals – coffee versus decaffeinated coffee.

Method:

The author has conducted many glucose experiments and research studies since mid-2019 by eating different kinds of food materials, nutritional ingredients, and cooking methods. During one of his multiple experiments of eating 138 meals with eggs only, he discovered the significant difference on glucose amount and peak glucose timing between 71 liquid meals (egg drop soup) and 67 solid meals (pan-fried egg). The biochemical interpretation could only provide a partial explanation of his results, while his math-physical methodology combined with a statistical "decision making using the elimination method" has provided a reasonable interpretation based on neuro-scientific considerations. While struggling to differentiate liquid food versus solid food, he thought about the possible existence of a neural communication model with a feedback loop where a "message is received and marching orders issued". He further hypothesized that the stomach treats the arrival of liquid food similar to drinking a cup of coffee or tea. But, in this research note, he has discovered that physical behavior of a liquid state food is different from the biochemical behavior from caffeine of a cup of coffee. A specific signal ascends from the stomach to the brain for decision making, where the brain issues a marching order to both the liver and pancreas regarding the production or release of glucose and insulin (both glucose amount and timing of peak glucose). Therefore, out of his curiosity regarding the possible similarity of glucose levels between egg drop soup and coffee, starting on 5/30/2020, he delved deeper into his meal-glucose research by drinking only coffee as his breakfast.

In 2010, he started his medical research work with a clear objective to control his severe type 2 diabetes conditions. Therefore, he needed to acquire knowledge on food nutrition along with managing his diabetes control and health improvement via a balanced food nutritional intake and a proper level of exercise. In fact, intermittent fasting is not his favorite method of controlling his weight and glucose; therefore, a coffee only breakfast option clearly violates the rules of his health program. He is not a clinical MD or a nutritionist with no "patients" under his care which can provide useful clinical data for his research work. In the end, his strong curiosity surpassed his health concern for a short period of time. For the past 17 days from 5/30/2020 to 6/15/2020, he had eight meals of decaffeinated coffee and seven with coffee for a total of 15 coffee only "breakfasts" (a rather small dataset but still representative).

Figure 1 illustrates the ingredients of his coffee only breakfasts. The green can contains 100% Arabica coffee which is 99.7% caffeine free, whereas the brown glass jar contains 100% caffeinated instant pure coffee. Combined with the cream and artificial sugar, Splenda, they contain less than 1 gram of carbs/sugar. Therefore, from a food nutritional viewpoint, the only difference between these two coffee meals is that the normal coffee with 100% caffeine, and the other decaffeinated coffee has only 0.3% caffeine.

The author researched other medical articles regarding the relationship between glucose and caffeine (see References 1, 2, 3). Although he gained some useful information, he became more confused about their conclusions. Here is a combined excerpt from References 1, 2, and 3:

Caffeine is arguably the most widely consumed drug in Western society. The annual world consumption of coffee exceeds 4 million tons. Caffeine constitutes 1–2% of roasted coffee beans and is present in many over-the-counter preparations for the treatment of cold and allergies, headaches, diuretics, and stimulants. In general, one cup of coffee is assumed to contain 100 mg of caffeine, and soft drinks contain ~10–50 mg of caffeine per 12-oz serving. The per capita consumption of caffeine averages ~200 mg/day, but in some countries, it can exceed 400 mg/day. Coffee consumption, which probably originated in northeast Africa, spread throughout the Middle East in the 15th century and thence to Europe, finally to USA and Asia. It is estimated that more than half of the US population now consumes coffee.

There has been great interest in defining the mechanism of action of caffeine and determining the health consequences of its consumption. Progress has been made on both accounts, but not without controversy.

The ability of decaffeinated coffee to achieve these effects is based on a limited number of studies, and the underlying biological mechanisms have yet to be elucidated.

Two human studies that distinguished between caffeinated and decaffeinated coffee suggest a possible resolution of the difference between caffeine's negative short-term effects on glucose metabolism and coffee's long-term ability to decrease diabetes risk.

In conclusion, some early evidence exists that decaffeinated coffee may be better suited for enhancing glucose tolerance and insulin sensitivity than is caffeinated coffee. More research is needed to elucidate both the short- and long-term effects of decaffeinated coffee on diabetes .

From ADA Editorial (Reference 2): Caffeine may reduce in insulin sensitivity by about 15% (obesity changes about 40%) which could elevate glucose level.

Though the author does not have a strong academic training in both biology and chemistry, most of his backgrounds are in mathematics, physics, computer science, and engineering. Those academic and professional trainings have prepared him on how to observe physical phenomena, collect relevant data, analyze and interpret results, and build up suitable computer models to simulate complex physical and mathematical problems.

Although the data amount is rather small with 15 coffee meals, he still can write up an intermediate research note based on what he has observed and analyzed to date. The results can speak for itself, regardless lacking of a proper interpretation for his observed physical phenomenon.

He has been a severe diabetes patient for 25 years and has suffered many metabolic disorder complications, including cardiovascular diseases, chronic kidney disease, bladder infection, foot ulcer, diabetic retinopathy, and hyperthyroidism. Therefore, his motivation for medical research is finding out what to eat and what to do in order to keep his glucose level on target. He has no interest into the research of the relationship between caffeine and the "risk" of having diabetes since he already is a severe diabetes patient.

Results:

The top table in Figure 3 along with Figure 4 provide a summary of the following: coffee has created a peak glucose (189 mg/dL) that is 175% higher than the decaffeinated coffee (108 mg/dL). In terms of the averaged sensor PPG over 3-hours, coffee produces 143 mg/dL average sensor glucose which is 140% higher than the decaffeinated coffee's averaged sensor glucose of 102 mg/dL. Both differences of the averaged PPG (40%) and peak PPG (75%) are noticeable and significant. The caffeine's energy associated with the peak PPG and averaged PPG are 306% and 196%, respectively, which are higher than the decaffeinated coffee. It is the energy associated with glucose that causes all the impact and damage on the human internal organs.

Figure 2 demonstrates detailed background information of these three coffee meals, including number of meals, finger PPG, and post-meal walking steps. The bottom curve diagram in Figure 3 puts these three sensor PPG waveforms on the same scale of mg/dL. We can clearly see the big difference between the decaffeinated (red curve) and caffeinated (blue curve) with the "total" (green curve) sitting in the middle. Figure 4, a conclusive diagram, repeatedly shows the significant difference between decaffeinated coffee and coffee (the big gap between these two curves).

Figure 5 shows that coffee (with caffeine) has much higher PPG value than both decaffeinated coffee and liquid egg drop soup (these two meal types have similar PPG levels)

Conclusions:

The significant averaged PPG difference of 40%, peak PPG difference of 75% and their associated "relative" energy difference of ~2x and ~3x between these two coffees can be easily observed from the research results.

It seems that caffeine is bad for diabetes control since it raises the glucose level by 40% and doubles the energy associated with the higher glucose.

The question here is why the glucose values are so different? So far, the author can detect the only differential factor which is "caffeine". But what kind of biochemical chain reactions in the organs or what kind of neural communication mechanism among the organs can cause this elevated glucose? The author needs to conduct additional research (hopefully with less personal experiments due to his long-term health concerns) in order to find a satisfactory answer. He wrote this intermediate research note regarding his findings in order to share it with other fellow research scientists and move forward to be able to get a clear answer about this mysterious phenomenon.

References:

1. Greenberg, JA, Boozer, CN & Geliebter, A (2006): "Coffee, diabetes, and weight control" American Journal of Clinical Nutrition 84, 682-693. CrossRef, Google Scholar, PubMed

2. ADA Editorial: Italo Biaggioni, MD and Stephen N. Davis, MD "Caffeine: A Cause of Insulin Resistance?" Diabetes Care 2002 Feb; 25(2): 399-400. https://doi.org/10.2337/diacare.25.2.399

3. Ming Ding, Shilpa N. Bhupathiraju1, Mu Chen, Rob M. van Dam1, and Frank B. Hu. ADA, Meta-analysis: "Caffeinated and Decaffeinated Coffee Consumption and Risk of Type 2 Diabetes: A Systematic Review and a Dose-Response Meta-analysis", Corresponding author: Frank B. Hu, nhbfh@channing.harvard.edu. Diabetes Care 2014 Feb; 37(2): 569-586. https://doi.org/10.2337/dc13-1203

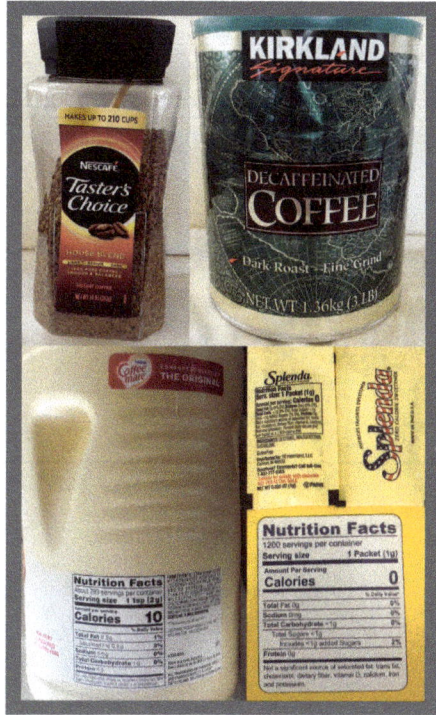

Figure 1: Two different coffee meals, cream, and artificial sugar

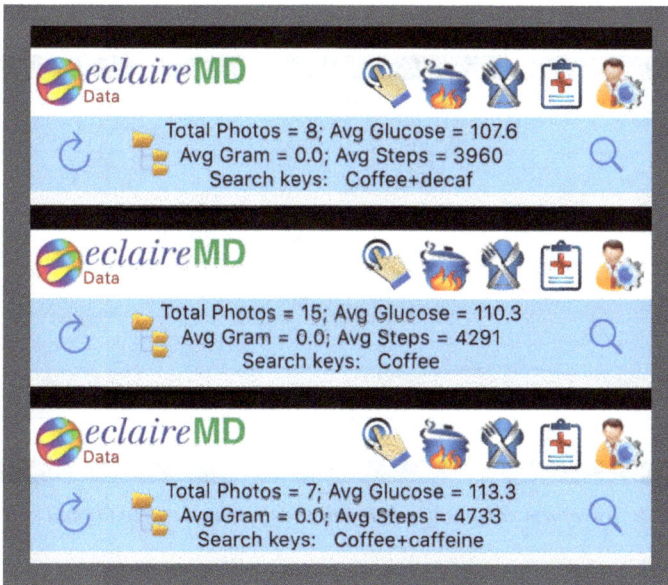

Figure 2: Three coffee meals data of numbers, finger PPG, and post-meal walking steps

PPG (Coffee only)	Finger PPG	Sensor PPG	Peak PPG (mg/dL)	Peak time (min)	Walking Steps
Coffee Decaf (8)	108	102	108	45	3,960
Coffee (Total 15)	110	121	145	60	4,291
Coffee Caffeine (7)	113	143	189	60	4,733

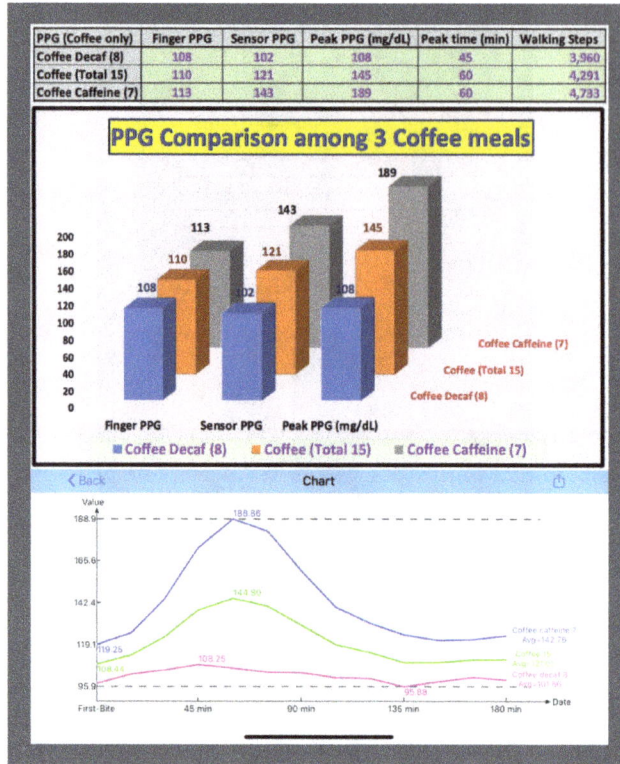

Figure 3: Three coffee meals Sensor PPG information (table and charts)

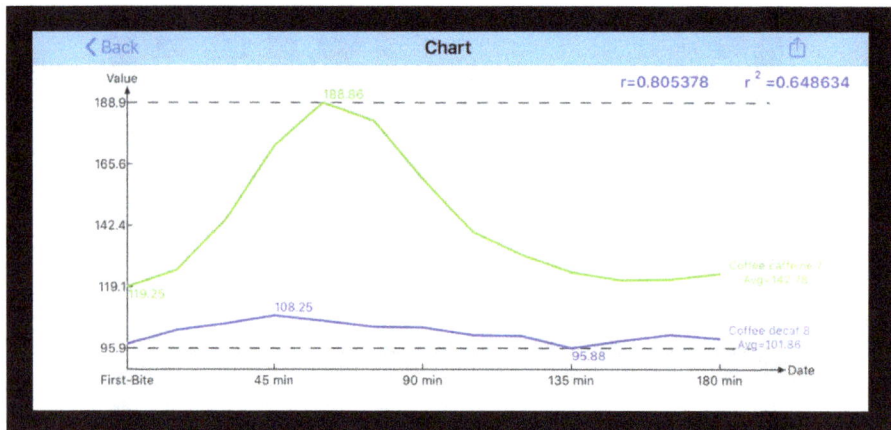

Figure 4: Waveform comparison between decaffeinated coffee (8) and coffee (7)

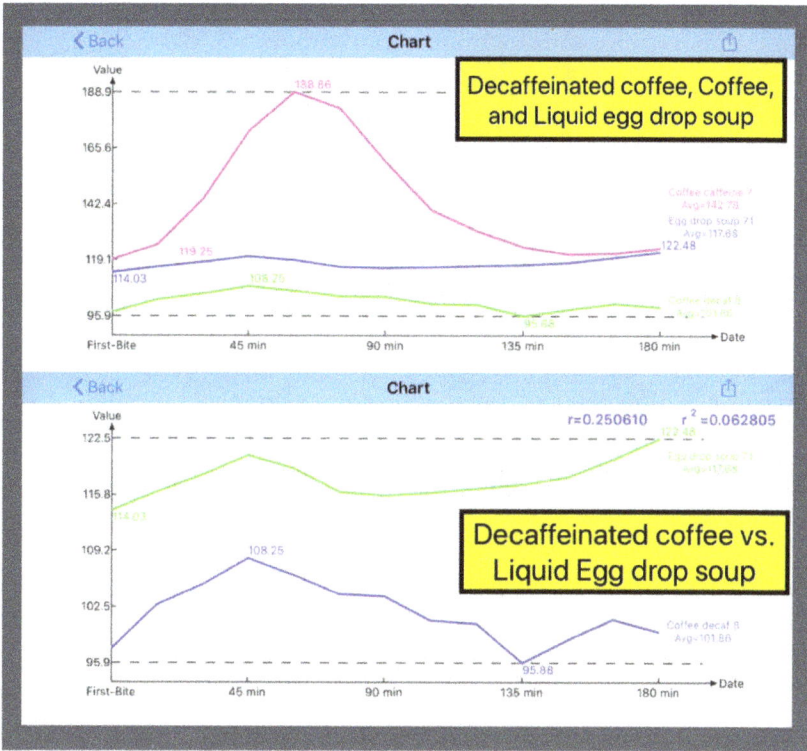

Figure 5: Coffee (with caffeine) has much higher PPG than both decaffeinated coffee and liquid egg drop soup (these two meal types have similar PPG levels)

A geriatric study of self-recovering diabetes conditions using GH-Method: Math-physical medicine (280)

By: Gerald C. Hsu
eclaireMD Foundation, USA
6/22/2020

Introduction:

The author, who is a 73-years-old male with type 2 diabetes (T2D), describes how he reversed his severe metabolic disorder conditions via a stringent lifestyle program which is based on his developed GH-Method: Math-physical medicine.

Method:

The author was diagnosed with T2D approximately 25 years ago in 1995. Fifteen years later, in 2010, his average glucose reached up to 280 mg/dL, where his peak glucose occasionally reached up to ~400 mg/dL, and his HbA1C was 10%. His diabetic complications included five cardiac episodes, without having a stroke, chronic kidney disease, bladder infection, foot ulcer, diabetic retinopathy, and hypothyroidisms. In 2010, when he was 63 years old, three physicians advised him to begin insulin injections which will eventually lead to dialysis treatment. This was his final wake up call. He then decided to rescue his own life through self-study and research on internal medicine, specifically obesity, diabetes, hypertension, hyperlipidemia, heart attack, and stroke; therefore, he focused on the common root cause, which is metabolism improvement and lifestyle change (Reference 1).

By the end of 2014, he developed a computerized mathematical model to evaluate his daily metabolism status. In 2015-2016, he further created four prediction tools of weight, fasting plasma glucose (FPG), postprandial plasma glucose (PPG), and HbA1C, with a prediction accuracy of 95% to 99%. He was able to successfully reduce his weight from 198 to 178 pounds, shorten his waistline from 44 to 34 inches, drop his glucose from above 200 mg/dL to approximately 120 mg/dL and decrease his HbA1C from 10% to 7%. His best accomplishment was discontinuing his three diabetes medications on 12/8/2015, which he never took them again.

By 2017, all of his previous diabetic complications have subsided and his medical examination reports have confirmed the same outcomes.

By having his diabetes and its complications under control is an important component; however, by trying to reverse his severe diabetes conditions would be more remarkable. The author is a senior citizen who does not have many years of life left. All of his medical doctors told him that diabetes is a non-reversible and a non-curable disease. He is an obstinate research scientist and engineer who does not listen to others casually or yield to situations easily; therefore, in early 2019, he decided to launch his own research and experiments with the possibility of self-recovery of pancreatic beta cells insulin production. He used seven different cutting angles as entry points to investigate this difficult subject. By the end of 2019, he already published his first medical paper based on his findings for this research project. Thus far, he has written seven additional medical papers related to this topic. He has finally proven that his pancreatic beta cells are actually repairing itself at a slow rate of ~2.3% per year. It is not much, but at least it is moving in the right direction. As a result, within the last six to eight years, the functions of his insulin production have been repaired and improved by 14% to 18% (Reference 3).

Since 1/1/2012, he measured his finger glucoses four times a day, once for FPG, and three times for PPG. In addition, from 5/5/2018, he utilized a CGM sensor device to collect ~80 glucoses per day. In summary, he has already collected ~75,000 glucose data and ~2 million data of his lifestyle detail for his medical research. Therefore, as of early 2020, he decided to further prove his findings on the pancreatic beta cells self-recovery by conducting one specific biophysical experiment on his own body.

During the early period of 2012-2014, whenever he ate a meal containing "starchy" ingredients, such as wheat, flour, bread, noodle, rice, grains, and potato, his PPG would increase to ~200 mg/dL, with no exceptions. Therefore, for the following 6-years from 2015 to 2020, he avoided them entirely. The past 5-months in the COVID-19 quarantine period (since 1/19/2020), he decided to conduct a special physical experiment on his body. He started to eat toast and kept all the related records about its biological behavioral and physical phenomena associated with this particular meal. He then utilized his GH-Method: math-physical medicine approach to analyze all of these specific dataset.

Results:

As shown in Figure 1, a photo of toast meals, he had a total of 30 meals with toast along with small quantity of vegetables which have a reasonable amount of carbs/sugar, or with high protein food, such as egg and seafood, with no carbs/sugar. These 30 toast meals have an average finger-pierced PPG of 110.6 mg/dL. His average carbs/sugar intake amount of 21.4 grams, and his post-meal walking of 4,208 steps.

Figure 2 shows primary characters of PPG, such as its waveform (i.e. a curve over three-hours period), maximum value, minimum value, and average value. The top diagram reveals a "synthesized" PPG waveform from 30 toast meals, whereas the bottom diagram depicts these 30 individual candlesticks (Reference 2). There are some small deviation existing between the primary values of these two diagrams which resulted from different numerical calculation process and different time instants. The most important characteristic is the maximum (i.e. highest) PPG values which are 136 mg/dL for synthesized PPG curve and 149 mg/dL for 30 individual PPG candlesticks *(from time domain over 172 days)*. ***These highest PPG values of 136-149 mg/dL are much lower than his previous highest PPG record of around 200 mg/dL resulted from starchy food during 2012-2014.***

As shown in Figure 3, a photo of total meals, he had a total of 517 meals with a variety of food ingredients. These 517 total meals during the period from 1/1/2020 to 6/21/2020 have an average finger-piercing PPG of 110.8 mg/dL. His average carbs/sugar intake amount of 13.4 grams, and his post-meal walking of 4,427 steps. These 517 total meals' finger PPG and post-meal walking steps are similar to those 30 toast meals, except for the carbs/sugar amounts which are 13.4 grams for total meals and 21.4 grams for toast meals. ***Toast meals carbs/sugar amount is 60% higher than average total meals. If using a linear amplification rate for his calculation, the toast meals finger PPG should be 110.6 * 1.6 = 177 mg/dL (with a condition associated with highly damaged pancreatic beta cells) which is fairly close to his early PPG records of around 200 mg/dL during 2012-2014. This finding proves that his beta*** *cells have been self-repaired during the past 6 to 8 years.*

Figure 4 illustrates a comparison among 30 toast meals, 517 total meals, and 9 decaffeinated coffee. First, in terms of PPG waveform comparison, both toast meals and total meals have remarkably similar waveforms (i.e. curve patterns) with a very high correlation coefficient of 91%. This phenomenon means that there are no differences between average toast meals and average total meals. The total meals' synthesized peak PPG is 135 mg/dL while the toast meals' synthesized peak PPG is 136 mg/dL. *This also means that toast does not have a significant impact on his recent synthesized PPG profile in 2020, or his body is starting to treat toast just like any other regular food. Any normal person without diabetes should have seen this observed "calm" physical phenomenon due to the existence, strength, and capability of a better situation of insulin production. This physical evidence further confirms self-recovery of his damaged pancreatic beta cells over the past 6 to 8 years.*

Furthermore, he places his recent PPG results from the 9 decaffeinated coffee meals (Reference 4), which is similar to water intake, along with 30 toast meals and 517 total meals. It is evident that the decaffeinated coffee serves as the "lower bound" of the other meals which have different degrees of carbs/sugar intake, including toast meals.

Conclusion:

This simple biophysical experiment and its related mathematical analysis have provided more physical evidence of reversing the diabetes disease, at least it can be improved through self-repair of the damaged pancreatic beta cells insulin function, even for a 73-year-old, the author himself.

Many senior citizens are suffering from diabetes and dying from its complications. The author's own experiences and research results have proven that seniors, like me, cannot give up. There is hope and available ways to improve our general health and medical conditions, which he believes is the underlying fundamental spirit of the geriatric research and practice that is to prolong one's life through health improvement.

Life is precious and good health is important. Having a long and healthy life is a dream for everyone. This article provides one more logical insight and practical ways to achieve longevity.

References:

1. Hsu, Gerald C., eclaireMD Foundation, USA, No. 223: "Effective health age resulting from metabolic condition changes and lifestyle maintenance program"

2. Hsu, Gerald C., eclaireMD Foundation, USA, No. 261: "Comparison study of PPG characteristics from candlestick model using GH-Method: Math-Physical Medicine"

3. Hsu, Gerald C., eclaireMD Foundation, USA, No. 252: "A summary report on partial regeneration of the pancreatic beta cells insulin regression using both FPG, PPG, and HbA1C data (GH-Method: math-physical medicine)"

4. Hsu, Gerald C., eclaireMD Foundation, USA, No. 277: "Different glucose levels produced by coffee versus decaffeinated coffee (GH-Method: Math-physical medicine)"

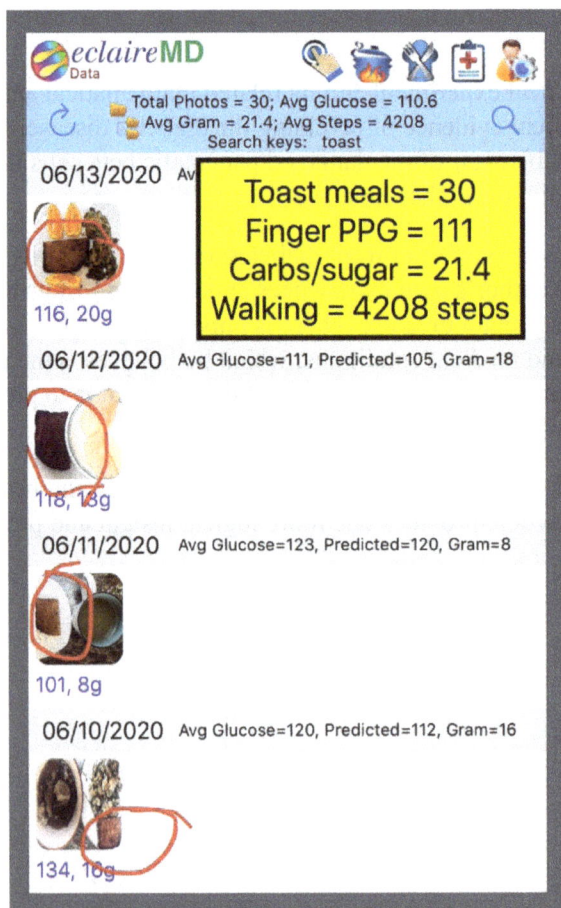

Figure 1: 30 toast meals (1/1/2020-6/21/2020)

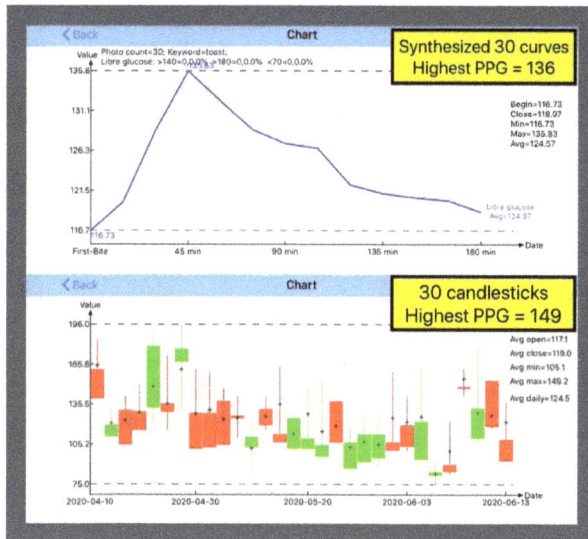

Figure 2: Synthesized PPG curve ad 30 Candlesticks Chart

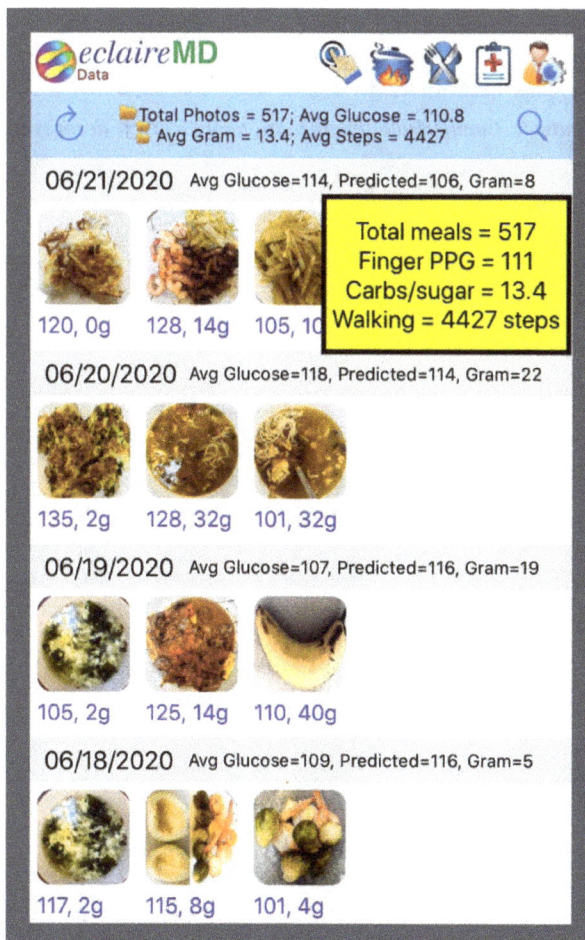

Figure 3: 517 total meals (1/1/2020 - 6/21/2020)

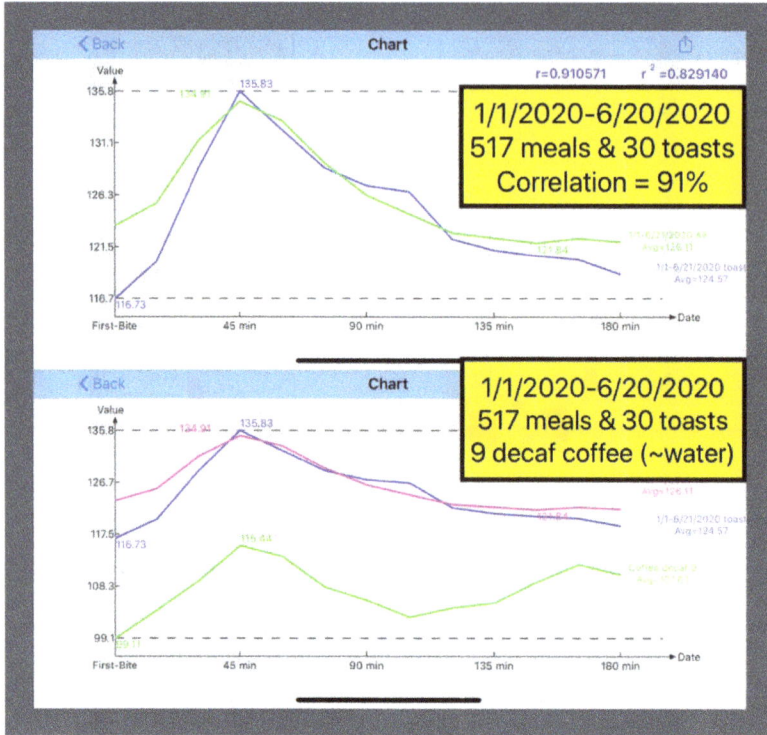

Figure 4: Comparison among toast, total meals, & decaf coffee

Estimation of organ impact by relative energy associated with higher-frequency glucose components using GH-Method: math-physical medicine (No. 290)

Gerald C. Hsu
eclaireMD Foundation, USA
7/5-6/2020

Abstract:

This paper describes the author's estimation of the relative energy associated with higher-frequency glucose components. During this research, he attempted to develop a simplified yet practical "equation" for calculating his estimated relative energy. His ultimate goal is to identify the degree of impact or damage on the human internal organs due to excessive energy caused by hyperglycemia of diabetes patients. He has applied his developed GH-Method: math-physical medicine approach to conduct this medical research.

By using his own ~33,000 glucose data for the past 129 days, he has identified ~20% of relative glucose energy associated with higher-frequency glucose components (67% of total frequency numbers).

The comparison ratios between low frequency with high amplitude glucoses versus high frequency with low amplitude glucoses are summarized as follows:

Energy (E) ratio:
4 to 1
Frequency numbers (n) ratio:
1 to 2
Frequency amplitude square (a*a) ratio:
8 to 1

This research project requires using Bluetooth technology to collect bigger sets of glucose data (3x more data) which allows him to identify ~20% of possible impact or damage on the internal organs resulting from those relative energy associated with high-frequency glucose components. This finding can serve as a starting point for his future research on various diabetic complications.

Introduction:

This paper describes the author's estimation of the relative energy associated with higher-frequency glucose components. During this research, he attempted to develop a simplified yet practical "equation" for his estimated relative energy. His ultimate goal is to identify the degree of impact or damage on the human internal organs due to excessive energy caused by hyperglycemia of diabetes patients. He has applied his developed GH-Method: math-physical medicine approach to conduct this medical research.

Methods:

Background:

The author majored in mathematics, physics, engineering, and computer science in college. After college, he worked in various industries, including space and defense, nuclear and power, computer and information technology (IT), semiconductors and artificial intelligence (AI), where he utilized many of his learned basic concepts and academic theories on different challenging industrial applications.

He has had type 2 diabetes (T2D) since 1995. In 2010, he suffered five cardiovascular episodes and many other diabetic complications, including bladder infections, kidney disorder, foot ulcer, neuropathy, diabetic retinopathy, and hyperthyroidism. Three physicians warned him about the severity of his chronic diseases and related conditions with the possibility of an early death around 65 years old. Facing the immediate threat of dialysis treatments, he finally woke up and decided to save his own life via his own efforts. Since 2010, he has immersed himself into self-study and research on diabetes and its complications with a special focus on glucose and metabolism. Based on his acquired medical knowledge, he realized that glucose is the primary criminal, while blood pressure and lipids are the accomplices. Combining them together would inflict different degree of damage on almost all of the internal organs through the blood circulatory system. However, another broad topic of "metabolism" is far more important than the individual factors related to health. In Figure 1, moving from the inner circle towards the outer rings, this depicts the stringent lifestyle management leading into a good metabolic state, and then converting into a strong immunity to fight against three major disease categories, chronic diseases and complications (~50% of death), cancers (~29% of death), and infectious diseases (~11% of death), except for the remaining ~10% of non-diseases related death cases. This is a logical pathway to achieve overall health conditions, including diabetes control (Reference 1).

Data Collection:
Since 1/1/2012, the author measured his glucose values using the finger-piercing method: once for FPG and three times for PPG each day. On 5/5/2018, he applied a continuous glucose monitoring (CGM) sensor device (Freestyle Libre) on his upper arm and checked his glucose measurements every 15 minutes, a total of ~80 times each day. After the first bite of his meal, he measured his postprandial plasma glucose (PPG) level every 15 minutes for a total of 3-hours or 180 minutes. He has maintained the same measurement pattern during all of his waking hours. However, during his sleeping hours (00:00-07:00), he measured his fasting plasma glucose (FPG) in one-hour intervals.

Starting from 2/19/2020, he has conducted a new experiment on his body. He utilized a hardware device based on Bluetooth technology and embedded with his customized application software to automatically transmit all of his CGM collected glucose data (both 5-minute and 15-minute intervals) from the Libre sensor directly into his developed research application program known as the "eclaireMD system". The data transmission of his glucose values at each "5-minute" time interval would continuously go through the entire day; therefore, he is able to collect ~240 glucose data within 24 hours. With such a bigger set of glucose data, it contains both lower frequency glucose components and higher frequency glucose components.

He used the past 4+ months from 2/19/2020 to 6/27/2020 (129 days), as his research period for analyzing the relative energy associated with both lower-frequency and higher-frequency glucose components.

Data Analysis using wave theory:
The biomedical glucose waves are similar to all kinds of waves in nature, such as earthquake, tsunami, light, sound, and electronics with their respective carried

energies. In his previous industrial work, he studied and investigated the damages to structures and equipments resulted from various earthquakes on many nuclear power plants worldwide. Earthquake wave itself is not the direct "murderer", but the energy associated with earthquake wave, i.e. forces, is the true killer which brings damage on structures and equipments. An initial impact from this wave, some of buildings or structures could suffer destruction or instant collapse. However, certain structures could still survive through the initial impact of force, i.e. energy, but have already suffered from internal damages, such as cracks. As a result, when more earthquake waves carried with their energies continuously hit on the damaged building or structure, eventually it could cause the ultimate structural collapse or equipment failures.

The structural damage from energy associated with earthquake wave is remarkably similar to the human organ impact and damage from the energy associated with the glucose wave. A diabetes patient who suffers from hyperglycemia for a long period of time, all of his internal organs have already sustained different degrees of damage resulted from his daily high glucose wave's energy. Sooner or later, some of these organs will face destruction and create serious problems.

Based on physics, the wave's energy is directly proportional to the square of the amplitude of a wave. Therefore, the author tried to develop a simple yet practical equation using the multiplication of "a2", i.e. square of amplitude" and "n", i.e. the number of data points within a range of glucose wave, to represent this "glucose energy".

Here is his proposed equation of estimated relative energy associated with glucose components within certain frequency range. *He calls it the "equation of glucose energy"*:

E = na2

Where "E" is relative glucose energy, "n" is the number of glucose components of a wave, and "a" is the "average amplitude" of frequency domain's Y-coordinates which is proportional to the square of glucose value. Here, the *"average amplitude, a"* is defined as follow:

$$a = (\sum_{i=1}^{n} Ai) / n$$

Where **"A"** is individual amplitude, and **"n"** is the upper limit of glucose component numbers.

The author further validated this theoretically derived simple "glucose energy equation" by using his real clinical data collected from his own body during the past 129 days (2/19/2020 - 6/27/2020).

Results:

Figure 2 shows his 15-minute "synthesized" sensor glucose wave over the course of a day (x-scale: 24 hours). Here "synthesized" means that the final wave is the combination of 129 days (from 2/19/2020 through 6/27/2020) average glucose waves. This Figure 2 also includes his synthesized 5-minute wave and the comparison chart of these two time-domain daily glucose waves (5-minutes vs. 15-minutes).

From this figure, it is obvious that there are more higher frequency glucose components in the 5-minute wave due to availability of three times more the collected number of glucose data points. The extremely high correlation coefficient of 99% existed between 5-minutes time-domain wave and 15-minutes time-domain wave means that these two measured waveforms are very similar in shape, except for the 5-minute wave containing more glucose components, especially including some higher-frequency glucose components.

The author than enhanced his customized applications program (the eclaireMD software system) to include Fourier transform operation, frequency domain analysis, wave theory applications, and relative glucose energy calculations using his developed "equation of glucose energy: E=na2". The conclusive results are shown in Figure 3, a bar chart of comparison of energy distribution percentages.

He has defined the frequency band of lower-frequency with higher amplitude (Lo f & Hi a) as 0 to 48 (n=48) and the frequency band of higher-frequency with lower amplitude (Hi f & Lo a) as 48 to 144 (n=96). The calculated **"distribution % of relative glucose energy"** for these two frequency bands are listed as follows:

Lo f & Hi a: 81%
Hi f & Lo a: 19%

Furthermore, he also calculated the following **"distribution percentages of values of glucose amplitude square (a*a)"**:

Lo f & Hi a: 89%
Hi f & Lo a: 11%

The comparison ratio between two relative glucose energies (E), 81% versus 19%, is about 4 to 1. The comparison ratio between the numbers of chosen higher-frequency component number ("n") of 96 (67% or two third) versus the lower-frequency component number ("n") of 48 (33% or one third), is exactly 2 to 1. The comparison ratio of glucose energy ("E"), 81% versus 19% is around 4 to 1.

The following simple arithmetic calculation can depict the relationships among these three sets of data.

Lo f & Hi a (Y%*X%) / Hi f & Lo a (Y%*X%): i.e. ratio of a2 * n
= (89*33.3) / (11*66.7)
= 4 / 1
= 81 /19 : i.e. ratio of energy

Glucose serves as the nutritional supply to the body by transforming into energy which body needs. In theory, hyperglycemia is elevated glucose that provides excess "energy" more than the body needs. When our body cannot burn off all of these produced and stored energy with glucose, the excessive "left-over" energy circulating in the bloodstream will eventually cause different degrees of damage to our internal organs. This is the author's interpretation based on physics regarding why senior people having excessive glucose energy are most likely suffering from diabetes complications. An effective way to control diabetes conditions for all aged people are two simple steps: first, eat less (provide less fuel), and second, exercise more (burn off more energy).

This math-physical medicine research approach is capable to provide some reasonable but accurate answers for various biomedical problems.

Conclusions:

By using his own ~33,000 glucose data for the past 129 days, he has identified ~20% of relative glucose energy associated with higher-frequency glucose components (67% of total frequency numbers).

The comparison ratios between low frequency with high amplitude glucoses versus high frequency with low amplitude glucoses are summarized as follows:

Energy (E) ratio:
4 to 1
Frequency numbers (n) ratio:
1 to 2
Frequency amplitude square (a*a) ratio:
8 to 1

This research project requires using Bluetooth technology to collect bigger sets of glucose data (3x more data) which allows him to identify ~20% of possible impact or damage on the internal organs resulting from those relative energy associated with high-frequency glucose components. This finding can serve as a starting point for his future research on various diabetic complications.

References:

1. Hsu, Gerald C. eclaireMD Foundation, USA. May 2020. No. 263: "Risk probability of having a metabolic disorder induced cancer (GH-Method: MPM)."

2. Hsu, Gerald C. eclaireMD Foundation, USA. May 2019. No. 82: "Using GH-Method: Math-Physical Medicine, Fourier Transform, and Frequency Segmentation Pattern Analysis to Investigate Relative Energy Associated with Glucose."

3. Hsu, Gerald C. eclaireMD Foundation, USA. December 2019. No. 152: "Applying first-order perturbation theory of quantum mechanics to predict and build a

postprandial plasma glucose waveform (GH-Method: math-physical medicine).”

4. Hsu, Gerald C. eclaireMD Foundation, USA. June 2020. No.281: ”Differences between 5-minute and 15-minute measurement time intervals of the CGM sensor glucoses device using GH-Method: math-physical medicine.”

5. Hsu, Gerald C. eclaireMD Foundation, USA. June 2020. No. 272: “Estimated relative energy level of four different Finger PPG ranges using wave theory and frequency domain analysis (GH-Method: math-physical medicine).”

6. Hsu, Gerald C. eclaireMD Foundation, USA. June 2020. No. 273: “Using glucose and its associated energy to study the risk probability percentage of having a stroke or cardiovascular diseases from 2018 through 2020 (GH-Method: math-physical medicine).”

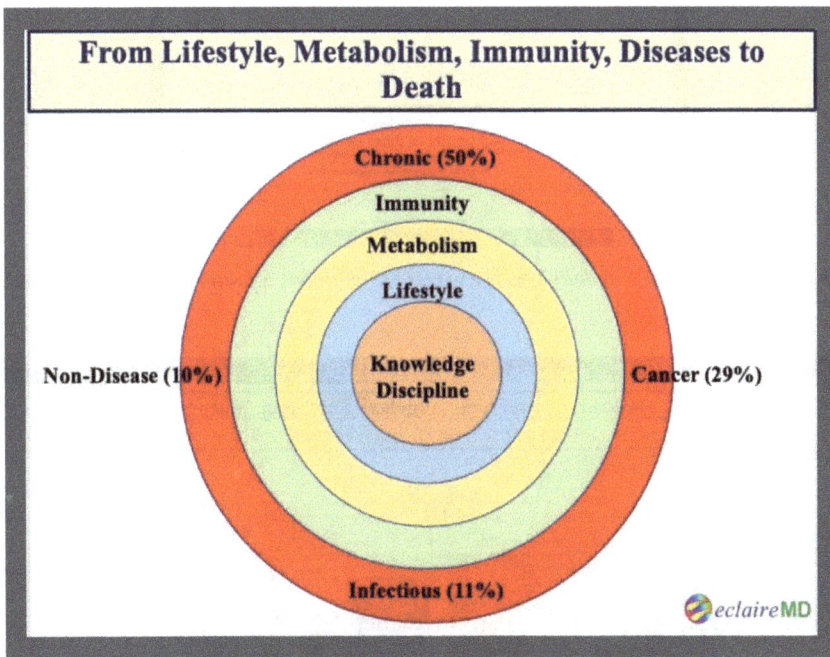

From Lifestyle, Metabolism, Immunity, Diseases to Death

Chronic (50%)

Immunity

Metabolism

Lifestyle

Non-Disease (10%)

Knowledge Discipline

Cancer (29%)

Infectious (11%)

eclaireMD

Figure 1: From lifestyle through metabolism, immunity, to diseases and death

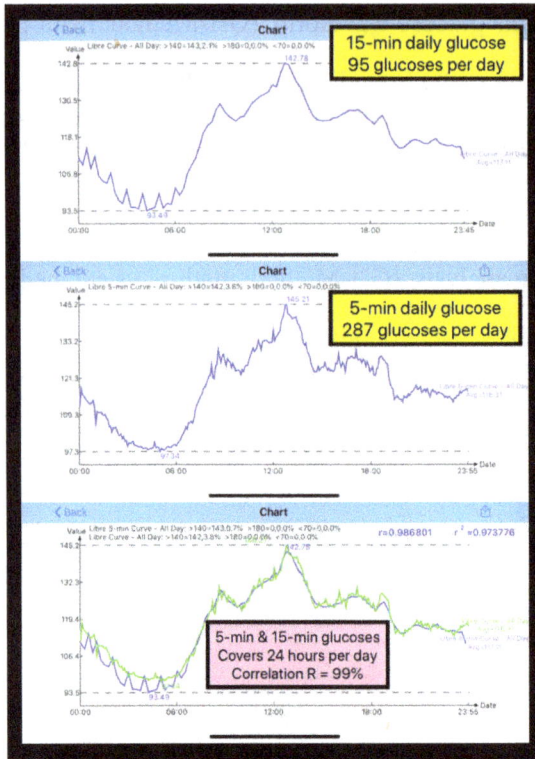

Figure 2: Time-domain daily glucose waves (15-minutes, 5-minutes, and comparison)

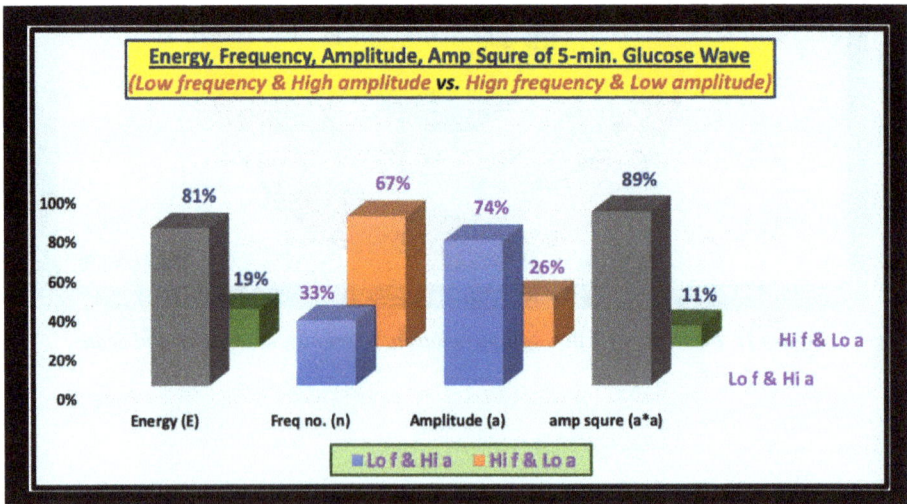

Figure 3: Distribution % of Energy, Frequency number, frequency domain Amplitude, & amplitude square

An investigation of continuous glucose monitor based PPG waves and results using GH-Method: math-physical medicine (No. 304)

Gerald C. Hsu
eclaireMD Foundation, USA
8/5/2020

Abstract:

This article is a study of postprandial plasma glucose (PPG) waveforms and results over a period of 822 days from 5/5/2018 to 8/4/2020. It consists of 29,592 continuous glucose monitor (CGM) sensor readings and 2,466 finger-piercing measurements for a total of 32,058 PPG values. The research methodology utilizes the author developed GH-Method: math-physical medicine (MPM) which has been applied for the past decade.

Listed below are the summarized key data in the order of CGM-15 min PPG, Finger PPG, carbs/sugar, and post-meal walking steps (Figure 1):

Breakfast:
134 mg/dL, 115 mg/dL, 9.8 g, 4,433 steps
Lunch:
138 mg/dL, 116 mg/dL, 17.1 g, 3,975 steps
Dinner:
128 mg/dL, 110 mg/dL, 14.7 g, 4,478 steps
Daily:
133 mg/dL, 113.8 mg/dL, 13.9 g, 4,294 steps

Applying his PPG prediction method (Reference 6), the calculation of predicted PPG using his formula-based approach on the status of fasting plasma glucose (FPG), carbs/sugar intake amount, and post-meal walking steps are shown:

Predicted Finger PPG
= 0.966* Finger FPG + (carbs/sugar grams * 2) - (post-meal walking steps in thousand * 5)

Predicted PPG
= 0.966 * 111.2 + (13.9 *2) - ((4294/1000)* 5)
= 107.5 + 27.7 - 21.5
= 113.7 mg/dL

The comparison of this formula-based finger PPG prediction of 113.7 mg/dL with the actual measured finger PPG of 113.8 mg/dL has shown ~100% of the PPG prediction accuracy.

The following five PPG values are arranged by their average glucose levels from high to low:

60-minutes: *141.96 mg/ dL*
Daily average: *133.39 mg/ dL*
120-minutes: *130.42 mg/ dL*
180-minutes: *129.08 mg/ dL*
0-minute: *127.87 mg/ dL*

In summary, there are four conclusive statements:

First, the author's lifestyle of having a heavier lunch results with the highest PPG value compared to the other meals of the day.

Second, the peak of PPG occurs around 60-minutes after the first bite of his meal, not the traditional standard of two-hours after.

Third, the differences between the higher CGM PPG and the lower Finger PPG are between 13% to 17%. However, with his ongoing lifestyle management improvements, these two PPG values are converging together.

Fourth, his formula-based Finger PPG prediction model can provide a near 100% prediction accuracy.

Introduction:

This article is a study of postprandial plasma glucose (PPG) waveforms and results over a period of 822 days from 5/5/2018 to 8/4/2020. It consists of 29,592 continuous glucose monitor (CGM) sensor readings and 2,466 finger-piercing measurements for a total of 32,058 PPG values. The research methodology utilizes the author developed GH-Method: math-physical medicine (MPM) which has been applied for the past decade.

Method:

GH-method: Math-physical medicine (MPM) methodology

The description below explains the MPM research methodology developed by the author utilized in his biomedical research.

Any system, whether medical, political, economic, engineering, biological, chemical, and even psychological have causes or triggers (inputs) and consequences (outputs). There are definitely some existing connections between inputs and outputs that can be either simple or complicated. The inputs and outputs of any type of system, including biomedical system, can be observed visually or measured by certain instruments. These physically observed phenomena, including features, images, incidents, or numbers are merely the partial "physical expression" of these underneath system structure. This system structure includes human organs for a biomedical system, the human brain for a neurological or mental system, or steel plate for structural or mechanical engineering system.

Once we have collected these readings of the physical phenomena (external expression, similar to a behavior, symptom, or response), through either incident, image, or data, we should be able to organize or categorize them in a logical manner. When we check or analyze these partial physical phenomena outputs and cannot figure out why they act or behave in certain way due to internal causes, reasons, or stressors, we can try to develop some guesses or formulate some reasonable hypotheses based on some available basic principles, theories, or concepts from physics. At this point, we just cannot pull out an existing equation from a physics textbook and insert these input variables in to conduct a "plug and play" game. An equation is an expression of a concept or a theory, which is usually associated with some existing conditions, either initial or boundary; however, a biomedical system usually has different kind of conditions from other systems.

After understanding the meaning of observed physical phenomena, the next step is to prove the hypothesis, guess, or interpretation of the phenomenon being correct or incorrect. At this stage, a solid understanding of mathematics becomes extremely useful to develop a meaningful model which could represent or interpret these observed physical phenomena and created hypothesis. In addition, some engineering modeling techniques, such as finite element method and computer science tools, including software, artificial intelligence (AI), and big data analytics can offer great assistance on verification of analysis results from these mathematical operations.

If the mathematical results cannot support the created hypothesis, then a new hypothesis needs to be formulated. When this new hypothesis is proven to be correct, then we can extend or convert this hypothesis into a useful mathematical equation or into a simpler arithmetical formula for others to adopt this easier way of thinking and understanding of the results. In the final stage, the derived mathematical equation or arithmetical formula can then be used to "predict" future outcomes of the selected system based on other different sets of inputs.

Diabetes Research

The author has been a severe type 2 diabetes (T2D) patient since 1995. He has developed many serious complications and finally, in 2010, they became life-threatening. Therefore, he has spent the next 10-years to self-study and research diabetes, metabolism, and endocrinology, in order to save his own life.

He spent his first four years, from 2010 to 2013, to self-study 6 chronic diseases, i.e. obesity, diabetes, hypertension, hyperlipidemia, cardiovascular diseases, stroke, as well as food nutrition. Food is probably the most important and also complicated input element to influence these chronic diseases. After his first 4-years of self-learning, he then spent the entire year of 2014 to develop a complex model of metabolism. This mathematical model contains 4 biomarkers of medical conditions (weight, glucose, blood pressure, and lipids) along with 6 lifestyle details (food portion and nutritional balance, water intake, exercise, sleep amount and quality, stress reduction, and daily life routines regularity). He applied the concept of topology and the approximation engineering modeling technique of finite element method to develop this metabolism mathematical model which became the cornerstone of his future research work.

Starting from 2015, he spent three consecutive years, from 2015 to 2017, to discover the characteristics and behaviors of this complex "wild beast" of glucose. His major objective is to truly understand the "inner characteristics" of the glucose, not just using medication's chemical power to control its "external biological symptoms". His research work is similar to a horseman trying to tame a horse by understanding its temperament first, not just giving a tranquilizer to calm it down. As a result, during this period of 3-years, he has developed 4 prediction models, which include Weight, PPG, FPG, and HbA1C with very high prediction accuracy (95% to 99%) to reach to his purpose of *understanding glucoses*.

The author estimated and proved that PPG contributes approximately 75% to 80% towards HbA1C formation. Therefore, he tried to unravel the mystery of PPG first. Through his diabetes research, he has identified at least 19 influential factors associated with PPG formation. Among those influential factors, diet (carbs/sugar intake amount) would provide ~38% and exercise (post-meal walking) would contribute ~41%. Combining these two primary influential factors, it gives ~80% of the PPG formation. Among the rest of the 17 secondary factors, a high weather temperature contributes ~5%, whereas stress and illness only make noticeable contributions when they occur.

For most T2D patients who take medications, its biochemical effect would become the most significant influential factor. However, as we know, medication cannot cure diabetes and only control its symptoms. Therefore, the author decided to focus on controlling diabetes at the most fundamental level by investigating its root cause. Previously, he has taken high doses of three prescribed diabetes medications for 18 years since 1997; however, in 2013, he started to reduce the number of prescriptions and dosages of his daily medications. By 12/8/2015, he finally ceased taking any diabetes medications.

From 2016 to 2017, he discovered a solid statistical connection between his FPG and his weight (>90% of correlation coefficient). In addition, similar to his PPG research, he also recognized that there are about 5 influential factors of FPG formation with weight alone contributing >85% and cold weather temperature influencing ~5%.

Since July 2019, he also launched a special investigation on the degree of damage to his pancreatic beta cells. During the past 12-months of research work, he noticed that both of his FPG and PPG have been decreased in the past 6 to 8 years at an annual rate of 2.2% to 3.2%. In other words, his pancreatic beta cells have been self-regenerating or self-repairing about 13% to 26% over these 6-8 years. He then thought about FPG as being a good indicator on how healthy his pancreatic beta cells are since there are no food intake and exercise while sleeping. During the last 5 years, his body weight has been maintained around 172 lbs. Besides, his body has been medication-free over the past 5-years as well. It makes sense that FPG carries a significant and clear message about his health status of pancreatic beta cells; therefore, it can be served as the baseline of his overall glucose predications.

The detailed explanation of his glucose research work is provided because this particular study is based on "glucoses".

Glucose Data Collection:

During this investigation period, he utilizes the Libre Freestyle CGM on his upper arm to collect glucose values at 15-minute time intervals. Therefore, the collection rate is comprised of 96 glucose data and 36 PPG data per day. The PPG data of each meal contain 12 data points, from 0-minute throughout 180 minutes with 15-minute time intervals. While no device is free of defects, the existing glucose measuring devices, both finger-piercing testing strip and CGM sensor have their respective inherent reliability issues.

At the same time, he has kept a complete record of his carbs/sugar intake amount in grams and post-meal walking steps associated with each of his 2,450 meals over these 822 days.

Results:

Figure 1 has a data table on its top diagram which includes all of his collected and calculated background data of this study. Its bottom diagram is a line chart that contains his 4 PPG curves of breakfast, lunch, dinner, and daily PPG. It is obvious that his lunch PPG waveform is the highest, next is breakfast, and then dinner is the lowest among these three waveforms. His eating times starting with Breakfast is at 07:00, Lunch at 12:00, and Dinner at 18:00. His eating patterns include good-protein and high-quality breakfast, then lunch with the largest volume with a variety of meal contents, and a simple and smaller volume for dinner (due to his weight control). Although he has strong knowledge about food nutrition and diet limitations for diabetes, it is inevitable to consume more amount of carbohydrates and sugar during lunch, which is his largest meal of the day. It should be mentioned that his post-meal walking steps have been consistent around 4,000 steps after each meal for the past 6 years.

This line chart depicts four curves (i.e. waveforms) of his synthesized PPG on a mealtime scale of 3-hours from the first bite at 0 minute to 180 minutes. This figure is generated by averaging all of the 36 measured glucoses for each meal per day over these 822 days. As a result, the author developed his data analysis software to use the average glucoses of these 36 data within 3 meal hours to be the patient's "average PPG".

Listed below are the summarized key data in the order of CGM-15 min PPG, Finger PPG, carbs/sugar, and post-meal walking steps (Figure 1):

Breakfast:
134 mg/dL, 115 mg/dL, 9.8 g, 4,433 steps
Lunch:
138 mg/dL, 116 mg/dL, 17.1 g, 3,975 steps
Dinner:
128 mg/dL, 110 mg/dL, 14.7 g, 4,478 steps
Daily:
133 mg/dL, 113.8 mg/dL, 13.9 g, 4,294 steps

Applying his PPG prediction method (Reference 6), the calculation of predicted PPG using his formula-based approach on the status of fasting plasma glucose (FPG), carbs/sugar intake amount, and post-meal walking steps are shown:

Predicted Finger PPG
= 0.966* Finger FPG + (carbs/sugar grams * 2) - (post-meal walking steps in thousand * 5)

Predicted PPG
= 0.966 * 111.2 + (13.9 *2) - ((4294/1000)* 5)

= 107.5 + 27.7 - 21.5
= 113.7 mg/dL

In Figure 1, the data table indicates his PPG rising due to his average carbs/sugar intake of 13.9 grams which would generate ~27.7 mg/dL PPG amount. Around 45 minutes after his first bite of meal, he starts to do his routine post-meal walking exercise at 4,294 steps which would reduce to ~21.5 mg/dL PPG. Therefore, the net gain of his PPG from his carbs/sugar intake and post-meal exercise would be ~6.2 mg/dL.

The comparison of this formula-based finger PPG prediction of 113.7 mg/dL with the actual measured finger PPG of 113.8 mg/dL has shown ~100% of PPG prediction accuracy. Even if he uses 100% of finger FPG as his baseline PPG, he still can obtain a predicted PPG of 117.5 mg/dL with ~97% of prediction accuracy.

Figure 2 shows the comparison among 5 PPG waveforms over the 822 days at the first bite at 0-minute, 60-minutes, 120-minutes, 180-minutes, and daily average PPG. The following five PPG values are arranged by their average glucose levels from high to low:

60-minutes: *141.96 mg/ dL*
Daily average: *133.39 mg/ dL*
120-minutes: *130.42 mg/ dL*
180-minutes: *129.08 mg/ dL*
0-minute: *127.87 mg/ dL*

The PPG wave moves from its lowest point at 0-minute then moves upward to reach its peak at 60-minutes, and later moves downward to its lowest positions between 120-minutes and 180-minutes. The standard advice given to diabetes patients in measuring their PPG at two hours after the first bite of their meal has no valid reason for it. At 120-minutes, it essentially catches their lowest PPG, not the highest PPG at 60-minutes.

In Figure 3, it demonstrates a comparison between CGM-15 min PPG and Finger PPG within two different periods. The top diagram shows a longer period of 2+ years, from 5/5/2018 to 8/4/2020, with CGM PPG of 133 mg/dL and Finger PPG of 114 mg/ dL. The bottom diagram reveals a shorter period of 6+ months, from 1/19/2020 to 8/4/2020, with CGM PPG of 124 mg/dL and Finger PPG of 110 mg/dL. These two diagrams prove that his PPG are improving based on both Finger PPG and CGM-15 min PPG. Furthermore, the CGM PPG is 17% higher than Finger PPG during the longer period, while the CGM PPG is only 13% higher than Finger PPG during the shorter period. This means that these two different measurements of PPG values are "converging" together.

Conclusions:

In summary, there are four conclusive statements:

First, the author's lifestyle of having a heavier lunch results with the highest PPG value compared to the other meals of the day.

Second, the peak of PPG occurs around 60-minutes after the first bite of his meal, not the traditional standard of two-hours after.

Third, the differences between the higher CGM PPG and the lower Finger PPG are between 13% to 17%. However, with his ongoing lifestyle management improvements, these two PPG values are converging together. Fourth, his formula-based Finger PPG prediction model can provide a near 100% prediction accuracy.

References:

1. Hsu, Gerald C. eclaireMD Foundation, USA. "A simplified yet accurate linear equation of PPG prediction model for T2D patients using GH-Method: math-physical medicine (No. 97)."

2. Hsu, Gerald C. eclaireMD Foundation, USA. "Application of linear equation-based PPG prediction model for four T2D clinic cases using GH-Method: math-physical medicine (No. 99)."

3. Hsu, Gerald C. eclaireMD Foundation, USA. "Using GH-Method: Math-Physical Medicine to Conduct the Accuracy Comparison of Two different PPG Prediction Methods (No. 89)."

4. Hsu, Gerald C. eclaireMD Foundation, USA. "Accuracy of Predicted PPG by using AI Glucometer and GH-Method: math-physical medicine (No. 106)."

5. Hsu, Gerald C. eclaireMD Foundation, USA. "A comparison of three glucose measurement results during COVID-19 period using GH-Method: math-physical medicine (No. 303)"

6. Hsu, Gerald C. eclaireMD Foundation, USA. "A simple formula based on postprandial plasma glucose prediction using 5,640 meals data via GH-Method: math-physical medicine (No. 301)"

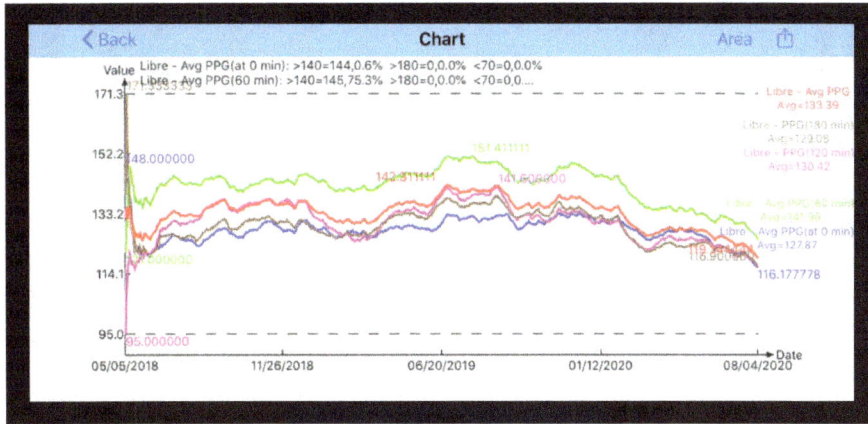

Figure 1: Data table and line chart of synthesized PPG waveforms of breakfast, lunch, dinner, and daily using CGM 15-minutes glucoses over 822 days (5/5/2018 - 8/4/2020)

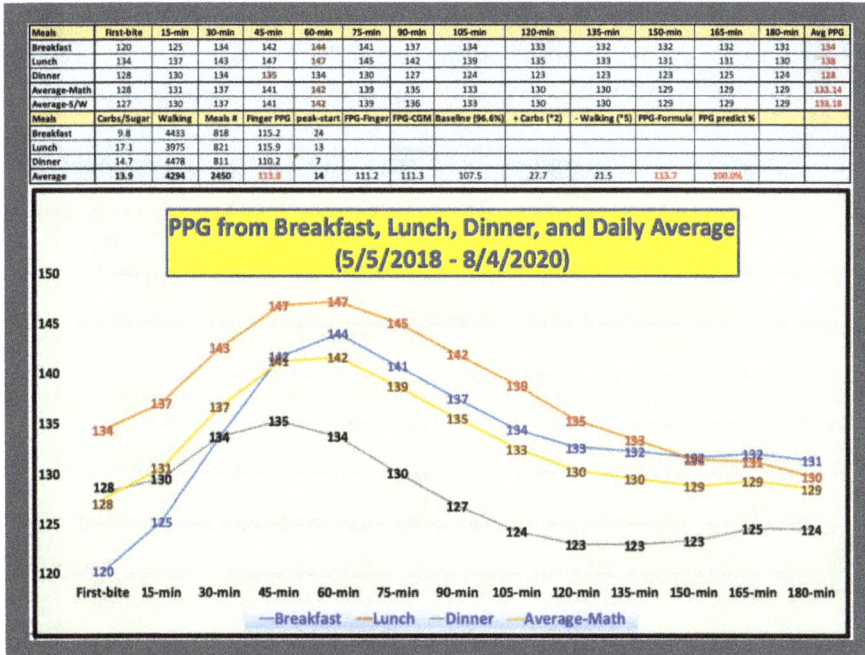

Figure 2: 90-days moving averaged PPG waveforms at 0-min, 60-min, 120-min, 180-min, and daily average using CGM 15-minutes glucoses over 822 days (5/5/2018 - 8/4/2020)

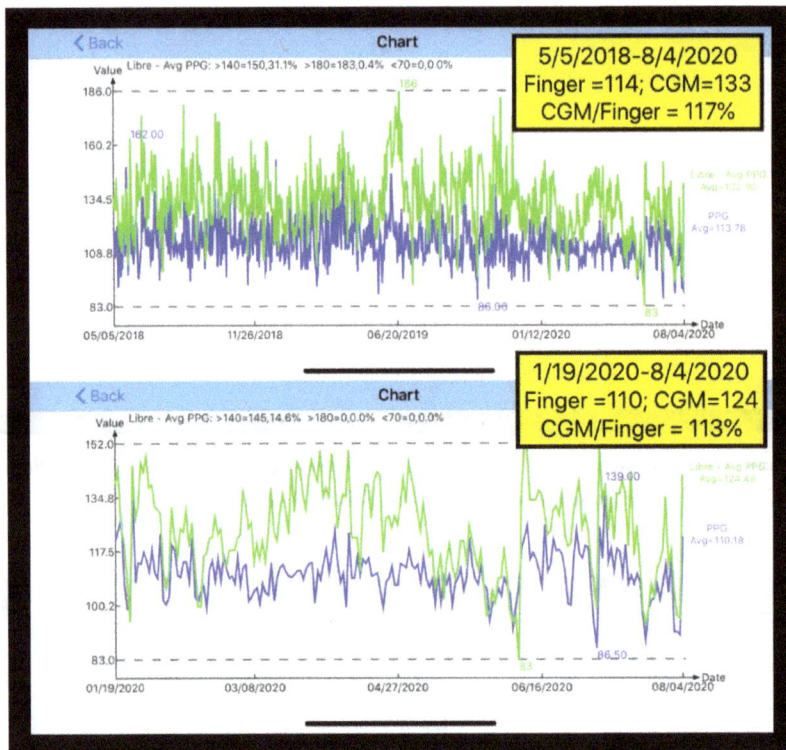

Figure 3: Daily averaged PPG waveforms of both Finger and CGM 15-min for two periods (longer period: 5/5/2018 - 8/4/2020 and shorter period: 1/19/2020 - 8/4/2020)

Glucose trend pattern analysis and progressive behavior modification of a T2D patient using GH-Method: math-physical medicine (No. 305)

By: Gerald C. Hsu
eclaireMD Foundation, USA
8/7-8/2020

Abstract:

In this article, the author used data based on 10-years' worth of glucoses and prominent lifestyle details such as diet and exercise to address his glucose trend pattern analysis and progressive lifestyle behavior modifications. The research methodology used is the GH-Method: math-physical medicine (MPM) approach which has been developed by the author over the past decade. This *Progressive Behavior Modification* concept is also a part of his Mentality-Personality Modeling (MPM). He addresses the quantitative linkage between diabetes physiological phenomena and behavior psychological influences of a type 2 diabetes (T2D) patient.

He has created a geometric presentation model with carbs/sugar intake amount as the x-axis, post-meal walking steps as the y-axis, and daily glucose as the z-axis (Figure 2). He decided to "fold over" the z-axis and superimpose it with the x-y planar space in a form of "radio wave" format. Under his created 3D presentation on a 2D planar space, the glucose trend pattern becomes ultra-clear. For over the past 10-years, his annual glucose movement path started in the upper right corner (subregion E5 in 2010), moving at a ~30 degree downward slope before arriving to the location near the upper middle but skewed to the left (subregion B3 in 2014), and then continuously dropping to the lower left corner (subregion B1 in 2020).

In summary, his glucose moving path is a 30-degree downward angle to the left and then straight downward to the bottom. His annualized average daily glucoses have been reduced from the starting point of 250 mg/dL in 2010 through the "reflection point" of 135 mg/dL in 2014, and then straight down to the ending point of 110 mg/dL in 2020. The triangular relationship among diet, exercise, and daily glucose can be easily observed on this "glucose trend pattern" diagram (Figure 2).

Through analyzing those distinctive daily glucose trend patterns, the personality traits and behavior psychological characteristics of this T2D patient can be revealed instantly and clearly. As a result, a more practical guidance of *"progressive behavior modification"* can be provided to other T2D patients in order to improve their medical conditions for chronic diseases.

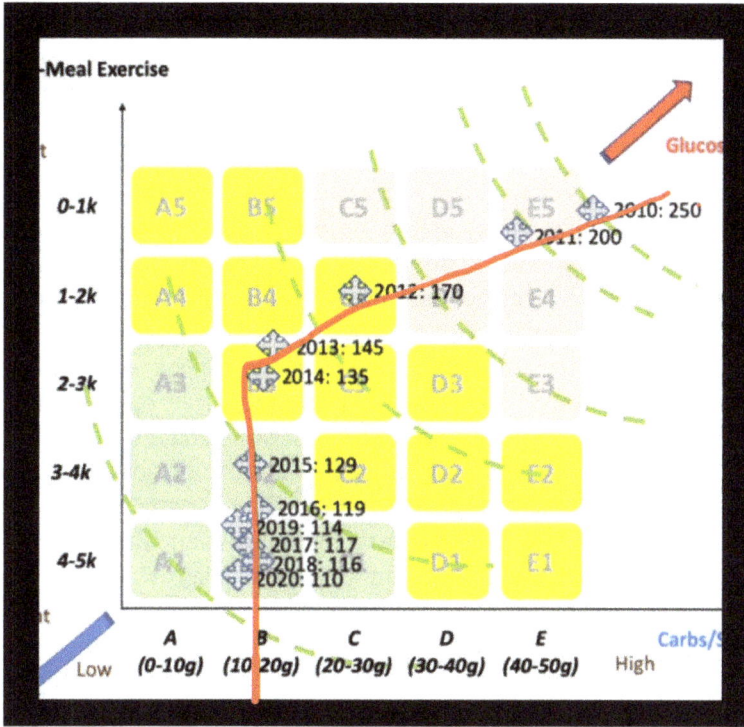

Figure 2: Glucose trend pattern diagram

Introduction:

In this article, the author used data based on 10-years' worth of glucoses and prominent lifestyle details such as diet and exercise to address his glucose trend pattern analysis and progressive lifestyle behavior modifications. The research methodology used is the GH-Method: math-physical medicine (MPM) approach which has been developed by the author over the past decade. This Progressive Behavior Modification concept is also a part of his Mentality-Personality Modeling (MPM). He addresses the quantitative linkage between physiological diabetes phenomena and behavior psychological influences of a type 2 diabetes (T2D) patient.

Method:

GH-method: Math-physical medicine (MPM) methodology

The description below explains the GH-Method: MPM research methodology developed by the author utilized in his biomedical research (Reference 1).

Any system, whether medical, political, economic, engineering, biological, chemical, and even psychological have causes or triggers (inputs) and consequences (outputs). There are definitely some existing connections between inputs and outputs that can be either simple or complicated. The inputs and outputs of any type of system, including biomedical system, can be observed visually or measured by certain instruments. These physically observed phenomena, including features, images, incidents, or numbers are merely the partial "physical expression" of these underneath system structure. This system structure includes human organs for a biomedical system, the human brain for a neurological or mental system, or steel plate for structural or mechanical engineering system.

Once we have collected these readings of the physical phenomena (external expression, similar to a behavior, symptom, or response), through either incident, image, or data, we should be able to organize or categorize them in a logical manner. When we check or analyze these partial physical phenomena outputs and cannot figure out why they act or behave in certain way due to internal causes, reasons, or stressors, we can try to develop some guesses or formulate some reasonable hypotheses based on some available basic principles, theories, or concepts from physics. At this point, we just cannot pull out an existing equation from a physics textbook and insert these input variables in to conduct a "plug and play" game. An equation is an expression of a concept or a theory, which is usually associated with some existing conditions, either initial or boundary; however, a biomedical system usually has different kind of conditions from other systems.

After understanding the meaning of observed physical phenomena, the next step is to prove the hypothesis, guess, or interpretation of the phenomenon being correct or incorrect. At this stage, a solid understanding of mathematics becomes extremely useful to develop a meaningful model which could represent or interpret these observed physical phenomena and created hypothesis. In addition, some engineering modeling techniques, such as finite element method and computer science tools, including software, artificial intelligence (AI), and big data analytics can offer great assistance on verification of analysis results from these mathematical operations.

If the mathematical results cannot support the created hypothesis, then a new hypothesis needs to be formulated. When this new hypothesis is proven to be correct, then we can extend or convert this hypothesis into a useful mathematical equation or into a simpler arithmetical formula for others to adopt this easier way of thinking and understanding of the results. In the final stage, the derived mathematical equation or arithmetical formula can then be used to "predict" future outcomes of the selected system based on other different sets of inputs.

Diabetes Research

The author has been a severe type 2 diabetes (T2D) patient since 1995. He has developed many serious complications and finally, in 2010, they became life-threatening. Therefore, he has spent the next 10-years to self-study and research diabetes, metabolism, and endocrinology, in order to save his own life.

He spent his first four years, from 2010 to 2013, to self-study 6 chronic diseases, i.e. obesity, diabetes, hypertension, hyperlipidemia, cardiovascular diseases, stroke, as well as food nutrition. Food is probably the most important and also complicated input element to influence these chronic diseases. After his first 4-years of self-learning, he then spent the entire year of 2014 to develop a complex model of metabolism. This mathematical model contains four biomarkers of medical conditions (weight, glucose, blood pressure, and lipids) along with six lifestyle details (food portion and nutritional balance, drinking water intake, adequate exercise, sufficient sleep amount and quality, stress reduction, and daily life routines regularity). He applied the concept of topology from mathematics and the approximation modeling technique of finite element method from engineering to develop this metabolism model which became the cornerstone of his future medical research work. As a result, his overall health conditions also started to be improved.

Starting from 2015, he spent three consecutive years, from 2015 to 2017, to discover the characteristics and behaviors of this complex "wild beast" of glucose. His major objective is to truly understand the "inner characteristics" of the glucose, not just using medication's chemical power to control the disease' external biological "symptoms". His research work is similar to a horseman trying to tame a horse by understanding its temperament first, not just giving a tranquilizer to calm it down. As a result, during this period of 3 years, he has developed four prediction models, which include Weight, PPG, FPG, and HbA1C with extremely high prediction accuracy (95% to 99%) to reach to his purpose of "understanding glucoses".

The author estimated and proved that PPG contributes approximately 75% to 80% towards HbA1C formation. Therefore, he tried to unravel the mystery of PPG first. Through his diabetes research, he has identified at least 19 influential factors associated with PPG formation. Among those influential factors, diet (carbs/sugar intake amount) would provide ~38% and exercise (post-meal walking) would contribute ~41%. Combining these two primary influential factors, it gives ~80% of the PPG formation. Among the rest of the 17 secondary factors, a high weather temperature contributes ~5%, whereas stress and illness only make noticeable contributions when they occur.

For most T2D patients who take medication, its biochemical effect would become the most significant influential factor of glucose. However, as we know, medication cannot cure diabetes and only control its symptoms. Therefore, the author decided to focus on controlling diabetes at the most fundamental core level by investigating its root cause. Previously, he has taken high doses of three prescribed diabetes medications for 18 years since 1997; however, in 2013, he started to reduce the number of prescriptions and dosages of his daily medications. By 12/8/2015, he finally ceased taking any diabetes medications.

From 2016 to 2017, he discovered a solid statistical connection between his FPG and his body weight with a >90% correlation coefficient. In addition, similar to his PPG research, he also recognized that there are about 5 influential factors of FPG formation with weight alone contributing >85% and cold weather temperature influencing ~5%.

Since July 2019, he also launched a special investigation on the degree of damage to his pancreatic beta cells. During the past 12-months of research work, he noticed that both of his FPG and PPG have been decreased in the past 6 to 8 years at an annual rate of 2.2% to 3.2%. In other words, his pancreatic beta cells have been self-regenerating or self-repairing about 13% to 26% over these 6-8 years. He then thought about FPG as being a good indicator on how healthy his pancreatic beta cells are since there are no food intake and exercise while sleeping. In addition, during the last 5 years, his body weight has been maintained around 172 lbs. Besides, his body has been medication-free over the past 5-years as well. It makes sense that FPG carries a significant and clear message about his health status of pancreatic beta cells; therefore, it can be served as the baseline of his overall glucose predications.

The detailed explanation of his glucose research work is provided because this particular study is based on "glucoses".

Glucose Trend-pattern Diagram:

A typical T2D patient faces three major challenges:

Availability of accurate and precise disease information with either physical evidences or quantitative proofs, not just some general qualitative descriptions that may include false or commercial driven news over the internet (a *knowledge* issue).
Awareness of his disease's specific status and overcome self-denial in order to take effective actions. The most difficult barrier to overcome is having determination, willpower, and persistence on lifestyle change (a *behavior* issues).
A non-invasive, effective, and ease of use technology-based tool to accurately predict biomedical outcomes and also guide patients (a *technology* issue).

The MPM methodology and its related diabetes research work covers the scope of this first issue, knowledge. The third issue, technology, has also been discussed in his previously published papers (Reference 2). This investigation report addresses the second issue, behavior, specifically, i.e. a patient's lifestyle behavior on his diet control and exercise. Beyond acquiring accurate and sufficient knowledge of diabetes, the resistance of food temptation and diligence on post-meal exercise occur with every patient at a frequency of three times a day. These lifestyle behaviors require strong determination, willpower, and persistence to achieve the goal of diabetes control. These concerns are related to a patient's personality traits.

The author has collected a total of two million data of his medical conditions and lifestyle details for the past ten years (2010 to 2020). In this study, he only utilized three subsets of his collected and stored data such as finger-piercing measured glucoses, carbs/sugar intake amount, and post-meal walking steps.

As he described in his diabetes research section, his learned knowledge and research results of diabetes control are progressively introduced and added into his data collection software from earlier years moving into later years. In short, he studied both diseases and nutrition from 2010 to 2013, then started collecting weight data since 2011, PPG data since 2014, carbs/sugar and post-meal walking data since 2015, and FPG data since 2016. Before accumulating this additional data, he already collected some partial data, but not on a daily basis and with an organized fashion similar to those periods after the starting years. However, his best guesstimated annualized data, prior to those starting years, are still able to provide an accurate annualized information. Therefore, in the data table, the red-colored data are his guesstimated annual data based on partial collected data, while the black-colored data are collected real data based on each meal and each day within an entire year (Figure 1).

In order to demonstrate the results of his *trend pattern analysis,* he created a modified two-dimensional (2D) planar space which can describe a three-dimensional (3D) data information. Initially, he set his x-coordinate as his carbs/sugar intake amount from low scale to high scale with the following 5 segments:

Segment A: 0-10 grams
Segment B: 10-20 grams
Segment C: 20-30 grams
Segment D: 30-40 grams
Segment E: 40-50 grams

Secondly, he set his y-coordinate as his post-meal walking steps from high scale to low scale with the following five segments:

Segment 1: 4-5k steps
Segment 2: 3-4k steps
Segment 3: 2-3k steps
Segment 4: 1-2k steps
Segment 5: 0-1k steps

Therefore, these x and y axes constitute a 2D planar space with a total of 25 sub-regions inside, such as A1 through E5.

Thirdly, he set his "pseudo" z-coordinate" as his daily glucose levels from low scale (lower left corner) to high scale (upper right corner) in a "radio-wave" format with the following six segments:

Segment 1: 100-130 mg/dL
Segment 2: 130-160 mg/dL
Segment 3: 160-190 mg/dL
Segment 4: 190-220 mg/dL
Segment 5: 220-250 mg/dL
Segment 6: 250-280 mg/dL - This segment is not used for his daily glucose, but useful for his PPG data.

However, for a better view, he "superimposes" his z-axis on his 2D planar x-y space with a "radio-wave" format to show their different levels (Figure 2). In this presentation, the reader of this article can easily observe the glucose trend pattern from 2010 to 2020 along with their respective relationship with carbs/sugar intake amount and post-meal walking steps.

From observing this trend pattern diagram, patients can modify their behavior one step at a time, by taking little steps on a smaller scale. This is what the author defined as a *progressive behavior modification.*

Results:

In Figure 1, it shows background data table and line chart of 5 values, daily glucose, FPG, PPG, carbs/sugar intake amount in grams, and post-meal walking step. Since PPG occupies 75% of daily glucose, both daily glucose and PPG move in a similar pattern on this line chart of time-series diagram. The author started with his daily glucose at 250 mg/dL (PPG at 280 mg/dL) in 2010 and moving forward to a lower daily glucose at 129 mg/dL in 2015 (PPG at 130 mg/dL), and finally reached 110 mg/dL in 2020 (PPG at 110 mg/dL). The bottom two curves of "decreasing" carbs/sugar and "increasing" post-meal walking steps demonstrate their significant influences on both of his daily glucose and PPG.

In the early mornings, the author measures his finger FPG once he wakes up. There is no influence from both food and exercise on FPG. From his previous research results, the relationship between his weight and FPG has a high correlation coefficient (>90%). In 2012, he weighed 220 lbs., then reduced his weight to 183 lbs. in 2013, and subsequently to 175 lbs. in 2015. Correspondingly, his FPG was 160 mg/dL in 2010, 135 mg/dL in 2013, and 124 mg/dL in 2015. It should be mentioned here again that he took three different diabetes medication before 2013, gradually reducing his dosages during 2013-2015, and completely ceased taking any medication on 12/8/2015. Obviously, the biological effect of taking medications produce strong influences on controlling glucose symptoms, in terms of the external appearance of diabetes, for both FPG and PPG. However, the most interesting fact is that his FPG levels continue to be reduced from 124 mg/dL in 2015 down to 107 mg/dL in 2020, while maintaining his weight at ~173 lbs. and living a total "medication-free" life. This FPG reduction could be interpreted as the health state of his pancreatic beta cells "self-repairing" between 13% to 26% over the past 6 to 8 years at an annual rate of 2.2% to 3.2% (Reference 3).

He decreased his carbs/sugar intake amount from 68 grams per meal in 2010 down to 13 grams per meal in 2020. During the same 10-year period, he increased his post-meal walking exercise from 400 steps per meal in 2010 up to 4,400 steps per meal in 2020. His glucose improvement in this trend pattern diagram demonstrates what the author has said previously is to *control diabetes from the most fundamental core level.*

In Figure 2, he created a presentation diagram of "radio-wave" glucose format on a 2D planar space. This diagram actually depicts his "glucose trend pattern analysis" with his lifestyle behavior modifications together. It is not an easy task to *reduce* one's carbs/sugar intake below 15 grams along with *maintaining* post-meal walking exercise of ~4,300 steps at a frequency of three times a day for many years. It takes an extraordinarily strong determination, willpower, and persistence for an individual to maintain this behavior for 8-years. The author has done this task successfully; therefore, he saved his own life from the life-threatening complications of diabetes, including five cardiovascular episodes and renal difficulties. In Figure 2, we can see clearly that these lifestyle behavior modification efforts finally paid off in the long run. ***There is nothing better than living a healthier and longer life.***

His daily glucoses (gray-colored star symbols in the pseudo z-axis data) starting from the upper right corner of 250 mg/dL at 2010, which moves toward the lower left direction with a ~30 degree downhill slope after acquiring correct knowledge and being persistent with his diet and exercise regimen. Regardless of his medication reduction process during this time frame of three years (2013-2015), his daily glucoses are further reduced from 145 mg/dL in 2013 to 129 mg/dL in 2015. During 2015-2019, he has mainly focused on increasing his post-meal walking steps from ~3,300 step to 4,400 steps. As a result, his daily glucoses dropped "straight downward" to the lower left corner of this planar space like a "free-falling" object. Finally, he reached to 110 mg/dL level in 2020 with an average glucose from 1/1/2020 to 8/6/2020. This case has demonstrated the patient's strong determination, willpower, and persistence along with his continuous struggle with maintaining his levels of diet and exercise over the past 10 years.

The author has written a few papers in 2019 with the subject of comparison and linkage between behavior psychology and diabetes physiology (References 4, 5, 6, 7, and 8). At that time, he considered his research work forward-thinking and foresaw big glucose data being easily collected from T2D patients with the availability of using a continuous glucose monitor (CGM) device (Reference 9). Therefore, in early 2019, he was laying the necessary groundwork for a future endeavor. On 5/5/2018, he applied a CGM sensor device on his arm to collect about 80-96 glucoses per day; however, by March of 2019, he has not yet collected sufficient CGM glucose data that could be utilized in his research purpose. Besides, he has discovered that his sensor glucoses are about 13% to 17% higher than his finger glucoses. That is the reason he chose to use his finger-piercing measured glucoses during the past 10-years as his background database in this particular study report, which is a long-term effect on his glucose from both diet and exercise.

Conclusion:

In summary, his entire glucose moving path is a 30-degree downward angle to the left and then straight downward to the bottom. His annualized average daily glucoses have been reduced from the starting point of 250 mg/dL in 2010 through the "reflection point" of 135 mg/dL in 2014, and then straight down to the ending point of 110 mg/dL in 2020. The triangular relationship among diet, exercise, and daily glucose can be easily observed on this "glucose trend pattern" diagram (Figure 2).

Through analyzing those distinctive daily glucose trend patterns, the personality traits and behavior psychological characteristics of this T2D patient can be revealed instantly and clearly. As a result, a more practical guidance of *progressive behavior modification* can be provided to other T2D patients in order to improve their medical conditions for chronic diseases.

References:

1. Hsu, Gerald C. (2019). eclaireMD Foundation, USA; "GH-Method: Methodology of math-physical medicine (No. 54)."

2. Hsu, Gerald C.(2019). eclaireMD Foundation, USA; "Controlling type 2 diabetes via artificial intelligence technology using GH-Method: math-physical medicine (No. 125)."

3. Hsu, Gerald C. (2019). eclaireMD Foundation, USA; "Guesstimate probable partial self-recovery of pancreatic beta cells using calculations of annualized glucose data using GH-Method: math-physical medicine (No. 139)."

4. Hsu, Gerald C. (2019). eclaireMD Foundation, USA; "Using wave characteristic analysis to study T2D patient's personality traits and psychological behavior using GH-Method: math-physical medicine (No. 52)."

5. Hsu, Gerald C. (2019). eclaireMD Foundation, USA; "Trending pattern analysis and progressive behavior modification of two clinic cases of correlation between patient psychological behavior and physiological characteristics of T2D Using GH-Method: math-physical medicine & mentality-personality modeling (No. 53)."

6. Hsu, Gerald C. (2019). eclaireMD Foundation, USA; "Using wave characteristic analysis to study T2D patient's personality traits and psychological behavior based on GH-Method: Math-Physical Medicine (No. 59)."

7. (Hsu, Gerald C. (2019). eclaireMD Foundation, USA; "Using GH-Method: math-physical medicine, mentality-personality modeling, and segmentation pattern analysis to compare two clinic cases about linkage between T2D patient's psychological behavior and physiological characteristics (No.72)."

8. Hsu, Gerald C. (2019). eclaireMD Foundation, USA; "Using artificial intelligence technology to overcome some behavioral psychological resistance for diabetes patients on controlling their glucose level using GH-Method: math-physical medicine & mentality-personality modeling (No. 93)."

9. Hsu, Gerald C. (2020). eclaireMD Foundation, USA; "A comparison of three glucose measurement results during COVID-19 period using GH-Method: math-physical medicine (No. 303)."

	Daily Glucose	FPG	PPG	Carbs/Sugar (g)	PM Walk (/100)
Y2010	250	160	280	68	4
Y2011	200	150	220	41	8
Y2012	170	140	180	25	12
Y2013	145	135	148	16	30
Y2014	135	127	137	15	34
Y2015	129	124	130	14	37
Y2016	119	117	120	15	41
Y2017	117	120	117	14	44
Y2018	116	114	117	15	45
Y2019	114	115	114	13	40
Y2020	110	107	110	13	44

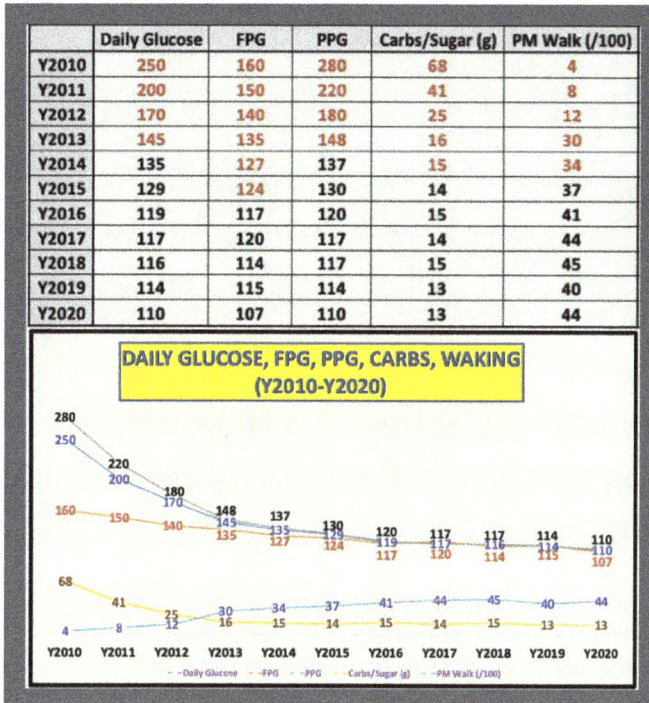

Figure 1: Background data table and line chart of daily glucose, FPG, PPG, carbs/sugar intake, and post-meal walking steps (2010-2020)

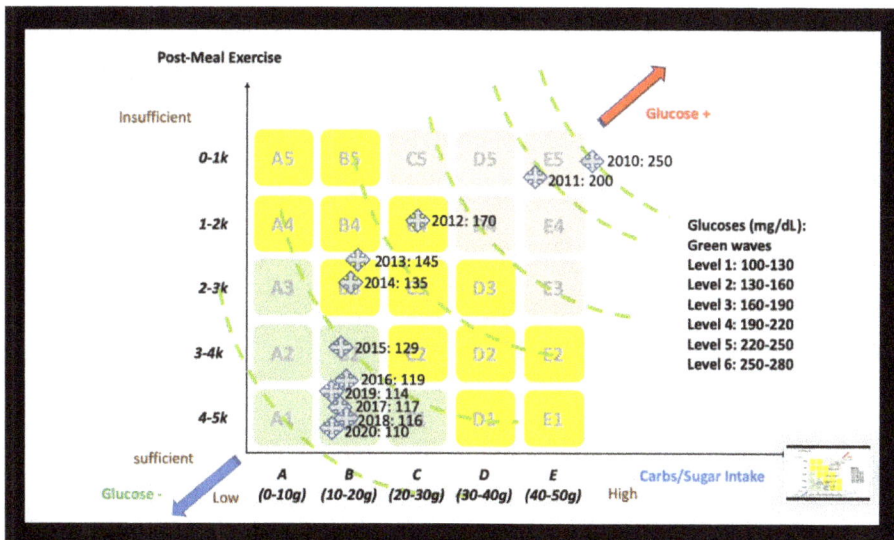

Figure 2: Glucose trend pattern diagram among daily glucoses, carbs/sugar intake amount, and post-meal walking steps in 10 years (2010-2020)

Glucose control and behavior psychology of a T2D patient using GH-Method: mentality-personality modeling via math-physical medicine (No. 306)

By: Gerald C. Hsu
eclaireMD Foundation, USA
8/8-9/2020

Abstract:

In this article, the author used 10-years' worth of data of glucoses and prominent lifestyle details such as diet and exercise to address his glucose trend pattern analysis and progressive lifestyle behavior modifications. This progressive lifestyle behavior modification is closely related to behavior psychology. The research methodology used is the GH-Method: math-physical medicine (MPM) approach which has been developed by the author over the past decade. This "Progressive Behavior Modification" concept is also a part of his Mentality-Personality Modeling (MPM). He addresses the quantitative linkage between diabetes physiological phenomena and behavior psychological influences of a type 2 diabetes (T2D) patient.

He has created a geometric presentation model with carbs/sugar intake amount as the x-axis, post-meal walking steps as the y-axis, and daily glucose as the z-axis (Figure 2). He decided to "fold over" the z-axis and superimpose it with the x-y plane space in a form of "radio wave" format. Under his created 3D data presentation on a 2D planar space, the glucose trend pattern becomes ultra-clear. These x-axis and y-axis values are a representation of his progressive lifestyle behavior modifications (mentality-personality model) over the past 10 years, while the z-axis values are a presentation of his diabetes physiological outcomes (math-physical medicine).

For over the past 10-years, his annual glucose movement path started in the upper right corner (subregion E5 in 2010), moving at a ~30 degree downward slope before arriving to the location near the upper middle but skewed to the left (subregion B3 in 2014), and then continuously dropping to the lower left corner (subregion B1 in 2020).

In summary, his entire glucose moving path is a 30-degree downward angle to the left and then straight downward to the bottom. His annualized average daily glucoses have been reduced from the starting point of 250 mg/dL in 2010 through the "reflection point" of 135 mg/dL in 2014, and then straight down to the ending point of 110 mg/dL in 2020. The triangular relationship among diet, exercise, and daily glucose can be easily observed on this "glucose trend pattern" diagram (Figure 2).

Through analyzing those distinctive daily glucose trend patterns, the personality traits and behavior psychological characteristics of this T2D patient can be revealed instantly and clearly. As a result, a more practical guidance of *"progressive behavior modification"* can be provided to other T2D patients in order to improve their medical conditions for chronic diseases.

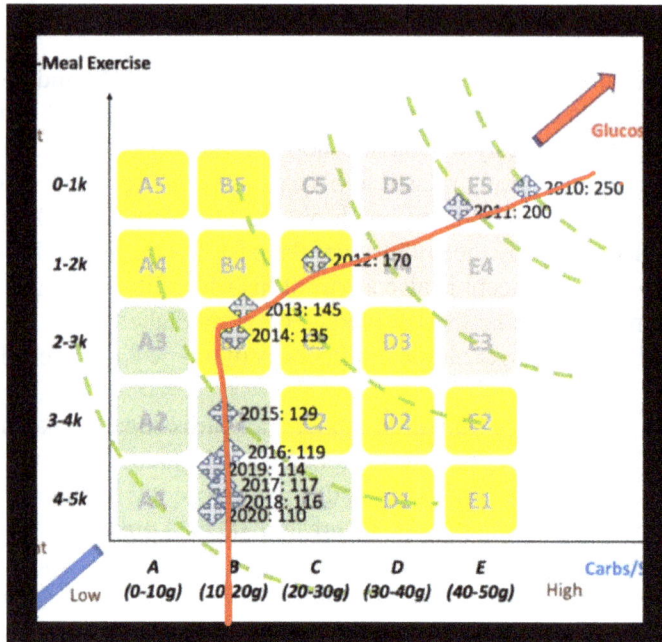

Figure 2:Glucose trend pattern diagram

Introduction:

In this article, the author used 10-years' worth of data of glucoses and prominent lifestyle details such as diet and exercise to address his glucose trend pattern analysis and progressive lifestyle behavior modifications. This progressive lifestyle behavior modification is closely related to behavior psychology. The research methodology used is the GH-Method: math-physical medicine (MPM) approach which has been developed by the author over the past decade. This "*Progressive Behavior Modification*" concept is also a part of his Mentality-Personality Modeling (MPM). He addresses the quantitative linkage between diabetes physiological phenomena and behavior psychological influences of a type 2 diabetes (T2D) patient.

Method:

GH-method: Math-physical medicine (MPM) methodology:

The description below explains the MPM research methodology developed by the author, which is utilized in his biomedical research (Reference 1).

Any system, whether medical, political, economic, engineering, biological, chemical, and even psychological have causes or triggers (inputs) and consequences (outputs). There are definitely some existing connections between inputs and outputs that can be either simple or complicated. The inputs and outputs of any type of system, including biomedical system, can be observed visually or measured by certain instruments. These physically observed phenomena, including features, images, incidents, or numbers are merely the partial "physical expression" of these underneath system structure. This system structure includes human organs for a biomedical system, the human brain for a neurological or mental system, or steel plate for structural or mechanical engineering system.

Once we have collected these readings of the physical phenomena (external expression, similar to a behavior, symptom, or response), through either incident, image, or data, we should be able to organize or categorize them in a logical manner. When we check or analyze these partial physical phenomena outputs and cannot figure out why they act or behave in certain way due to internal causes, reasons, or stressors, we can try to develop some guesses or formulate some reasonable hypotheses based on some available basic principles, theories, or concepts from physics. At this point, we just cannot pull out an existing equation from a physics textbook and insert these input variables in to conduct a "plug and play" game. An equation is an expression of a concept or a theory, which is usually associated with some existing conditions, either initial or boundary; however, a biomedical system usually has different kind of conditions from other systems.

After understanding the meaning of observed physical phenomena, the next step is to prove the hypothesis, guess, or interpretation of the phenomenon being correct or incorrect. At this stage, a solid understanding of mathematics becomes extremely useful to develop a meaningful model which could represent or interpret these observed physical phenomena and created hypothesis. In addition, some engineering modeling techniques, such as finite element method and computer science tools, including software, artificial intelligence (AI), and big data analytics can offer great assistance on verification of analysis results from these mathematical operations.

If the mathematical results cannot support the created hypothesis, then a new hypothesis needs to be formulated. When this new hypothesis is proven to be correct, then we can extend or convert this hypothesis into a useful mathematical equation or into a simpler arithmetical formula for others to adopt this easier way of thinking and understanding of the results. In the final stage, the derived mathematical equation or arithmetical formula can then be used to "predict" future outcomes of the selected system based on other different sets of inputs.

Diabetes Research:
The author has been a severe type 2 diabetes (T2D) patient since 1995. He has developed many serious complications and finally, in 2010, they became life-threatening. Therefore, he has spent the next 10-years to self-study and research diabetes, metabolism, and endocrinology, in order to save his own life.

He spent his first four years, from 2010 to 2013, to self-study 6 chronic diseases, i.e. obesity, diabetes, hypertension, hyperlipidemia, cardiovascular diseases, stroke, as well as food nutrition. Food is probably the most important and also complicated input element to influence these chronic diseases. After his first 4-years of self-learning, he then spent the entire year of 2014 to develop a complex model of metabolism. This mathematical model contains 4 biomarkers of medical conditions (weight, glucose, blood pressure, and lipids) along with 6 lifestyle details (food portion and nutritional balance, drinking water intake, adequate exercise, sufficient sleep amount and quality, stress reduction, and daily life routines regularity). He applied the concept of topology from mathematics and the approximation modeling technique of finite element method from engineering to develop this metabolism model which became the cornerstone of his future medical research work. As a result, his overall health conditions also started to be improved.

Starting from 2015, he spent three consecutive years, from 2015 to 2017, to discover the characteristics and behaviors of this complex "wild beast" of glucose. His major objective is to truly understand the "inner characteristics" of the glucose, not just using medication's chemical power to control the disease' external biological "symptoms". His research work is similar to a horseman trying to tame a horse by understanding its temperament first, not just giving a tranquilizer to calm it down. As a result, during this period of 3-years, he has developed 4 prediction models, which include Weight, PPG, FPG, and HbA1C with very high prediction accuracy (95% to 99%) to reach to his purpose of "understanding glucoses".

The author estimated and proved that PPG contributes approximately 75% to 80% towards HbA1C formation. Therefore, he tried to unravel the mystery of PPG first. Through his diabetes research, he has identified at least 19 influential factors associated with PPG formation. Among those influential factors, diet (carbs/sugar intake amount) would provide ~38% and exercise (post-meal walking) would contribute ~41%. Combining these two primary influential factors, it gives ~80% of the PPG formation. Among the rest of the 17 secondary factors, a high weather temperature contributes ~5%, whereas stress and illness only make noticeable contributions when they occur.

For most T2D patients who take medication, its biochemical effect would become the most significant influential factor of glucose. However, as we know, medication cannot cure diabetes and only control its symptoms. Therefore, the author decided to focus on controlling diabetes at the most fundamental level by investigating its root cause. Previously, he has taken high doses of three prescribed diabetes medications for 18 years since 1997; however, in 2013, he started to reduce the number of prescriptions and dosages of his daily medications. By 12/8/2015, he finally ceased taking any diabetes medications.

From 2016 to 2017, he discovered a solid statistical connection between his FPG and his weight (>90% of correlation coefficient). In addition, similar to his PPG research, he also recognized that there are about 5 influential factors of FPG formation with weight alone contributing >85% and cold weather temperature influencing ~5%.

Since July 2019, he also launched a special investigation on the degree of damage to his pancreatic beta cells. During the past 12-months of research work, he noticed that both of his FPG and PPG have been decreased in the past 6 to 8 years at an annual rate of 2.2% to 3.2%. In other words, his pancreatic beta cells have been self-regenerating or self-repairing about 13% to 26% over these 6-8 years. He then thought about FPG as being a good indicator on how healthy his pancreatic beta cells are since there are no food intake and exercise while sleeping. In addition, during the last 5 years, his body weight has been maintained around 172 lbs. Besides, his body has been medication-free over the past 5-years as well. It makes sense that FPG carries a significant and clear message about his health status of pancreatic beta cells; therefore, it can be served as the baseline of his overall glucose predications.

The detailed explanation of his glucose research work is provided because this particular study is based on "glucoses" and lifestyle habits.

Glucose Trend Pattern Diagram:

A typical T2D patient faces three major challenges:

Availability of accurate and precise disease information with either physical evidence or quantitative proof, not just some general qualitative descriptions that may include false or commercial driven news over the internet (a ***knowledge*** issue).
Awareness of his disease's specific status and overcome self-denial in order to take effective actions. The most difficult barrier to overcome is to have determination, willpower, and persistence on lifestyle change (a ***behavior*** issues).
A non-invasive, effective, and ease of use technology-based tool to accurately predict biomedical outcomes and to guide patients (a ***technology*** issue).

The MPM methodology and its related diabetes research work covers the scope of this first issue, knowledge. The third issue, technology, has also been discussed in his previously published papers (e.g. Reference 2). This investigation report addresses the second issue, behavior, specifically, i.e. a patient's lifestyle behavior on his diet control and exercise. Beyond acquiring accurate and sufficient knowledge of diabetes, the resistance of food temptation and diligence on post-meal exercise occur with every patient at a frequency of three times a day. These lifestyle behaviors require strong determination, willpower, and persistence to achieve the goal of diabetes control. These concerns are related to a patient's personality traits.

The author has collected a total of two million data of his medical conditions and lifestyle details for the past ten years (2010 to 2020). In this study, he only utilized three subsets of his collected and stored data such as finger-piercing measured glucoses, carbs/sugar intake amount, and post-meal walking steps.

As he described in his diabetes research section, his learned knowledge and research results of diabetes control are progressively introduced and added into his data collection software from earlier years moving into later years. In short, he studied both diseases and nutrition from 2010 to 2013, then started collecting weight data since 2011, PPG data since 2014, carbs/sugar and post-meal walking data since 2015, and FPG data since 2016. Before accumulating this additional data, he already collected some partial data, but not on a daily basis and with an organized fashion similar to those periods after the starting years. However, his best guesstimated annualized data, prior to those starting years, are still able to provide an accurate annualized information. Therefore, in the data table, the red-colored data are his guesstimated annual data based on partial collected data, while the black-colored data are collected real data based on each meal and each day within an entire year (Figure 1).

In order to demonstrate the results of his *"trend pattern analysis"*, he created a modified two-dimensional (2D) planar space which can describe a three-dimensional (3D) data & information. At first, he set his x-coordinate as his carbs/sugar intake amount from low scale to high scale with the following 5 segments:

Segment A: 0-10 grams
Segment B: 10-20 grams
Segment C: 20-30 grams
Segment D: 30-40 grams
Segment E: 40-50 grams

Secondly, he set his y-coordinate as his post-meal walking steps from high scale to low scale with the following 5 segments:

Segment 1: 4-5k steps
Segment 2: 3-4k steps
Segment 3: 2-3k steps
Segment 4: 1-2k steps
Segment 5: 0-1k steps

Therefore, these x- and y-axes constitute a 2D planar space with a total of 25 sub-regions inside, such as A1 through E5.

Thirdly, he set his "pseudo" z-coordinate" as his daily glucose levels from low scale (lower left corner) to high scale (upper right corner) in a "radio-wave" format with the following 6 segments:

Segment 1: 100-130 mg/dL
Segment 2: 130-160 mg/dL
Segment 3: 160-190 mg/dL
Segment 4: 190-220 mg/dL
Segment 5: 220-250 mg/dL
Segment 6: 250-280 mg/dL - This segment is not used for his daily glucose, but useful for his PPG data.

However, for a better view, he "superimposes" his z-axis on his 2D planar x-y space with a "radio-wave" format to show their different levels of glucoses (Figure 2). In this presentation, the reader of this article can easily observe the glucose trend pattern from 2010 to 2020 and their respective relationship with carbs/sugar intake amount and post-meal walking steps.

From observing this trend pattern diagram, patients can modify their behavior one step at a time, by taking little steps on a smaller scale. This is what the author defined as a *"progressive behavior modification"*.

Behavior Psychology:

On August 28th, 2018, Dr. Bryn Farnsworth stated that *"Behavioral psychology is the study of how our behaviors relate to our mind – it looks at our behavior through the lens of psychology and draws a link between the two."*

FPM is an editorially independent, peer-reviewed journal published by American Academy of family physicians. Here is an excerpt from the March-April 2018 edition, *"Using these brief interventions, you can help your patients make healthy behavior changes"* (Reference 10).

"Effectively encouraging patients to change their health behavior is a critical skill for primary care physicians. Modifiable health behaviors contribute to an estimated 40 percent of deaths in the United States. Tobacco use, poor diet, physical inactivity, poor sleep, poor adherence to medication, and similar behaviors are prevalent and can diminish the quality and length of patients' lives. Research has found an inverse relationship between the risk of all-cause mortality and the number of healthy lifestyle behaviors a patient follows.

KEY POINTS (See Figure 3):
(1) Modifiable health behaviors, such as poor diet or smoking, are significant contributors to poor outcomes.
(2) Family physicians can use brief, evidence-based techniques to encourage patients to change their unhealthy behaviors.
(3) Working with patients to develop health goals, eliminate barriers, and track their own behavior can be beneficial.
(4) Interventions that target specific behaviors, such as prescribing physical activity for patients who don't get enough exercise or providing patient education for better medication adherence, can help patients to improve their health."

From articles in References 10-13, we can see the close relationship between health and lifestyle behavior psychology.

Results:

In Figure 1, it shows background data table and line chart of 5 values, daily glucose, FPG, PPG, carbs/sugar intake amount in grams, and post-meal walking step in a hundred steps. Since PPG occupies 75% of daily glucose, both daily glucose and PPG move in a similar pattern on this line chart of time-series diagram. The author started with his daily glucose at 250 mg/dL (PPG at 280 mg/dL) in 2010 and moving forward to a lower daily glucose at 129 mg/dL in 2015 rapidly (PPG at 130 mg/dL), and finally reached 110 mg/dL in 2020 (PPG at 110 mg/dL). The bottom two curves of "decreasing" carbs/sugar and "increasing" post-meal walking steps demonstrate their significant influences on both of his daily glucose and PPG.

In the early mornings, the author measures his finger FPG once he wakes up. There is no influence from both food and exercise on FPG. From his previous research results, the relationship between his weight and FPG has a high correlation coefficient (>90%). In 2012, he weighed 220 lbs., then reduced his weight to 183 lbs. in 2013, and subsequently to 175 lbs. in 2015. Correspondingly, his FPG was 160 mg/dL in 2010, 135 mg/dL in 2013, and 124 mg/dL in 2015. It should be mentioned that he took three different diabetes medication before 2013, gradually reducing his dosages during 2013-2015, and completely ceased taking any medication on 12/8/2015. Obviously, the biological effect of taking medications produce strong influences on controlling glucose symptoms, in terms of the external appearance of diabetes, for both FPG and PPG. However, the most interesting fact is that his FPG levels continue to be reduced from 124 mg/dL in 2015 down to 107 mg/dL in 2020, while maintaining his weight at ~173 lbs. and living a total "medication-free" life. This FPG reduction could be interpreted as the health state of his pancreatic beta cells "self-repairing" between 13% to 26% over the past 6 to 8 years at an annual rate of 2.2% to 3.2% (Reference 3).

He decreased his carbs/sugar intake amount from 68 grams per meal in 2010 down to 13 grams per meal in 2020. During the same 10-year period, he increased his post-meal walking exercise from 400 steps per meal in 2010 up to 4,400 steps per meal in 2020. His glucose improvement in this trend pattern diagram demonstrates what the author has said previously is to *"control diabetes from the most fundamental core level"*.

In Figure 2, he created a presentation diagram of "radio-wave" glucose format on a 2D planar space. This diagram actually depicts his "glucose trend pattern analysis" with his lifestyle behavior modifications together. It is not an easy task to reduce one's carbs/sugar intake below 15 grams along with maintaining post-meal walking exercise of ~4,300 steps at a frequency of three times a day for many years. It takes an extraordinarily strong determination, willpower, and persistence for an individual to maintain this behavior for 8-years. The author has done this task successfully; therefore, he saved his own life from the life-threatening complications of diabetes, including five cardiovascular episodes and renal difficulties. In Figure 2, we can see clearly that these lifestyle behavior modification efforts finally paid off in the long run. *There is nothing better than living a healthier and longer life.*

His daily glucoses (the grey-colored star signs of the pseudo z-axis data) started from upper right corner of 250 mg/dL at 2010, and moving toward the lower left direction with a ~30 degree downhill slope via acquiring correct knowledge and being persistent with his diet and exercise regimen. Regardless of his medication reduction process during this time frame of three years (2013-2015), his daily glucoses are further reduced from 145 mg/dL in 2013 to 129 mg/dL in 2015. During 2015-2019, he has mainly focused on increasing his post-meal walking steps from ~3,300 step to 4,400 steps. As a result, his daily glucoses dropped "straight downward" to the lower left corner of this planar space like a "free-falling" object. Finally, he reached to 110 mg/dL level in 2020 (an average glucose from 1/1/2020 to 8/6/2020). This case has demonstrated the patient's strong determination, willpower, and persistence along with his continuous struggle with maintaining his levels of diet and exercise over the past 10 years.

The author has written a few papers in 2019 with the subject of comparison and linkage between behavior psychology and diabetes physiology (References 4, 5, 6, 7, and 8). At that time, he considered his research work forward-thinking and foresaw big glucose data being easily collected from T2D patients with the availability of using a continuous glucose monitoring (CGM) device (Reference 9). Therefore, in early 2019, he was laying the necessary groundwork for a future endeavor. On 5/5/2018, he applied a CGM sensor device on his arm to collect about 96 glucoses per day; however, by March of 2019, he has not yet collected sufficient CGM glucose data that could be utilized in his research purpose. Besides, he has discovered that his sensor glucoses are about 13% to 17% higher than his finger glucoses. That is the reason he chose to use his finger-piercing measured glucoses during the past 10-years as his background database in this particular study report, which is a long-term effect on his glucose from both diet and exercise.

Conclusion:

In summary, his entire glucose moving path is a 30-degree downward angle to the left and then straight downward to the bottom. His annualized average daily glucoses have been reduced from the starting point of 250 mg/dL in 2010 through the "reflection point" of 135 mg/dL in 2014, and then straight down to the ending point of 110 mg/dL in 2020. The triangular relationship among diet, exercise, and daily glucose can be easily observed on this "glucose trend pattern" diagram (Figure 2).

Through analyzing those distinctive daily glucose trend patterns, the personality traits and behavior psychological characteristics of this T2D patient can be revealed instantly and clearly. As a result, a more practical guidance of "progressive behavior modification" can be provided to other T2D patients in order to improve their medical conditions for chronic diseases.

References:

1. Hsu, Gerald C. eclaireMD Foundation, USA. "GH-Method: Methodology of math-physical medicine (No. 54)."

2. Hsu, Gerald C. eclaireMD Foundation, USA. "Controlling type 2 diabetes via artificial intelligence technology using GH-Method: math-physical medicine) (No. 125)."

3. Hsu, Gerald C. eclaireMD Foundation, USA. "Guesstimate probable partial self-recovery of pancreatic beta cells using calculations of annualized glucose data using GH-Method: math-physical medicine (No. 139)."

4. Hsu, Gerald C. eclaireMD Foundation, USA. "Using wave characteristic analysis to study T2D patient's personality traits and psychological behavior using GH-Method: math-physical medicine (No. 52)"

5. Hsu, Gerald C., eclaireMD Foundation, USA; "Trending pattern analysis and progressive behavior modification of two clinic cases of correlation between

patient psychological behavior and physiological characteristics of T2D Using GH-Method: math-physical medicine & mentality-personality modeling, No. 53"

6. Hsu, Gerald C., eclaireMD Foundation, USA; "Using wave characteristic analysis to study T2D patient's personality traits and psychological behavior (Based on GH-Method: Math-Physical Medicine), No. 59"

7. Hsu, Gerald C., eclaireMD Foundation, USA; "Using GH-Method: math-physical medicine, mentality-personality modeling, and segmentation pattern analysis to compare two clinic cases about linkage between T2D patient's psychological behavior and physiological characteristics, No.72"

8. Hsu, Gerald C., eclaireMD Foundation, USA; "Using artificial intelligence technology to overcome some behavioral psychological resistance for diabetes patients on controlling their glucose level using GH-Method: math-physical medicine & mentality-personality modeling, No. 93"

9. Hsu, Gerald C., eclaireMD Foundation, USA; "A comparison of three glucose measurement results during COVID-19 period using GH-Method: math-physical medicine (No. 303)"

10. FPM, AAFP: "Encouraging Health Behavior Change: Eight Evidence-Based Strategies", by Stephanie A. Hooker, PhD, MPH, Anjoli Punjabi, PharmD, MPH, Kacey Justesen, MD, Lucas Boyle, MD, and Michelle D. Sherman, PhD, ABPP; Family Practice Management. 2018 Mar-Apr;25(2):31-36.

11. American Psychological Association, "Making lifestyle changes that last: Starting small, focusing on one behavior at a time and support from others can help you achieve your exercise or other health-related goals.

12. Florence-Health, "The Psychology of Adhering to a Treatment Plan: Why Patients Fail and How Providers Can Help"

13. Harvard Women's Health Watch, "Why behavior change is hard - and why you should keep trying: Successful change comes only in stages. How long it takes is an individual matter." Published: March 2012

	Daily Glucose	FPG	PPG	Carbs/Sugar (g)	PM Walk (/100)
Y2010	250	160	280	68	4
Y2011	200	150	220	41	8
Y2012	170	140	180	25	12
Y2013	145	135	148	16	30
Y2014	135	127	137	15	34
Y2015	129	124	130	14	37
Y2016	119	117	120	15	41
Y2017	117	120	117	14	44
Y2018	116	114	117	15	45
Y2019	114	115	114	13	40
Y2020	110	107	110	13	44

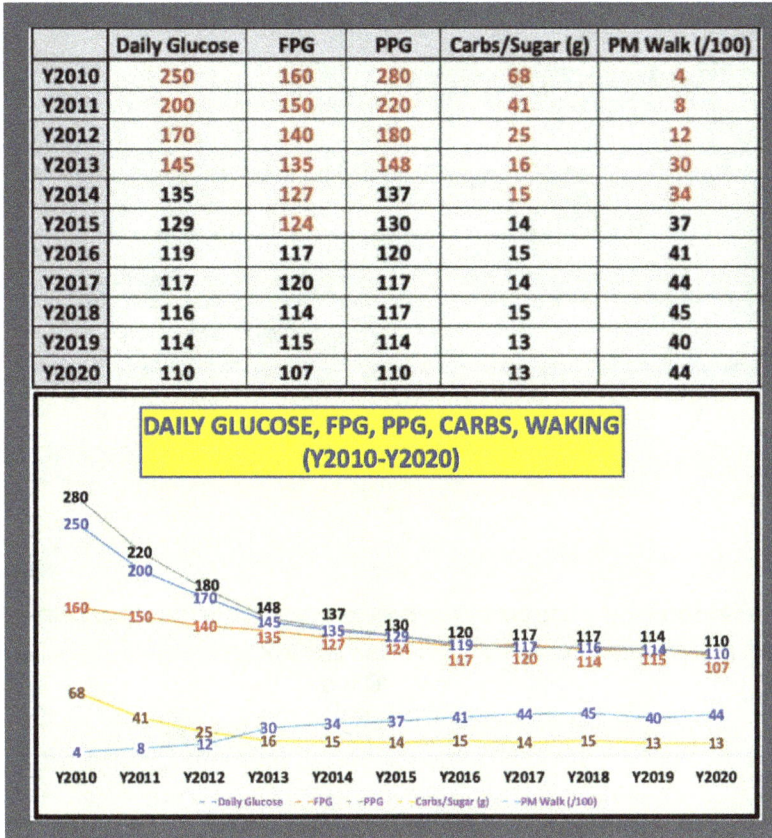

Figure 1: Background data table and line chart of daily glucose, FPG, PPG, carbs/sugar intake, and post-meal walking steps (2010-2020)

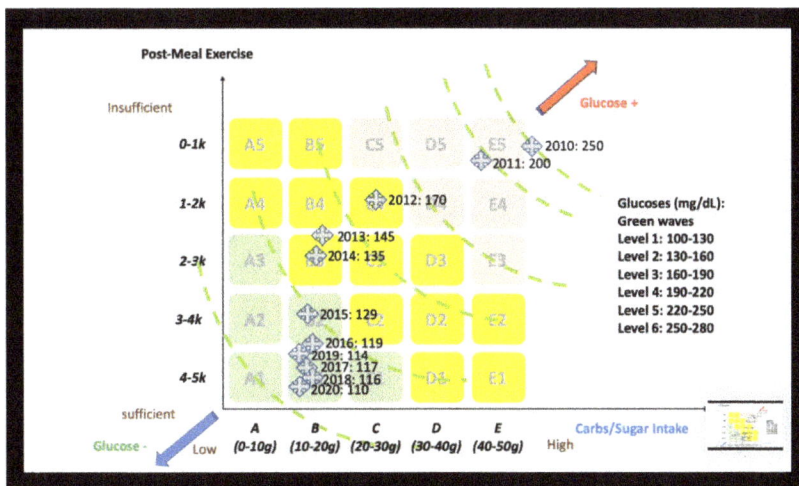

Figure 2: Glucose trend pattern diagram among daily glucoses, carbs/sugar intake amount, and post-meal walking steps in 10 years (2010-2020)

BRIEF EVIDENCE-BASED INTERVENTIONS FOR HEALTH BEHAVIOR CHANGE

BEHAVIOR	TECHNIQUE	DESCRIPTION
All	SMART goal setting	Ensure that goals are specific, measurable, attainable, relevant, and timely.
	Problem-solving barriers	Identify possible barriers to change and develop solutions.
	Self-monitoring	Have patients keep a record of the behavior they are trying to change.
Physical inactivity	Physical activity prescription	Collaboratively work with the patient to pick an activity type, amount, and frequency.
Unhealthy eating	Small changes	Have patients choose small, attainable goals to change their diets, such as reducing the frequency of desserts or soda intake or increasing daily fruit and vegetable consumption.
	Plate Method	Encourage patients to design their plates to include 50 percent fruits and vegetables, 25 percent lean protein, and 25 percent grains or starches

Figure 3: Using brief evidence-based interventions can help chronic diseases patients make healthy behavior changes

Biomedical research methodology based on GH-Method: math-physical medicine (No. 310)

By: Gerald C. Hsu
eclaireMD Foundation, USA
8/11-12/2020

Abstract:

This paper discusses the author's biomedical research work based on the *GH-Method: math-physical medicine (MPM)* approach over the past decade. This is significantly different from the traditional medical research using biochemical approach and simple statistical methods. He uses his own type 2 diabetes (T2D) metabolic conditions as a case study including several application examples as illustrations and explanations of the MPM methodology.

The MPM methodology will be described, then followed by 10 application examples to show how he applied his knowledge and disciplines in mathematics, physics, engineering modeling, computer science tools, and psychology during his 10-years of biomedical research, especially in the domain of lifestyle, metabolism, chronic diseases, diabetes, cardiovascular diseases, and renal complications.

The following list highlights the math-physical concepts, theories, principles, or equations used in the 10 application examples:

(1) Topology, finite element method
(2) Time-domain analysis, correlation and regression model, pattern recognition, segmentation analysis
(3) Signal processing, trial and error method, regression analysis
(4) Artificial intelligence (AI) auto-correction, quantum mechanics, safety margin of engineering design
(5) Optical physics, AI, perturbation theory of quantum mechanics
(6) Wave theory, Fourier transform, frequency-domain analysis
(7) Structural engineering modeling, solid mechanics (both elastic and plastic), fluids dynamics, energy theory
(8) Pattern recognition, behavior psychology
(9) Spatial analysis, time-series analysis
(10) Big data analytics, AI, software engineering

Using MPM, a non-traditional medical research methodology, provides many quantitative proofs with a high degree of accuracy (higher precision) compared to other disease research results. Medicine is based on biology and chemistry, while biology, chemistry, and engineering are based on physics, and physics is based on mathematics. Logically, mathematics is the mother of all sciences. When we explore our application problems down to the foundation level, we can discover more facts and deeper truths. This is the logical essence of "math-physical medicine." Using this MPM model, the accuracy of medical evaluations, along with the precision of predictive models can be greatly improved, with dramatic benefits to the patients.

Introduction:

This paper discusses the author's biomedical research work based on the *GH-Method: math-physical medicine (MPM)* approach over the past decade. This is significantly different from the traditional medical research using biochemical approach and simple statistical methods. He uses his own type 2 diabetes (T2D) metabolic conditions as a case study including several application examples as illustrations and explanations of the MPM methodology.

Methods:

Overview of MPM:

Diabetes is a disease that affects the endocrine system, cardiovascular system, nervous system, body metabolism, and including the psychological well-being of patients. Understanding and controlling glucoses is the cornerstone of diabetes control. Newer medications focus on glycemic control for the symptoms in T2D, but do not address the origin of diabetes, which is the progressive loss of ß-cell function and effectiveness. (Reference 1). Liu from University of Virginia School of Medicine, and Yang from the Center for Drug Evaluation and Research, Food and Drug Administration, advance the notion that *one of the most important factors in developing Type II diabetes (T2D) is "positive energy balance," e.g. surplus energy intake (over-eating) over expenditure (exercise), which is at the core for developing metabolic syndrome and T2D.*

Other factors complicating the management of T2D are the discrepancies between HbA1C and self-monitoring of blood glucose data, which led Hirsch et al to advocate the value of using patients' own glucose data to consolidate therapeutic, educational, and behavior-change objectives (Reference 2).

This particular paper presents a scientific system approach to achieve a more accurate prediction of glucose and measurement of HbA1C glycohemoglobin. This will lead to better control of the disease processes of T2D, which can predict untoward cardiovascular events and other major diabetic complications.

The author describes his MPM as a tool to reach more accurate predictions of glucose, HbA1C, and risk probability of having a cardiovascular disease, stroke, or chronic kidney disease utilizing mathematics, physics, engineering modeling, and computer science tools, instead of the current biochemical medicine approach (BCM) that mainly utilizes biology and chemistry. A comparison between the fundamental differences of the traditional BCM methodology and the non-traditional MPM methodology is reflected in Table 1. The inverse relationship can be observed between the accuracy and replicability of a measurement and the objective nature of a scientific field (Table 3). Pure math provides precise measurements with results that are nearly 100% replicable from one researcher to another, while on the other extreme, psychology is an empirical science that tends to be more subjective, producing a greater variance with inter-rater reliability. Everything else in between has different degrees of accuracy and replicability, but the higher it is in the hierarchy, the higher its applicability and the lower its accuracy (Table 3).

One of the most valuable tools for physicians is having a method that allows them to give advice to patients on improving treatment outcome. This requires a predictive analytic method, which can only be derived from a retrospective analysis of multiple data points, looking for a pattern common to a certain outcome. After conducting a retrospective analysis of pattern recognition, prospective testing is required to confirm the accuracy of the predictive model. However, this process is complicated by the multi-factorial origins of a medical event.

GH-Method: math-physical medicine (MPM)

The GH-Method: math-physical medicine (MPM) research methodology was developed by the author and utilized in his biomedical research over the past decade.

Here is a general description of the MPM:

Any system, whether medical, political, economic, engineering, biological, chemical, and even psychological, have causes or triggers (inputs) and consequences (outputs). There are some existing connections between inputs and outputs that can be either simple or complicated. The inputs and outputs of any type of system, including biomedical system, can be observed visually, or measured quantitatively by certain instruments. These physically observed phenomena, including features, images, incidents, or numbers are merely the partial "physical expression" from these underneath system structures. This system structures include human organs for a biomedical system, the human brain for a neurological or mental system, or steel plate/ pipe for a structural or mechanical system.

Once we have collected these readings of the physical phenomena (external expression, similar to a behavior, symptom, or response), through either incident, image, or data, we should be able to organize or categorize them in a logical manner. When we check or analyze these partial physical phenomena outputs and cannot figure out why they act or behave a certain way due to internal causes, reasons, or stressors, we can come up with certain guesses or formulate some reasonable hypotheses based on available basic principles, theories, or concepts from physics. At this point, we just cannot pull out an existing equation from a physics textbook and insert the input variables to conduct a "plug and play" game. An equation is an expression of a concept or a theory, which is usually associated with some existing conditions, either initial conditions or boundary conditions; however, a biomedical system usually has different kind of conditions from other systems.

After understanding the meaning of observed physical phenomena, the next step is to prove the hypothesis, guess, or interpretation of the phenomenon being correct or incorrect. At this stage, a solid understanding of mathematics becomes extremely useful to develop a meaningful model which could represent or interpret these observed physical phenomena and created hypothesis. In addition, some physics method, such as perturbation theory of quantum mechanics, energy theory, wave theory, and optical physics; engineering modeling techniques, such as finite element method and computer science tools, including software, AI, and big data analytics can offer great assistance on the verification of analysis results from these mathematical operations.

If the mathematical results cannot support the created hypothesis, then a new one needs to be formulated. When the new hypothesis is proven to be correct, then we can extend or convert it into a useful mathematical equation or a simpler arithmetical formula for others to adopt as an easier way of thinking and operation, as well as understanding of the output results. In the final stage, the derived mathematical equation or arithmetical formula can then be used to "predict" future outcomes of the selected system based on other different sets of inputs.

Results:

Application Examples of MPM

This article only selects the following 10 biomedical examples or real applications by using the developed GH-Method: math-physical medicine methodology.

The attached 19 figures are associated with each application example respectively from Figures 1 through 10.

Example No. 1: The term "metabolism" should be considered as a nonlinear, dynamic, and organic mathematical system having at least 10 categories with ~500 elements as many as 500 ! possible relationships defined by the author for his endocrinology research. This multi-factorial origin of metabolism equation can be better derived with the use of a mathematical concept of topology with partial differential equation, nonlinear algebra from mathematics, and approximation modeling technique of finite element method from engineering to construct a complex mathematical model of metabolism. (*Topology studies properties of spaces that are invariant under any continuous deformation. Similarly, human body's metabolic properties remain unchanged despite of the variance and deformation of human body's physical shapes and conditions*). The effect from the "metabolism model" can be calculated and clearly expressed using two new measuring variables: metabolism index (MI), and general health status unit (GHSU) as defined by the author. If both MI and GHSU results are below 73.5%, then the patient is "healthy", and when the index is above 73.5%, the patient is "unhealthy".

Example No. 2: For the past 10 years, the author spent 30,000 hours to self-study and research 6 chronic diseases as well as food nutrition. Furthermore, he has collected and processed more than 2 million data of his health conditions and lifestyle details. Based on these big data, he developed four biomarker prediction models, i.e. equations (not relying on statistics like BCM approach), for weight, postprandial plasma glucose (PPG), fasting plasma glucose (FPG), and hemoglobin A1C (HbA1C). All of these four prediction models have reached 95% to 99% of prediction accuracy. These 4 biomarkers have complex correlations with food, exercise, sleep, stress, and other lifestyle details.

In his previous engineering training, he was taught to always look for relationships between inputs and outputs of a system. However, on 3/17/2017, he discovered an interesting finding of the existing high correlation between his body weight and his FPG, where both of them are outputs from his human metabolism system.

Example No. 3: He applied "signal processing" technique of electronics engineering and geophysics to decompose a PPG wave into multiple sub-wave components. Nineteen influential factors were identified for PPG formation and five factors for FPG formation. Primary influential factors according to their respective contribution margin are summarized below:

PPG Influential factors and their relative contribution margin:
1) Post-meal exercise (~41%),
2) Carbs & sugar intake amount (~38%),
3) Ambient weather temperature (~5% to 10%).
4) All other 16 secondary factors, such as stress, sleep, sickness, water, life routine regularities, and others (combined ~11%).

FPG Influential factors and their relative contribution margin:
1) Body weight in the morning (~80% to 85%)
2) Ambient weather temperature (~5% to 10%)
3) All other 3 secondary factors, i.e. stress, sleep, disease, (~5% to 10%).

Each factor has a different contribution percentage (weighting factor) or degree of significance in terms of its impact to the formation of glucose. The weight assigned to each factor was retrospectively derived along with pattern recognition to allow a predictive component and equation to be developed. The initial weighting factors designated to influential factors for the calculation of predictive values are further modified or enhanced via mathematical and computer science tools, such as big data analytics and AI. For example, a finger-piercing measured PPG can be predicted via a simple linear arithmetical formula with a prediction accuracy of 98% to 99%, as follows:

either Formula 1:
Predicted PPG =
FPG*0.97+(carbs/sugar*1.8
(post-meal walking steps in thousand *5.0)

or Formula 2:
Predicted PPG =
FPG*0.95+(carbs/sugar*2.0
- (post-meal walking steps in thousand *5.0)

either Formula 1:
Predicted PPG =
FPG*0.97+(carbs/sugar*1.8
(post-meal walking steps in thousand *5.0)

or Formula 2:

Predicted PPG =
FPG*0.95+(carbs/sugar*2.0
- (post-meal walking steps in thousand *5.0)

This example for the two linear arithmetical formulas of the predicted PPG shows the existence of a range of multipliers for the FPG value and Carbs/sugar amount. This kind of uncertain phenomenon is a typical finding from his biomedical research.

Example No. 4: During the development of HbA1C, the author applied the concept of "safety margin" from his nuclear power design experience on his predicted HbA1C. Although this extra 5% to 10% of safety margin would lower its prediction accuracy somewhat (~4%), but it provides extra attention and pre-warning to T2D patients regarding their forthcoming HbA1C level.

The author was a trained mathematician and computer scientist who focuses on precision, but also a professional engineer and high-tech industrialist who concentrates on solving practical problems with the best approximated answers that combines concerns of accuracy, cost, and effectiveness. He applied his industrial experience from aerospace, ocean, nuclear, computer hardware and software, electronic hardware, and semiconductors fields. A professional engineer or practical industrialist would not waste too much time and energy investigating some minor influence factors once they have achieved a fairly accurate and acceptable answer for the problem. This is the reason the author applied many engineering modeling techniques in his MPM research work. The mechanical and structural engineering disciplines and electronic engineering training have helped him to fine-tune and enforce his many developed biomedical models.

Example No. 5: The PPG prediction model was developed using optical physics with artificial intelligence (AI) at the front-end and perturbation theory of quantum mechanics with wave theory of physics at the back-end. He used his developed algorithm using AI and precision from meal photos that contained big volume of data (with 20 million pixels or 160 million alpha-numerical digits per picture) to estimate the internal carb/sugar amount of the meal. He then applied the perturbation theory of quantum mechanics and wave theory of physics to a 3-hour long predicted PPG waveform before the T2D patients eat their meals with a 95% to 99% prediction accuracy.

These various theories and concepts of physics, geophysics, and electronics engineering (EE) tools helped the author to understand and calculate the relationship between food and glucose as well as the other detailed characteristics of PPG waves with their formation variances.

Example No. 6: The author has collected 80-96 glucose data per day using a continuous glucose monitoring (CGM) sensor device since 5/5/2918. Thus far, he has collected more than 66,400 data within 830 days. During a data processing task, many different waveforms (i.e. curves) would appear. In general, they represent the data amplitudes over time scale (i.e. time-domain). In fact, any fluctuation of physical representation (either causes or symptoms of a disease) can be presented via a "wave" format. These time-domain waves (e.g. EKG, glucose, or BP curves) are generated by different medical devices to represent prominent characteristics of certain diseases, including cardiovascular disease, diabetes, or hypertension. These output waves not only reveal the specific disease symptoms but also possess certain specific inner physical characteristics (hidden or apparent) such as wavelength, period, frequency, amplitude, and others.

Through the Fourier Transform operation from mathematics, we can convert a "time-domain" wave into a "frequency-domain" wave. The expressions or shapes of these two waves are vastly different since they express various hidden information. Through this frequency-domain wave, we can then conduct calculations to decipher the energy associated with this wave within certain range of frequencies, for example a glucose wave's low frequency and high amplitude. From these numerical operations, we can determine the different associated "energy" level generated by certain frequency ranges of the originally collected glucose time-domain wave. Our body needs energy to maintain its normal operating functions; however, the excessive "leftover" energy circulating within the human body can cause damages to the internal organs. Based on energy theory, the author developed a program to calculate this excessive leftover energy from *energy infusion minus energy consumption,* and then find ways to achieve a "metabolism balance" state. When our metabolism is in a good state, our immunity will be strong accordingly. Immune system is our body's defensive army against external diseases' invasion, including chronic diseases and complications (~50%), cancers (~29%), ineffectual diseases and virus (~11%). In theory, these body energy calculations can also shed a light on the estimation of longevity. Therefore, the wave theory can be a useful tool in his studies of many other chronic diseases, including cancer, dementia, and central nervous system disease along with metabolic disorders such as diabetes, hypertension, and hyperlipidemia.

Example No. 7: By combining both wave theory and energy theory, a mathematical model was derived to use as an assessment for the risk probability of cardiovascular disease (CVD), stroke, chronic kidney disease (CKD), and cancer. All of these chronic diseases are resulted from metabolic disorders, directly or indirectly. In his detailed calculation for the assessments of risk probability, he established some proper "structural engineering" models of the human blood vessels including arteries and micro-vessels. He applied structural solid mechanics concepts such as elasticity, dynamic plastic behavior, and fracture mechanics, in combination with effects due to aging, high glucose, and high blood pressure to simulate artery rupture situation with approximately 20% to 30% of CVD/Stroke occurrence rate. He also utilized fluid dynamics concepts combined with blood vessel inflammation due to high glucose and high cholesterol deposits to simulate artery blockage situation with around 70% to 80% of CVD/Stroke occurrence rate. The micro-vessel related risks mainly involved leakage through the tiny vessel wall, instead of blockage due to micro-vessel's smaller size in comparison with general lipid plaques.

Example No. 8: In order to link behavior psychological factors such as disciplines of diet and exercise along with disease physiological characteristics such as obesity and diabetes, the author decomposed ~2,500 PPG waveforms with ~32,000 glucose data points, and then re-integrated them into 3 distinctive PPG waveform types, i.e. Himalaya (too much carbs/sugar intake and inactivity), Grand Canyon (diet control and sufficient post-meal exercise), and Twin-Peaks (too much carbs/sugar intake combined with certain insufficient activity to breakdown the energy infusion). These three distinctive PPG waveform shapes could reveal different personality traits and psychological behaviors of a T2D patient. After identifying these three distinctive PPG waveforms and their associated contribution percentages, he then created a customized "progressive behavior modification" plan for diabetes patients to gradually modify their lifestyle behaviors in order to change or improve their lifestyle progressively - an evidence-based lifestyle change technique. This research begins to provide an understanding of the linkage between patient's psychological behaviors and disease's physiological characters in a quantitative manner, rather than using only qualitative descriptions in the traditional psychotherapy approach or semi-quantitative treatments in the traditional internal medicine approach. By having an in-depth knowledge of glucose can reduce the sole dependency on diabetes medication for T2D patients to control their diabetes. Diabetes cannot be cured by medication alone because it only manages the external "symptoms" of the disease, not changing patient's pancreatic beta cells health state.

Example No. 9: For a single time-stamped variable, traditional time-series analysis was used, which is similar to the EKG cardiology chart with time as its X- or horizontal axis. For interactions between two variables, such as weight and glucose, the author used a 2D spatial analysis to identify some hidden characteristics or relationships among two different sets of variables (e.g. metabolic symptom). This spatial analysis using two different variables as two axes has not been widely utilized in medical research. Dr. John Snow of London, UK, was one the first to apply this application showing clusters of cholera cases in the 1854 Broad Street cholera outbreak. This was an initial use of map-based 2D spatial analysis in medicine; however, from a statistical viewpoint, it was not considered as a spatial analysis. The author found this tool to be quite powerful for biomedical data analysis, especially to identify the close relationship among multiple variables such as weight and FPG, diet/exercise and PPG, blood pressure, and glucose. He has published numerous medical papers using this technique. For example, in one of his articles, he identified high correlations exited among weight, glucose and blood pressure via a triple dual-components analysis.

Weight vs. Glucose: 89%
Glucose vs. Blood Pressure: 83%
Weight vs. Blood Pressure: 76%

Example No. 10: The author expands the scope of his Example No. 5 (PPG & AI) to include the utilization of more computer science tools, specifically artificial intelligence and big data analytics, for wider applications. He developed an AI-based Glucometer software in 2015 installed on mobile phones, which required entering the following data via an iPhone or web-based APP on a PC:

(1) Entering the quantity of food intake and bowel movement to get a predicted body weight.

(2) Based on morning body weight to get a predicted FPG value.

(3) Taking a meal photo and entering into a customized APP along with post-meal walking time or steps. These two inputs will provide a predicted PPG value. If the predicted PPG level is too high, the individual can either reduce the carbs/sugar intake or increase the post-meal walking steps or exercise time in order to obtain a lower measured PPG.

(4) Based on predicted FPG value and three PPG values, plus past four months glucose data with different weighting factors, an estimated daily HbA1C value will be instantly shown on mobile phone. The author has published 8 medical papers regarding his predicted HbA1C values that included 8 consecutive periods with a time frame of 5-months each. His eight mathematically predicted HbA1C values have matched 100% with his eight lab-tested HbA1C measured values.

This AI-based Glucometer was developed utilizing various computer science IT tools, including big data analytics, machine learning (including self-learning, self-modification, and self-simplification), and AI based tool containing ~8 million pre-stored food nutritional data. This database includes 6 million food material data from the United States Department of Agriculture, 1.6 million data from 500 chain restaurants, and the author's own 0.6 million data from his collected ~6,000 meal photos data.

Results of T2D case study:

As shown in Table2, in 2010, the author had an average glucose of 280 mg/dL along with his A1C above 10%. He weighed 220 lbs. (100 kg), with a BMI above 32, and a waistline of 44 inches (112 cm). From 1994 to 2006, he suffered five cardiac episodes, renal complications, bladder infection, foot ulcer, diabetic retinopathy, and hypothyroidism.

Currently, in 2020, after using these 5 prediction models and his developed AI Glucometer software, his average glucose reduced to 108 mg/dL and his A1C is 6.2% without taking any diabetes medications. He weighs 170 lbs. (77 kg), with a BMI at 24.7, and a waistline of 32 inches (82 cm). Since his health condition is stable, he does not have any recurrent cardiovascular incidents and all of the other diabetes complications have subsided. In summary, he has saved his own live through his GH-Method: math-physical medicine research efforts (Table 2).

Discussion:

Physicians always search for ways to encourage people to adopt a healthier lifestyle by exercising more and/or decreasing caloric intake (Reference 1). However, they are compromised by the accuracy of testing methods. Patients with diabetes rely on blood glucose monitoring devices to manage their condition. As some self-monitoring devices are becoming more accurate, it becomes critical to understand the relationship between system accuracy and clinical outcomes, and the potential benefits of analytical accuracy. However, without the knowledge of wave theory and energy theory, a traditional medical researcher may have some difficulties to truly understand the characteristics and behaviors of the glucose waveforms. Instead, they may rely on simple statistics to study average values. As a result, this would reduce the benefits of collecting a big amount of glucose data from measuring devices such as the CGM.

In one study of simulated meter models derived from the published characteristics of 43 commercial meters, researchers isolated the differences in clinical performance that are directly associated with the meter characteristics (Reference 3). They reported that a meter's systematic bias has a significant and inverse effect on HbA1C (P < .01), while also affecting the number of severe hypoglycemic events. On the other hand, an error is defined as the fraction of measurements beyond 5% of the true value, which is a predictor of severe hypoglycemic events (P < .01). Both bias and error have significant effects on the total daily insulin (TDI) and the number of necessary glucose measurements per day (P < .01). Furthermore, these relationships can be accurately modeled using linear regression on meter bias and error (Reference 3). Two components of meter accuracy, bias and error clearly affect clinical outcomes. While error has little effect on HbA1C, it tends to increase episodes of severe hypoglycemia. Meter bias has significant effects on all considered metrics: a positive systemic bias will reduce HbA1C, but increase the number of severe hypoglycemic attacks, TDI use, and number of finger-sticks per day (Reference 3).

The author published his research results on the comparison of glucose measurements between finger-piercing and a particular brand of continuous glucose monitoring (CGM) sensor (References 4, 5, 6, and 7). The sensor measurement results in comparison with finger-piercing measurements reveal that using the sensor measurements, the average PPG is +17% higher and peak PPG is +38% higher in some time periods, compared to the finger stick method. The most shocking finding is PPG peaks occur around 45 minutes to 75 minutes (approximately 60 minutes) after the "first bite" of meal, not the traditional standard of two hours after. In addition, the "lowest' PPG value usually occurs about 120 minutes after the first bite of meal which is the same timing of finger-piercing measurement recommended by many physicians. The author published many articles regarding this subject due to his serious concerns regarding hypoglycemic incidents, or the so called "insulin shocks" which can lead to sudden death.

The use of the AI Glucometer testing software provides physicians a mechanism to assist their patients to gain better control of their A1C glycohemoglobin, and lessen the cardiovascular risk associated with diabetes, while motivating them to engage in a healthier lifestyle. This is done without the need for finger-sticks or even a CGM sensor device, which most patients find objectionable (Reference 8).

The MPM methodology used in the author's research is compared and contrasted to current mechanisms in common use today as in BCM with an achieved accuracy level of ~99% (Table 1). As a result, a non-invasive technique using AI Glucometer software, with high degree of accuracy, is preferable to current BCM method.

As of 8/12/2020, the author has written 310 medical papers and published more than 250 of them in various medical journals, with the majority of them using the MPM method. If interested in reading other MPM associated papers, the author recommends using Google to search for the related topics.

Conclusion:

Using MPM, a non-traditional medical research methodology, provides many quantitative proofs with a high degree of accuracy (higher precision) compared to other disease research results. Medicine is based on biology and chemistry, while biology, chemistry, and engineering are based on physics, and physics is based on mathematics. Logically, mathematics is the mother of all sciences. When we explore our application problems down to the foundation level, we can discover more facts and deeper truths. This is the logical essence of "math-physical medicine." Using this MPM model, the accuracy of medical evaluations, along with the precision of predictive models can be greatly improved, with dramatic benefits to the patients.

References

1. Liu, Z, Yang, B, Drug Development Strategy for Type 2 Diabetes: Targeting Positive Energy Balances, Curr Drug Targets. 2018 Dec 16. doi: 10.2174/1389450 120666181217111500. [Epub ahead of print]

2. Hirsch IB1, Amiel SA, Blumer IR, Bode BW, Edelman SV, Seley JJ, Verderese CA, Kilpatrick ES, Using multiple measures of glycemic to support individualized diabetes management: recommendations for clinicians, patients, and payers. Diabetes Technol Ther. 2012 Nov;14(11):973-83; quiz 983. doi: 10.1089/dia.2012.0132. Epub 2012 Oct 15.

3. Campos-Náñez E1, Fortwaengler K2, Breton MD1, Clinical Impact of Blood Glucose Monitoring Accuracy: An In-Silico Study. J Diabetes Sci Technol. 2017 Nov;11(6):1187-1195. doi: 10.1177/1932296817710474. Epub 2017 Jun 1.

4. Hsu, Gerald C. (2018). Using Math-Physical Medicine to Control T2D via Metabolism Monitoring and Glucose Predictions. Journal of Endocrinology and Diabetes, 1(1), 1-6.

5. Hsu, Gerald C. (2018). Using Signal Processing Techniques to Predict PPG for T2D. International Journal of Diabetes & Metabolic Disorders, 3(2),1-3.

6. Hsu, Gerald C. (2018). Using Math-Physical Medicine and Artificial Intelligence Technology to Manage Lifestyle and Control Metabolic Conditions of T2D. International Journal of Diabetes & Its Complications, 2(3),1-7.

7. Hsu, Gerald C. (2018). Using Math-Physical Medicine to Study the Risk Probability of having a Heart Attack or Stroke Based on 3 Approaches, Medical Conditions, Lifestyle Management Details, and Metabolic Index. EC Cardiology, 5(12), 1-9.

8. Jin's A1, Tierney MJ2, Tamada JA2, McGill S2, Desai S2, Chua B2, Chang A3, Christiansen M4. Design, development, and evaluation of a novel microneedle array-based continuous glucose monitor. J Diabetes Sci Technol. 2014 May;8(3):483-7. doi: 10.1177/1932296814526191. Epub 2014 Mar 6.

9.

Comparison of Methodology	Bio-Chemical Medicine (BCM)	Math-Physical Medicine (MPM)
Academic Foundation	Based on both Biology and Chemistry, which are both based on Physics and Math	Based on Engineering and Physics, which are both based on Mathematics
Precision and Accuracy of Results	It appears that most likely the results are less precise and less accurate than MPM	Most likely more precise and accurate than BCM due to mathematics and physics
Data Size	It seems that most of the data size is smaller (hundreds to thousands)	Most of the data size are larger (thousands to millions)
Application of Mathematics	It appears that mostly utilizing statistics (an extension of mathematics)	Mostly utilizing mathematical equations, including many branches of mathematics
Distinguish by Importance Level (Weighting Factors)	It appears that mostly no weighting factors are considered before analysis	Figuring out various weighting factors and then assigned to key influential factors (Engineering Concept for approximation)
Data Collection and Cleaning	It seems that most of work spends 50% to 80% on data collection, cleaning, and organization	Spend only 10% to 30% on data collection, cleaning, and organization by utilizing computer technology, including AI

Table 1: Comparison of BCM versus MPM

Health Examination Record	2010	2017	2020	Disease
FPG (<120 mg/dL)	185	119	107	Diabetes
PPG (<120 mg/dL)	350	116	110	Diabetes
Lab-testedA1C (<6.4%)	10	6.5	6.3	Diabetes
eclaireMD predicted A1C (<6.4%)	10.0	6.84	6.31	Diabetes
90-days Average Glucose (<120 mg/dL)	279	117	109	Diabetes
Triglyceride (<150)	1161	69	110	Hyperlipidemia
HDL (>40)	24	48	49	Hyperlipidemia
LDL (<130)	174	74	123	Hyperlipidemia
Total Cholesterol (<200)	253	118	168	Hyperlipidemia
Blood Pressure: SBP/DBP (< 120 / 80)	140 / 100	100 / 60	108 / 60	Hypertension
ACR (<30)	116.4	12.3	19	Kidney Problem
BMI (<25.0)	31.0	24.9	25.3	Obesity
Weight (lbs)	210	172	172	Obesity
Waistline (inch)	44	34	33	Obesity
Matabolism Index (MI / GHSU: <73.5%)	140% / 103%	49% / 55%	53.6% / 54.1%	Complications
Heart episodes (1994 - 2006)				5 times
Kidney Complications				Yes
Blader Infection				Yes
Thyroid Problems				Yes
Foot Ulcer				Yes

Table 2: Comparison of health conditions

Hierarchy of Science

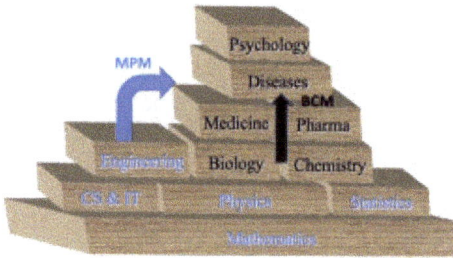

The higher lever in hierarchy, the lower accuracy

Diseases Treatment is based on Medicine & Pharmacy

Current Medicine is based on Biology & Chemistry,
Bio-Chemical Medicine (BCM)

Engineering, Biology, Chemistry are Applied Physics

Computer Science and Statistics are Applied Math;
CS&IT includes Big Data, Machine Learning (AI)

Mathematics is the "Mother of Science"

GH-Method: Math-Physical Medicine (MPM)
Based on mathematics (includes CS&IT and statistics), physics, & engineering modeling

Table 3: Hierarchy of Science

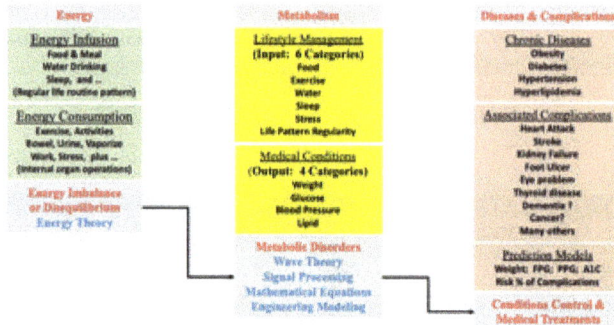

Table 4: From energy via Metabolism to chronic diseases

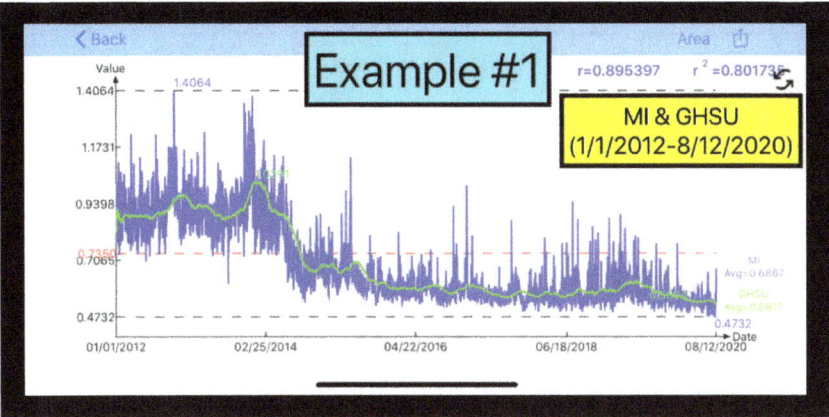

Figure 1: Application example #1

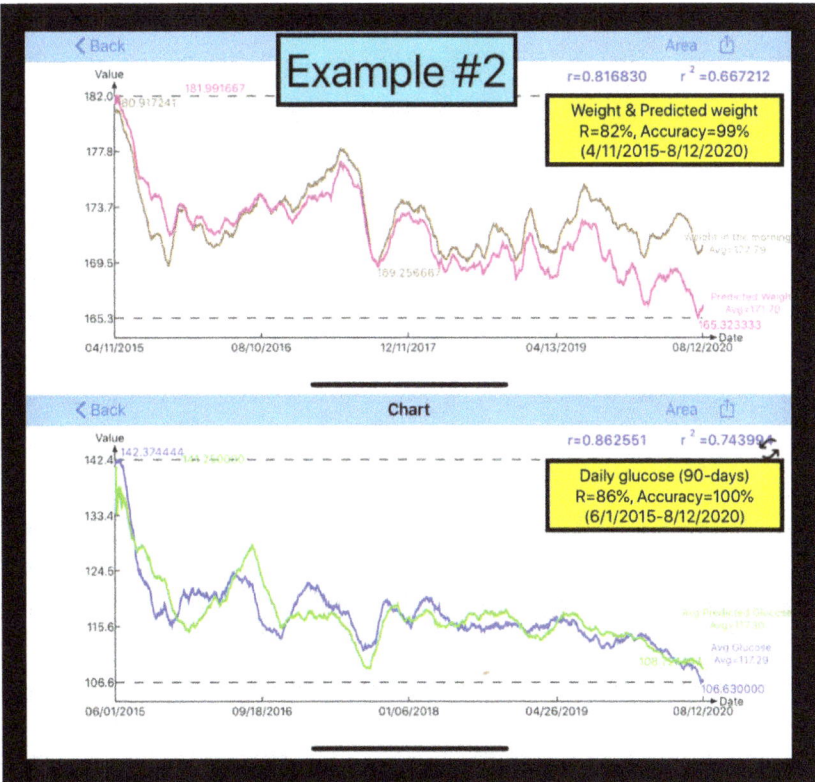

Figure 2: Application example #2

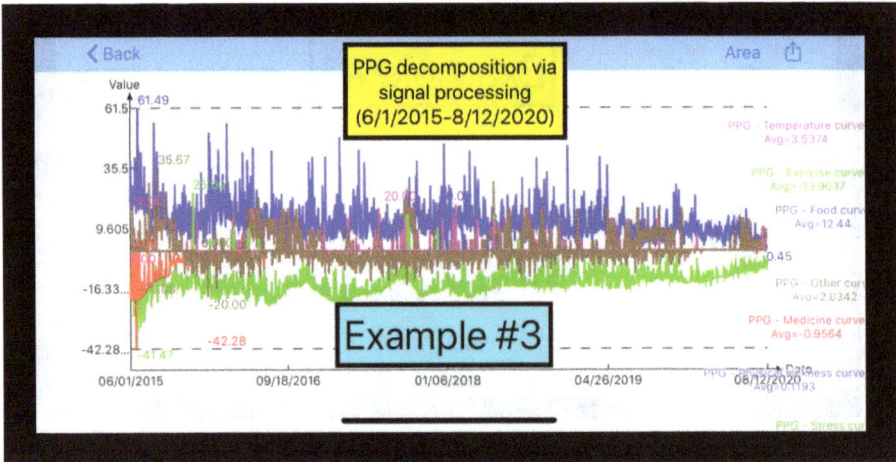

Figure 3: Application example #3

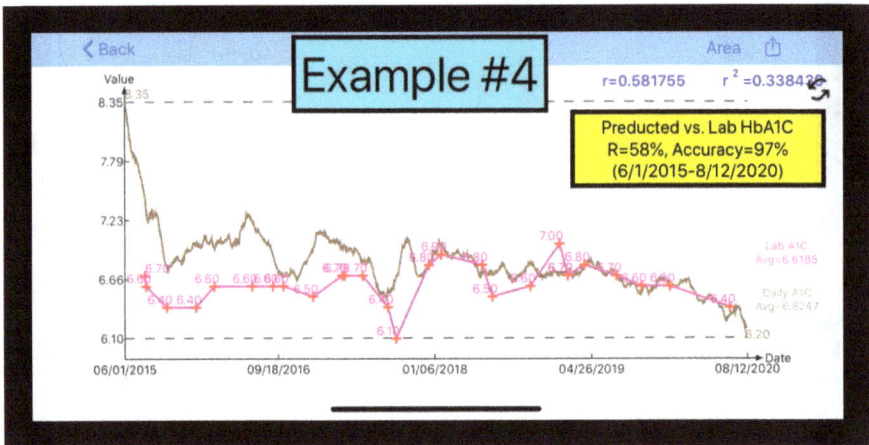

Figure 4: Application example #4

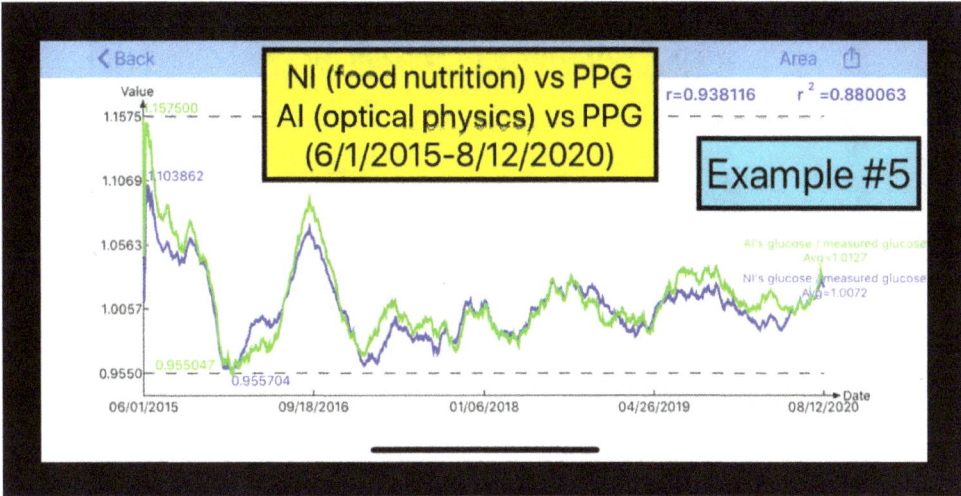

Figure 5: Application example #5

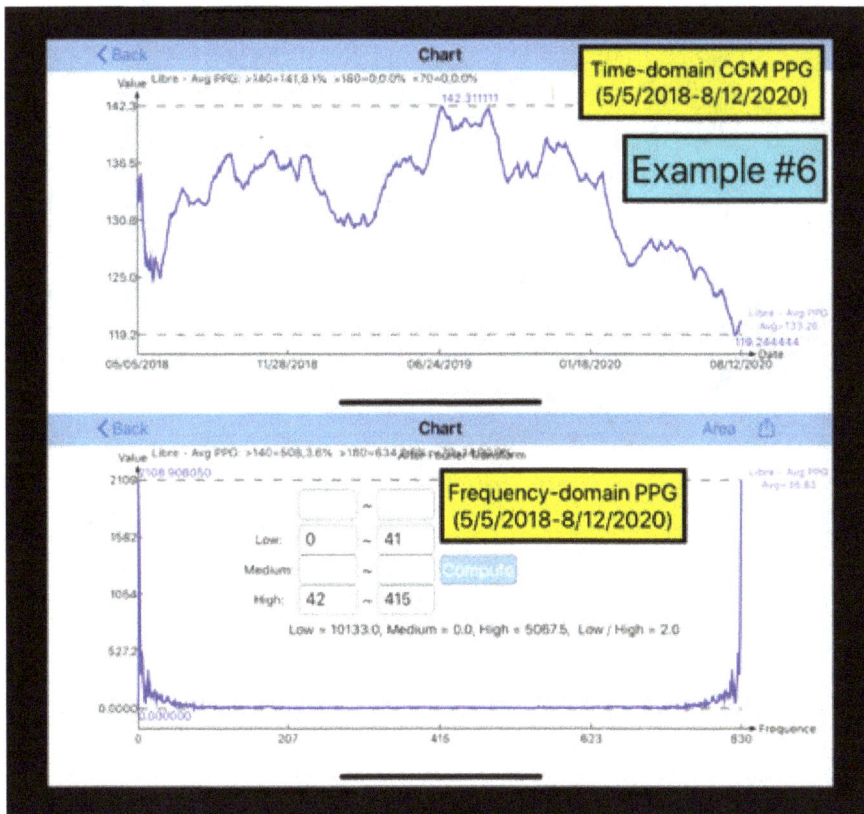

Figure 6: Application example #6

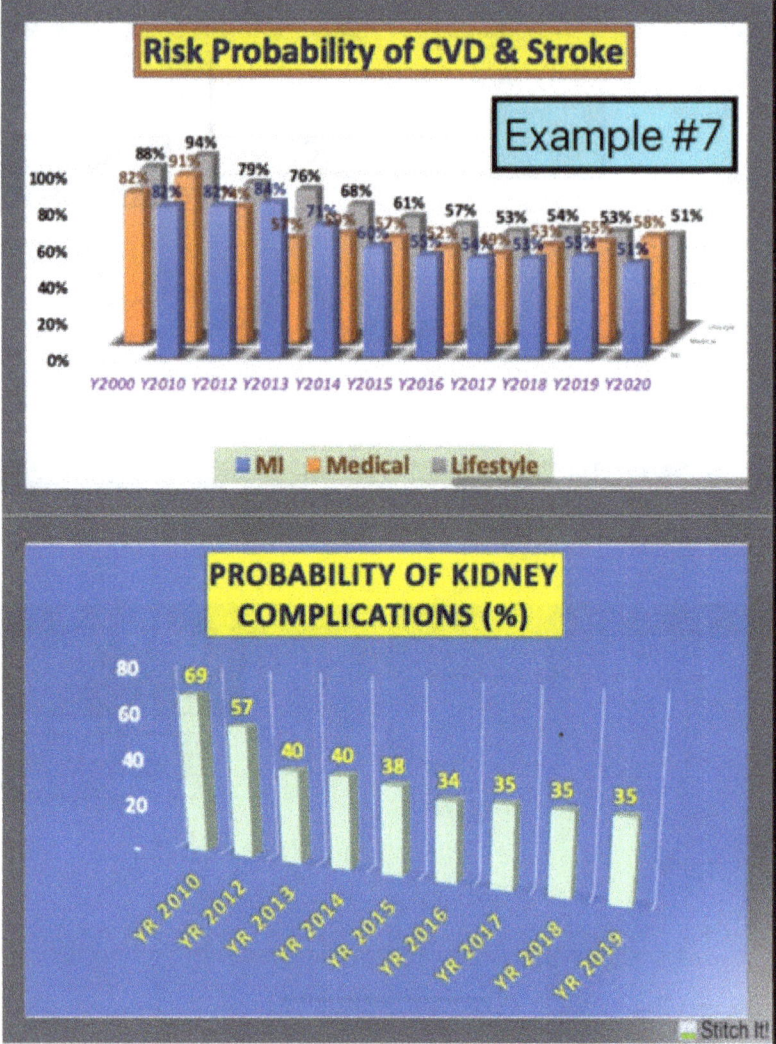

Figure 7: Application example #7

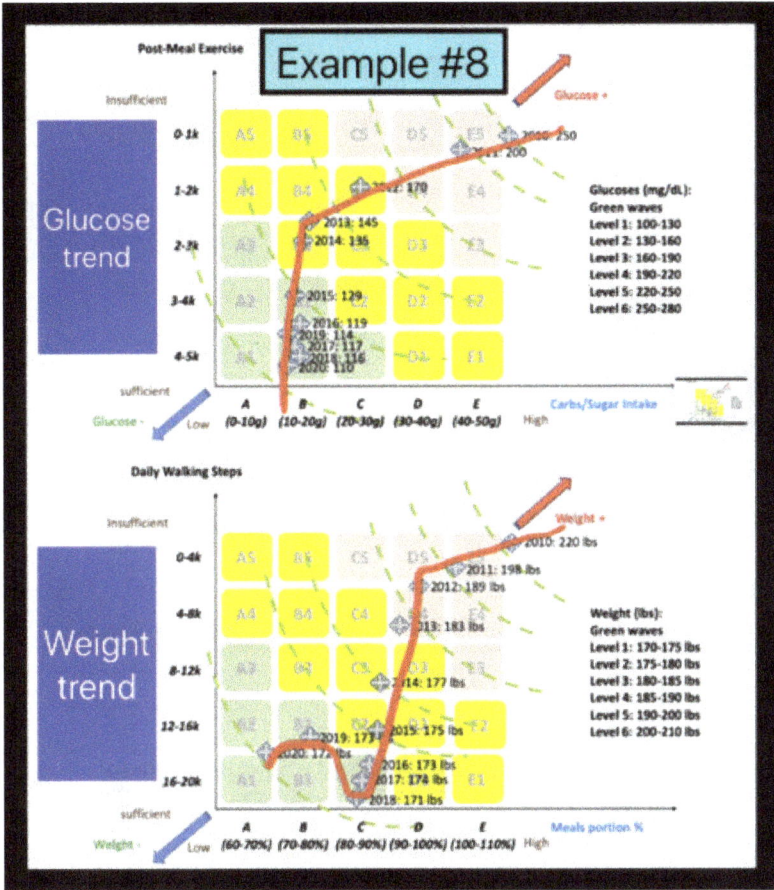

Figure 8: Application example #8

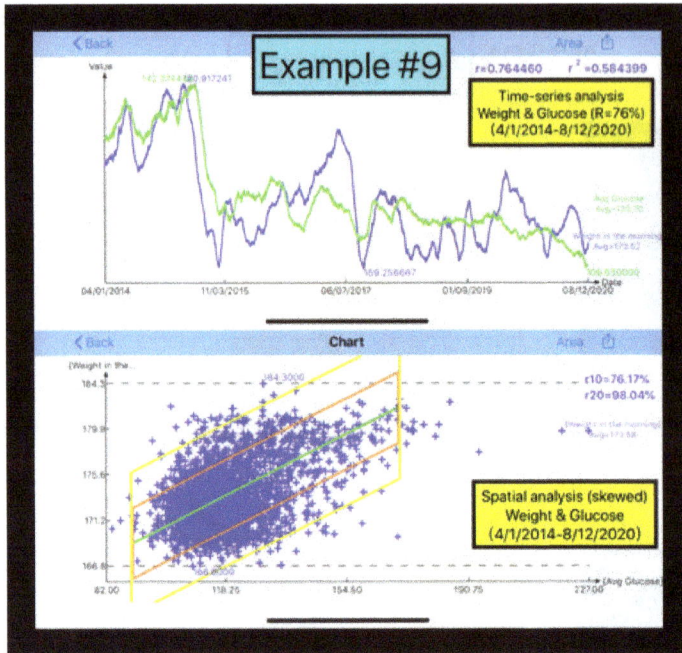

Figure 9: Application example #9

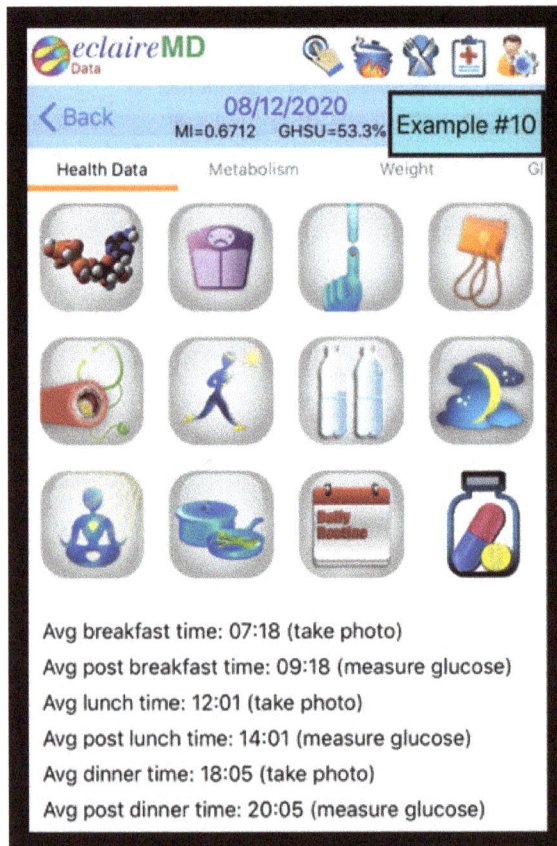

Figure 10: Application example #10

A neural communication model between brain and internal organs via postprandial plasma glucose waveforms study based on 95 liquid egg meals and 110 solid egg meals (No. 311)

By: Gerald C. Hsu
eclaireMD Foundation, USA
8/13/2020

Abstract:

In this paper, the author described the progress on his two-year long special research project, from 5/5/2018 through 8/13/2020, to identify a neural communication model between the brain's cerebral cortex and certain internal organs such as the stomach, liver, and pancreas. He used a continuous glucose monitor (CGM) sensor collected postprandial plasma glucose (PPG) data to investigate the glucose production amount at different timing and waveform differences between 95 liquid egg meals and 110 solid egg meals.

The significant PPG differences between these two food types can be easily observed (Figure 5). In addition, the PPG peak value differences are 20 mg/dL in Phase 2 study and Phase 3 study, with almost identical inputs of carbs/sugar intake amounts and post-meal walking steps.

The author conducted this special investigative experiment in three phases. All of the findings from these research phases are extremely similar to each other, with minor deviations, even though his collected experimental data size nearly doubled in each phase.

From a neuroscientific point of view, the author utilized his developed math-physical medicine methodology (MPM) and his learned biomedical knowledge *to "trick" the cerebral cortex of the brain into producing or releasing a "lesser" amount of PPG,* without altering or disturbing the required food nutritional balance. If this idea works, by changing the cooking method, it can then help many type 2 diabetes (T2D) patients to lower their peak PPG and average PPG levels without reducing or changing their food nutritional contents. Obviously, T2D patients must avoid overeating foods with high carbohydrates and sugar contents at all times.

By sharing his research findings with other fellow medical research scientists, he hopes that they can provide some better explanations, more proof, or further justifications by using a different or traditional research methodology, such as the biochemical medicine (BCM) approach.

Introduction:

In this paper, the author described the progress on his two-year long special research project, from 5/5/2018 through 8/13/2020, to identify a neural communication model between the brain's cerebral cortex and certain internal organs such as the stomach, liver, and pancreas. He used a continuous glucose monitor (CGM) sensor collected postprandial plasma glucose (PPG) data to investigate the glucose production amount at different timing and waveform differences between 95 liquid egg meals and 110 solid egg meals.

Method:

Since 1/1/2012, the author developed a research-oriented software on his iPhone to collect all of his diabetes-related medical data and lifestyle details. In addition, he started to collect his glucose data using a CGM sensor device from 5/5/2018. He accumulated approximately 80 to 96 glucose data per day with 13 glucose data per meal over a 3-hour timeframe. On 9/25/2019, he launched a special investigation regarding the relationship between food preparation method and PPG level using his own body to conduct the necessary experiments.

He described the results from his Phase 1 in his research work, from 9/25/2019 to 2/11/2020, by utilizing the collected data from his 30 egg drop soup meals and 30 pan-fried egg meals during phase one (Reference 1).

For the Phase 2 in his research work, he further collected an additional 36 liquid meals and 39 solid meals with identical food material and cooking method (Reference 5). During this phase, from 9/25/2019 to 5/29/2020, he accumulated a total of 69 liquid meals (egg drop soup) and 66 solid meals (pan-fried egg). He also enhanced his software program to be able to present these glucose data using the Candlestick K-Line chart (References 2 and 3). Through the Candlestick chart, it clearly reflects five key PPG values at different time instants between liquid food and solid food.

For his experimental Phase 3, from 9/25/2019 through 8/13/2020, he accumulated additional data from a total of 95 liquid egg meals (egg drop soup) and 110 solid egg meals (including 68 pan-fried eggs and 42 hardboiled eggs). In comparison with the Phase 2 data, he collected additional 26 liquid meals and 44 solid meals over these 76 days.

He focused on investigating the relationships among different food inputs such as meal nutritional contents, cooking methods, physical phases, and different glucose outputs, i.e. PPG "waveforms". When he observed those different physical phenomenon of glucose waves from liquid and solid meals, he wondered why these two different cooking methods would end up with two varying PPG waveforms with identical food nutritional ingredients input. Most of his medical associates in the fields of internal medicine and food nutrition have mentioned that food nutritional components, particularly carbohydrates and sugar amount, and exercise influence PPG values. Therefore, he decided to conduct an experiment of eating the same food ingredients but with two different cooking or preparation methods. It should be noted that he kept the intensity and duration of his post-meal exercise at the same level.

By 2/11/2020 with ~30 meals in each liquid and solid category, he discovered the vast differences existing between these two types of meals. At that moment, he came up with a neural communication "hypothesis" between the brain and certain internal organs via our nervous system. He then decided to extend his experiments in order to verify this neural communication model with the path of *sending messages from the stomach to the brain and then forwarding the feedback message to the liver and pancreas,* which determines the PPG production amount at different time instance by using a bigger experimental database and additional mathematical tools.

On 5/29/2020, his friend, Dr. Deborah Zelinsky, a research scientist and a clinical doctor, who specializes in the area of interaction among the ear, eye, and brain, forwarded him an article (Reference 4).

Here is an excerpt:

Published May 18th in the Proceedings of the National Academy of Sciences, an important world first, a study co-authored by Dr. Levinthal and Dr. Peter Strick, both from the Pitt School of Medicine, has explained what parts of the brain's cerebral cortex influence stomach function and how it can impact health. Dr. Peter Strick is a world leader in establishing evidence that internal organs are strongly modulated at the highest levels by the cerebral cortex. It's been traditional in biology and medicine that the internal organs are self-regulatory through the autonomic nervous system, largely independent of higher brain regions. Dr. Strick's previous research, for instance, also showed that similar areas of the cerebral cortex also control kidney and adrenal function. That course of research now could extend to "the heart, liver and pancreas to discover more about how the brain coordinates control of internal organs," said Mr. Sterling who holds a Ph.D. in neuroscience. When it comes to trusting your gut, it already is well-established that the stomach and gut send "ascending" signals to the brain in a way that influences brain function. But the study has found that the "central nervous system both influences and is influenced by the gastrointestinal system." What people haven't understood to date, Dr. Strick said, is that the brain also has "descending influences on the stomach" with various parts of the brain involved in that signaling, including those areas that control movement and emotions. Those areas control the stomach "as directly as cortical control of movement. These are not trivial influences."

On May 27, 2020, David Templeton, a writer for the Pittsburgh Post-Gazette presented this excellent medical discovery report. It described exactly what the author, for almost a year, guessed and felt about the neural communication model between the brain and other internal organs. By training, he is a mathematician, physicist, and engineer, but not a medical doctor or a neuroscientist. However, during his research work in this area since 9/15/2019, he has discovered and proved his *"gut-feel"* of these "ascending" messages from the stomach to brain regarding food entry, and also "descending" messages from the brain to liver and pancreas regarding glucose production or release. He also verified these observations via his examination of specific physical phenomena, established a few mathematical models, and then confirmed with big data analytics. In 2019, he cautiously selected words, such as *hypotheses, guess*, and *might be*, to describe his gut-feelings generated from his findings, but now he has found the support and proof from the neuroscientific work done by other brain experts (Reference 4).

Since he published a few articles along this line of thought in early 2020, by using various food and glucose data, he will forgo some explanations and come to the same conclusion based on a relatively "larger" size of experimental data.

Results:

In this phase three study, he focused on the following two specific meal groups which involved eggs only. The main difference between these two "egg alone" meals is the cooking or preparation method. In Figure 1, one large egg contains mainly proteins (6.3g) and fat (5g) with a small amount of carbohydrates (0.38g) and sugar (0.38g). It should be noted that he occasionally takes two eggs, or adds chopped spring onions in his pan-fried egg for flavor, or a small amount of seaweed in his egg drop soup for iodine.

Here is some important data from Figures 2 and 3. To date, the author has eaten 95 liquid egg meals and 110 solid egg meals without any other food materials including carbs/sugar ingredients. The average carbs/sugar intake amounts are 2.7 grams for liquid meals and 2.2 grams for solid meals. His average post-meal walking steps are 4,390 for liquid meals and 4,604 for solid meals. His average finger PPG is 107 mg/dL for liquid meals and 112 mg/dL for solid meals. (Note: finger PPG has no value in his study due to its limited data size and measurement timing at 120-minutes after first bite of meal).

His average sensor PPG is 114 mg/dL for liquid meals (7% higher than finger PPG), and 129 mg/dL for solid meals (15% higher than finger PPG). **Their average sensor PPG difference is 15 mg/dL.** But his average peak sensor PPG is 115 mg/dL for liquid meals, and 135 mg/dL for solid meals. **Their peak sensor PPG difference is 20 mg/dL.**

His personal target for post-meal walking is 4,000 steps. Each 1,000 post-meal steps decreases PPG value by approximately 5 mg/dL. Since his post-meal exercise for these two food categories are almost equal between 4,400 steps and 4,600 steps, he can just focus on the influence from food intake on his PPG values. Based on his previous research results, each gram of carbs/sugar intake amount increases his PPG value by 1.8 mg/dL to 2.0 mg/dL. Therefore, his finger PPG values would increase about 4 to 5 mg/dL due to the carbs/sugar intake amount, which is in small quantities and almost negligible. This finding not only proves that the finger-piercing PPG values are insignificant to his research work, it provides a hint that *"something-else"* is occurring.

In this particular study, the food nutritional ingredients are almost identical, but the cooking methods are completely different. Therefore, he decided to focus on his cooking method that yields two different *physical states*, liquid versus solid. His first exposure to physics and chemistry occurred in his second year of middle school, at age 11. He was taught the three states of matter: "solid, liquid, and gas/steam". After 62 years, this basic knowledge of physics came to mind in assisting him to discover these neurological related phenomenon.

The two 3-hour PPG waveforms with their respective candlestick K-Line charts are illustrated for liquid meals and solid meals, respectively (Figures 2 and 3).

In Figure 4, it shows 5 key values of PPG from his candlestick K-Line chart technique

(References 2 and 3). Each candlestick chart has five key characteristics, which includes opening glucose at 0-minute, close glucose at 180-minutes, maximum glucose usually around 45-minutes to 75-minutes, minimum glucose usually around 120-minutes, and average glucose over a time period of 180 minutes. These five key values for liquid meals and solid meals are quite different as well.

The most important figure in this article is shown in Figure 5. The author put two waveforms of both liquid meals and solid meals together in the same diagram.

The significant PPG differences between these two food types can be easily observed. In addition, the PPG peak value differences are 20 mg/dL from both Phase 2 study and Phase 3 study, with almost identical inputs of carbs/sugar intake amounts and post-meal walking steps.

Discussion:

With the same food ingredient, why do they have different PPG values? Both food's physical appearances have the same nutritional ingredient inputs; however, their different cooking or preparation methods result into different physical states, liquid or solid. Maybe the message (or signal) ascending from the stomach to the cerebral cortex is not food ingredients, but rather the food's arrival and its physical state. Therefore, the brain misinterprets soup as an equivalent to a cup of decaf-coffee, tea, or water and then the brain descends a message to the liver for producing or releasing a lesser amount of glucose.

Another point is, during the period of 5/5/2018 to 8/13/2020, his diabetes conditions were already under control without taking any medication. This means that these results are strictly the internal biological outcomes by his stringent lifestyle management program and without any external medication's chemical intervention.

The author analyzed his 2,493 meals with 32,409 PPG data for the past 831 days. The first evidence is that the stomach takes about 10-15 minutes to inform the food entry message to the brain. The second indication is that, for both liquid egg meals and solid egg meals, it takes about 45 minutes for the liver to release glucose at its peak amount. Based on his findings from his previous research work, the peak PPG occurring time instants are between 45 minutes to 75 minutes (in average, around 60 minutes) after eating.

When the author could not locate a satisfactory explanation from professional knowledge of either food nutrition or clinical internal medicine, he started to delve deeper into the source of this problem: "the creation of glucose". He realized that glucose is *not directly converted* from food nutritional ingredients. Instead, the glucose was *directly produced* by the liver. Of course, the human body and all of its internal organs, including the stomach, liver, and pancreas are dependent on the food supply for their needed energy.

As a result, he came up with his *first hypothesis* that the glucose difference is probably due to the physical state of consumed food, such as liquid or solid, that is decided by the brain.

Furthermore, the author has learned three basic facts from his past 9-years of biomedical research work. First, 70% of our daily energy intake are consumed by our brain and nervous system. Second, the brain is the only internal organ which has the power of cognition, judgement, information processing, decision making, and marching order issuance. Third, all of the internal organs work closely together but under the orders from a single command center, which is the brain.

Based on the above acquired biomedical knowledge, the author further developed his *second hypothesis*. When one particular food type enters into the gastrointestinal system, the stomach will immediately send a message (or a signal) to inform the brain about the arrival of food and its physical state. After receiving this input signal from the stomach, the brain will then start to process information, make proper judgements, and then issues its feedback message (descending marching order) to the liver regarding how much glucose amount should be produced or released at what time instant, as well as within what time frame to reach to the peak of glucose. At the same time, the brain will also inform the pancreas regarding how much insulin should be produced or released when an excessive amount of glucose has been produced or released by the liver. However, for severe diabetes patients whose pancreatic beta cells were damaged to a certain degree, each patient's insulin capabilities and qualities (i.e. production quantity and insulin resistance) will not be the same to influence the final PPG reading.

These two particular hypotheses support the author's view on how his neural communication model between the cerebral cortex of the brain and internal organs, specifically stomach, liver, and pancreas regarding the PPG production (during the 180 minutes period) after the first bite of meal.

Perhaps the difference in PPG readings may also be affected by the absorption factors of chyme, which is a semiliquid digested food that passes from the stomach to small intestine, consisting of gastric juices and some leftover food. In theory, chyme from solid meals is relatively dense and may take more time passing through the absorptive surface area of the small intestine, while chyme from liquid meals is mostly liquid shape and may pass through the absorptive surface more quickly. *However, the author is not convinced about the absorption speed of chyme affecting the timing of peak PPG.* In his findings during the Phase 2 experiments, he found that peak PPG occurred at 45 minutes for liquid meals and at 60 minutes for solid meals, while his Phase 3 experimental findings indicate that both meal type's peak PPG values took place at the same 45 minutes after eating. From his previous research findings, he has already found that the peak PPG usually occurred approximately 45 minutes to 75 minutes after eating.

Conclusions:

The author conducted this special investigative experiment in three phases. All of the findings from these research phases are extremely similar to each other, with minor deviations, even though his collected experimental data size nearly doubled in each phase.

From a neuroscientific point of view, the author utilized his developed math-physical medicine methodology (MPM) and his learned biomedical knowledge **to "trick" the cerebral cortex of the brain into producing or releasing a "lesser" amount of PPG,** without altering or disturbing the required food nutritional balance. If this idea works, by changing the cooking method, it can then help many type 2 diabetes (T2D) patients to lower their peak PPG and average PPG levels without reducing or changing their food nutritional contents. Obviously, T2D patients must avoid overeating foods with high carbohydrates and sugar contents at all times.

By sharing his research findings with other fellow medical research scientists, he hopes that they can provide some better explanations, more proof, or further justifications by using a different or traditional research methodology, such as the biochemical medicine (BCM) approach.

References:

1. Hsu, Gerald C., eclaireMD Foundation, USA, 9/25/2019 - 2/11/2020, No. 229: "Hypothesis on glucose production communication model between the brain and internal organs via investigating the PPG values of pan-fried solid egg meal vs. egg drop liquid soup meal"

2. Hsu, Gerald C., eclaireMD Foundation, USA, No. 76: "Using Candlestick Charting Techniques to Investigate Glucose Behaviors (GH-Method: Math-Physical Medicine)"

3. Hsu, Gerald C., eclaireMD Foundation, USA, No. 261: "Comparison study of PPG characteristics from candlestick model using GH-Method: Math-Physical Medicine"

4. Templeton, David, Pittsburgh Post-Gazette, May 27, 2020: "Pitt study shows brain and stomach connections are a two-way street" dtempleton@post-gazette.com https://www.post-gazette.com/news/health/2020/05/27/Peter-Strick-David-Levinthal-Pittsburgh-School-of-Medicine-PNAS-cerebral-cortex-microbiome-stomach/stories/202005190088.

5. Hsu, Gerald C., eclaireMD Foundation, USA, No. 266: "Physical evidence of neural communication among brain, stomach, and liver via PPG waveform differences between liquid food and solid food"

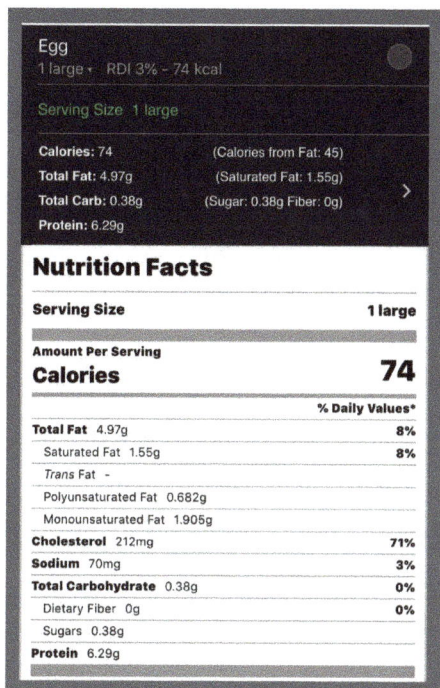

Figure 1: Nutrition ingredients of one large egg

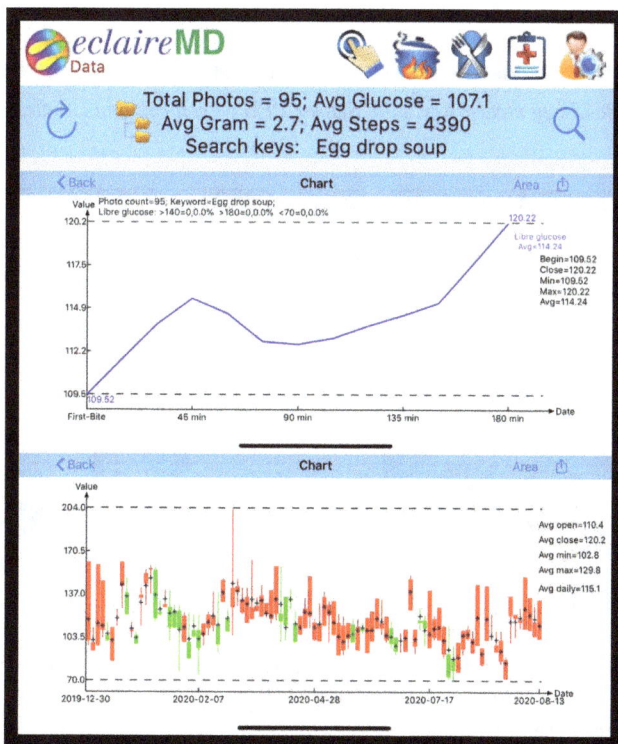

Figure 2: 95 Liquid egg meals:
Key data, Sensor PPG waveform, and candlestick K-Line chart

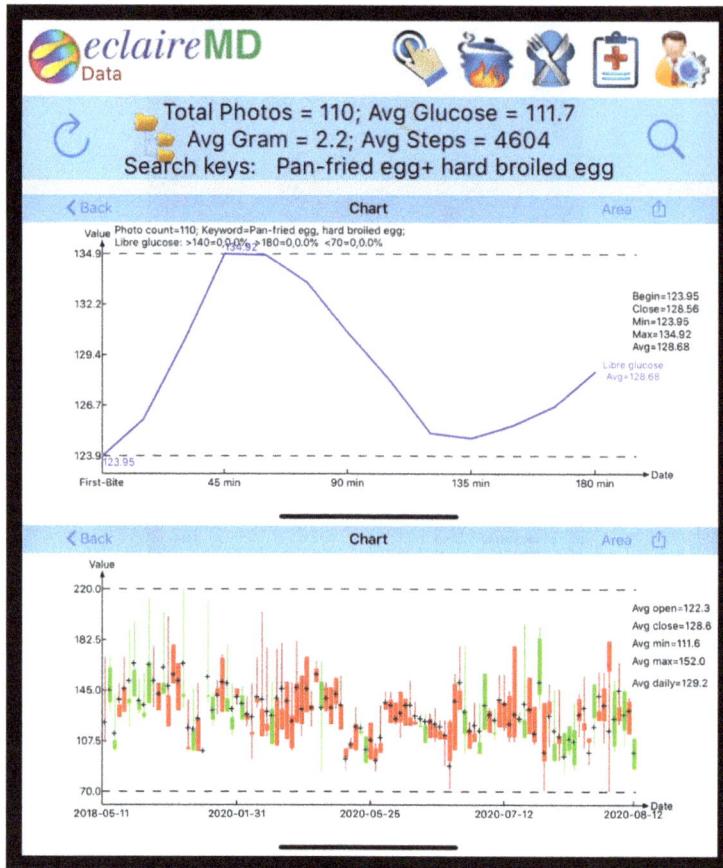

Figure 3: 110 Solid egg meals: Key data, Sensor PPG waveform, and candlestick K-Line chart

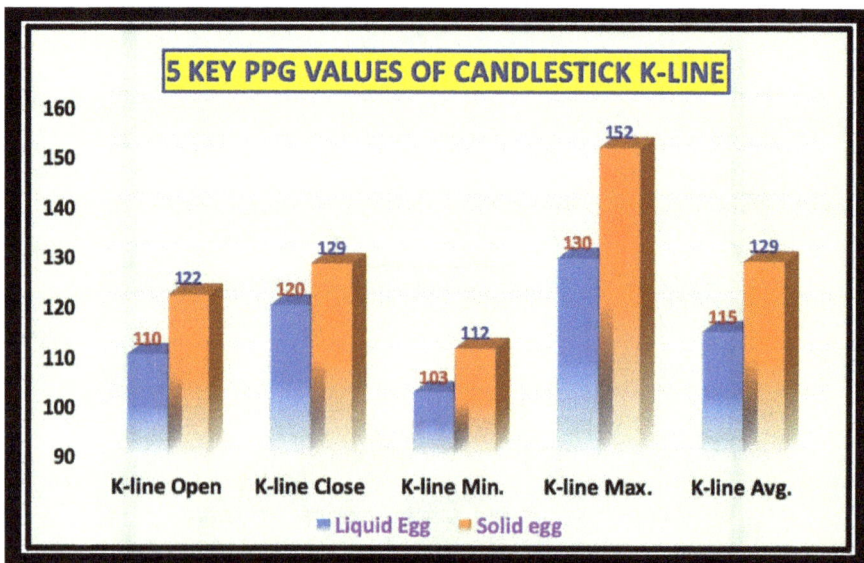

Figure 4: Comparison of 5 key values of Candlestick K-Line charts between 95 liquid egg meals and 110 solid egg meals

Sensor PPG (mg/dL)	Liquid Egg	Solid egg
No. of meals	95	110
Average Sensor PPG	114	129
Post-meal Walking	4390	4604
Carbs/Sugar (grams)	2.7	2.2
Finger PPG (mg/dL)	107	112
K-line Open	110	122
K-line Close	120	129
K-line Min.	103	112
K-line Max.	130	152
K-line Avg.	115	129

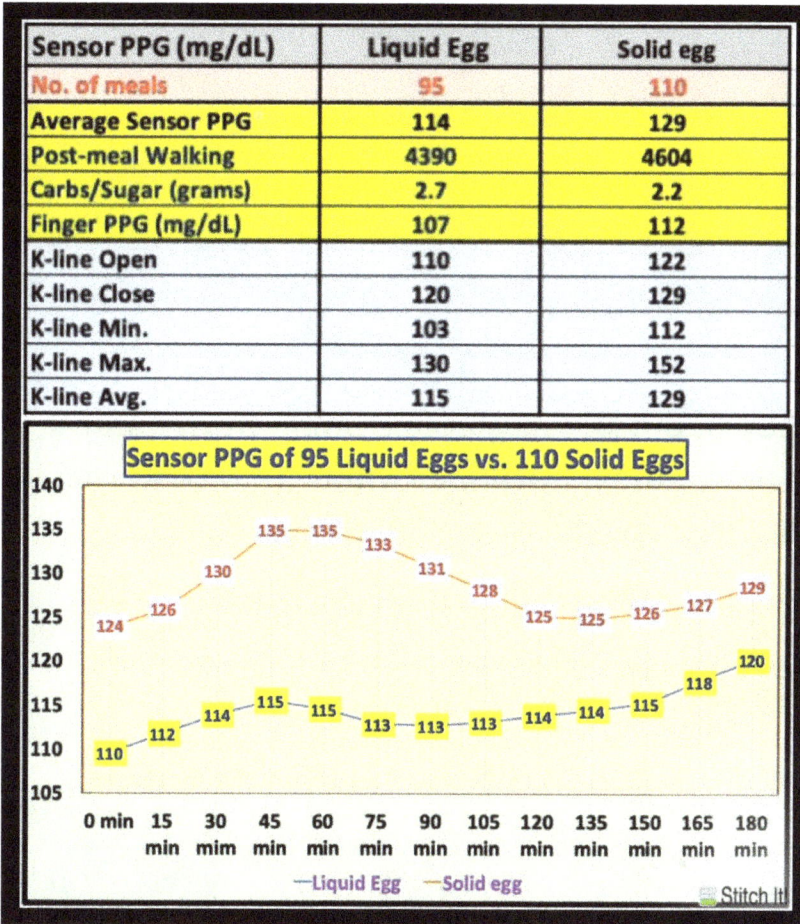

Figure 5: PPG Data and waveform Graphics Comparison between 95 Liquid egg meals and 110 Solid egg meals

Accuracy of predicted glucose using both natural intelligence (NI) and artificial intelligence (AI) via GH-Method: math-physical medicine (No. 320)

Gerald C. Hsu
eclaireMD Foundation, USA
8/28/2020

Abstract:

This paper describes the accuracy of using natural intelligence (NI) and artificial intelligence (AI) methods to predict three glucoses, including fasting plasma glucose (FPG), postprandial plasma glucose (PPG), and daily average glucose, in comparison with the actual measured PPG by using the finger-piercing (Finger) method. The entire glucose database contains 7,652 glucoses (4 glucose data per day) over 1,913 days from 6/1/2015 through 8/27/2020.

The most significant three conclusions are listed as follows:

(1) NI-based PPG prediction has an accuracy of 99.8%.
(2) NI-based daily glucose prediction has an accuracy of 100%, which is the most important factor for diabetes control.
(3) Overall, NI predicted glucose vs. finger measured glucose has an accuracy of 99.3%, while AI predicted glucose vs. finger measured glucose has an accuracy of 98.8%. NI prediction is better than AI prediction by 0.5%.

The author developed this tool with built-in AI capabilities, including auto-learning and auto-correction to make the system smarter and more accurate with additional data input. As a result, his AI prediction accuracy has reached to 98.8% and NI prediction accuracy has reached to 99.3% based on a relatively large dataset from a period of 1,913 days with 7,652 glucoses. The author observed AI and NI curves with a remarkably similar pattern (correlation of 94%), but the NI accuracy is still 0.5% better than the AI accuracy. This makes sense since his brain's NI knowledge created his AI tool.

In summary, this article demonstrates the power and usefulness of GH-Method: math-physical medicine, including AI to win the war against diabetes. He believes that these glucose prediction methods can be used as a practical tool for other T2D patients to control their daily conditions of diabetes without the cumbersome, painful, and costly traditional glucose finger-piercing test method. This is a good example of what and how mathematics, physics, and AI technology can contribute to medicine.

Introduction:

This paper describes the accuracy of using natural intelligence (NI) and artificial intelligence (AI) methods to predict three glucoses, including fasting plasma glucose (FPG), postprandial plasma glucose (PPG), and daily average glucose, in comparison with the actual measured PPG by using the finger-piercing (Finger) method. The entire glucose database contains 7,652 glucoses (4 glucose data per day) over 1,913 days from 6/1/2015 through 8/27/2020.

Methods:

To learn more about the GH-Method: math-physical medicine (MPM) methodology, readers can review the article in Reference 1 to understand his MPM analysis method.

Food database:

Starting in 2010, the author self-studied food nutrition science and four chronic diseases, including obesity, diabetes, hypertension, and hyperlipidemia.

He spent his first two years from 2011 to 2013 to build a large food database containing 6 million USDA food nutrition data and ~1.6 million re-organized franchise restaurant nutritional database from different public sources. Beginning on 5/1/2015, he kept all of his meal data with three meal photos per day. To date, he collected a total of 5,739 meal photos which have ~0.5 million personal meal nutritional data. In total, his food database contains ~8 million data. It should be noted that each photo taken by an iPhone contains 20 million pixels and each lighting pixel is expressed by a unique 8 alpha-numerical digits combination. Therefore, each meal picture contains 160 million digits and 5,739 meal pictures equate to 57.39 billion digits. This kind of mathematical calculation is indeed a " big data" operation.

NI and AI:

The author then defined a new terminology of natural intelligence as "NI" in comparison with artificial intelligence or "AI". NI uses his eyes to receive various observed food information from the meal photos, then his brain processes the information based on the past 10-years of study and learning this subject.

The author learned the subject of "machine learning" before the term "artificial intelligence" was invented. He dedicated most of his professional career on AI technology development and its various applications in different industries, including spending 14 years on the auto-design of semiconductor chips using AI. It is his opinion that human brain power is always superior to computer power, at least in the arena of logical judgement and decision making, in the foreseeable future. Therefore, he hopes that his NI-based prediction results would be more accurate than his AI-based prediction results. Of course, if there is a discrepancy of prediction accuracy between the NI and AI result, with continuous efforts to improve his AI algorithm, this discrepancy of prediction accuracy will shrink to within a negligible range.

Methodology and Tools:

Since 2014, the author has conducted his research on metabolism and glucose, including both FPG and PPG. Initially, he utilized signal processing techniques of wave theory to decompose a synthesized glucose wave (i.e. curve of data) into 19 sub-waves (influential factors) for PPG and 5 influential factors for FPG. He also calculated the contribution percentage of each influential factor of glucose. For example, he found that carbs/sugar intake amount contributes ~39% and post-meal exercise contributes ~41%, hit weather temperature contributes ~5%, and all of the remaining 16 factors contribute ~15% on PPG formation. He also identified body weight as the primary factor of FPG with a contribution ratio up to 90%, cold weather temperature contributes ~5%, and the rest of the three factors contribute 5% of FPG formation.

In early 2015, he developed an AI product via computer software program containing all of his learned knowledge of food and diabetes in the past, collected NI information from his food database, plus many other AI features, such as machine-learning, auto-judging, and self-correction capabilities.

Initially, he applied optical physics (e.g. amplitude, frequency, period, and wavelength of optical waves) to identify the physical characteristics of food and link those optical wave characteristics (i.e. color of food) with the food's molecular structural characteristics (i.e. nutritional ingredients), specifically carbs and sugar content. Next, he was able to calculate glucose generation through food intake amount based on his previous diabetes research results.

By using his MPM approach, he could bypass the necessity of detailed learning and research work of botanical molecular structures and their chemical interactions with food components. In other words, he can apply just physics and mathematics and bypass biology and chemistry to study a biomedical problem.

Based on his 10 years of diabetes research and these two different approaches of using AI and NI, he was able to develop an end-user oriented APP, known as the "AI Glucometer" (Figure 1), for diabetes patients to use in their daily life. One example of this AI Glucometer is shown in Figure 2. The yellow rectangular area in the left diagram of Figure 2 shows the high carbs/sugar area, mainly rice, and its original AI-predicted PPG was 119.0 mg/dL. After removing a small portion of this high carbs/sugar food, white rice, his AI-predicted PPG would drop down to 117.6 mg/dL.

In 2017, he developed another AI-based software (APP and software for both a smartphone and PC) using only a portion of those identified influential factors of glucose, for example 8-factors for PPG and 2-factors for FPG, to predict FPG, PPG, and daily glucose. Since PPG contributes around 75% to 80% of HbA1C, obviously, he placed more emphasis on monitoring PPG fluctuations.

Results:

In Figure 3, it reflects the conclusive data table for this article.

In Figure 4, it depicts the comparison of three PPG among breakfast, lunch, and dinner which are expressed in the following format of (measured PPG mg/dL, Predicted PPG mg/dL, Accuracy in %):

Breakfast: (118.3, 115.0, 97.3%)
Lunch: (120.0, 120.8, 99.3%)
Dinner: (113.4, 116.8, 97.1%)

In Figure 5, it shows the comparison of three glucose among FPG, PPG, and daily glucose which are expressed in the following format of (measured PPG mg/dL, Predicted PPG mg/dL, Accuracy %, correlation R %):

FPG: (115.8, 115.7, 97.3%, 99%)
PPG: (117.3, 117.6, 99.8%, 87%)
Daily glucose: (117.2, 117.2, 100%, 87%)

It should be mentioned that both Figure 4 and Figure 5 use NI-based prediction results which are slightly more accurate than AI-based prediction results as shown in Figure 6.

In Figure 6, it illustrates the comparison between predicted glucose using NI and AI, respectively. The results are as follows:

NI vs. measured glucose: 99.3%
AI vs. measured glucose: 98.8%

The top diagram in Figure 6 uses daily data which provides a more accurate average value. The bottom diagram uses 90-days moving average data which gives better views regarding curve pattern and trend while sacrificing a small amount of accuracy.

Conclusions:

The most significant three conclusions are listed as follows:

(1) NI-based PPG prediction has an accuracy of 99.8%.
(2) NI-based daily glucose prediction has an accuracy of 100%, which is the most important factor for diabetes control and HbA1C prediction.
(3) Overall, NI predicted glucose vs. finger measured glucose has an accuracy of 99.3%, while AI predicted glucose vs. finger measured glucose has an accuracy of 98.8%. *NI prediction is better than AI prediction by 0.5%.*

The author developed this tool with built-in AI capabilities, including auto-learning and auto-correction to make the system smarter and more accurate with additional data input. As a result, his AI prediction accuracy has reached to 98.8% and NI prediction accuracy has reached to 99.3% based on a relatively large dataset from a period of 1,913 days with 7,652 glucoses. The author observed AI and NI curves with a remarkably similar pattern (correlation of 94%), but the NI accuracy is still 0.5% better than the AI accuracy. This makes sense since *his brain's NI knowledge created his AI tool.*

In summary, this article demonstrates the power and usefulness of GH-Method: math-physical medicine, including AI to win the war against diabetes. He believes that these glucose prediction methods can be used as a practical tool for other T2D patients to control their daily conditions of diabetes without the cumbersome, painful, and costly traditional glucose finger-piercing test method. This is a good example of what and how mathematics, physics, and AI technology can contribute to medicine.

References:

1. Hsu, Gerald C., eclaireMD Foundation, USA, No. 310 "Biomedical research methodology based on GH-Method: math-physical medicine",

2. Hsu, Gerald C., eclaireMD Foundation, USA, No. 89: "Using GH-Method: Math-Physical Medicine to Conduct the Accuracy Comparison of Two different PPG Prediction Methods"

3. Hsu, Gerald C., eclaireMD Foundation, USA, No. 125: "Controlling type 2 diabetes via artificial intelligence technology (GH-Method: math-physical medicine)"

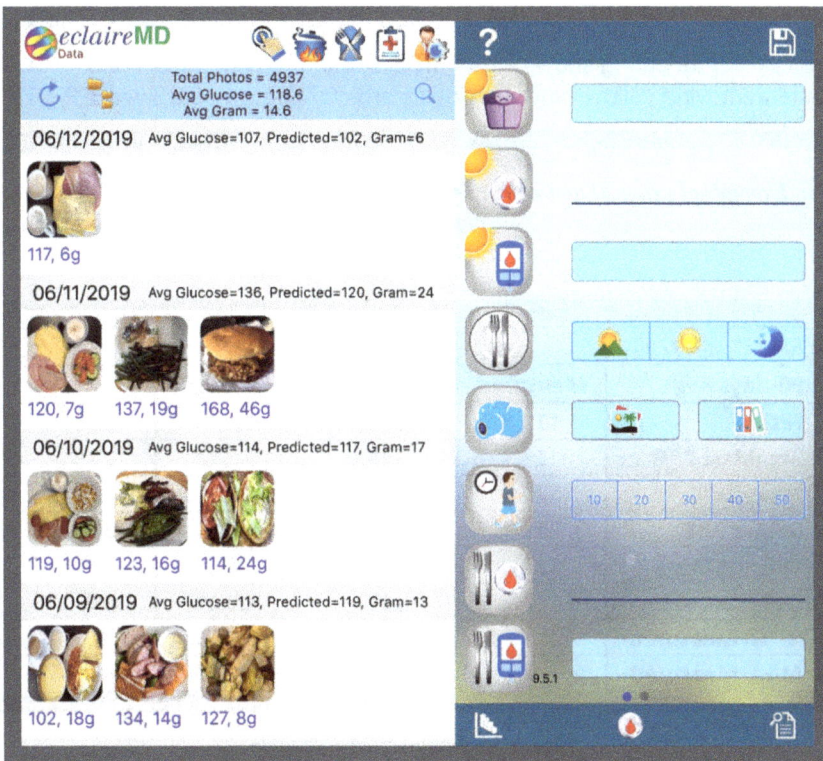

Figure 1: AI Glucometer tool

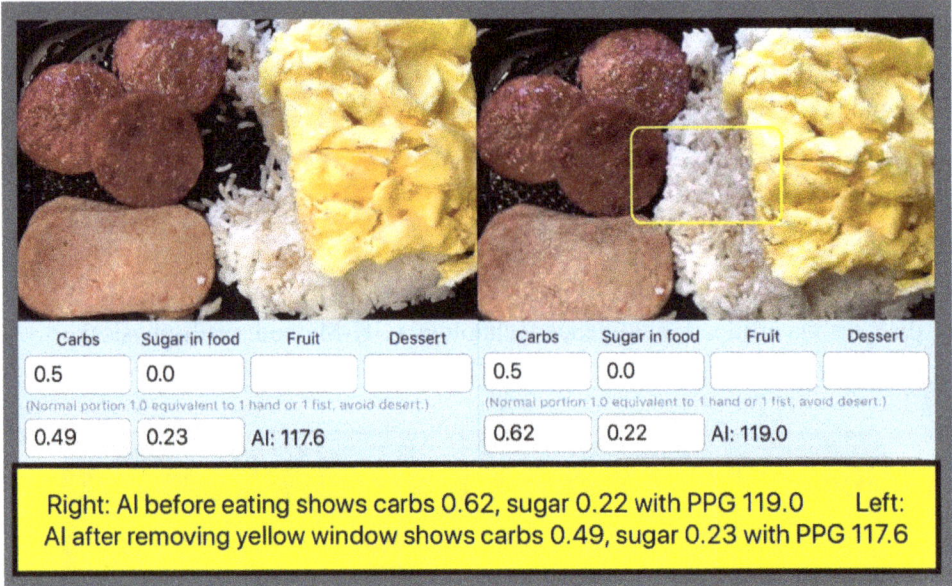

Carbs	Sugar in food	Fruit	Dessert	Carbs	Sugar in food	Fruit	Dessert
0.5	0.0			0.5	0.0		
(Normal portion 1.0 equivalent to 1 hand or 1 fist, avoid desert.)				(Normal portion 1.0 equivalent to 1 hand or 1 fist, avoid desert.)			
0.49	0.23	AI: 117.6		0.62	0.22	AI: 119.0	

Right: AI before eating shows carbs 0.62, sugar 0.22 with PPG 119.0   Left: AI after removing yellow window shows carbs 0.49, sugar 0.23 with PPG 117.6

Figure 2: Example of using AI to predict PPG (removing a small portion of white rice to reduce 1.4 mg/dL of PPG)

6/1/15-8/27/20				
90-days Avg.	**Measured**	**NI Predicted**	**1+(P-M)/M**	**Accuracy**
FPG	115.8	115.7	99.9%	99.9%
Breakfast PPG	118.3	115.0	97.3%	97.3%
Lunch PPG	120.0	120.8	100.7%	99.3%
Dinner PPG	113.4	116.8	102.9%	97.1%
PPG	117.3	117.6	100.2%	99.8%
Daily Glucose	117.2	117.2	100.0%	100.0%
NI vs. Measured			100.7%	99.3%
AI vs. Measured			101.2%	98.8%

Figure 3: Summarized data table

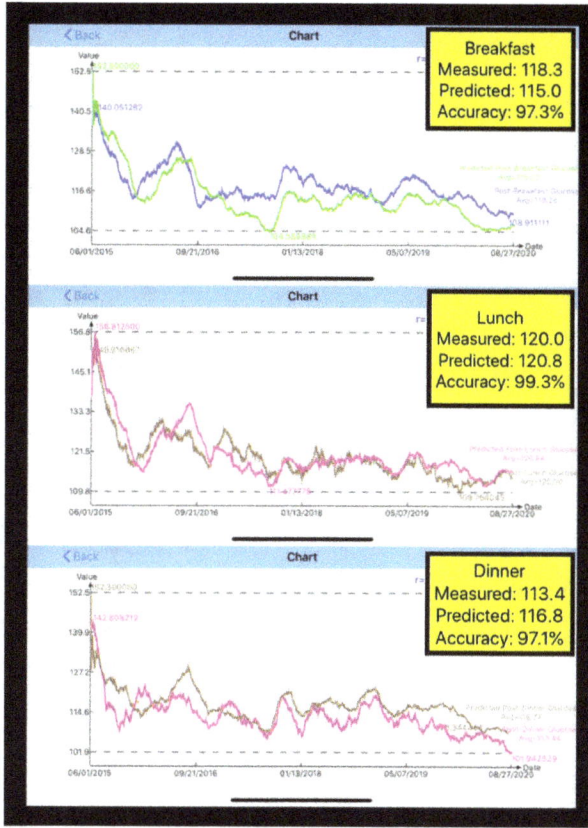

Figure 4: NI predicted PPG for Breakfast, Lunch, & Dinner

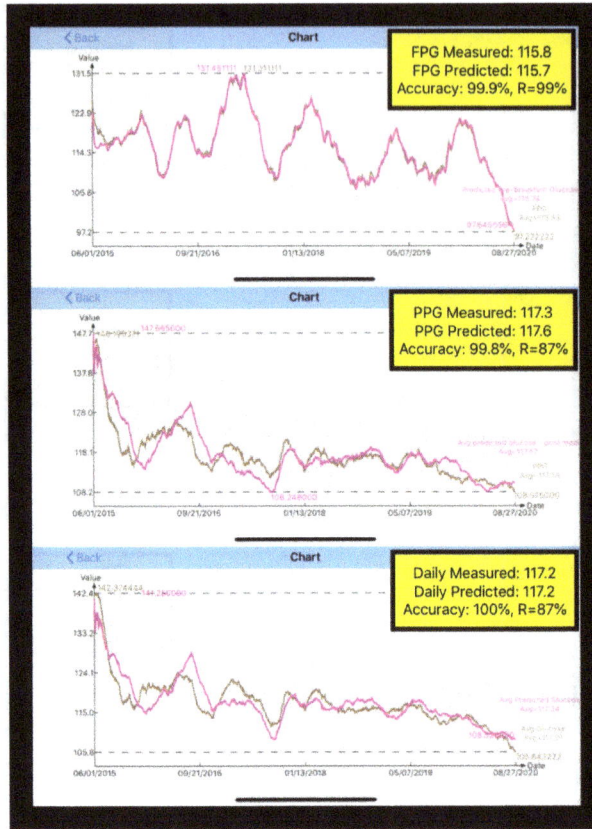

Figure 5: NI predicted PPG for FPG, PPG, & Daily glucose

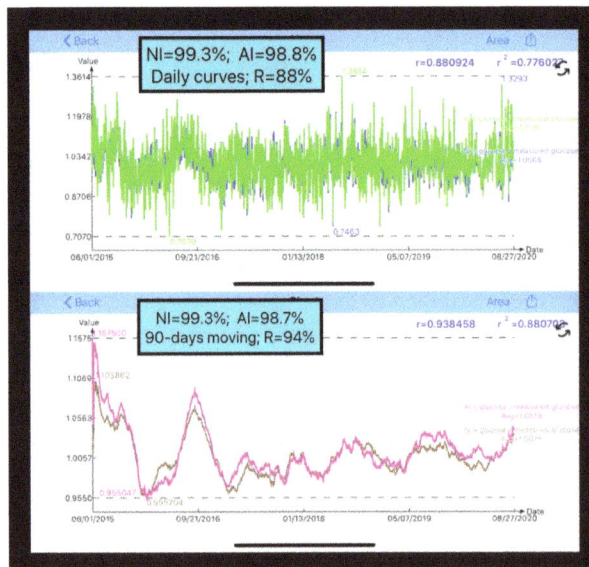

Figure 6: NI and AI Comparison against Finger measured PPG

A neurocommunication model between the brain and liver regarding glucose production and secretion in early morning using GH-Method: math-physical medicine (No. 324)

Gerald C. Hsu
eclaireMD Foundation, USA
9/5-6/2020

Abstract:

This article address the author's hypothesis on the neurocommunication model existing between the brain and liver regarding production and glucose secretion in the early morning. This is based on the observation of the difference between glucose at wake up moment in the morning for the fasting plasma glucose (FPG), and glucose at the first bite of breakfast for the glucose at 0-minute or "open glucose" of postprandial plasma glucose (PPG).

All of the eight identified glucoses of breakfast PPG are **higher** than the eight glucoses at time of wake up by a difference of an average of 8 mg/dL.
The value difference using Method B of CGM sensor glucoses during the COVID-19 period offers the most accurate picture and credible glucose difference of 8 mg/dL between his FPG at wake-up moment and PPG at the first bite of breakfast.

The author believes that the brain senses when a person wakes up due to different kinds of stimuli from many sources, including eye, environment, and even internal organs, which will alert the body to be in "active" mode requiring "energy" through glucose. Even though the person has not eaten anything or is not actively moving, the brain issues a marching order to the liver to produce or release glucose for the body to use in the forthcoming day. This hypothesis can currently explain why his glucose of eating his breakfast is ~8 mg/dL higher than his FPG at wakeup.

Introduction:

This article address the author's hypothesis on the neurocommunication model existing between the brain and liver regarding production and glucose secretion in the early morning. This is based on the observation of the difference between glucose at wake up moment in the morning for the fasting plasma glucose (FPG), and glucose at the first bite of breakfast for the glucose at 0-minute or "open glucose" of postprandial plasma glucose (PPG).

Method:

Data Collection:

The author started measuring his glucose since 1/1/2012 using traditional finger-piercing and test strip (Finger glucose) 4 times each day, once in early morning (FPG) when he just wakes up from his sleep, and three times at two-hours after each meal (PPG).

In addition, since 5/5/2018, he applied a continuous glucose monitoring (CGM) device on his upper arm and collect ~96 glucoses each day at a time interval of each 15 minutes. With this CGM-based sensor collected glucoses (Sensor glucose), he has defined his Sensor FPG as the average glucose of 28 values between 00:00 am (midnight) and 07:00 am (around the time of first bite of breakfast). In this particular analysis, he will not use the average FPG within 7 hours of nocturnal sleep time. In addition, he selected a 3-hour (180 minute) timespan after the first bite of meal as his standard Sensor PPG timeframe. As a result, he will only use his glucose at the first bite of breakfast, which is 0-minute of his breakfast PPG waveform, and disregard all of the other glucose data.

Background:

To learn more about the GH-Method: math-physical medicine (MPM) research methodology, readers can review his article, *Biomedical research methodology based on GH-Method: math-physical medicine (No. 310),* to understand his MPM analysis method.

For the past 12 months, he has researched and written approximately 10 medical papers, see an example in Reference 2, regarding the specific neurocommunication model existing between the brain and some internal organs, specifically the stomach, liver, and pancreas via observing and analyzing his glucose variances from his nearly 2 million collected data.

For the past ~8 months during the COVID-19 quarantined period (Virus period), he has achieved better results on his glucose control and metabolism maintenance due to his non-traveling, peaceful, and regular routine lifestyle (Reference 3). His average daily glucose was 115 mg/dL over a period of ~20 months, from 5/5/2018 through 1/18/2020 (Pre-Virus period), in comparison with an average daily glucose of 108 mg/dL for the recent ~8 months of Virus period.

Recently, during the Virus period, he noticed a specific phenomenon of glucose rapidly rising after his wake-up moment until the first bite of breakfast. Usually, he measures his FPG after he wakes up from his sleep, then measures his blood pressure and body weight to input these biomarker data into his APP software. Finally, he prepares his simple breakfast, normally containing egg and coffee. During this entire time period, usually within 30 to 45 minutes, he does not eat anything else or has any physical activity (his total walking steps is around 100 steps on average). Surprisingly, he noticed that his *fast-rising glucose* makes his glucose at the moment from the first bite of his meal higher than the glucose at his wake-up moment. The timespan between these two moments is within ~45 minutes without any external influences from diet and exercise; therefore, he wonders why this occurred and what is the difference in glucose over a longer period of time?

Results:

First, he chose three different periods:

Virus period:
(1/19/2020 - 9/6/2020)

Pre-Virus period:
(5/5/2018 - 1/18/2020)

Total period:
(5/5/2018 - 9/6/2020)

Secondly, he chose three different analytical methods described below to calculate the glucose values he desired:

Method A: He uses time series analysis to calculate his average FPG value measured at wake-up moment. Please note that he used finger FPG for Pre-Virus period and CGM sensor FPG at wake-up moment for Virus period. Therefore, his glucose data comparison during Pre-Virus period has deteriorated on data accuracy due to data inconsistency between finger FPG and sensor PPG. In his previous research papers, he already identified his average sensor glucose as being higher than his average finger glucose. As a result, his glucose data comparison during the Virus period has the highest degree of data accuracy due to data consistency between sensor FPG and sensor PPG.

Method B: He uses segmented pattern analysis to calculate and generate a "synthesized" PPG waveform of breakfast and then single out the breakfast PPG at 0-minute. He also applies the "Candlestick K-line" model (Reference 4) to double check his breakfast PPG at 0-minute (i.e. "open" glucose of breakfast candlestick) to make sure these two values are identical. Please note that this second step uses CGM data only since Finger glucose contains one-point data which cannot represent a curve or waveform.

Method C: He uses synthesized *all-day glucose waveform* from 00:00 throughout 23:45 with a total of 96 glucose data-points for each day. He then summarized those 231 days' data for Virus period, 620 days' data for Pre-Virus period, and 851 days' data for Total period to generate a *synthesized* all-day glucose waveform. He chose two glucose values at 06:00 am as his "approximate" wake up moment and 07:00 am as his "approximate" first bite moment of breakfast. Although he is a very disciplined person, he cannot wake up every morning consistently at 06:15 and eats his breakfast at 07:00 every day. Therefore, the glucose data comparison using Method C has the highest margin of error, i.e. lowest data accuracy.

Figures 1, 2, and 3 show the resulting diagrams of his measured FPG at wake up moment, breakfast PPG waveform, breakfast PPG K-line, PPG at first bite of breakfast, and the glucose difference between these two different moments in the three respective periods using Method A and Method B.

Summarized glucose differences are listed below:

Virus: 8 mg/dL (most accurate)
Pre-virus: 10 mg/dL (less accurate)
Total: 9 mg/dL (hybrid in-between)
Average: 9 mg/dL

Figures 4, 5, and 6 show the diagram results of his synthesized daily glucose curve over 24 hours with a data table containing his FPG at wake up moment and his PPG at first bite of his breakfast, and the glucose difference between these two different moments in the three respective periods using Method C. As mentioned above, this set of glucose comparison has the lowest data accuracy due to his exact wake-up time is not consistently at 06:15 am (usually between 5:30 am and 7:30 am), and the time of first bite of breakfast is not consistently at 07:00 am (about 80% at 7:00 am).

The summarized glucose differences are listed below:

Virus: 10 mg/dL (higher than A & B)
Pre-virus: 4 mg/dL (longer period)
Total: 7 mg/dL (hybrid in-between)
Average: 7 mg/dL

By analyzing the above observations of 8 glucose difference values, except the 4 mg/dL glucose difference during pre-virus period using Method C (i.e. using a synthesized daily glucose curve and two fixed time instants), all of the other 7 glucose difference values are between 7 mg/dL to 10 mg/dL. However, *the result of 8 mg/dL glucose difference value using Method B of CGM sensor glucoses during virus period offers the most accurate picture and reliable glucose difference of 8 mg/dL between his FPG at wake up moment and PPG at the first bite (i.e. 0-minute) of his breakfast.*

Figure 7 contains the most important and conclusive information for this article because it shows the background data table and its associated bar charts. *It is obvious that all of the glucoses of breakfast PPG at first bite are higher than those glucoses at the wake-up moment, by a difference of an average amount of 8 mg/dL.*

Now the question is why this phenomenon occurred.

The author believes that the brain senses when a person wakes up due to different kinds of stimuli from many sources, including eye, environment, and even internal organs, which will alert the body to be in "active" mode requiring "energy" through glucose. Even though the person has not eaten anything or is not actively moving, the brain issues a marching order to the liver to produce or release glucose for the body to use in the forthcoming day. As a result, this currently explains why his glucose of eating his breakfast is higher than his FPG at wake-up moment.

The author developed his hypothesis using a method he learned in business statistics, decision making through elimination. In order to explain his observed phenomenon of higher glucose, he collected 8 possible sources or inputs: A is diet, B is exercise, C is body weight, D is weather temperature, E is stress, F is illness, G is sleep condition, and H is un-identified source. For two glucose values occurring within ~45 minutes on the same day and in the same living environment, he could rule out possible inputs of C, D, E, F, and G. Besides, C for body weight and D for weather temperature are already identified as the two major influential factors in his predicted FPG. In addition, he does not have any influences from A for diet and B for exercise before eating his breakfast. As a result, the remaining factor is H for the un-identified source or input factor. The unknown factor is the brain through the nervous system communicating with the internal organs. This is how the author established his hypothesis via the specific evidence of glucose difference value for the early morning.

Conclusions:

This article is slightly different from the author's earlier research work focusing on the same subject of neuro-communication models between the brain and organs, such as the stomach, liver, and pancreas. His previous papers were based on the observation of PPG differences using the same food material and different cooking methods, resulting with food in different physical states. For this article, it has nothing to do with food but addresses the same neurological phenomenon through observation of his two glucoses in the early morning.

As he conduct more research on neuroscience, the more fascinated he gets with this particular subject . In the body, all of the organs are interconnected with the brain via the nervous system and blood system. Lifestyle affects the entire body; therefore, lifestyle is linked to metabolism which further affects the immune system to defend the body from many diseases. As a result, we must manage our lifestyle extremely well in order to maintain good health.

References:

1. Hsu, Gerald C. (2020). eclaireMD Foundation, USA. "Biomedical research methodology based on GH-Method: math-physical medicine (No. 310)."

2. Hsu, Gerald C. (2020). eclaireMD Foundation, USA. "Self-recovery of pancreatic beta cell's insulin secretion based on annualized fasting plasma glucose, baseline postprandial plasma glucose, and baseline daily glucose data using GH-Method: math-physical medicine (No. 297)."

3. Hsu, Gerald C. (2020). eclaireMD Foundation, USA. "Diabetes control and metabolism maintenance during COVID-19 period in comparison to three other periods using GH-Method: math-physical medicine (No.288)."

4. Hsu, Gerald C. (2020). eclaireMD Foundation, USA. "Comparison study of PPG characteristics from candlestick model using GH-Method: Math-Physical Medicine (No. 261)."

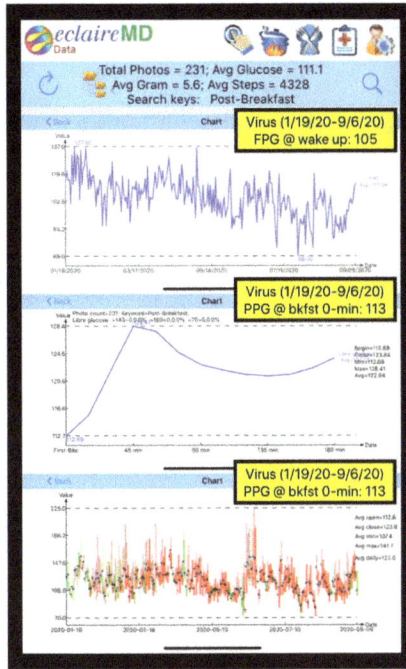

Figure 1: Virus period (Method A and Method B)

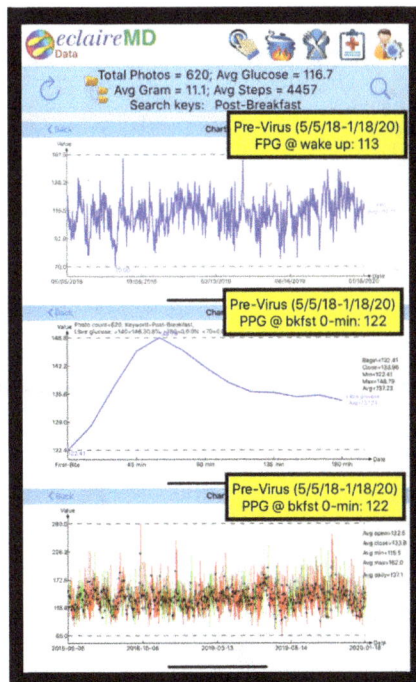

Figure 2: Pre-Virus period (Method A and Method B)

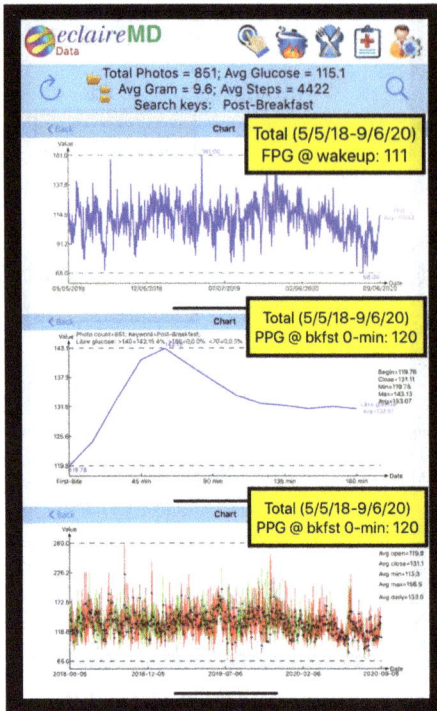

Figure 3: Total period (Method A and Method B)

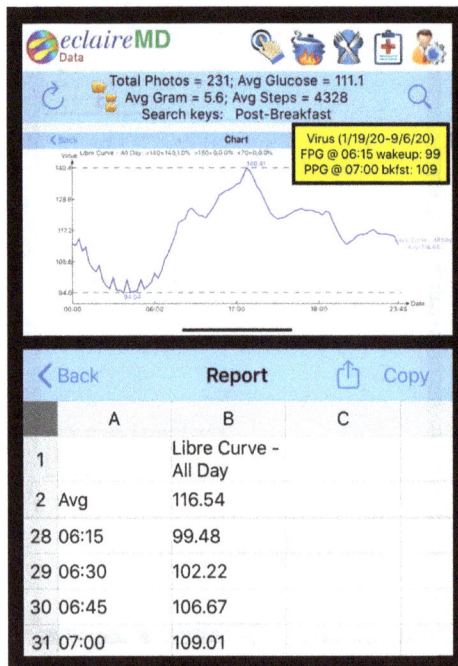

Figure 4: Virus period (Method C)

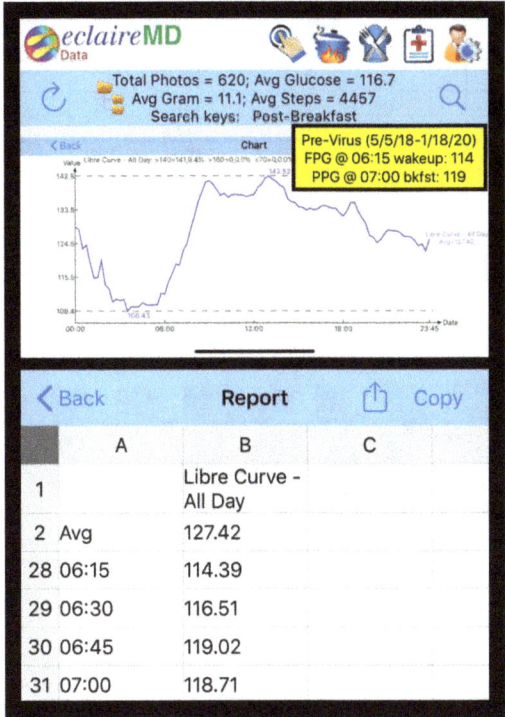

Figure 5: Pre-Virus period (Method C)

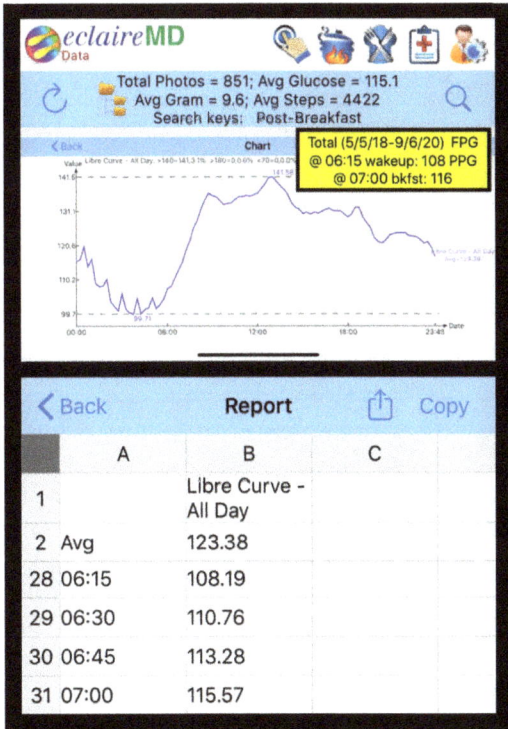

Figure 6: Total period (Method C)

	Difference (mg/dL)	FPG at wakeup	PPG at first bite of breakfast
Virus period	8	105	113
Pre-Virus period	10	113	122
Total period	9	111	120
Average (measured)	9	109	118
Virus period	10	99	109
Pre-virus period	4	114	119
Total period	7	108	116
Average (daily curve)	7	107	114

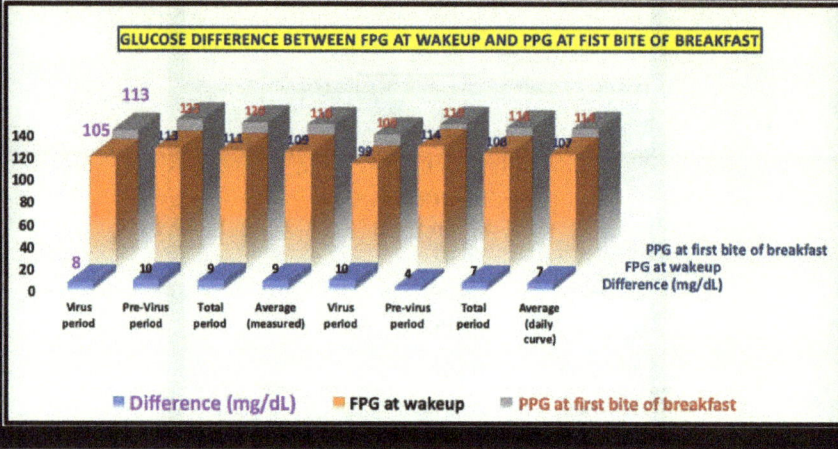

Figure 7: Data table and Bar chart of three periods (~8 mg/dL of glucose difference in early morning)

Investigating the influential factors on body weight and its impact on glucoses using GH-Method: math-physical medicine (No. 327)

Gerald C. Hsu
eclaireMD Foundation, USA
9/11/2020

Abstract:

The author attempts to identify three major and two secondary influential factors of body weight along with its impact on six different glucose components using Pearson correlation coefficient "R" of statistics to calculate different degree of association between two datasets. This investigation utilized the daily weight and glucose data in conjunction with six lifestyle details, including food, exercise, water, sleep, and weather temperature, during a period of ~6 years from 1/1/2015 to 9/11/2020.

Weight's influential factors:
Food quantity: + 47% (the more you eat, the higher your weight)
Daily walking steps: - 52% (the more you exercise, the lower your weight, recommend walking within 20,000 steps per day)
Water intake: - 48% (the more water you drink, the lower your weight, recommend within 3,000 cc per day)
Sleep hours: +24% (low moderate R)
Sleep quality: +16% (low moderate R)

Obesity is the root cause of three chronic diseases such as diabetes, hypertension, and hyperlipidemia. They can cause many other complications including, but not limited to, cardiovascular disease (CVD), stroke, chronic kidney disease (CKD), foot ulcer, diabetic retinopathy, hypothyroidism, dementia, and even cancer. As a result, individuals should focus on weight control as their first priority to be able to control other chronic diseases.

In the United States, approximately 36.5% of adults are obese and another 32.5% are overweight. In other words, there are only 31% of American adults within the normal range of body weight (BMI < 25). The author weighed 220 lbs. (110 kg) with a BMI of 32 in 2010. From 2015 to 2020, his average weight was reduced to 173 lbs. (78.6 kg) with a BMI of 25.54. Recently, his weight has further decreased to 169 lbs. (76.8 kg) with a BMI of 24.95. From his 10-year journey, he definitely understands how hard it is to reduce his body weight. During the past decade, he conducted research on metabolism, endocrinology, and various complications induced by chronic diseases; however, he was not able to identify a clear and significant influential factor for weight control. Occasionally, he feels that weight seems to have a mind on its own randomly fluctuating according to its will. Of course, he also realized that weight must have certain controlling factors within itself

At least, in this study, he is able to prove his intuitive feeling that "**meal portion**" or **"food quantity"** is one of the most important contributing factors, even with a moderate R of 47%. In addition, adequate exercise and sufficient water intake assisted with his weight reduction.

With the higher correlation coefficients between weight and glucose components have been demonstrated many times in his previous published papers, he discovered the most efficient way to control his glucose is to concentrate on his body weight first.

Introduction:

The author attempts to identify three major and two secondary influential factors of body weight along with its impact on six different glucose components using Pearson correlation coefficient "R" of statistics to calculate different degree of association between two datasets. This investigation utilized the daily weight and glucose data in conjunction with six lifestyle details, including food, exercise, water, sleep, and weather temperature, during a period of ~6 years from 1/1/2015 to 9/11/2020.

Method:

Background:
To learn more about the GH-Method: math-physical medicine (MPM) research methodology, readers can review his specific article, *Biomedical research methodology based on GH-Method: math-physical medicine (No. 310),* to understand his MPM analysis method.

Data Collection:
The author started measuring his body weight since 1/1/2012. He measures weight twice a day, once in early morning when he wakes up and at night when he is ready to go to sleep. In addition, he uses the traditional finger-piercing and test strip (Finger glucose) to measure his daily glucoses. He measures his glucoses four times each day, once in early morning (FPG) when he wakes up from sleeping, and three times at two-hours after each meal (PPG).

In order to estimate his metabolism situation using his developed mathematical metabolism index (MI) model, he needs to collect many of his lifestyle details. Most of his lifestyle data collection started approximately on 1/1/2015. The following six items are required to conduct this particular study.

(1) Food quantity: percentage of his normal meal portion
(2) Daily walking steps
(3) Daily water intake amount
(4) Sleep hours
(5) Sleep quality: includes 9 elements
(6) Ambient weather temperature: using the highest temperature around noon time each day

Correlation coefficients:
Here is an excerpt from Wikipedia:

*A **correlation coefficient** is a numerical measure of some type of correlation, meaning a statistical relationship between two variables. The variables may be two columns of a given data set of observations, often called a sample, or two components of a* multivariate random variable with a known distribution. Several types of correlation coefficient exist, each with their own definition and own range of usability and characteristics.

The Pearson product-moment correlation coefficient, also known as r, R, or Pearson's r, is a measure of the strength and direction of the linear relationship between two variables that is defined as the covariance of the variables divided by the product of their standard deviations. This is the best-known and most commonly used type of correlation coefficient. When the term "correlation coefficient" is used without further qualification, it usually refers to the Pearson product-moment correlation coefficient. Sometimes, it is also called the "bivariate correlation" which is a statistic that measures linear correlation between two variables X and Y. It has a value between +1 and −1. A value of +1 is total positive linear correlation, 0 is no linear correlation, and −1 is total negative linear correlation.

Time series analysis:
All of the variables mentioned above including weight, glucose, and six lifestyle details are expressed in a form of the "time-series curve". These curves have two axes. The horizontal x-axis is time (date) from 1/1/2015 throughout 9/11/2020 and the vertical y-axis is the amount of weight, glucose, or lifestyle details corresponding to different date on the x-axis. In order to avoid the "over-presentation" of the graphic results, the author does not include all of these time-series curves in the graphs section in this paper. As an alternative, he presents a summarized data table that includes all of the important and conclusive data related to the variables such as weight, glucose, lifestyles, and their corresponding correlation coefficients.

Results:

In Figure 1, it shows the summarized background data of this study. As a result, Figures 2, 3, and 4 are produced based on this background data table.

Figure 2 only shows the R between Weight and six lifestyle inputs. The correlation coefficient R can only be calculated between two variables. The objectives are to identify what influential factors that actually control his body weight. With this purpose in mind, his weight variable becomes the common denominator of this entire analysis. Consequently, he went through many calculations of R to search for the significant influential factors of weight. At the end, he only identified five significant factors. The R of the ambient weather temperature is almost zero percent (-5%); therefore, it does not have a noticeable influence on weight. During the process of searching and calculation, he also discovered some more evidences regarding the impact of his weight on his glucoses associated with his three daily meals. As shown in Figure 3, his body weight has different degrees of influences on all of the six glucose components, including breakfast PPG, lunch PPG, dinner PPG, daily PPG, FPG, and daily average glucose.

The following descriptions highlight the conclusions drawn from Figures 1, 2, and 3. It is expressed in terms of individual correlation coefficient percentage of R.

(A) Weight's influential factors:
Food quantity: +47% (the more you eat, the higher your weight)
Daily walking steps: -52% (the more you exercise, the lower your weight, recommend

walking within 20,000 steps per day)
Water intake: -48% (the more water you drink, the lower your weight, recommend within 3,000 cc per day)
Sleep hours: +24%
(low moderate R)
Sleep quality: +16%
(low moderate R)
Weather temperature: -5% (negligible R)

Food quantity, exercise level, and water intake amount have moderate influences on body weight. In contrast, sleep has a low moderate influence on weight, while weather temperature has a negligible influence on weight (-5%).

(B) Weight's impact on glucoses:
Breakfast PPG: 58%
Lunch PPG: 73%
Dinner PPG: 67%
PPG: 70%
FPG: 67%
Daily average glucose: 74%

Body weight has quite high correlation coefficients with all of the six glucose components; therefore, weight definitely has a strong impact on glucoses. This conclusion can be observed via the two time-series curves between weight vs. FPG and weight vs. PPG (Figure 4).

In Figure 5, it depicts an interesting finding in this weight study. His average weight gain is +2.51 lbs. during the daytime and his average weight loss is -2.47 lbs. during his sleep time over this ~6-year period. These two values almost cancel out each other. As a result, his weight has been maintained around 173 lbs. with a BMI of ~25 for the past ~6 years. This fact further demonstrate an important message regarding his satisfaction with the overall metabolism situation because body weight contains many vital information for both medical conditions and lifestyle details.

Conclusions:

Obesity is the root cause of three chronic diseases such as diabetes, hypertension, and hyperlipidemia. They can cause many other complications including, but not limited to, cardiovascular disease (CVD), stroke, chronic kidney disease (CKD), foot ulcer, diabetic retinopathy, hypothyroidism, dementia, and even cancer. As a result, individuals should focus on weight control as their first priority to be able to control other chronic diseases.

In the United States, approximately 36.5% of adults are obese and another 32.5% are overweight. In other words, there are only 31% of American adults within the normal range of body weight (BMI < 25). The author weighed 220 lbs. (110 kg) with a BMI of 32 in 2010. From 2015 to 2020, his average weight was reduced to 173 lbs. (78.6

kg) with a BMI of 25.54. Recently, his weight has further decreased to 169 lbs. (76.8 kg) with a BMI of 24.95. From his 10-year journey, he definitely understands how hard it is to reduce his body weight. During the past decade, he conducted research on metabolism, endocrinology, and various complications induced by chronic diseases; however, he was not able to identify a clear and significant influential factor for weight control. Occasionally, he feels that weight seems to have a mind on its own randomly fluctuating according to its will. Of course, he also realized that weight must have certain controlling factors within itself

At least, in this study, he is able to prove his intuitive feeling that **"meal portion"** or **"food quantity"** is one of the most important contributing factors, even with a moderate R of 47%. In addition, adequate exercise and sufficient water intake assisted with his weight reduction.

With the higher correlation coefficients between weight and glucose components have been demonstrated many times in his previous published papers, he discovered the most efficient way to control his glucose is to concentrate on his body weight first.

References:

1. Hsu, Gerald C., eclaireMD Foundation, USA, No. 310: "Biomedical research methodology based on GH-Method: math-physical medicine"

2. Hsu, Gerald C., eclaireMD Foundation, USA, No. 320: "Accuracy of predicted glucose using both natural intelligence (NI) and artificial intelligence (AI) via GH-Method: math-physical medicine"

3. Hsu, Gerald C., eclaireMD Foundation, USA, No. 307: "Weight control trend analysis and progressive behavior modification of a T2D patient using GH-Method: math-physical medicine"

4. Hsu, Gerald C., eclaireMD Foundation, USA, No. 288: "Diabetes control and metabolism maintenance during COVID-19 period in comparison to three other periods using GH-Method: math-physical medicine"

5. Hsu, Gerald C., eclaireMD Foundation, USA, No. 11: "Relationship Between Weight and Glucose Using Math-Physics Medicine"

6. Hsu, Gerald C., eclaireMD Foundation, USA, No. 321: "Postprandial plasma glucose segmentation analysis of influences from diet and exercise between the pre-COVID-19 and COVID-19 periods"

7. Hsu, Gerald C., eclaireMD Foundation, USA, No. 312: "Segmentation analysis of impact on glucoses via diet, exercise, and weather temperature during COVID-19 quarantine period"

8. Hsu, Gerald C., eclaireMD Foundation, USA, No. 325: "Segmentation and pattern analyses of three meals' PPG using GH-Method: math-physical medicine"

(1/1/2015 - 9/11/2020)		Morning Weight = 173.21 lbs	
Weight inputs:	**Correlation**	**Real Data**	**Note:**
Food quantity	47%	83%	Moderate association
Daily Exercise	-52%	16652 steps	Moderate association
Water drinking	-48%	2898 cc (5.8 bottles)	Moderate association
Sleep hours	24%	7.1 hours	Negligible association
Sleep Quality	16%	63%	Negligible association
Weather temperature	-5%	73 degree F	Almost no association
Weight Impacts:	**Correlation**	**Real Data**	**Note:**
Breakfast PPG	58%	119.49 mg/dL%	Moderate association
Lunch PPG	73%	121.92 mg/dL%	Moderate association
Dinner PPG	67%	115.01 mg/dL%	Moderate association
PPG	70%	118.98 mg/dL%	Moderate association
FPG	67%	116.78 mg/dL%	Moderate association
Daily Glucose	74%	118.66 mg/dL%	Moderate association
Glucose, Food, Weight	**Correlation**	**Real Data**	**Note:**
FPG & Food quantity	53%	116.78 mg/dL & 83%	Moderate association
PPG & Food quantity	82%	118.98 mg/dL & 83%	Very strong association
weight loss & gain	-96%	Weight loss in sleep: -2.47 lbs	Weight gain in day: +2.51 lbs

Figure 1: Background data table (1/1/2015 - 9/11/2020)

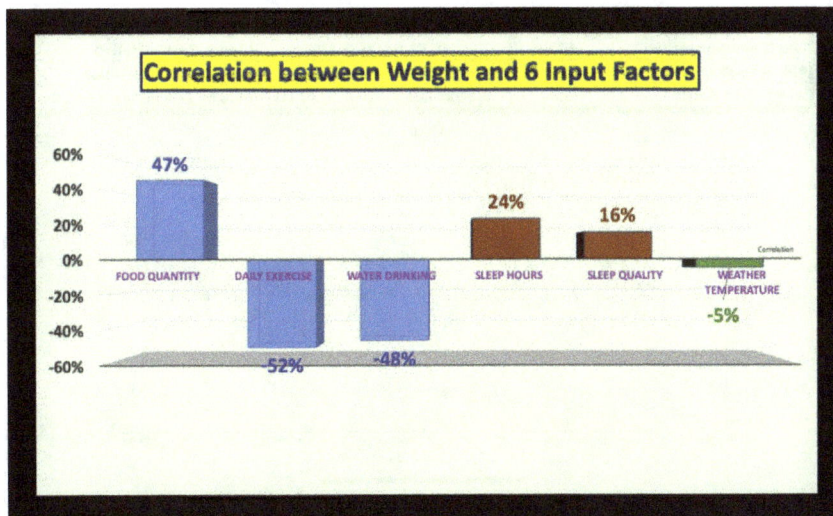

Figure 2: 6 R values between weight and 6 influential factors (1/1/2015 - 9/11/2020)

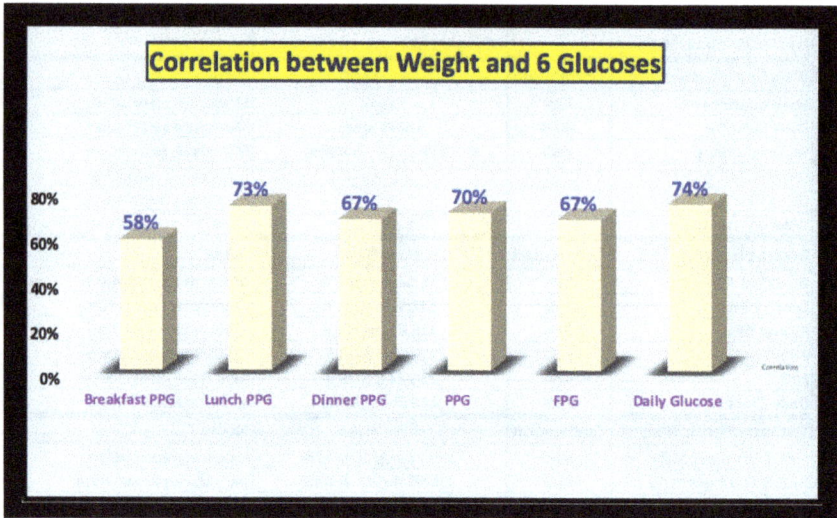

Figure 3: 6 R values of weight impact on 6 glucose components (1/1/2015 - 9/11/2020)

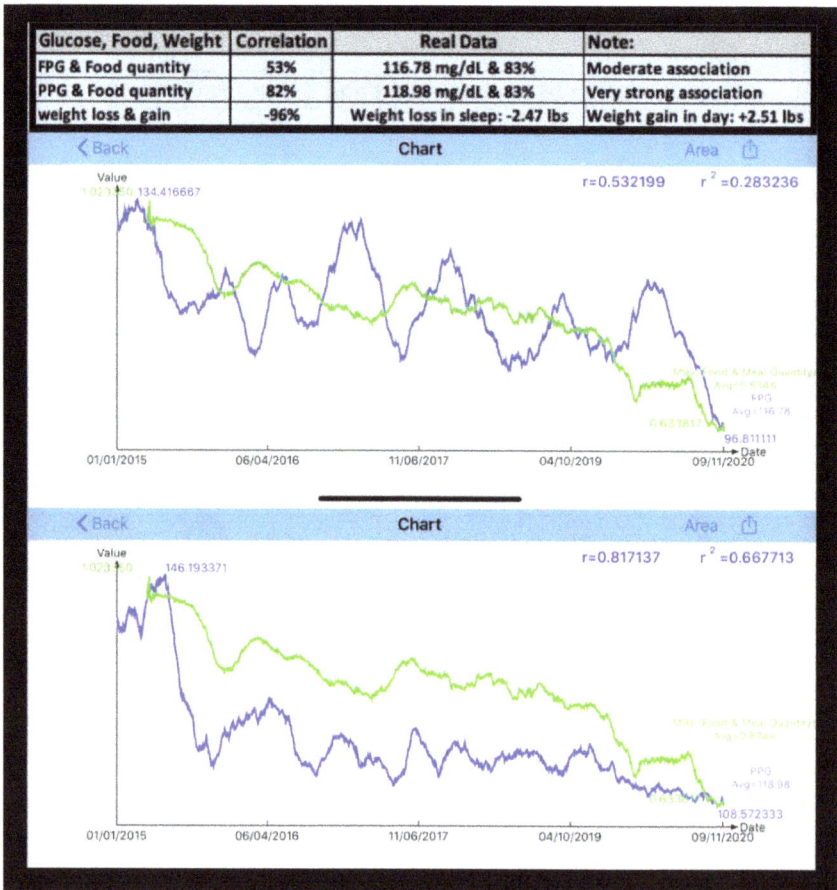

Figure 4: Time-series curves of weight vs. FPG and weight vs. PPG (1/1/2015 - 9/11/2020)

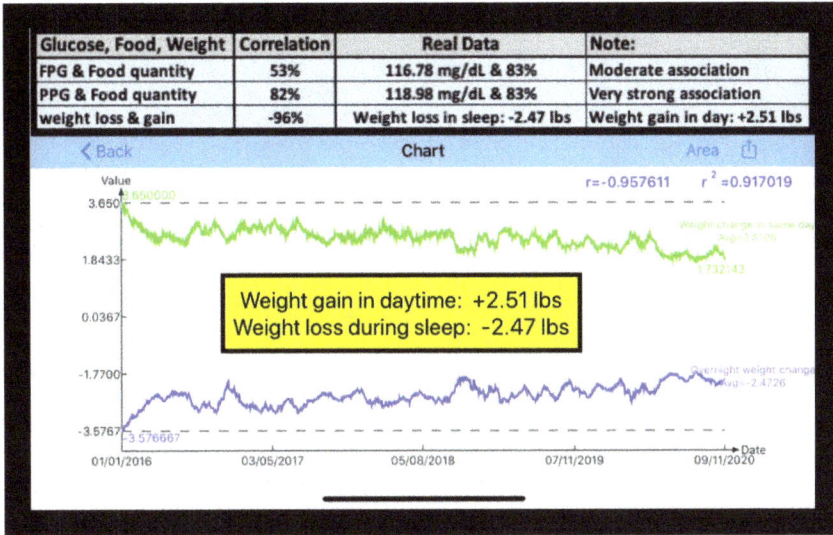

Glucose, Food, Weight	Correlation	Real Data	Note:
FPG & Food quantity	53%	116.78 mg/dL & 83%	Moderate association
PPG & Food quantity	82%	118.98 mg/dL & 83%	Very strong association
weight loss & gain	-96%	Weight loss in sleep: -2.47 lbs	Weight gain in day: +2.51 lbs

Figure 5: Averaged weigh gain in daytime and averaged weight loss during sleep time (1/1/2015 – 9/11/2020)

Self-recovery of pancreatic beta cell's insulin secretion based on 10+ years annualized data of food, exercise, weight, and glucose using GH-Method: math-physical medicine (No. 339)

By: Gerald C. Hsu
eclaireMD Foundation, USA
10/1-2/2020

Abstract:

The author was inspired from reading two recently published medical papers regarding pancreatic beta cells insulin secretion or diabetes reversal via weight reduction. The weight reduction is directly related to the patient's lifestyle improvement through diet and exercise. He has published six medical papers on beta cells based on different stages in observations of his continuous glucose improvements; therefore, in this article, he will investigate food ingredients, meal portions, weight, and glucose improvement based on his 10+ years of collected big data.

Here are the summaries of his findings:

1. His successful weight reduction, from 220 lbs. in 2010 to 171 lbs. in 2020, comes from his food portion reduction and exercise increase.
2. His lower carbs/sugar intake amount, from 40 grams in 2010 to 12 grams in 2020, is resulted from his learned food nutrition knowledge and meal portion reduction, from 150% in 2010 to 67% in 2020.
3. His weight reduction contributes to his FPG reduction, from 220 mg/dL in 2010 to 104 mg/dL in 2020. His carbs/sugar control and increased walking steps, from 2,000 steps in 2010 to ~16,000 steps in 202, have contributed to his PPG reduction, from 300 mg/dL in 2010 to 109 mg/dL in 2020. When both FPG and PPG are reduced, his daily glucose is decreased as well, from 280 mg/dL in 2010 to 108 mg/dL in 2020.
4. His damaged beta cell's insulin production and functionality, most likely, have been repaired about 16% for the past 6 years or 27% in the past 10 years at a self-repair rate of 2.7% per year.

The conclusion from this paper is a *2.7% annual beta cells self-repair rate* which is similar to his previously published papers regarding his range of pancreatic beta cells self-recovery of insulin secretion with an annual rate between 2.3% to 3.2%.

To date, the author has written seven papers discussing his pancreatic beta cell's self-recovery of insulin secretion. In his first six papers (see References 2 through 7), he used several different "cutting angles" or "analysis approaches" to delve deeper into this complex biomedical subject and achieved consistent results within the range of 2.3% to 3.2% of annual self-recovery rate.

He used a quantitative approach with precision to discover and reconfirm his pancreatic beta cell's health state by linking it backwards step-by-step with his collected data of glucose, weight, diet, and exercise. He has produced another dataset for a self-repair rate of 2.7% which is located right in the middle between 2.3% and 3.2% from his previous findings.

In his opinion, type 2 diabetes (T2D) is no longer a non-reversible or non-curable disease. Diabetes is not only "controllable" but it is also "self-repairable", even though at a rather slow rate. He would like to share his research findings and his persistent efforts from the past decade with his medical research colleagues and to provide encouragement to motivate other T2D patients like himself to reverse their diabetes conditions.

Introduction:

The author was inspired from reading two recently published medical papers regarding pancreatic beta cells insulin secretion or diabetes reversal via weight reduction. The weight reduction is directly related to the patient's lifestyle improvement through diet and exercise. He has published six medical papers on beta cells based on different stages in observations of his continuous glucose improvements; therefore, in this article, he will investigate food ingredients, meal portions, weight, and glucose improvement based on his 10+ years of collected big data.

Methods:

Background:

To learn more about his developed GH-Method: math-physical medicine (MPM) research methodology, readers can review his article, Biomedical research methodology based on GH-Method: math-physical medicine (No. 54 and No. 310), in Reference 1 to understand his MPM analysis method.

Diabetes history:

In 1995, the author was diagnosed with severe type 2 diabetes (T2D). His daily average glucose reached 280 mg/dL with a peak glucose at 398 mg/dL and his HbA1C was at 10% in 2010. Since 2005, he has suffered many kinds of diabetes complications, including five cardiac episodes (without having a stroke), foot ulcer, renal complications, bladder infection, diabetic retinopathy, and hypothyroidism.

As of 9/30/2020, his daily average glucose is approximately 106 mg/dL and HbA1C at 6.1%. It should be mentioned that he started to reduce the dosage of his three different diabetes medications (maximum dosages) in early 2013 and finally stop taking them on 12/8/2015. In other words, his glucose record since 2016 to the present is totally "medication-free".

Beginning on 1/1/2012, he started to collect his weight value in the early morning and his glucose values four times a day: FPG x1 in the early morning and PPG x3 at two hours after the first bite of each meal. Since 1/1/2014, he also started to collect his carbs/sugar amount in grams and post-meal walking steps. Prior to these two dates, especially during the period of 2010 to 2012, the manually collected biomarkers and lifestyle details were scattered and unorganized. Therefore, those annualized data from 2010 to 2012 or 2014 were guesstimated values with his best effort. It should be further mentioned that on 1/1/2013, he began to reduce his dosages of three diabetes educations step by step. By 1/1/2015, he was only taking 500 mg of Metformin for controlling his diabetes conditions. Finally, he completely ceased taking Metformin on 12/8/2015; therefore, since 1/1/2016, his body has been completely free of any diabetes medications.

Other research results:

Recently, a Danish medical research team has published an article on JAMA which emphasizes a strengthen lifestyle program can "reverse" T2D. This program includes a weekly exercise (5-6 times and 30-60 minutes each time), daily walking more than 10,000 steps using smart phone to keep a record, personalized diet and nutritional guidance by healthcare professionals, etc. The observed results from this Danish report are patients' overall HbA1C reduction of 0.31%, and their diabetes medication dosage reduction from 73% to 26%.

DiRECT research report from UK also indicated that an aggressive weight reduction program can induce improvement on diabetes conditions. This UK program includes low-calories diet for 3-5 months with 825-853 K-calories per day, plus daily walking of 15,000 steps per day. The observed results from this UK report are patients' overall HbA1C reduction of 0.9%, weight reduction of 10 kg (or 22 lbs.), and reduced diabetes medication dosage as well.

The author's approach:

Inspired by the results from the two European studies and based on his own collected big data over the past 10+ years, from 2010 to 2020, he decided to conduct a similar research on his own. He has separated his 10+ years data into two periods. The first period of 5 years, from 2010 to 2014, with partially collected and partially guesstimated data under different degrees of medication influence, and the second period of 6 years, from 2015 to 2020, with a complete set of collected raw data stored in software and sever without any medication influence.

His trend of thoughts include a sequence from cause to consequence as listed below from top to bottom:

Food and meal's portion %
K-calories per day
Weight (lbs.)
FPG (mg/dL)
Carbs/sugar intake (grams)
Walking
PPG (mg/dL)
Daily glucose (mg/dL)

He has further conducted nine calculations of correlation coefficient based on the above parameters to examine the degree of connections between any 2 elements of these total 8 parameters. It should be mentioned that the correlation coefficients can only be done between two data sets, or two curves.

More importantly, in addition to examining the raw data, he also placing an emphasis on the *annual change rate percentage*, its trend, and their comparisons of these 8 parameters.

Results:

Figure 1 shows his background data table which includes his calculated annual averages of the 8 parameters plus proteins, fat, and daily K-calories, based on his daily data collected during 2010 to 2020.

Figure 2 depicts the annual change rate percentage of his food (meal portion %, K-calories, and carbs/sugar) and his weight. In this figure, meal portion and weight have similar change rates which means the less he eats, the lighter his weight. Also, carbs/sugar amount and K-calories have similar change rates which means the less his K-calories, the less his carbs/sugar intake amount.

Figure 3 illustrates the similar trend of annual data of his weight and three food components (meal portion, K-calories, and carbs/sugar amount).

Exercise is a missing component from this figure which is also essential on weight reduction. The more he eats, the higher intake amounts of his K-calories and his carbs/sugar as well. During the past decade on his effort for weight reduction, he has focused on reducing both of his meal portion percentage and carb/sugar intake amount. As a result, he was able to reduce his weight from 220 lbs. (100 kg) and his average glucose from 280 mg/dL in 2010 to 171 lbs. (78 kg) and 106 mg/dL in 2020 (without any medication).

Figure 4 reflects the annual change rate percentage of his daily glucose, weight and carbs/sugar amount. In this figure, the change rates of his glucose and weight are remarkably similar, almost a mirror image, which indicates the lower his weight, the lower his glucose. This finding matches the two European studies and the common knowledge possessed by healthcare professionals. The reason for the obviously mismatched change rates between carbs/sugar and glucose or weight is due to the missing component of exercise which is equally important on glucose reduction.

Figure 5 focuses exclusively on the relationships among data of glucose, carbs/sugar, and exercise. The positive correlation coefficient between glucose and carbs/sugar is expressed by these two similar moving trends. On the other hand, the negative correlation coefficient between glucose and exercise (walking) is expressed by these two opposite moving trends.

Figures 6, 7, and 8 collectively collective together to show the 9 sets of calculated correlation coefficients among those 8 listed elements in above section of Methods. A better illustration of these three figures can be found in a table, where all of the calculated correlations are above 90%, which means they are highly connected to each other (Figure 9). Even the correlation of -89% between glucose and walking exercise is also extremely high in a negative manner.

Figure 10 reveals the detailed annual change rates of 8 elements for a 10+ year period from 2010 to 2020. It should be pointed out that his average change rates within 6 years from 2015 through 2020 are 2.7% per year for both FPG and PPG, and 3.4%

for daily glucose. This conclusion is similar to his six previously published papers regarding his pancreatic beta cell's self-recovery rate of insulin secretion. Most likely, his beta cells insulin production and functionality have been repaired about 16% during the past 6 years or 27% during the past 10 years at a self-repair rate of 2.7% per year.

Here are the summaries of his findings:

His successful weight reduction, from 220 lbs. in 2010 to 171 lbs. in 2020, comes from his food portion reduction and exercise increase.
His lower carbs/sugar intake amount, from 40 grams in 2010 to 12 grams in 2020, is resulted from his learned food nutrition knowledge and meal portion reduction, from 150% in 2010 to 67% in 2020.
His weight reduction contributes to his FPG reduction, from 220 mg/dL in 2010 to 104 mg/dL in 2020. His carbs/sugar control and increased walking steps, from 2,000 steps in 2010 to ~16,000 steps in 202, have contributed to his PPG reduction, from 300 mg/dL in 2010 to 109 mg/dL in 2020. When both FPG and PPG are reduced, his daily glucose is decreased as well, from 280 mg/dL in 2010 to 108 mg/dL in 2020.
His damaged beta cell's insulin production and functionality, most likely, have been repaired about 16% for the past 6 years or 27% in the past 10 years at a self-repair rate of 2.7% per year.

Summary:

To date, the author has written seven papers discussing his pancreatic beta cell's self-recovery of insulin secretion. In his first six papers (see References 2 through 7), he used several different "cutting angles" or "analysis approaches" to delve deeper into this complex biomedical subject and achieved consistent results within the range of 2.3% to 3.2% of annual self-recovery rate.

He used a quantitative approach with precision to discover and reconfirm his pancreatic beta cell's health state by linking it backwards step-by-step with his collected data of glucose, weight, diet, and exercise. He has produced another dataset for a self-repair rate of 2.7% which is located right in the middle between 2.3% and 3.2% from his previous findings.

In his opinion, type 2 diabetes (T2D) is no longer a non-reversible or non-curable disease. Diabetes is not only "controllable" but it is also "self-repairable", even though at a rather slow rate. He would like to share his research findings and his persistent efforts from the past decade with his medical research colleagues and to provide encouragement to motivate other T2D patients like himself to reverse their diabetes conditions.

References:

1. Hsu, Gerald C., eclaireMD Foundation, USA; "GH-Method: Methodology of math-physical medicine, No. 54 and No. 310"

2. Hsu, Gerald C. eclaireMD Foundation, USA. "Changes in relative health state of pancreas beta cells over eleven years using GH-Method: math-physical medicine (No. 112)."

3. Hsu, Gerald C. eclaireMD Foundation, USA. "Probable partial recovery of pancreatic beta cells insulin regeneration using annualized fasting plasma glucose via GH-Method: math-physical medicine (No. 133)."

4. Hsu, Gerald C. eclaireMD Foundation, USA. "Probable partial self-recovery of pancreatic beta cells using calculations of annualized fasting plasma glucose using GH-Method: math-physical medicine (No. 138)."

5. Hsu, Gerald C. eclaireMD Foundation, USA. "Guesstimate probable partial self-recovery of pancreatic beta cells using calculations of annualized glucose data using GH-Method: math-physical medicine (No. 139)."

6. Hsu, Gerald C. eclaireMD Foundation, USA. "Relationship between metabolism and risk of cardiovascular disease and stroke, risk of chronic kidney disease, and probability of pancreatic beta cells self-recovery using GH-Method: Math-Physical Medicine (No. 259)."

7. Hsu, Gerald C. eclaireMD Foundation, USA. "Self-recovery of pancreatic beta cell's insulin secretion based on annualized fasting plasma glucose, baseline postprandial plasma glucose, and baseline daily glucose data using GH-Method: math-physical medicine (No. 297)"

	Y2010	Y2011	Y2012	Y2013	Y2014	Y2015	Y2016	Y2017	Y2018	Y2019	Y2020	11-yrs Avg	6-yrs Avg
Carbs/Sugar (g)	40	35	33	30	25	20	15	14	15	13	12	23	15
Protein (g)	40	35	33	30	25	20	15	16	15	16	15	24	16
Fat (g)	40	35	33	30	22	18	11	11	9	11	7	21	11
K-Calories	2720	2380	2244	2040	1601	1288	885	860	829	844	706	1491	902
Meals Portion (%)	150	133	120	115	105	94	88	85	84	76	67	102	82
Weight (lbs)	220	198	189	183	177	175	173	174	171	173	171	182	173
Walking (Steps)	2000	3000	4000	7564	11767	14997	17017	17863	18458	15742	15882	13663	16660
Glucose (mg/dL)	280	230	165	132	135	129	119	117	116	114	108	150	117
PPG (mg/dL)	300	250	170	133	137	130	120	117	117	114	109	154	118
FPG (mg/dL)	220	170	150	135	128	121	117	120	114	115	104	136	115
Calculated Glucose	280	230	165	133	135	128	119	117	116	114	108	150	117
Calculated / Measured	100%	100%	100%	101%	100%	99%	100%	100%	100%	100%	100%	100%	100%
Note:	Start	Food	Data	Walking	MI Model	PPG, drug	FPG, carbs	CVD	CKD	Beta Cell	Neuro	with guess	more precise

	Y2010	Y2011	Y2012	Y2013	Y2014	Y2015	Y2016	Y2017	Y2018	Y2019	Y2020	11-yrs Avg	6-yrs Avg
Carbs/Sugar (g)	40	35	33	30	25	20	15	14	15	13	12	23	15
K-Calories (/10)	272	238	224	204	160	129	88	86	83	84	71	1491	902
Meals Portion (%)	150	133	120	115	105	94	88	85	84	76	67	102	82
Weight (lbs)	220	198	189	183	177	175	173	174	171	173	171	182	173

	Y2010	Y2011	Y2012	Y2013	Y2014	Y2015	Y2016	Y2017	Y2018	Y2019	Y2020	11-yrs Avg	6-yrs Avg
Carbs/Sugar (g)	40	35	33	30	25	20	15	14	15	13	12	23	15
Walking (100 Steps)	20	30	40	76	118	150	170	179	185	157	159	117	167
Glucose (mg/dL)	280	230	165	132	135	129	119	117	116	114	108	150	117
PPG (mg/dL)	300	250	170	133	137	130	120	117	117	114	109	154	118
FPG (mg/dL)	220	170	150	135	128	121	117	120	114	115	104	136	115

Figure 1: Background data table

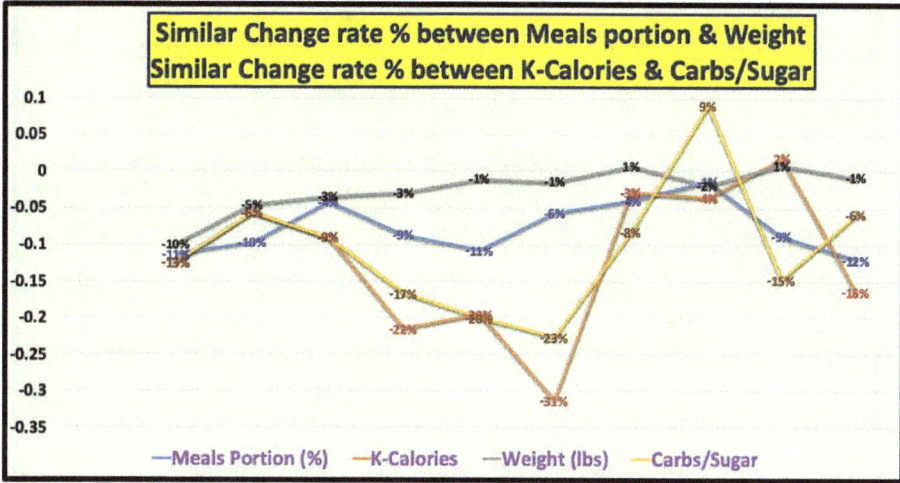

Figure 2: Annual change rates of Weight and Food (meal portion, K-calories, carbs/sugar)

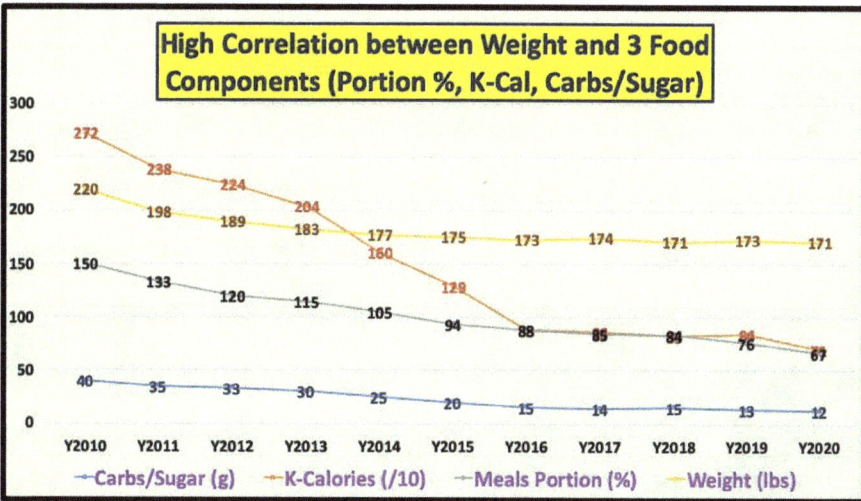

Figure 3: Annual change rates of
Weight and Food (meal portion, K-calories, carbs/sugar)

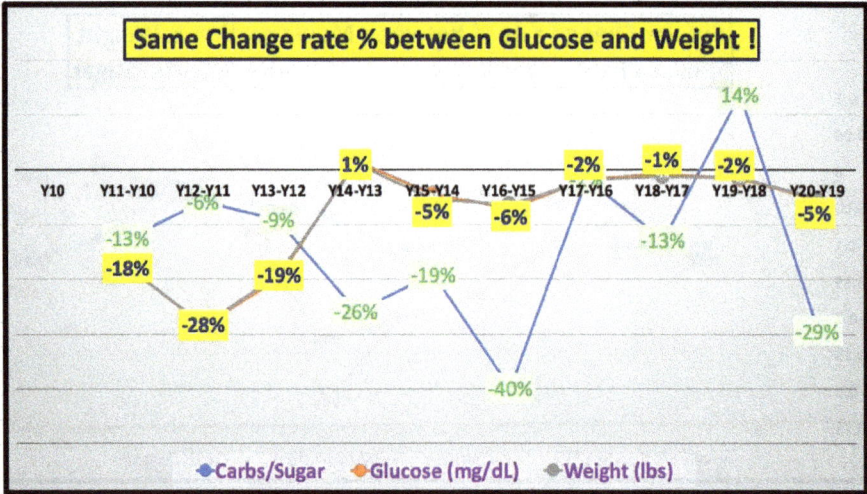

Figure 4: Annual change rates of
Weight, Glucose, and Carbs/sugar

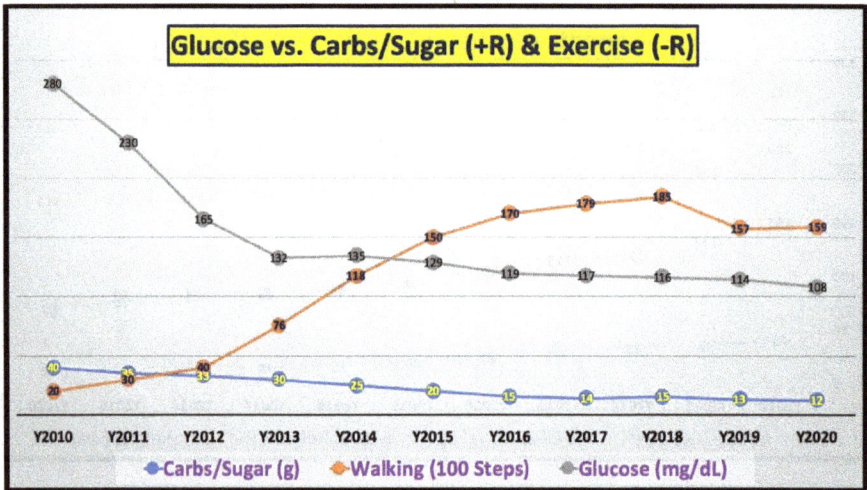

Figure 5: Annual data of Weight, Glucose, and Carbs/sugar

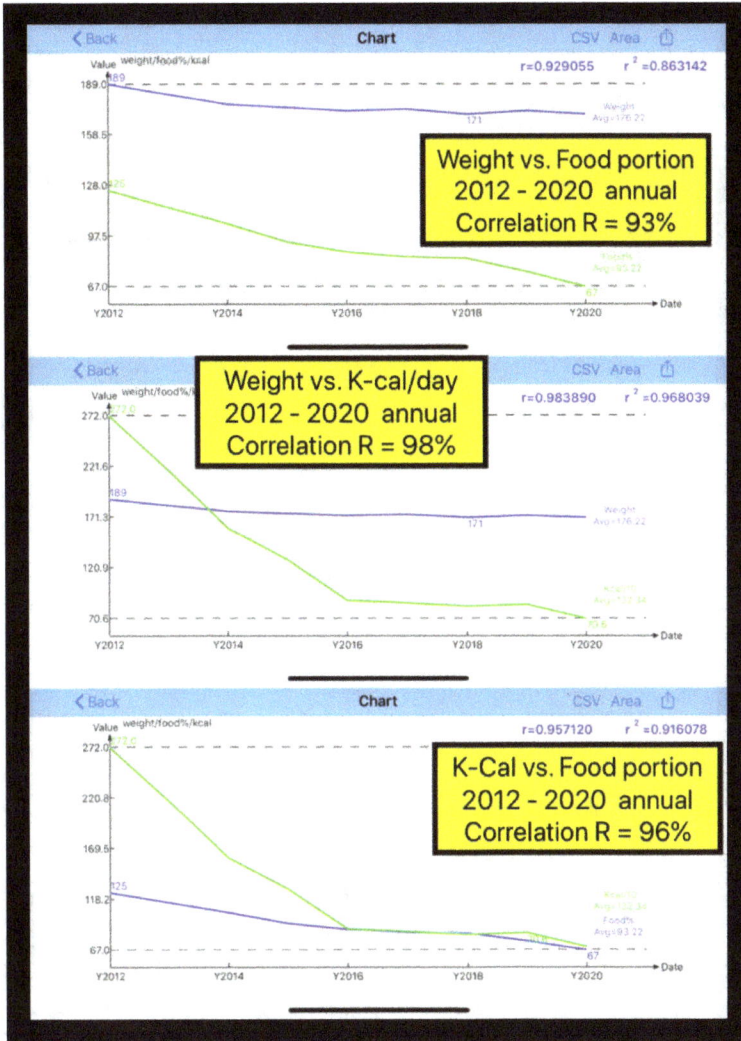

Figure 6: Correlation coefficients among Weight, K-calories, meal portion

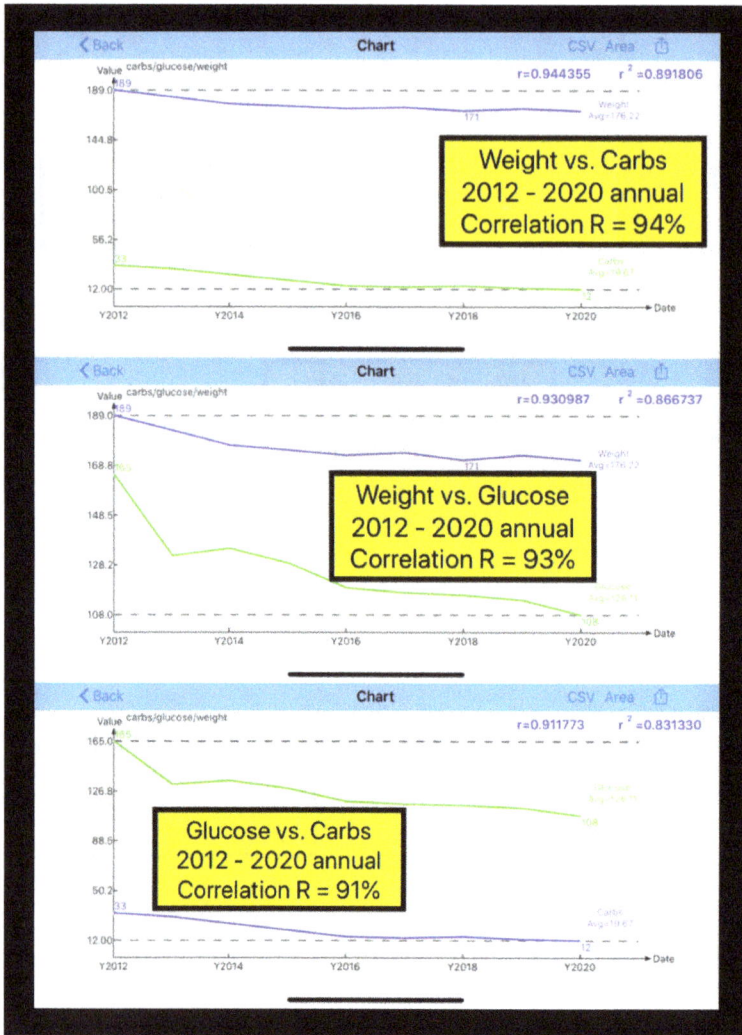

Figure 7: Correlation coefficients among Weight, Glucose, Carbs/sugar

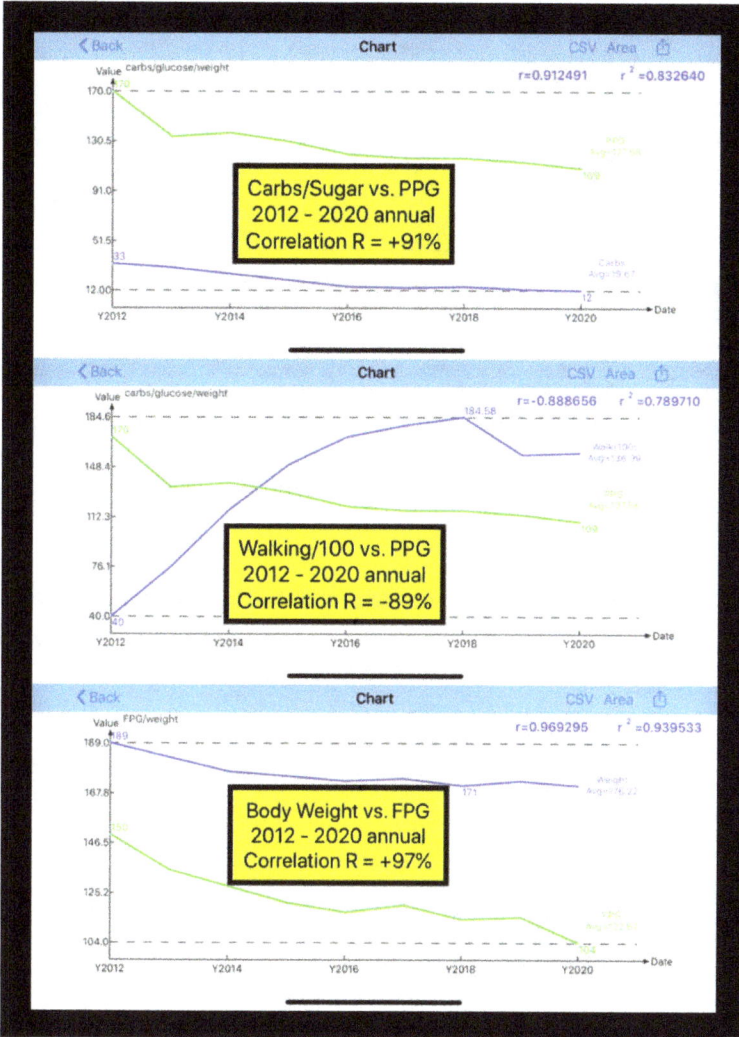

Figure 8: Correlation coefficients among PPG, Carb/sugar, Walking, FPG, Weight

Correlation *	Weight	Food Portion	K-Cal / day	Carbs/Sugar	Glucose	PPG	FPG	Walking
Weight		93%	98%	94%	93%		97%	
Food Portion	93%		96%					
K-Cal / day	98%	96%						
Carbs/Sugar	94%				91%	91%		
Glucose	93%			91%				
PPG				91%				-89%
FPG	97%							
Walking Steps						-89%		

Figure 9: A combined data table of 9 correlation coefficients among 8 elements

Reduction %	Y10	Y11-Y10	Y12-Y11	Y13-Y12	Y14-Y13	Y15-Y14	Y16-Y15	Y17-Y16	Y18-Y17	Y19-Y18	Y20-Y19	10-yrs Rate	5-yrs Rate
Meals Portion (%)		-11%	-10%	-4%	-9%	-11%	-6%	-4%	-1%	-9%	-12%	-8%	-6%
K-Calories		-13%	-6%	-9%	-22%	-20%	-31%	-3%	-4%	2%	-16%	-12%	-10%
Weight (lbs)		-10%	-5%	-3%	-3%	-1%	-1%	1%	-2%	1%	-1%	-2%	-0.5%
Carbs/Sugar		-13%	-6%	-9%	-17%	-20%	-23%	-8%	9%	-15%	-6%	-11%	-8%
Reduction %	Y10	Y11-Y10	Y12-Y11	Y13-Y12	Y14-Y13	Y15-Y14	Y16-Y15	Y17-Y16	Y18-Y17	Y19-Y18	Y20-Y19	10-yrs Rate	5-yrs Rate
Carbs/Sugar		-13%	-6%	-9%	-26%	-19%	-40%	-2%	-13%	14%	-29%	-14%	-14%
Glucose (mg/dL)		-18%	-28%	-20%	2%	-4%	-7%	-2%	-1%	-2%	-5%	-9%	-3.4%
Weight (lbs)		-18%	-28%	-19%	1%	-5%	-6%	-2%	-1%	-2%	-5%	-9%	-3.2%
FPG (mg/dL)		-23%	-12%	-10%	-6%	-6%	-3%	2%	-5%	1%	-9%	-7%	-2.7%
PPG (mg/dL)		-23%	-12%	-10%	-6%	-6%	-3%	2%	-5%	1%	-9%	-7%	-2.7%

Figure 10: A combined data table of annual change rates of 7 elements, especially glucose change rates of 2.7%

Cancer prevention through improvements on lifestyle and metabolism using GH-Method: math-physical medicine (No. 342)

Gerald C. Hsu
eclaireMD Foundation, USA
10/6-7/2020

Abstract:

This paper describes the author's investigation into the prevention from having various cancers and his risk probability based on improvements on lifestyle and metabolism.

His risk probabilities percentage of having cancer over the past 11 years with lower risk percentages (<50%) during 2014 - 2020 and higher risk percentages (>50%) during 2010 - 2013. It should be noted that the higher prediction accuracy existed during 2015-2020 due to his collection of more completed data.

(1) Year of 2010: 88%
(2) Year of 2011: 74%
(3) Year of 2012: 58%
(4) Year of 2013: 55%
(5) Year of 2014: 50%
(6) Year of 2015: 48%
(7) Year of 2016: 46%
(8) Year of 2017: 45%
(9) Year of 2018: 45%
(10) Year of 2019: 45%
(11) Year of 2020: 43%

It seems that 50% is a reasonable "cut-off" line between higher risk versus lower risk. The trend of the past 11 years risk probability percentages of having cancer from the viewpoint of cancer prevention is being reduced year after year, which is an encouraging fact.

The calculated cancer prevention and risk probability results via lifestyle and metabolism have been validated by his many health examination reports from the past 20 years. This big data based on a dynamic simulation model and data-mining using GH-Method: math-physical medicine approach can provide an early warning to which factors or areas to monitor in order to continuously improve his health conditions.

The author wrote this article to share with other people, who may have similar interest in reducing their risk probability of getting cancer. As stated previously, he is not an expert on oncology but a research scientist in both lifestyle and metabolism. Metabolism and cancer have a strong relationship with one another; therefore, hopefully, his research method and preliminary findings would have some merit to help others to prevent them from getting cancer.

Introduction:

This paper describes the author's investigation into the prevention from having various cancers and his risk probability based on improvements on lifestyle and metabolism.

Method:

Background:

To learn more about his developed GH-Method: math-physical medicine (MPM) research methodology, readers can review his article, *Biomedical research methodology based on GH-Method: math-physical medicine (No. 310),* in Reference 1 to understand his developed GH-Method: math-physical medicine.

Using the same methodology, he has developed, written, and published numerous articles regarding the risk probability of having a stroke, cardiovascular disease (CVD), or chronic kidney disease (CKD) over the past two years (Reference 3).

Data collection:

He has spent ten years collecting big data (~2 million data) of his health and lifestyle details in order to conduct his biomedical research on chronic diseases and their various complications. Since 1995, he has suffered three chronic diseases, including diabetes, hyperlipidemia, and hypertension. He has also endured five CVD from 1994 to 2006, CKD in 2010, bladder infection, foot ulcer, diabetic retinopathy (DR), and hypothyroidism over the past decade. By 2017, most of his metabolic disorders induced chronic diseases and complications have been well controlled. During the same year, he started to self-study cancer diseases with a particular interest on its causes and preventive ways via the improvement on lifestyle and metabolism.

Mathematical model:

Since 2014, by using topology concept and finite element engineering modeling, he developed a complex mathematical metabolism model to calculate and check his overall metabolism state on a daily basis. This developed mathematical model of metabolism includes two specific areas. For the first area, the medical conditions has four categories, weight (m1), glucose (m2), blood pressure (m3), lipid and others (m4). Only m1 of weights and m2 of glucoses are utilized in this cancer prevention study. For the second area, the lifestyle details has six categories, exercise (m5), water drinking (m6), sleep (m7), stress (m8), diet (m9), and life routine regularity (m10). All six lifestyle categories are utilized in this cancer study.

Furthermore, he subdivided diet (m9) into food quantity (m9a) and food quality (m9b) along with subdividing life routine regularity (m10) into life habits (m10a) and cancer-related habits (m10b). In these two categories, he emphasized food quality (m9b) and cancer-related habits (m10b). He continues to add detailed elements into the mathematical model of metabolism during his self-study and research process. This model has the capability to automatically calculate the combined sub-group scores of medical conditions (m1 through m4) and lifestyle details (m6 through m10), as well as the total combined score of metabolism or metabolism index (MI). It should be mentioned that the 10 categories also contain around 500 detailed elements. He utilized artificial intelligence (AI) technology for auto-judgement and auto-correction to assist with the daily data collection.

From 2015 to 2017, he applied optical physics, wave theory, energy theory, quantum mechanics, big data analytics, AI, segmented analysis, pattern recognition, and various statistics tools such as time-series, spatial analysis, and frequency domain analysis to his method. As a result, he developed four prediction models for body weight, fasting plasma glucose (FPG), postprandial plasma glucose (PPG), and HbA1C as biomarkers. All of these models have achieved greater than 95% prediction accuracy. From 2018 to 2019, he also developed two risk assessment models for having CVD/ Stroke or CKD (Reference 3).

The author spent 10 years to develop and continuously enhance a sophisticated and customized software program to collect all types of input data and process them dynamically in order to provide a daily guideline for the purpose of improving his overall metabolism and health. Once his metabolism is in good condition, then his immune system will be strong enough to defend against three major groups that lead to death (reference 4). They include chronic diseases with various complications (50%), cancers (29%), infectious diseases (11%), along with another special group of non-diseases related death (10%), from the data observed in Figure 1.

This section has described the backbone of his mathematical model for calculating his risk probability of having various cancers closely related to the prevention via improvements on lifestyle and metabolism.

Cancer data:
Cancer is an exceedingly difficult and complicated disease that can affect any organ within the body, where abnormal cells divide and mutate rapidly, destroying healthy normal cells in the process. The possible cause of cancer can result from a combination of many different reasons. The author has dedicated the past decade on researching endocrinology and metabolism. He considers that both endocrinology and cancer are quite similar from the viewpoint of "digging into the black box of science". However, based on his rudimentary understanding of cancer, he also feels that the diseases caused by cancer are probably at least 10 times more complicated than endocrinology. Although he is not an oncology expert, only a veteran and research scientist on chronic diseases and their complications, he still has a strong curiosity and motivation in wanting to know what his risk probability percentage is of having cancer. This reason inspires his cancer research work by using his strength of lifestyle management and metabolism knowledge to conduct his assessment on the relationship between metabolism and cancer. An example of his research work can be seen in Reference 2. This particular article only serves as the beginning of his long journey in studying cancer using his research methodology, the GH-Method: math-physical medicine.

In reference 5, the article indicates that there are 23 cancer factors in the area of metabolic disorders which cause a total of 45.2% of the entire cancer cases in China (around 2.3 million cases per year). In addition, Harvard Health has also mentioned certain cancer prevention information listed in the following excerpt.

"About one of every three Americans will develop some form of malignancy during his or her lifetime. Despite these grim statistics, doctors have made great progress in understanding the biology of cancer cells, and they have already been able to improve the diagnosis and treatment of cancer.

*But instead of just waiting for new breakthroughs, you can do a lot to protect yourself right now. Screening tests can help detect malignancies in their earliest stages, but you should always be alert for symptoms of the disease. The American Cancer Society developed this simple reminder (**CAUTION**) years ago:*

- *C: Change in bowel or bladder habits*
- *A: A sore that does not heal*
- *U: Unusual bleeding or discharge, unexpected weight loss or fatigue*
- *T: Thickening or lump in the breast or elsewhere*
- *I: Indigestion or difficulty in swallowing*
- *O: Obvious change in a wart or mole*
- *N: Nagging cough or hoarseness*

*Early diagnosis is important, but can you go one better? Can you reduce your risk of getting cancer in the first place? It sounds too good to be true, but it's not. **Scientists at the Harvard School of Public Health estimate that up to 75% of American cancer deaths can be prevented.** You don't have to be an international scientist to understand how you can try to protect yourself and your family. The 10 commandments of cancer prevention are...."*

The author compiled the following list of 18 specific cancer prevention recommendations from five reputable sources, including the American Institute of Cancer Research (AICR), American Cancer Society (ACS), Harvard Medical, Mayo Clinic, and UCLA. He then links each of these 18 recommendations with his 10 established metabolism categories (i.e. mi where i = 1 through 10) from his mathematical metabolism model as shown below:

m1: Be a healthy weight (AICR)
m5: Be physically active, exercise regularly, and stay lean (AICR, Harvard)
m9b: Eat a diet rich in whole grains, vegetables, fruits, and beans (AICR, Harvard)
m2, m9a, m9b: Limit consumption of "fast foods" and other processed foods that are high in fat, starches, or sugars (AICR, Harvard)
m9a, m9b: Limit consumptions of red and processed meat (AICR, Harvard)
m2, m9a, m9b: Limit consumption of sugar-sweetened drinks (AICR); this also related to diabetes, glucose, and meal quantity
m10b: Genetic & basic habits: Limit alcohol consumption (AICR, Harvard)
m10b: Genetic & basic habits: Do not smoke cigarettes and avoiding other exposure to tobacco (AICR, Harvard)
m7: Make quality sleep a priority (Harvard)
m9b: Get enough vitamin D, but don't count on other supplements for cancer

prevention (AICR, Harvard)

m10b: Avoid risky behaviors, e.g. safe sex, don't use illicit drugs, don't share needles, and avoid infections that contribute to cancer (Mayo, Harvard)

m4b and m10b: Get vaccinated and have regular checkups to receive medical care (Mayo)

m9b: Lower risks via dietary patterns rich in plant foods and low in animal products and refined carbohydrates; and the Mediterranean diet pattern. Consumption of non-starchy vegetables and/or vegetables rich in carotenoids may lower risk for estrogen receptor-negative breast tumors; diets higher in calcium/calcium□rich dairy may reduce risk (ACS, Harvard).

m10b: Avoid unnecessary exposure to radiation, and excessive sun radiation (AICR, Harvard).

m10b: Avoid exposure to industrial and environmental toxins (Harvard)

m10b: Beware and stay away from air and water pollution (UCLA)

m10b: Don't get food poison or eat polluted food (UCLA)

m10b: For mothers, breastfeed your baby, if you can; this is for 99% of women who get breast cancer - not having children, not breastfeeding, birth control (hormones content), hormone therapy after menopause, breast implant (AICR)

In this article, he omits the genetic and basic habits, such as smoking tobacco and alcohol intake, which may result in an additional ~10% to his calculation of cancer risk probability. These findings are remarkably similar to his research findings regarding chronic diseases and their complications, such as CVD or stroke, which have ~80% or more preventable via lifestyle and metabolism.

Results:

In Figure 1, it shows the number of US deaths in 2017 due to three chronic diseases and their complications (50%), various cancers (29%), infectious diseases (11%), and non-diseases death (10%). Cancer deaths total almost 600,000 cases in 2017. If only 33% to 50% of these American cancer patients paid attention to cancer prevention via improvements on lifestyle and metabolism, it could save at least 200,000 to 300,000 lives per year.

Figure 2 is the background data table of this study. It should be pointed out in the medical conditions group, weight and glucose data during 2010 and 2011 were guesstimated numbers based on partially collected data. In the lifestyle group, its data during 2010 through 2014 were also guesstimated data based on partially collected data. Nevertheless, all the data after 1/1/2015 have been based on daily collected raw data. In addition, since his medical conditions only used weight and glucose, he assigned a weighting factor of 20% for weight (overweight or obesity) and glucose (diabetes). Since this study is more focused on lifestyle, he assigned a weighting factor of 60% for the six lifestyle categories (m5 through m10). The author is currently expanding the scope of his software to include more influential factors related to cancer prevention, especially in the two sub-categories of food quality (m9b) and cancer related daily life routines (m10b which includes environmental factors). His follow-up cancer investigations will further improve its cancer risk prediction accuracy and effectiveness of cancer prevention methods.

Figure 3 shows his risk probabilities percentage of having cancer over the past 11 years with lower risk percentages (<50%) during 2014 - 2020 and higher risk percentages (>50%) during 2010 - 2013. It should be noted again that the higher prediction accuracy existed during 2015-2020 due to his collection of more completed data.

Year of 2010: 88% (obesity BMI 31, 3 chronic diseases, 5 cardiac episodes)
Year of 2011: 74% (still bad condition on both weight, glucose, and lifestyle)
Year of 2012: 58% (weight reduction started, more careful about diet, started daily exercise, CKD)
Year of 2013: 55% (making progress on lifestyle, but still not good enough)
Year of 2014: 50% (developed metabolism model and started his lifestyle management program)
Year of 2015: 48% (BMI 25, FPG under control due to his weight reduction)
Year of 2016: 46% (both PPG and HbA1C under control due to his development of PPG and HbA1C prediction models)
Year of 2017: 45% (overall lifestyle, medical conditions, and metabolism were under control)
Year of 2018: 45% (heavy traveling for attending medical conferences)
Year of 2019: 45% (heavy traveling for attending medical conferences)
Year of 2020: 43% (from 1/1/2020 to 10/6/2020, already reaches to the best state within past 25 years due to COVID-19 quarantined life)

It should be noted that the risk probability percentages are expressed on a relative scale, not on an absolute scale, with an emphasis on lifestyle management. It seems that ~50% is a reasonable "cut-off" line between higher risk versus lower risk. The trend of his 11 years risk probability percentages of having cancer is being reduced year after year, which is an encouraging fact. Cancer by definition can also be a chronic disease and its listed prevention recommendations are highly similar to diabetes prevention.

Conclusion:

The calculated cancer prevention and risk probability results via lifestyle and metabolism have been validated by his many health examination reports from the past 20 years. This big data based on a dynamic simulation model and data-mining using GH-Method: math-physical medicine approach can provide an early warning to which factors or areas to monitor in order to continuously improve his health conditions.

The author wrote this article to share with other people, who may have similar interest in reducing their risk probability of getting cancer. As stated previously, he is not an expert on oncology but a research scientist in both lifestyle and metabolism. Metabolism and cancer have a strong relationship with one another; therefore, hopefully, his research method and preliminary findings would have some merit to help others to prevent them from getting cancer.

References:

1. Hsu, Gerald C., eclaireMD Foundation, USA; No. 310: "Biomedical research methodology based on GH-Method: math-physical medicine".

2. Hsu, Gerald C., eclaireMD Foundation, USA; No. 263: "Risk probability of having a metabolic disorder induced cancer (GH-Method: MPM)

3. Hsu, Gerald C., eclaireMD Foundation, USA, No. 258: "Relationship between metabolism and probability risks of having cardiovascular diseases or renal complications using GH-Method: Math-Physical Medicine."

4. Hsu, Gerald C., eclaireMD Foundation, USA, No. 235: "Linkage among metabolism, immune system, and various diseases using GH-Method: math-physical medicine (MPM)."

5. Chen, Wanqing, Feb. 2019 "Disparities by province, age, and sex in site-specific cancer burden attributable to 23 potentially modifiable risk factors in China: a comparative risk assessment."

6. www.health.harvard.edu; Published: April, 2009, Updated: October 1, 2019

2017 Death	Category	percentage
Heart	647,457	31%
Cancer	599,108	29%
Accidents	169,936	8%
Respiratory	160,201	8%
Stroke	146,383	7%
Alzheimer's	121,404	6%
Diabetes	83,564	4%
Pneumonia	55,672	3%
Kidney	50,633	2%
Suicide	47,173	2%
Total	2,081,531	100%
Chronic Related	1,049,441	50%
Cancer	599,108	29%
Infectious	215,873	11%
Accidents & Suicide	217,109	10%

Figure 1: 2017 death case % of cancers which has 599,108 death cases and 29% of total death cases

Cancer Prevention Study	Y2010	Y2011	Y2012	Y2013	Y2014	Y2015	Y2016	Y2017	Y2018	Y2019	Y2020
Weight	220	200	189	183	177	175	173	174	171	173	171
Weight / 167.61	1.2941	1.1765	1.1119	1.0739	1.0425	1.0465	1.0228	1.0352	1.0167	1.0222	1.0135
Glucose	180	175	128	132	135	129	119	117	116	114	108
Glucose / 120	1.5000	1.4583	1.0644	1.1041	1.1218	1.0726	0.9958	0.9791	0.9705	0.9537	0.8991
Cancer Prevention Study	Y2010	Y2011	Y2012	Y2013	Y2014	Y2015	Y2016	Y2017	Y2018	Y2019	Y2020
Averaged Medical	1.3971	1.3174	1.0882	1.0890	1.0821	1.0596	1.0093	1.0072	0.9936	0.9880	0.9563
Weighted Medical (20%)	0.2794	0.2635	0.2176	0.2178	0.2164	0.2119	0.2019	0.2014	0.1987	0.1976	0.1913
Averaged Lifestyle	1.0000	0.8000	0.6000	0.5500	0.4800	0.4480	0.4341	0.4132	0.4174	0.4254	0.3921
Weighted Lifestyle (60%)	0.6000	0.4800	0.3600	0.3300	0.2880	0.2688	0.2605	0.2479	0.2504	0.2552	0.2353
Cancer Prevention Study	Y2010	Y2011	Y2012	Y2013	Y2014	Y2015	Y2016	Y2017	Y2018	Y2019	Y2020
Total Weighted Risk Score	88%	74%	58%	55%	50%	48%	46%	45%	45%	45%	43%
Weighted Medical (20%)	28%	26%	22%	22%	22%	21%	20%	20%	20%	20%	19%
Weighted Lifestyle (60%)	60%	48%	36%	33%	29%	27%	26%	25%	25%	26%	24%

Figure 2: Background data table

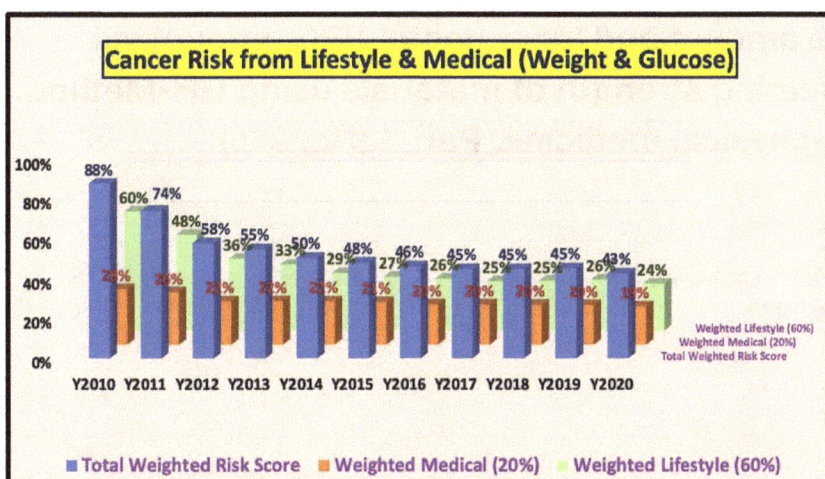

Figure 3: Risk probability % of having cancer based on lifestyle, medical conditions, and combined metabolism categories

Linear relationship between carbohydrates & sugar intake amount and incremental PPG amount via engineering strength of materials using GH-Method: math-physical medicine, Part 1 (No. 346)

Gerald C. Hsu
eclaireMD Foundation, USA
10/14-16/2020

Abstract:

This article is a special research on the linear elasticity behavior of glucose using his defined GH-modulus (or M2) to link the input of carbs/sugar intake amount and output of incremental PPG amount.

Here is the formula he used in his previously published papers:

Predicted PPG
= (FPG* 0.97) + (carbs/sugar grams * M2) - (post-meal waking K-steps * 5)

He has connected this biomedical equation with a basic concept of stress and strain, along with the Young's modulus of strength of materials in structural and mechanical engineering. Using his collected 11,580 data of glucose, food, and exercise, he has demonstrated that a "pseudo-linear" relationship indeed existing between the carbs/sugar intake amount multiplied with a "GH modulus (i.e. M2)", which is similar to the "stress" on an engineering system; and the incremental PPG amount, which is similar to the "strain" of an engineering system. A newly defined coefficient of "GH-modulus" as the value of M2 multiplier is similar to the Young's modules of stress-strain relationship in the subject of engineering strength of materials.

This investigation has proven the existing pseudo-linear relationship between food as stress on the liver and incremental glucose as strain from the liver, particularly during his better controlled period of diabetes from 7/1/2015 to 10/13/2020.

This article is a special research on the linear elasticity of glucose with his defined GH-modulus (or M2) and engineering modeling methodologies to investigate various biomedical problems. This methodology and approach are resulted from his specific academic background and different professional experiences prior to his medical research work beginning in 2010. Therefore, he has been trying to link his newly acquired biomedical knowledge over the past decade with his previously acquired mathematics, physics, computer science, and engineering knowledge over 40 years.

The human body is the most complex system he has dealt with. However, by applying his previous acquired knowledge to his newly found interest of medicine, he can discover many hidden facts or truths inside the biomedical systems. Many basic concepts, theoretical frame of thoughts, and practical modeling techniques from his fundamental disciplines in the past can be applied to his medical research endeavor. After all, science is based on theory via creation and proof via evidence, and as long as we can discover hidden truths, it does not matter which method we use and which way we take. This is the foundation of the GH-Method: math-physics medicine.

Introduction:

This article is a special research on the linear elasticity behavior of glucose using his defined GH-modulus (or M2) to link the input of carbs/sugar intake amount and output of incremental PPG amount.

Here is the formula he used in his previously published papers:

Predicted PPG
= (FPG* 0.97) + (carbs/sugar grams * M2) - (post-meal waking K-steps * 5)

He has connected this biomedical equation with a basic concept of stress and strain, along with the Young's modulus of strength of materials in structural and mechanical engineering. Using his collected 11,580 data of glucose, food, and exercise, he has demonstrated that a "pseudo-linear" relationship indeed existing between the carbs/sugar intake amount multiplied with a "GH modulus (i.e. M2)", which is similar to the "stress" on an engineering system; and the incremental PPG amount, which is similar to the "strain" of an engineering system. A newly defined coefficient of "GH-modulus" as the value of M2 multiplier is similar to the Young's modules of stress-strain relationship in the subject of engineering strength of materials.

This investigation has proven the existing pseudo-linear relationship between food as stress on the liver and incremental glucose as strain from the liver, particularly during his better controlled period of diabetes from 7/1/2015 to 10/13/2020.

Methods:

Background:
To learn more about the author's GH-Method: math-physical medicine (MPM) methodology, readers can refer to his article to understand the developed MPM analysis method in Reference 1.

Highlights of his previous research:
In 2015, the author decomposed the PPG waveforms (data curves) into 19 influential components and identified carbs/sugar intake amount and post-meal walking exercise contributing to approximately 40% of PPG formation, respectively. Therefore, he could safely discount the importance of the remaining ~20% contribution by the 16 other influential components.

In 2016, he utilized optical physics, big data analytics, and artificial intelligence (AI) techniques to develop computer software to predict PPG based on the patient's food pictures or meal photos. This sophisticated AI approach and iPhone APP software product have reached to a 98.8% prediction accuracy based on ~6,000 meal photos.

In 2017, he also detected that body weight contributes to over 85% to fasting plasma glucose (FPG) formation. Furthermore, in 2019, he identified that FPG could serve as a good indicator of the pancreatic beta cells' health status; therefore, he can apply the FPG value (more precisely, 97% of FPG value) to serve as the baseline PPG value of his predicted PPG.

In 2018, based on his collected ~2,500 meals and associated sensor PPG waveforms, he applied the perturbation theory from quantum mechanics at first-bite moment of his meal to further predict the PPG waveform (i.e. PPG curve) covering the entire follow-on 180 minutes with a 95% of PPG prediction accuracy.

In 2019, all of his developed PPG prediction mathematical models have achieved high percentages of prediction accuracy, but he also realized that his prediction models are too difficult to use by the general public. The above-mentioned sophisticated math-physical medicine methods would be difficult for healthcare professionals and diabetes patients to understand, let alone use them in their daily life for diabetes control. Therefore, he tried to supplement his complex models with a simple linear equation of predicted PPG (References 2, 3, and 4).

Here is the simple linear formula:

Predicted PPG
= FPG * M1 + (carbs-sugar * M2) - (post-meal walking k-steps * M3)

Where M1, M2, M3 are 3 multipliers.

After lengthy research, trial and error, and data tuning, he finally identified the best multipliers for FPG and exercise as 0.97 for M1 and 5.0 for M3. In comparison with PPG, the FPG is a more stabilized biomarker since it is directly related to body weight. Weight reduction is a hard undertaking but is a far calmer and more stabilizing biomarker in comparison to glucose which fluctuate from moment to moment. The influence of exercise (specifically, post-meal walking steps) on PPG (41% contribution and >80% negative correlation with PPG) is almost equal to the influence from the carbs/sugar intake amount on PPG (39% contribution and >80% positive correlation with PPG). In terms of intensity and duration, exercise is a much simpler subject to study and deal with. On the other hand, the relationship between food nutrition and glucose is an exceedingly complex and difficult subject to fully understand and effectively manage, since there are many types of food and their associated carbs/sugar contents. For example, the author's food nutrition database has already contained over six million data. As a result, he decided to implement two multipliers, i.e. M1 for FPG and M3 for exercise, as two "constants" and keep M2 as the only "variable" in his PPG prediction equation.

This further simplified his linear equation for predicted PPG as follows:

Predicted PPG
= (0.97*FPG)+(Carbs&sugar * M2) - (post-meal walking k-steps * 5)

He also defines the following three new terms in Equations 2, 3, and 4:

Term 1:
GH modulus = M2

Term 2:
The incremental PPG amount

= Predicted PPG - PPG baseline
 (i.e. 0.97 * FPG) + exercise effect
 (i.e. walking k-steps * 5)

Term 3:
GH modulus (i.e. M2)
= (Incremental PPG) / (Carbs&sugar)

Stress, Strain, & Young's modulus:
Prior to the past decade in his self-study and medical research work, he was an engineer in the fields of structural (aerospace and naval defense), mechanical (nuclear power plants and computer-aided-design), and electronics (computers and semiconductors). The following excerpt comes from the public domain, e.g. Google, Wikipedia.

"Strain - ε:
Strain is the "deformation of a solid due to stress" - change in dimension divided by the original value of the dimension - and can be expressed as
$\varepsilon = dL / L$
where
ε = strain (m/m, in/in)
dL = elongation or compression (offset) of object (m, in)
L = length of object (m, in)

Stress - σ:
Stress is force per unit area and can be expressed as
$\sigma = F / A$
where
σ = stress (N/m2, lb/in2, psi)
F = applied force (N, lb)
A = stress area of object (m2, in2)

Stress includes tensile stress, compressible stress, shearing stress, etc.

E, Young's modulus:
It can be expressed as:
E = stress / strain
  = σ / ε
  = (F / A) / (dL / L)
where

E = Young's Modulus of Elasticity (Pa, N/m2, lb/in2, psi) was named after the 18th-century English physicist Thomas Young.

Elasticity:
Elasticity is a property of an object or material indicating how it will restore it to its original shape after distortion. A spring is an example of an elastic object - when

stretched, it exerts a restoring force which tends to bring it back to its original length (Figure 1).

Plasticity:
When the force is going beyond the elastic limit of material, it is into a "plastic' zone which means even when force is removed, the material will not return back to its original state (Figure 1)."

In this particular study, the above-mentioned Equation 4 is remarkably similar in "concept and format" to the stress-strain equation as shown below *except GH modules and Young's modulus are reverse to each other.*

GH modulus (i.e. M2)
=(Incremental PPG)/(Carbs&sugar)

Young's modulus E
= stress / strain
= σ / ε

The author visualizes the carbs/sugar intake amount as the stress (the force, cause, or stimulator) on his liver and the incremental PPG amount as the strain (the response, consequence, or stimulation) from the liver. The GH modulus (i.e. 1/M2) is similar to the Young's modulus (i.e. E) which describes the "pseudo-linear" relationship existed between the carbs/sugar (stress) and incremental PPG (strain).

Finally, conceptually, he is able to connect together the subject of liver glucose production in endocrinology with the subject of strength of materials in structural & mechanical engineering.

Results:

The author has recorded his glucoses and weight data since 1/1/2012 and then began collecting carbs/sugar intake amount and post-meal walking steps on 7/1/2015. This period coincides with his "best-controlled" diabetes period, where his average daily glucoses reduced to around or under 120 mg/dL (i.e. near a normal range) without any medications. He named this as his "linear elastic zone" of diabetes health. It should also be noted that in 2010, his average glucose was 280 mg/dL and HbA1C was 10%, while taking three diabetes medications (i.e. strong chemical interventions). Prior to 2015, he called that period as his "nonlinear plastic zone" of diabetes health.

From 7/15/2015 to 10/13/2020 (1,930 days), he has collected 6 data per day, 1 FPG, 3 PPG, carb/sugar, and post-meal walking steps. He utilized these 11,580 data and then organized them into 6 years to conduct his annual calculations.
The collected raw data and two sets of calculations are shown in Figure 2. The calculations in this figure have used two different sets of M2 values.

In Case A, calculation is based on different M2 values (i.e. variables) each year in order to obtain 100% of the PPG prediction accuracy for every year in this period. The 100% accuracy indicates that the annual predicted PPG is identical to the annual measured PPG. In Case B, calculation is based on a constant value of 1.82 for M2 (using the 6-years' average) to obtain six different annual PPG prediction accuracies ranging from 93% to 103%. Figure 3 illustrates calculated data table of these two cases, Case A with different M2 and Cade B with constant M2.

Figure 4 and Figure 5 show the graphic results of Case A and Case B reflectively, based on the calculated data table in Figure 3.

Figure 4 depicts the results from using variable M2 values to achieve a 100% match between the predicted PPG and measured PPG of each year.

Listed below are the values for the M2 multiplier (GH-modulus) for each year:

Year 2015 -   1.56
Year 2016 -   1.76
Year 2017 -   1.59
Year 2018 -   1.87
Year 2019 -   1.75
Year 2020 -   2.41
Averaged -   1.82

In Figure 5, it reflects the results from using a constant GH-modulus (M2) of 1.82 to achieve different predicted PPG values from the measured PPG values, with different prediction accuracy for each year (from 93% to 103%).

Listed below are the values of the prediction accuracy for each year:

Year 2015 - 103%
Year 2016 - 101%
Year 2017 - 103%
Year 2018 - 99%
Year 2019 - 101%
Year 2020 - 93%
Averaged - 100%

In fact, the prediction accuracies varying between 93% to 103% with a 6-years averaged accuracy of 100% are acceptable for the purpose of practical glucose control. This is equivalent to a diabetes patient's situation of glucose prediction accuracy ranging from 112 mg/dL (93%) to 124 mg/dL (103%) using a normal dividing line of 120 mg/dL (100%).

Figure 6 shows an x-y data diagram with a "pseudo-linear" relationship between x-values of carbs/sugar multiplied by M2, and y-values of the incremental PPG due to FPGand exercise as defined in the following Equation:

The incremental PPG amount
= Predicted PPG - (FPG * 0.97) + (walking k-steps * 5)

The data ranges of x-axis and y-axis are from 20 to 32. It is obvious that the six-annual data "almost" form a straight line with a slope of 45% and a very small degree of deviations which is why the author calls it a "pseudo-linear" relationship. This is similar to the "elastic zone" of the stress-strain-Young's modulus diagram in strength of materials of structural and mechanical engineering (Figure 1). This linear relationship makes the task of PPG prediction and diabetes control much easier.

Discussion:

The author was a severe type 2 diabetes patient since 1995. He suffered many life-threatening diabetic complications during the period of Y2000 to Y2012. He started to self-study and research on diabetes and food nutrition since 2010 when his average glucose value was 280 mg/dL and HbA1C 10%, and suffered 5 cardiovascular episodes. He collected his diet and exercise data since 6/1/2015. After 2015, his diabetes conditions have been under control via a stringent lifestyle program without taking any diabetes medications; therefore, in this study, he used his collected big data of lifestyle details and glucoses to conduct his rather completed numerical analysis. From 7/1/2015 to 10/13/2020, his diabetes conditions are more or less falling into a linear "elastic" zone which suggests that his PPG would fall off to a reasonable range (around 120 mg/dL or below) when he consumes less amounts of carbs/sugar and exercise adequately.

On the other hand, during the period of 2000-2010, when his diabetes was totally out of control, he believes that he should belong to a "nonlinear plastic" zone, or at least a "bi-linear plastic" zone, meaning his PPG would remain at a certain elevated level even if he reduced or stopped the intake of carbs/sugar. Worse than just having "elevated glucoses"
(hyperglycemia i.e. >180 mg/dL), he could suffer from hypoglycemia (glucose <70 mg/dL) leading to insulin shock and eventually sudden death. However, due to the lack of sufficient data collection, he cannot conduct a similar detailed and completed numerical analysis to prove his suspicion of "nonlinear plastic" zone. He can only try to use his scattered data collection from 2010 to 2014 to obtain a guesstimated observation and some partial conclusions.

As shown in Figure 7, he displayed an x-y diagram of predicted PPG versus measured PPG over both periods, the smaller area of linear elastic period of 2015-2020 and lager area of nonlinear plastic period of 2010-2014. The comparison between these two "strength of materials" zones are interesting, but yet he needs to find other ways to prove his suspicion on the linkage between his glucose spikes and fluctuations (i.e. nonlinearity) of glucoses in the plastic zone and carbs/sugar intake amount in order to compare against his controlled glucoses situations of the pseudo-linear elastic zone.

In his research papers published since 2019, he has proven that his pancreatic beta cells' insulin capability of production and quality have been self-repaired at a rather slow speed of an annual rate of 2.7% (References 5 and 6). It means that at least 16% of his insulin production and quality problems have been repaired since 2015 which is in the elastic zone and may be even 27% of his insulin production and quality problems have been repaired since 2011 which covers both partial plastic and elastic zones. This type of "organic" cells' regeneration capability and biomedical phenomena was unknown to him when he was an engineer and only dealing with various "inorganic" materials, such as metal, concrete, and silicon. As a result, since 2010, he has been fascinated and worked with the various stimulators and complex stimulations of the biomedical system. The more research work he performs, the more unknown phenomena enter into his eyes and the more questions enter into his mind, causing him to search for more problems and seek for better answers.

Conclusions:

This article represents the author's special interest in using math-physical and engineering modeling methodologies to investigate various biomedical problems. This methodology and approach are resulted from his specific academic background and different professional experiences prior to his medical research work beginning in 2010. Therefore, he has been trying to link his newly acquired biomedical knowledge over the past decade with his previously acquired knowledge in mathematics, physics, computer science, and engineering over 40 years.

The human body is the most complex system he has ever dealt with. However, by applying his previous acquired knowledge to his newly found interest of medicine, he can discover many hidden facts or truths inside the biomedical systems. Many basic concepts, theoretical frame of thoughts, and practical modeling techniques from his previously acquired fundamental disciplines can be applied to his medical research endeavor. After all, science is based on theory via creation and proof via evidence, and as long as we can discover hidden truths, it does not matter which method we use and which way we take. This is the foundation of the GH-Method: math-physics medicine.

References:

1. Hsu, Gerald C., eclaireMD Foundation, USA, No. 310: "Biomedical research methodology based on GH-Method: math-physical medicine"

2. Hsu, Gerald C., eclaireMD Foundation, USA, No. 345: "Application of linear equations to predict sensor and finger based postprandial plasma glucoses and daily glucoses for pre-virus, virus, and total periods using GH-Method: math-physical medicine"

3. Hsu, Gerald C., eclaireMD Foundation, USA, No. 97: "A simplified yet accurate linear equation of PPG prediction model for T2D patients (GH-Method: math-physical medicine)"

4. Hsu, Gerald C., eclaireMD Foundation, USA, No. 99: "Application of linear equation-based PPG prediction model for four T2D clinic cases (GH-Method: math-physical medicine)"

5. Hsu, Gerald C., eclaireMD Foundation, USA, No. 339: "Self-recovery of pancreatic beta cell's insulin secretion based on 10+ years annualized data of food, exercise, weight, and glucose using GH-Method: math-physical medicine)

6. Hsu, Gerald C., eclaireMD Foundation, USA, No. 340: "A neural communication model between brain and internal organs, specifically stomach, liver, and pancreatic beta cells based on PPG waveforms of 131 liquid egg meals and 124 solid egg meals)

7.

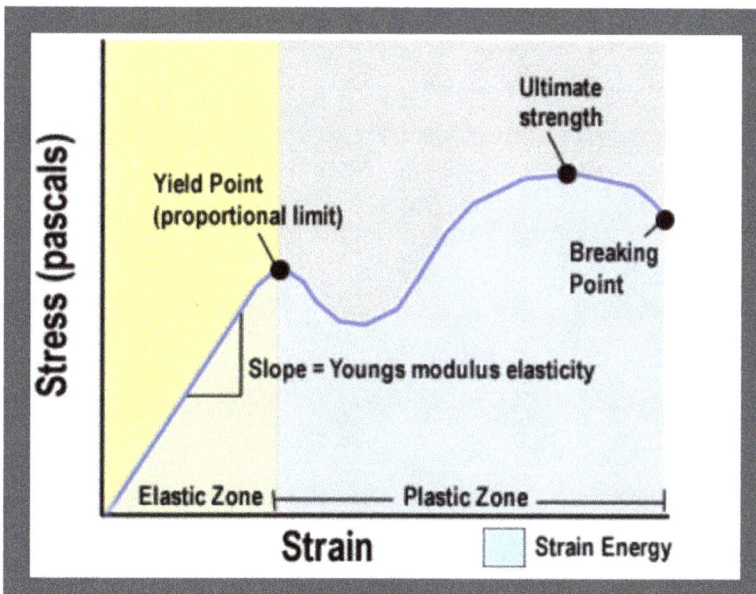

Figure 1: Stress-Strain-Young's modulus, Elastic Zone vs. Plastic Zone

(5/5/18-1/18/20) & (1/19/20-10/10/20)	Y2015 (7/1)	Y2016	Y2017	Y2018	Y2019	Y2020 (10/13)	Average
Carb/Sugar (grams)	14.46	15.47	14.19	15.47	13.19	12.40	14.20
Post-meal Walking (k-steps)	3.681	4.110	4.440	4.538	4.038	4.296	4.184
(5/5/18-1/18/20) & (1/19/20-10/10/20)	Y2015 (7/1)	Y2016	Y2017	Y2018	Y2019	Y2020 (10/13)	Average
Finger FPG	119	117	120	114	115	104	115
Finger PPG	119	120	117	117	114	109	116
Finger Daily	119	119	117	116	114	108	116
Predicted PPG = (FPG*0.97)+(Carbs*M2)-(Steps*5)	Y2015 (7/1)	Y2016	Y2017	Y2018	Y2019	Y2020 (10/13)	Average
Predicted Finger PPG	119	120	117	117	114	109	116
Measured Finger PPG	119	120	117	117	114	109	116
Equation Multipliers (5/5/18-10/10/20)	M2	M2	M2	M2	M2	M2	Average
Prediction Accuracy (Finger PPG)	100%	100%	100%	100%	100%	100%	100%
M2 for Finger PPG Prediction Equation	1.6	1.8	1.6	1.9	1.8	2.4	1.8
Predicted PPG = (FPG*0.97)+(Carbs*M2)-(Steps*5)	Y2015 (7/1)	Y2016	Y2017	Y2018	Y2019	Y2020 (10/13)	Average
Predicted Finger PPG	123	121	120	116	115	102	116
Measured Finger PPG	119	120	117	117	114	109	116
Equation Multipliers (5/5/18-10/10/20)	M2	M2	M2	M2	M2	M2	Average
Prediction Accuracy (Finger PPG)	103%	101%	103%	99%	101%	93%	100%
M2 for Finger PPG Prediction Equation	1.8	1.8	1.8	1.8	1.8	1.8	1.8

Figure 2: Raw data for the period of 7/1/2015 - 10/13/2020

Predicted PPG = (FPG*0.97)+(Carbs*M2)-(Steps*5)	Y2015 (7/1)	Y2016	Y2017	Y2018	Y2019	Y2020 (10/13)	Average
Predicted Finger PPG	119	120	117	117	114	109	116
Finger PPG	119	120	117	117	114	109	116
Prediction Accuracy (Finger PPG)	100%	100%	100%	100%	100%	100%	100%
Predicted Finger Daily Glucose	119.28	119.42	117.41	116.40	114.37	107.70	116
Finger Daily Glucose	119.28	119.42	117.38	116.36	114.38	107.74	116
Predicted Accuracy (Finger Daily)	100%	100%	100%	100%	100%	100%	100%
Equation Multipliers (5/5/18-10/10/20)	M2	M2	M2	M2	M2	M2	Average
Finger PPG Prediction Equation	1.56	1.76	1.59	1.87	1.75	2.41	1.82
Finger Daily Prediction Equation	1.52	1.56	1.82	1.70	1.79	1.99	1.73
Predicted PPG = (FPG*0.97)+(Carbs*M2)-(Steps*5)	Y2015 (7/1)	Y2016	Y2017	Y2018	Y2019	Y2020 (10/13)	Average
Predicted Finger PPG	123	121	120	116	115	102	116
Finger PPG	119	120	117	117	114	109	116
Prediction Accuracy (Finger PPG)	103%	101%	103%	99%	101%	93%	100%
Predicted Finger Daily Glucose	122	122	116	117	114	104	116
Finger Daily Glucose	119	119	117	116	114	108	116
Predicted Accuracy (Finger Daily)	103%	102%	99%	100%	99%	97%	100%
Equation Multipliers (5/5/18-10/10/20)	M2	M2	M2	M2	M2	M2	Average
Finger PPG Prediction Equation	1.82	1.82	1.82	1.82	1.82	1.82	1.82
Finger Daily Prediction Equation	1.73	1.73	1.73	1.73	1.73	1.73	1.73

Figure 3: Calculated PPG prediction using
both Case A (variable M2) and Case B (constant M2) for the period of 7/1/2015 - 10/13/2020

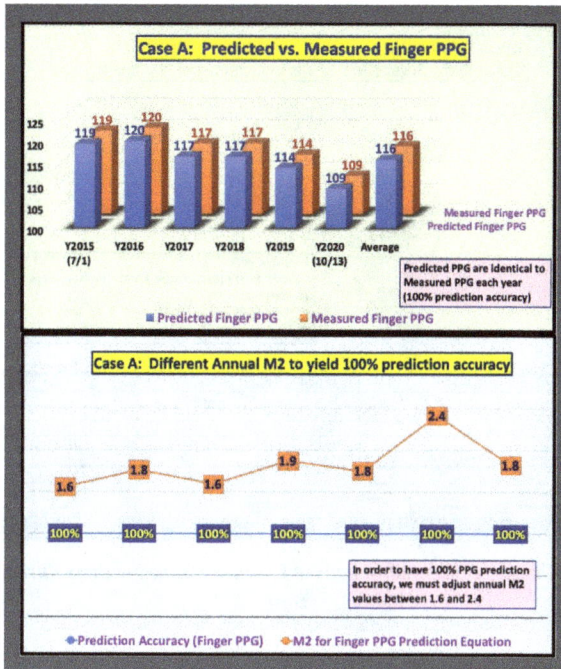

Figure 4: Calculated PPG prediction using Case A (variable M2) to have 100% prediction accuracy for each year of the period of 7/1/2015 - 10/13/2020

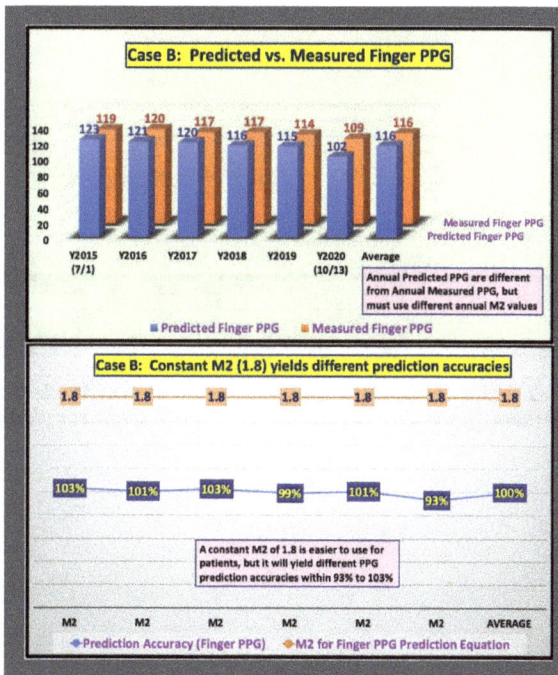

Figure 5: Calculated PPG prediction using Case A (constant M2) to have different prediction accuracy for each year (between 93% and 103%) of the period of 7/1/2015 - 10/13/2020

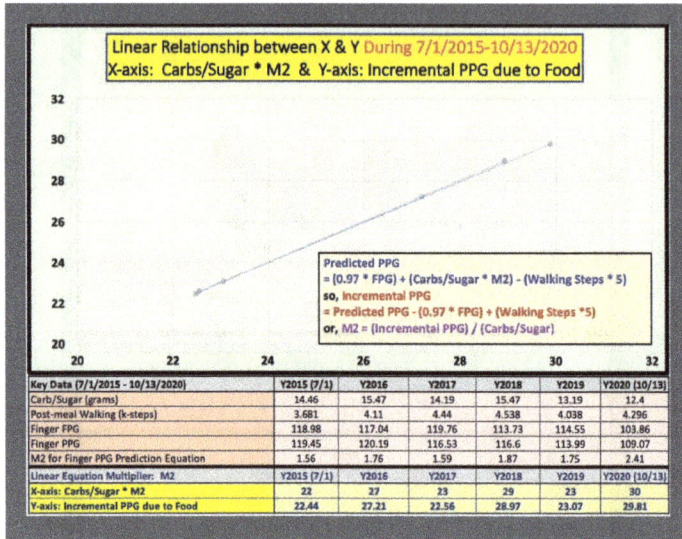

Figure 6: A "pseudo-linear" relationship between x-values and y-values during the "linear elastic" zone

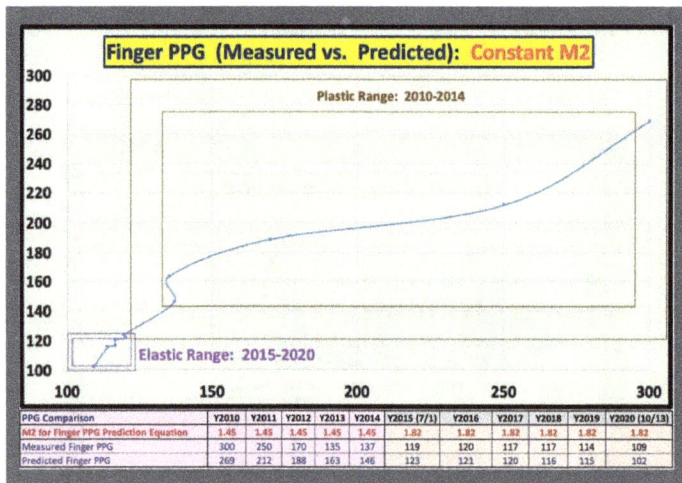

Figure 7: Discussion of variety of relationship between predicted PPG and measured PPG during 2010-2020 (both "pseudo-linear elastic" zone and "nonlinear plastic" zone)

Three cases using lifestyle medicine to control diabetes conditions via GH-Method: math-physical medicine (No. 347)

Gerald C. Hsu
eclaireMD Foundation, USA
10/17/2020

Abstract:

The author applies the diabetes research methodology and prior findings to examine the glucose control situations of three type 2 diabetes (T2D) patients from 2020 lifestyle viewpoints. The key methods involve the glucose data and their associated waveforms to check for curve shapes, changing patterns, and behavior interpretations. Glucoses are the direct outcomes of lifestyle details, such as diet, exercise, and medication. Instead of delving into carbs/sugar intake amounts and the intensity and duration of walking exercise, he can quickly assess a patient's overall health by examining the lifestyle details hidden behind the glucose data and curves. It should be noted that the three T2D patients are not taking any diabetes medications; therefore, this case study excludes the medication's chemical effect.

The method described above is called "lifestyle medicine" in addition to the traditional internal medical practice of relying on medications.

Case A has the worst diabetes conditions among these 3 patients (25 years history). His stringent carbs/sugar intake amount control (12.3 grams) and diligent post-meal walking exercise (4,300 steps) have brought down his sharp rising PPG peak very rapidly to a healthy state. Combined his regular schedule and good quality of sleep with his 9 lbs weight reduction in 2020, have directly contributed to his low averaged FPG at 100 mg/dL. His averaged PPG is at 123 mg/dL. Therefore, his averaged daily glucose is 116 mg/dL (<120 mg/dL).

Case B has a medium level of diabetes conditions among these 3 patients (22 years of history). Her diet is similar to the diet of Case A, except she loves to consume meat which has caused her hypertension and hyperlipidemia conditions. The intensity and duration of her exercise are at half amount of Case A (~2,000 steps and 30 minutes). However, her irregular sleep pattern of wakening up around 4am and then going back to sleep around 6am has raised not only her FPG to 103 mg/dL (in comparison with 100 mg/dL of Case A), but also pushed up her post-breakfast PPG around 8:00am to be the highest peak in her daily glucose waveform. Nevertheless Case B has the lowest daily averaged glucose at 111 mg/dL among these 3 patients.

Case C has the lightest diabetes conditions due to his 4 years history of T2D. However, he is an extremely obese patient (BMI 44 on 1/1/2020 and BMI 39 on 10/17/2020). This 34 lbs weight reduction and BMI 5 reduction in 2020 have assisted his glucose control tremendously. His inactivity after eating his breakfast has continuously pushed his glucose waveform to the peak of his daily glucose around 13:00 when he starts his post-lunch exercise. Case C has an averaged daily glucose of 114 mg/dL which is located in the middle among these 3 patients.

Overall speaking, these three T2D patients sensor glucoses are within the normal range of 120 mg/dL. But, many important facts of their lifestyle details can still be revealed via examination of glucose data and waveforms. These are examples of "lifestyle medicine".

This article demonstrates that lifestyle details, including diet, exercise, and sleep directly change the numerical values of glucose data and influence the physical shapes of the glucose waveforms. Through these three clinical cases, the author's role is like a physician, except that he uses lifestyle details to perform his interpretation, diagnosis, problem solving, and treatment instead of prescribing drugs to control the symptoms. He does not use medications himself because he believes that lifestyle is 80% of the root cause for T2D. Medication only suppresses the external symptoms of the chronic diseases; consequently, it does not cure it internally within the body. He firmly believes that the body is a wonderful machine which can repair itself in many ways; however, it would not be able to cure everything. Of course, a stringent lifestyle management program requires vast knowledge, useful tools, strong willpower, and persistence that unfortunately many patients are lacking. It is the most effective way of controlling diabetes and, to some degree, even self-repairing certain parts of the body, for example my pancreatic beta cells.

He has named his approach as "lifestyle medicine" which should be included in the scope of internal medicine. That is why he spent the past decade and ~30,000 hours to self-study and research chronic diseases and their complications. To date, he has written 347 articles or research notes over the past 10.25 years. Through presentations at medical conferences and publications in medical journals, he hopes to promote his math-physical medicine methodology, knowledge of lifestyle and metabolism, and discoveries from case studies to inspire other healthcare professionals and patients to join him in saving people's lives.

Introduction:

The author applies the diabetes research methodology and prior findings to examine the glucose control situations of three type 2 diabetes (T2D) patients from 2020 lifestyle viewpoints. The key methods involve the glucose data and their associated waveforms to check for curve shapes, changing patterns, and behavior interpretations. Glucoses are the direct outcomes of lifestyle details, such as diet, exercise, and medication. Instead of delving into carbs/sugar intake amounts and the intensity and duration of walking exercise, he can quickly assess a patient's overall health by examining the lifestyle details hidden behind the glucose data and curves. It should be noted that the three T2D patients are not taking any diabetes medications; therefore, this case study excludes the medication's chemical effect.

The method described above is called "lifestyle medicine" in addition to the traditional internal medical practice of relying on medications.

Methods:

Background:

To learn more about the author's developed GH-Method: math-physical medicine (MPM) methodology, readers can refer to his article to understand this MPM analysis method in Reference 1.

Highlights of his related research:

In his published medical papers, he has outlined the following key research findings:

(1) FPG and body weight have a high correlation (>77% based on 7-years data) between them. FPG has 5 influential components with weight contributing >85% of FPG formation.
(2) PPG has 19 influential components. Both carbs/sugar intake amount and post-meal walking exercise contribute ~40% of PPG formation, individually.
(3) He has identified that FPG could serve as a good indicator for pancreatic beta cells' health status in a diabetes patient.
(4) He proved that his pancreatic beta cells have been self-repairing at an annual rate of 2.7%.
(5) Sensor glucoses are ~14% to 18% higher than finger glucoses.

Three T2D patients' information:

Case A is the author himself. He is 73-year-old male with a 25-year history of T2D. His average glucose was 280 mg/dL and HbA1C 10% in 2010. He started his stringent lifestyle management program in 2014 and stopped taking his diabetes medication on 12/8/2015.

Case B is a 72-years-old female with a 22-year history of T2D. Her average glucose was 183 mg/dL and HbA1C 8% in 2010. She has followed the author's lifestyle management program since 2019 and stopped taking her diabetes medication on 1/1/2019.

Case C is a 47-year-old male with a 4-year history of T2D. His average glucose was 150 mg/dL and HbA1C 6.9% in 2017. He did not follow the author's lifestyle management program. His BMI was 44 in early 2020 and since 4/1/2020, he started a weight reduction program and has lost 34 lbs. He has never taken any diabetes medication.

Data in this case study:

All three patients are using a continuous glucose monitoring (CGM) device to collect their glucoses at 15-minutes time interval (Sensor glucoses). Therefore, each patient would collect 96 glucose data each day which are stored on a cloud server to be processed via iPhone. For data consistency concern, all of the patients' glucoses are sensor glucose data. The starting date for Cases A and B is 1/1/2020 and for Case C is 4/1/2020. The ending date of glucose data for this study is 10/17/2020.

Results:

Figure 1 shows the collected raw data of weight, daily average glucose, FPG, PPG, and their calculated weigh change, PPG rising and dropping speed, which is mg/dL per 10-minutes.

The first key observation is that the weight reductions are 9 lbs. (5%), 7 lbs. (4%), and 34 lbs. (12%), for the three cases, respectively. Weight reduction directly helps their FPG reduction and indirectly helps their PPG reduction during this research period. The second key observation is that the daily average glucoses are 116 mg/dL, 111 mg/dL, 114 mg/dL, for the three cases, respectively. This indicates that they have glucoses within the normal range (<120 mg/dL) from a diabetes standpoint. The third key observation is that their PPG rising speed / dropping speed (mg/dL per each 10 minutes) are 2.0/1.1, 0.6/0.6, and 0.3/0.3, for the three cases, respectively. Case A's highest PPG rising speed of 2.0 means his T2D conditions is the worst; his highest dropping speed of 1.1 means he has been diligently doing his post-meal walking exercise. This can be confirmed in Figure 5, reflecting his average carbs/sugar intake amount of 12.44 grams and his post-meal walking of 4,296 steps (1.8 miles or 2.9 km).

After examining the numerical data, he will then focus on checking the PPG waveforms (curves) which can disclose more hidden truth for each patient's lifestyle details.

Figure 2 depicts the synthesized or the assembly of glucose data together, FPG curve within 7 hours, from 00:00 through 07:00 with 15-minute time intervals, of the three cases, respectively. Case A's FPG waveform is almost identical to Case C's FPG waveform. Not only are their curve shape similar to a "salad bowl" with the highest value, 113 mg/dL for Case A and 111 mg/dL for Case C, on the rim of the bowl at 00:00; and with the lowest value of 93 mg/dL for both, at the bottom of the bowl around 03:00. However, Case B is a different story. Her peak FPG of 112 mg/dL occurs around 06:00 instead of 00:00. The author discovered that she usually wakes up around 04:00 with her FPG was 102 mg/dL, and then go back to sleep again around 06:00, where her FPG raised to 112 mg/dL. During this two-hour period, her FPG increased approximately 10 mg/dL. The author's previous neuroscience research based on his 2.5 years data also disclosed that between his wake-up moment and the first bite of breakfast, his FPG would increase around 10 mg/dL (Reference 7). Therefore, Case B's unique FPG waveform is a result from a disturbance in her sleep pattern.

Figure 3 illustrates the synthesized PPG curve within 3 hours or 180 minutes, with 15-minute time intervals, of three cases, respectively. Three PPG waveforms are similar in pattern with peak PPG values occurring around 45 to 60-minutes after the first bite of meals, except their peak PPG values are 131 mg/dL, 121 mg/dL, and 109 mg/dL, respectively. Their average PPG values are 123 mg/dL, 117 mg/dL, and 108 mg/dL, respectively. These differences in peak PPG and average PPG also reflect the severity of T2D in each patient: Case A being the worst, Case B in the middle, and Case C as the best. The three PPG waves are trending down at around

150 to 180-minutes. Actually, at the 120-minute time instant, all three PPG values are extremely low, at least lower than the PPG at 0-minute at the moment of first bite. This observed phenomena proves that the long-standing advice from healthcare professionals to diabetes patients of measuring their finger-piercing PPG at 2-hour post meal is inaccurate and useless. To match the author's statement in data observation from the Figure 1 table, the PPG waveforms indicate the same findings. The "cliff" shape with a sharp rise to the higher peak value and then a sharp drop in Case A have confirmed the severity of his diabetes (sensitivity of carbs/sugar) and the effectiveness of his stringent post-meal exercise. However, the "not-so-sharp lump" shapes of the PPG waveforms in Cases B and C reveal that they have room for improvement in their post-meal exercise.

The synthesized daily glucose curve within 24 hours with 15-minute time interval, of the three cases, respectively, is shown in Figure 4. At first glance, the three waveforms have similar shapes, except for Case B's peak occurring daily around post-breakfast time, whereas Cases A and C occur around post-lunch time. As mentioned earlier, Case B's sleep pattern disturbance in early morning from 04:00 - 06:00, combined with her carbs/sugar intake during breakfast at 07:00 pushes her glucose trend to the highest point, around 08:00.

For Case A, his heaviest meal is lunch, followed by breakfast, and then dinner as the lightest for weight control; therefore, his daily peak glucose occurs around 13:00, one hour after lunch. Due to smaller portions for breakfast and dinner, his two PPG peaks for breakfast and dinner are not as severe as the post-lunch peak.

The three meal portion sizes for Case B are similar, and her post-meal walking is about 2,000 steps (0.8 miles or 1.3 km). Therefore, her waveforms of lunch and dinner are quite similar.

When observing the curve for Case C, the author can tell that he eats his breakfast around 08:00; therefore, his breakfast peak occurs at 09:00 and does not walk or exercise at all after his meal. That is why his glucose wave continues to trend upward (despite a small dip between 09:00 and 10:00) to reach the lunch peak at 13:00. The sharp decline after 13:00 is resulting from his physical activities, probably some sort of exercise, until the wave reaches the valley between 15:00 to 18:00. His weight reduction program limits him to a light dinner, usually just a small salad. That is why there is no sharp rise after 18:00. In addition, he exercises again to bring his wave to a downward trend until sleep time.

Despite of their individual daily peak glucose values of 140 mg/dL (lunch), 129 mg/dL (breakfast), 139 mg/dL (lunch), respectively, the 3 patients average daily glucose values are 116 mg/dL, 111 mg/dL, 114 mg/dL, respectively. Therefore, their T2D severity ranking are Case A being the worst, Case C in the middle, and Case B being the best. It is important that the 3 T2D patients have done well on controlling their glucoses without any medication intervention. However, by examining their lifestyles with a magnifying glass, the author can still identify room of improvement for each individual.

From the above explanations, many lifestyle details can be seen and identified in the glucose data and waveforms. The body does not lie. Energy enters into the body via food and one must consume energy via exercise and activities; otherwise, the excessive unburned energy stored in the body will lead into obesity, diabetes, and other chronic diseases.

In Figure 5, it displays Case A's PPG waveforms, carbs/sugar intake amount, along with post-meal walking steps for breakfast, lunch, and dinner. Unfortunately, Cases B and C do not keep their detailed records of diet and exercise like Case A. As mentioner earlier, similar observations and interpretations can be applied to this diagram, for example, the author stated medium breakfast, heavy lunch, and light dinner from carbs/sugar intake amount of 8.7 grams, 18.9 grams, and 13.8 grams, respectively. His post-meal walking steps are 4,401, 3,844, and 4,895, respectively. The least amount of walking steps for post-lunch exercise is due to the hot weather temperature around noon time from the months of May through September. These five months of scorching temperature, consisting 50% of the total period, have directly lowered his willingness to walk outside in the heat.

Summary:

Case A has the worst diabetes conditions among these 3 patients (25 years history). His stringent carbs/sugar intake amount control (12.3 grams) and diligent post-meal walking exercise (4,300 steps) have brought down his sharp rising PPG peak very rapidly to a healthy state. Combined his regular schedule and good quality of sleep with his 9 lbs weight reduction in 2020, have directly contributed to his low averaged FPG at 100 mg/dL. His averaged PPG is at 123 mg/dL. Therefore, his averaged daily glucose is 116 mg/dL (<120 mg/dL).

Case B has a medium level of diabetes conditions among these 3 patients (22 years of history). Her diet is similar to the diet of Case A, except she loves to consume meat which has caused her hypertension and hyperlipidemia conditions. The intensity and duration of her exercise are at half amount of Case A (~2,000 steps and 30 minutes). However, her irregular sleep pattern of wakening up around 4am and then going back to sleep around 6am has raised not only her FPG to 103 mg/dL (in comparison with 100 mg/dL of Case A), but also pushed up her post-breakfast PPG around 8:00am to be the highest peak in her daily glucose waveform. Nevertheless Case B has the lowest daily averaged glucose at 111 mg/dL among these 3 patients.

Case C has the lightest diabetes conditions due to his 4 years history of T2D. However, he is an extremely obese patient (BMI 44 on 1/1/2020 and BMI 39 on 10/17/2020). This 34 lbs weight reduction and BMI 5 reduction in 2020 have assisted his glucose control tremendously. His inactivity after eating his breakfast has continuously pushed his glucose waveform to the peak of his daily glucose around 13:00 when he starts his post-lunch exercise. Case C has an averaged daily glucose of 114 mg/dL which is located in the middle among these 3 patients.

Overall speaking, these three T2D patients sensor glucoses are within the normal range of 120 mg/dL. But, many important facts of their lifestyle details can still be revealed via examination of glucose data and waveforms. These are examples of "lifestyle medicine".

Conclusions:

This article demonstrates that lifestyle details, including diet, exercise, and sleep directly change the numerical values of glucose data and influence the physical shapes of the glucose waveforms. Through these three clinical cases, the author's role is like a physician, except that he uses lifestyle details to perform his interpretation, diagnosis, problem solving, and treatment instead of prescribing drugs to control the symptoms. He does not use medications himself because he believes that lifestyle is 80% of the root cause for T2D. Medication only suppresses the external symptoms of the chronic diseases; consequently, it does not cure it internally within the body. He firmly believes that the body is a wonderful machine which can repair itself in many ways; however, it would not be able to cure everything. Of course, a stringent lifestyle management program requires vast knowledge, useful tools, strong willpower, and persistence that unfortunately many patients are lacking. It is the most effective way of controlling diabetes and, to some degree, even self-repairing certain parts of the body, for example my pancreatic beta cells.

He has named his approach as "lifestyle medicine" which should be included in the scope of internal medicine. That is why he spent the past decade and ~30,000 hours to self-study and research chronic diseases and their complications. To date, he has written 347 articles or research notes over the past 10.25 years. Through presentations at medical conferences and publications in medical journals, he hopes to promote his math-physical medicine methodology, knowledge of lifestyle and metabolism, and discoveries from case studies to inspire other healthcare professionals and patients to join him in saving people's lives.

References:

1. Hsu, Gerald C., eclaireMD Foundation, USA, No. 310: "Biomedical research methodology based on GH-Method: math-physical medicine"

2. Hsu, Gerald C., eclaireMD Foundation, USA, No. 345: "Application of linear equations to predict sensor and finger based postprandial plasma glucoses and daily glucoses for pre-virus, virus, and total periods using GH-Method: math-physical medicine"

3. Hsu, Gerald C., eclaireMD Foundation, USA, No. 97: "A simplified yet accurate linear equation of PPG prediction model for T2D patients (GH-Method: math-physical medicine)"

4. Hsu, Gerald C., eclaireMD Foundation, USA, No. 99: "Application of linear equation-based PPG prediction model for four T2D clinic cases (GH-Method: math-physical medicine)"

5. Hsu, Gerald C., eclaireMD Foundation, USA, No. 339: "Self-recovery of pancreatic beta cell's insulin secretion based on 10+ years annualized data of food, exercise, weight, and glucose using GH-Method: math-physical medicine)

6. Hsu, Gerald C., eclaireMD Foundation, USA, No. 340: "A neural communication model between brain and internal organs, specifically stomach, liver, and pancreatic beta cells based on PPG waveforms of 131 liquid egg meals and 124 solid egg meals)

7. Hsu, Gerald C., eclaireMD Foundation, USA, No. 324: "A neuro-communication model between the brain and liver regarding glucose production and secretion in early morning using GH-Method: math-physical medicine"

Lifestyle Medicine Cases	4/1-10/17/2020	1/1-10/17/2021	4/1-10/17/2022
T2D history	25 years	22 years	4 years
Data of Weight & Glucose	Case A	Case B	Case C
Weight (Average)	171	155	295
Weight (Reduction)	9	7	34
Weight reduction %	5%	4%	12%
Daily Glucose (Sensor)	116	111	114
FPG (Sensor)	100	103	99
PPG (Sensor)	123	117	108
Sensor PPG (Start, 0-min)	122	118	107
Sensor PPG (Max, 45/45/60 min)	131	121	109
Sensor PPG (Min, 150/180/150min)	119	113	107
PPG rising speed (every 10 min)	2.0	0.6	0.3
PPG dropping speed (every 10 min)	1.1	0.6	0.3
T2D conditions comparison	Worst	Medium	Lightest

Figure 1: Background data table and calculations of weight change and PPG speeds

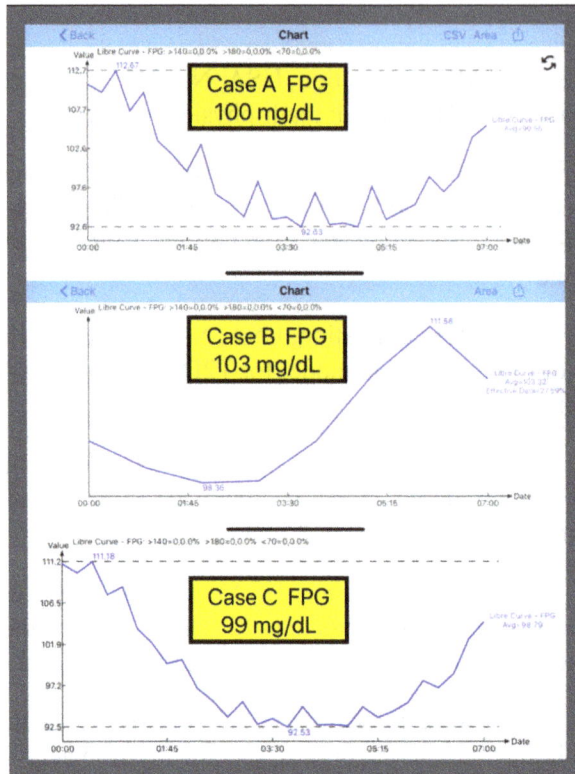

Figure 2: Synthesized FPG waveforms of 3 cases (7 hours)

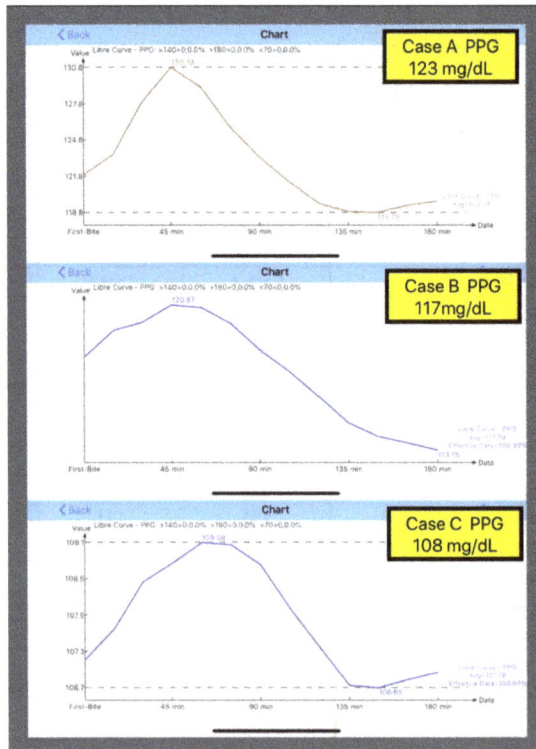

Figure 3: Synthesized PPG waveforms of 3 cases (3 hours)

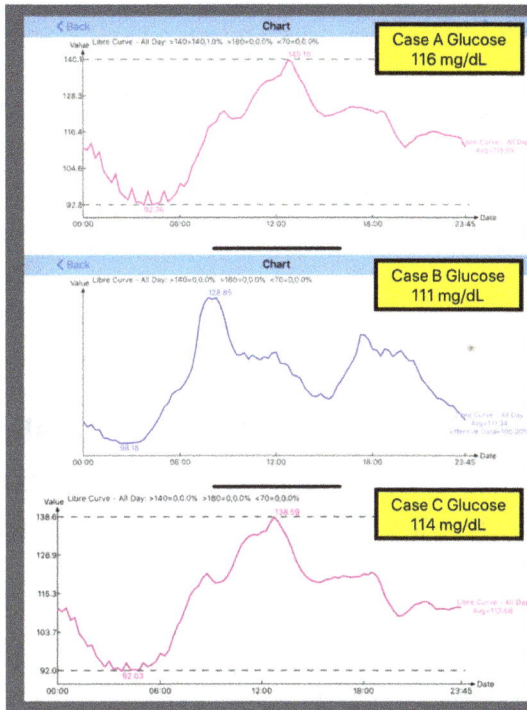

Figure 4: Synthesized daily glucose waveforms of 3 cases (24 hours)

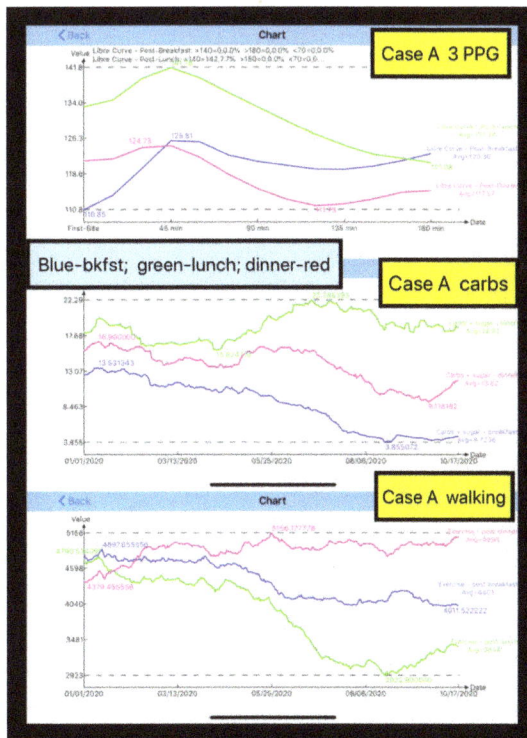

Figure 5: Case A's 3 meals PPG waveforms and carbs/sugar intake & post-meal walking step

Investigation on GH modulus of linear elastic glucose behavior with two diabetes patients data using GH-Method: math-physical medicine, Part 2 (No. 349)

Gerald C. Hsu
eclaireMD Foundation, USA
10/17-21/2020

Abstract:

This article is an extended research on the linear elasticity of glucose with the author's defined GH-modulus or M2 cited in Reference 7 (Part 1 or his paper no. 346). The main purpose of this study is twofold. First, it is to study the biomedical meaning of the GH modulus which depends on a patient's severity of type 2 diabetes (T2D) over a period of time. Second, it is to discover when its linear elastic features would appear, under what kind of conditions, and which easier path for patients to utilize this for their daily glucose control.

Here is the simple linear formula previously defined in References 2, 3, and 4 for predicting the postprandial plasma glucose (PPG):

Predicted PPG
= (FPG* 0.97) + (carbs/sugar intake grams * M2) - (post-meal waking K-steps * 5)

In Reference 7 (paper No. 346), the author connected the biomedical glucose prediction equation with a basic concept of stress and strain in engineering, along with the Young's modulus of engineering strength of materials. Using his collected 11,580 data of glucose, food, and exercise, he has demonstrated that a "pseudo-linear" relationship existing between the carbs/sugar intake amount which is similar to the "stress" part on the engineering system; and the incremental PPG amount which is similar to the "strain" part of the engineering system. A newly defined coefficient of "GH-modulus" (the M2 multiplier for carbs/sugar intake amount) is remarkably similar to the role of Young's modules on relating stress and strain on the subject of engineering strength of materials.

During his "better controlled" period of diabetes from 7/1/2015 to 10/13/2020, his averaged PPG is 116 mg/dL which is below 120 mg/dL and located within the normal range from diabetes concerns. Only within this "better-controlled" glucose range, the relationship between carbs/sugar intake and incremental PPG would then be "linear" or "pseudo-linear". Otherwise, for severe T2D patients who has elevated PPG level above 180 mg/dL (hyperglycemia) most of the time and then suddenly decreased to below 70 mg/dL (hypoglycemia or insulin shock), the relationship between food and PPG would then follow a nonlinear plastic pattern where the defined linear relationship would not be applicable.

By 2019, approximately 6% of worldwide population (or 463 million people) have diabetes. Although he believes that his linear elastic glucose behavior of GH modulus is only applicable for patient's glucose levels below 180 mg/dL and above 70 mg/dL, but it is already a wide enough range for lots of diabetes patients to use. In regard to nonlinear plastic zone, more hyperglycemic cases and associated data are required to collect and then conduct a further complex analysis. At least, this linear elastic glucose behavior is the first stage of getting sufficient information to move further into a more complicated nonlinear plastic glucose zone.

Based on two diabetes patients data, for either fixed M2 or variable M2 values, a linear relationship between carbs/sugar intake amount and incremental PPG amount have been oobserved. This defined GH-modulus (i.e. M2 value) is easier to be applied over a reasonable long period, for example, either 3 months or 4 months in order to match with the lab-tested HbA1C value. Since blood and liver cells are organic material, the GH-modulus changes according to the severity of a patient's diabetes conditions. However, the author would like to recommend using a fixed GH-modules or M2 value within a period of 3 to 4 months due to the simplicity of calculation and practical usage.

The author has spent four decades as a practical engineer, but he does understand the importance of basic concepts, sophisticated theories, and practical equations which serve as the necessary background of all kinds of applications. Therefore, he focused his time and energy to investigate glucose related subjects using a variety of methods he learned in the past, including this particularly interesting stress-strain approach. In addition, he understood the importance and urgency in helping diabetes patients to control their glucoses. That is why, over the past few years, he has continuously simplified his findings regarding diabetes and derived more useful formulas or practical tools in meeting the general public's interest on controlling chronic diseases and their complications to reduce pain and death probability.

Introduction:

This article is an extended research on the linear elasticity of glucose with the author's defined GH-modulus or M2 cited in Reference 7 (Part 1 or his paper no. 346). The main purpose of this study is twofold. First, it is to study the biomedical meaning of the GH modulus which depends on a patient's severity of type 2 diabetes (T2D) over a period of time. Second, it is to discover when its linear elastic features would appear, under what kind of conditions, and which easier path for patients to utilize this for their daily glucose control.

Here is the simple linear formula previously defined in References 2, 3, and 4 for predicting the postprandial plasma glucose (PPG):

Predicted PPG
= (FPG* 0.97) + (carbs/sugar intake grams * M2) - (post-meal waking K-steps * 5)

In Reference 7 (paper No. 346), the author connected the biomedical glucose prediction equation with a basic concept of stress and strain in engineering, along with the Young's modulus of engineering strength of materials. Using his collected 11,580 data of glucose, food, and exercise, he has demonstrated that a "pseudo-linear" relationship existing between the carbs/sugar intake amount which is similar to the "stress" part on the engineering system; and the incremental PPG amount which is similar to the "strain" part of the engineering system. A newly defined coefficient of "GH-modulus" (the M2 multiplier for carbs/sugar intake amount) is remarkably similar to the role of Young's modules on relating stress and strain on the subject of engineering strength of materials.

During his "better controlled" period of diabetes from 7/1/2015 to 10/13/2020, his averaged PPG is 116 mg/dL which is below 120 mg/dL and located within the normal range from diabetes concerns. Only within this "better-controlled" glucose range, the relationship between carbs/sugar intake and incremental PPG would then be "linear" or "pseudo-linear". Otherwise, for severe T2D patients who has elevated PPG level above 180 mg/dL (hyperglycemia) most of the time and then suddenly decreased to below 70 mg/dL (hypoglycemia or insulin shock), the relationship between food and PPG would then follow a nonlinear plastic pattern where the defined linear relationship would not be applicable.

By 2019, approximately 6% of worldwide population (or 463 million people) have diabetes. Although he believes that his linear elastic glucose behavior of GH modulus is only applicable for patient's glucose levels below 180 mg/dL and above 70 mg/dL, but it is already a wide enough range for lots of diabetes patients to use. In regard to nonlinear plastic zone, more hyperglycemic cases and associated data are required to collect and then conduct a further complex analysis. At least, this linear elastic glucose behavior is the first stage of getting sufficient information to move further into a more complicated nonlinear plastic glucose zone.

Methods:

Background:
To learn more about the author's GH-Method: math-physical medicine (MPM) methodology, readers can refer to his article to understand the developed MPM analysis method in Reference 1.

Highlights of his previous research:
In 2015, the author decomposed the PPG waveforms (data curves) into 19 influential components and identified carbs/sugar intake amount and post-meal walking exercise contributing to approximately 40% of PPG formation, respectively. Therefore, he could safely discount the importance of the remaining ~20% contribution by the 16 other influential components.

In 2016, he utilized optical physics, big data analytics, and artificial intelligence (AI) techniques to develop a computer software to predict PPG based on the patient's food pictures or meal photos. This sophisticated AI approach and iPhone APP software product have reached to a 98.8% prediction accuracy based on ~6,000 meal photos.

In 2017, he also detected that body weight contributes to over 85% to fasting plasma glucose (FPG) formation. Furthermore, in 2019, he identified that FPG could serve as a good indicator of the pancreatic beta cells' health status; therefore, he can apply the FPG value or more precisely, 97% of the FPG value, to serve as the baseline PPG value to calculate the PPG incremental amount in order to obtain the predicted PPG.

In 2018, based on his collected ~2,500 meals and associated sensor PPG waveforms, he further applied the perturbation theory from quantum mechanics, using the first bite of his meal as the initial condition and then extend and build an entire PPG waveform covering a period of 180 minutes, with a 95% of PPG prediction accuracy.

In 2019, all of his developed PPG prediction mathematical models have achieved high percentages of prediction accuracy, but he also realized that his prediction models are too difficult to use by the general public. The above-mentioned sophisticated methods would be difficult for healthcare professionals and diabetes patients to understand, let alone use them in their daily life for diabetes control. Therefore, he tried to supplement his complex models with a simple linear equation of predicted PPG (see References 2, 3, and 4).

Here is his simple linear formula:

Predicted PPG
= FPG * M1 + (carbs&sugar * M2) - (post-meal walking k-steps * M3)

Where M1, M2, M3 are 3 multipliers.

After lengthy research, trial and error, and data tuning, he finally identified the best multipliers for FPG and exercise as 0.97 for M1 and 5.0 for M3.

In comparison with PPG, the FPG is a more stabilized biomarker since it is directly related to body weight. We know that weight reduction is a hard task, but weight is a far calmer and more stabilizing biomarker in comparison to glucose which fluctuates from minute to minute.

The influence of exercise, specifically post-meal walking steps on PPG (41% contribution and >80% negative correlation with PPG), is almost equal to the influence from the carbs/sugar intake amount on PPG (39% contribution and >80% positive correlation with PPG). In terms of intensity and duration, exercise is a much simpler and straightforward subject to study and deal with.

Therefore, for the author, these two parameters, FPG and walking, have a lower chance of variation. However, for other diabetes patients, it is best to keep the multiplier M3 as a variable if they constantly change their exercise patterns.

On the other hand, the relationship between food nutrition and glucose is an exceedingly complex and difficult subject to fully understand and effectively manage, since there are many types of food and their associated carbs/sugar contents. For example, the author's food nutritional database contains over six million data. As a result, he decided to implement two multipliers, M1 for FPG and M3 for exercise, as the two "constants" and keep M2 as the only "variable" in his PPG prediction equation and the linear elastic glucose study in this article.

Here is his simplified linear equation for predicted PPG as follows:

Predicted PPG
= (0.97*FPG)+(Carbs&sugar * M2) - (post-meal walking k-steps * 5)

He also defines the following three new terms in terms 1, 2, and 3:

Term 1:
GH modulus = M2

Term 2:
The incremental PPG amount
= Predicted PPG - PPG baseline
  (i.e. 0.97 * FPG) + exercise effect
  (i.e. post-meal walking k-steps * 5)

Term 3:
GH modulus
= (Incremental PPG)/(Carbs&sugar)

Stress, Strain, & Young's modulus:
Prior to the past decade in his self-study and medical research work, he was an engineer in the fields of structural (aerospace and naval defense), mechanical (nuclear power plants and computer-aided-design), and electronics (computers and semiconductors).

The following excerpts come from Internet, e.g. Google and Wikipedia:

Strain - ε:
Strain is the "deformation of a solid due to stress" - change in dimension divided by the original value of the dimension - and can be expressed as
$\varepsilon = dL / L$
where
ε = strain (m/m, in/in)
dL = elongation or compression (offset) of object (m, in)
L = length of object (m, in)

Stress - σ:
Stress is force per unit area and can be expressed as
$\sigma = F / A$
where
σ = *stress (N/m2, lb/in2, psi)*
F = applied force (N, lb)
A = stress area of object (m2, in2)

Stress includes tensile stress, compressible stress, shearing stress, etc.

E, Young's modulus:
It can be expressed as:
E = stress / strain
  = σ / ε

$= (F / A) / (dL / L)$

where

E = Young's Modulus of Elasticity (Pa, N/m2, lb/in2, psi) was named after the 18th-century English physicist Thomas Young.

Elasticity:

Elasticity is a property of an object or material indicating how it will restore it to its original shape after distortion. A spring is an example of an elastic object - when stretched, it exerts a restoring force which tends to bring it back to its original length (Figure 1).

Plasticity:

When the force is going beyond the elastic limit of material, it is into a "plastic' zone which means even when force is removed, the material will not return back to its original state (Figure 1).

Based on various experimental results, the following table lists some Young's modulus associated with different materials:

Nylon: 2.7 GPa
Concrete: 17-30 GPa
Glass fibers: 72 GPa
Copper: 117 GPa
Steel: 190-215 GPa
Diamond: 1220 GPa

Young's modules in above table are ranked from soft material (low E) to stiff material (higher E)."

Professor James Andrews taught the author linear elasticity at the University of Iowa and Professor Norman Jones taught him nonlinear plasticity at Massachusetts Institute of Technology. These two great academic mentors provided him with the foundation knowledge of these two important subjects.

In this study, he uses the analogy of relationship among stress, strain, and Young's modulus to illustrate a similar relationship among carbs/sugar intake amount, incremental predicted PPG, and GH modulus (i.e. M2). They are listed below for a closer comparison.

GH modulus (i.e. M2)
= (Incremental PPG)/(Carbs&sugar)

Young's modulus E
= stress / strain
= σ / ε

Where Incremental PPG is the incremental amount of predicted PPG (note: the predicted PPG is also replaced by the measured PPG for one of the sensitivity study of glucose behaviors in this article).

The author visualizes the carbs/sugar intake amount as the stress (the force, cause, or stimulator) on his liver and the incremental PPG amount as the strain (the response, consequence, or stimulation) from the liver. The GH modulus (i.e. M2) is similar to the Young's modulus (i.e. E) which describes the "pseudo-linear" relationship existed between the carbs/sugar (stress) and incremental PPG (strain).

Finally, conceptually, he is able to connect together the subject of liver glucose production in endocrinology with the subject of strength of materials in structural & mechanical engineering.

Data collection:
The author (male case) is a 73-year-old male with a 25-year history of T2D. He began collecting his carbs/sugar intake amount and post-meal walking steps on 7/1/2015. From 7/15/2015 to 10/18/2020 (1,935 days), he has collected 6 data per day, 1 FPG, 3 PPG, carb/sugar, and post-meal walking steps. He utilized these 11,610 data of 1,935 days to conduct his prior research work on the subject of linear elastic glucose study (Reference 7). In addition, on 5/5/2018, he started to use a continuous glucose monitoring (CGM) sensor device to collect 96 glucose data each day.

The period of 7/1/2015 to 10/18/2020 is his "best-controlled" diabetes period, where his average daily glucoses is maintained at 116 mg/dL (<120 mg/dL). He named this as his "linear elastic zone" of diabetes health. It should also be noted that in 2010, his average glucose was 280 mg/dL and HbA1C was 10%, while taking three diabetes medications. Please note that the strong chemical interventions from various diabetes medications would seriously alter glucose physical behaviors. He called the period prior to 2015 as his "nonlinear plastic zone" of diabetes health.

The second set of data comes from his wife (female case) with a 22-year history of T2D. She began to collect her glucose data via finger-piercing method (finger glucose) since 1/1/2014. However, she does not keep a detailed record of her diet and exercise. Both patients eat almost the same meals prepared by the author, except that she consumes more meat which partially affects her hyperlipidemia and hypertension conditions. From the diabetes research viewpoint, he decided to use 80% of the male case's carbs/sugar amount for her and use 50% of the male case's post-meal walking steps for her. On 1/1/2020, she began using the same CGM device to collect her sensor glucose data at the same rate of 96 data per day since 1/1/2020.

In order to maintain data consistency for a fair and accurate comparison, the author took both male data and female data from 1/18/2020 through 10/18/2020 and subdivided them into 9 equal-length monthly sub-periods to study their glucose fluctuation patterns and data.

Results:

Fixed M2 Case:
Figure 2 shows the collected raw data with a fixed M2 values for calculating both predicted PPG and prediction accuracy percentages. In this table, the author utilized two different fixed values of M2 for male case and female case individually to calculate both x- and y- components of his "linear elastic glucose" equation. The comparison between the male case M2 value of 3.6 and the female case M2 of 2.6 revealed the individual severity of their respective T2D conditions. The male case indicates a more severe diabetes patient who requires higher M2 value to increase his predicted PPG in order to match his higher measured PPG value.

Again, the linear elastic glucose equation using predicted PPG is listed below:

Predicted PPG = (FPG * 0.97) + (carbs&sugar * M2) - (post-meal walking k-steps * 5)

The "x-component" of the linear elastic glucose equation is:
*(carbs&sugar * M2);*
While the "y-component" of the linear elastic glucose equation is:
*(**Predicted** PPG - (FPG * 0.97) + (post-meal walking k-steps * 5)*

Due to the linearity characteristics of this equation, the relationship between the x-component and y-component is always guaranteed to be "linear". However, the different M2 values would result into different data ranges of x and y components. Figures 3 and 4 show these different M2 values and data ranges for male case and female case, respectively.
The male case with the fixed M2 of 3.6, both x and y are within the range of 35 to 58 with an average value of 44 is shown in Figure 3. The female case with the fixed M2 of 2.6, both x and y are within the range of 22 to 34 with an average value of 26 is observed in Figure 4.

In summary, the higher M2, the higher x and y values become, and the higher predicted and measured PPG values are. The key point from these two figures is that the M2 values are varying based on a patient's body conditions. This is similar to the different organic materials from the different Young's modules (E) values, such as nylon'E ~3 versus steel's E ~200.

Listed below are the values of the prediction accuracy for male and female for each month. Please note that the prediction accuracy percentage varies with the fixed M2 input, however, their prediction accuracies are 100% for the total period of 9 months for both male case and female case which is the purpose of selecting these two fixed M2 values.

1/18 - 2/18: 101% & 97%
2/18 - 3/18: 97% & 99%
3/18 - 4/18: 98% & 95%
4/18 - 5/18: 111% & 108%

5/18 - 6/18: 101% & 107%
6/18 - 7/18: 88% & 93%
7/18 - 8/18: 100% & 95%
8/18 - 9/18: 102% & 101%
9/18 - 10/18: 98% & 106%
2020 Average: 100% & 100%

Variable M2 Case:

Figure 5 illustrates the collected raw data to be used in his variable M2 case of calculations. In this table, the author utilized variable value of M2 for each month in order to make the calculated x-component values to match with the calculated y-components values during each monthly sub-period; therefore, to "force" the predicted PPG value to match with the measured PPG value in each month. As a result, a "pseudo-linear" relationship between x-component and y-component could be created and observed. However, this approach will cause some degree of sacrifice on PPG prediction's accuracy.

This forced "pseudo-linear" relationship makes sense in the biomedical field since red blood cells and liver cells are organic materials which are different from those inorganic materials in the engineering systems, such as rubber, concrete, or steel. The human organ cells are not only organic but also have different lifespans, where they can mutate, change, repair, or die. For example, the lifespan of the red blood cells is 115 to 120 days, the lifespan of liver cells is 300 to 500 days, and the lifespan of pancreatic beta cells is unknown with slightly adaptive change (this is why pancreatic beta cells self-repair process is very slow, about 2.7% per year for the author). Not all of the body cells die at the same moment. At any given instance, an organ would have combinations of new cells, sick cells, dying cells, and mutated cells, mixing together. It is a very complex and extraordinarily situation; therefore, the author has chosen different M2 values for different months in order to achieve his 100% prediction accuracies for all sub-periods. This would be a reasonable approach in proceeding with his biomedical research.

In the previous paragraph (Figures 2, 3, and 4), the fixed M2 difference between the male case of 3.6 versus the female case of 2.6 is based on the severity of their T2D between patients. Furthermore, in this paragraph (Figures 5, 6, and 7), it has demonstrated that the variable M2 value differences of different months are resulted from the T2D conditions varying month to month for each patient. This means that glucose is a "dynamic" function instead of being a "static" function.
The above discussions are the major differences between the linear elasticity organic glucoses and the traditional linear elasticity of strength of inorganic engineering materials.

Again, for conducting his sensitivity analysis, the linear elastic glucose equation using **measured** PPG is modified and listed below:

Measured PPG = (FPG * 0.97) + (carbs&sugar * M2) - (post-meal walking k-steps * 5)

The "x-component" of the linear elastic glucose equation is:
(carbs&sugar * M2);
While the "y-component" of the linear elastic glucose equation is:
(**Measured** PPG - (FPG * 0.97) + (post-meal walking k-steps * 5)

By examining the variable M2 values, over 9 monthly sub-periods, the male case has M2 range from 2.8 to 5.2 with an average of 3.7 value, and the female case has M2 range from 1.9 to 3.6 with an average of 2.7 value (Figure 5). Please note the minor difference between fixed M2 of 3.6 versus 2.6 and variable M2 of 3.7 versus 2.7 which are caused by rounding off in the numerical analysis.

For the male case with variable M2, both x and y components are within the range of 37 to 51 with an average value of 45 (Figure 6). The female case with variable M2, both x and y components are within the range of 18 to 32 with an average value of 26 (Figure 7).

In summary, similar to the fixed M2 case, for most of the months, the higher variable M2, the higher x and y values become, and the higher predicted and measured PPG values are. The key point from these two figures is that the monthly M2 values are dependent on the patient's body conditions (combination of blood, liver, and pancreas) for that particular month. Figures 6 and 7 have graphically demonstrated the linear elastic glucoses data from Figure 5.

Listed below are the values of the individual M2 multiplier (i.e. GH-modulus) for each month in 2020, in the order of (male case vs. female case).

1/18 - 2/18:   3.5 vs. 3.0
2/18 - 3/18:   3.9 vs. 2.7
3/18 - 4/18:   3.8 vs. 3.1
4/18 - 5/18:   2.8 vs. 1.9
5/18 - 6/18:   3.5 vs. 1.9
6/18 - 7/18:   5.2 vs. 3.6
7/18 - 8/18:   3.6 vs. 3.2
8/18 - 9/18:   3.4 vs. 2.5
9/18 - 10/18:   3.8 vs. 1.9
2020 Average: 3.7 vs. 2.7

The purpose in selecting variable M2 values for each of the 9 monthly sub-periods is to achieve 100% match between x- component and y-component for both male case and female case.

Discussion:

This "linear elastic glucose" study started from the verification and improvement for the predicted PPG through his previously defined simple formula of PPG prediction. The author has learned from his engineering background that a linear system approach would be the easiest way to study a relationship between causes and consequences. Therefore, he started to investigate the similarity between elastic glucose system and elastic engineering system using Young's modulus and GH-modulus as his pair of analogy models. Nevertheless, he has never forgotten his ultimate objective is to identify an easier application model with a higher PPG prediction accuracy in order to help other diabetes patients while maintain the basic requirement of science to seek for truth with high precision.

Either using a fixed M2 value to achieve a high accuracy over a total period of 9 months or using monthly variable M2 values to achieve high accuracies for every monthly sub-period, he has observed a linear relationship existing between carbs/sugar intake amount and incremental PPG amount (including predicted or measured PPG, FPG, and exercise). More importantly, he still maintains an extremely high PPG prediction accuracy from using both approaches.

One important viewpoint is that glucose is an organic material which consists of nonlinear and dynamic functional behaviors in its nature. Therefore, in order to fully understand and be able to describe its behavior accurately, a research using a nonlinear plastic model is needed. However, at present time, similar to linear elasticity engineering applications, this linear elastic glucose behavior study already covers a sufficient scope of biomedical applications, and it is useful. As a counterpart example, many T2D patients are either in the pre-diabetes range (PPG value at 120 to 140 mg/dL) or their glucose levels fall below the hyperglycemia range (i.e., glucose at 180 mg/dL or lower). This simpler "linear glucose model" can be extremely useful for many diabetes patients worldwide already.

Depending on the approach, either the overall period's fixed M2 or sub-period's variable M2, it would be easier for diabetes patient to use this linear elastic glucose behavior for their glucose control. The author prefers the fixed M2 model since traditional internal medicine utilizes the HbA1C model. The HbA1C value is remarkably close to the average glucose over a 90-day period (conventionally) or over 120-day period (the author's defined model based on red blood cells life span). Besides, calculating or guess-estimating a single M2 value is much easier and acceptable by patients than using multiple M2 values for every sub-period calculations.

Conclusions:

The author has spent four decades as a practical engineer, but he does understand the importance of basic concepts, sophisticated theories, and practical equations which serve as the necessary background of all kinds of applications. Therefore, he has focused his time and energy to investigate glucose related subjects using a variety of methods he learned in the past, including this particularly interesting stress-strain approach. In addition, he understood the importance and urgency in helping diabetes patients to control their glucoses. That is why, over the past few years, he has continuously simplified his findings regarding diabetes and derived more useful formulas or practical tools in meeting the general public's interest on controlling chronic diseases and their complications to reduce pain and death probability.

References:

1. Hsu, Gerald C., eclaireMD Foundation, USA, No. 310: "Biomedical research methodology based on GH-Method: math-physical medicine"

2. Hsu, Gerald C., eclaireMD Foundation, USA, No. 345: "Application of linear equations to predict sensor and finger based postprandial plasma glucoses and daily glucoses for pre-virus, virus, and total periods using GH-Method: math-physical medicine"

3. Hsu, Gerald C., eclaireMD Foundation, USA, No. 97: "A simplified yet accurate linear equation of PPG prediction model for T2D patients (GH-Method: math-physical medicine)"

4. Hsu, Gerald C., eclaireMD Foundation, USA, No. 99: "Application of linear equation-based PPG prediction model for four T2D clinic cases (GH-Method: math-physical medicine)"

5. Hsu, Gerald C., eclaireMD Foundation, USA, No. 339: "Self-recovery of pancreatic beta cell's insulin secretion based on 10+ years annualized data of food, exercise, weight, and glucose using GH-Method: math-physical medicine)

6. Hsu, Gerald C., eclaireMD Foundation, USA, No. 340: "A neural communication model between brain and internal organs, specifically stomach, liver, and pancreatic beta cells based on PPG waveforms of 131 liquid egg meals and 124 solid egg meals)

7. Hsu, Gerald C., eclaireMD Foundation, USA, No. 346: "Interpretation of relationship between carbohydrates & sugar intake amount and incremental PPG via strength of materials of Structural and Mechanical Engineering using GH-Method: math-physical medicine"

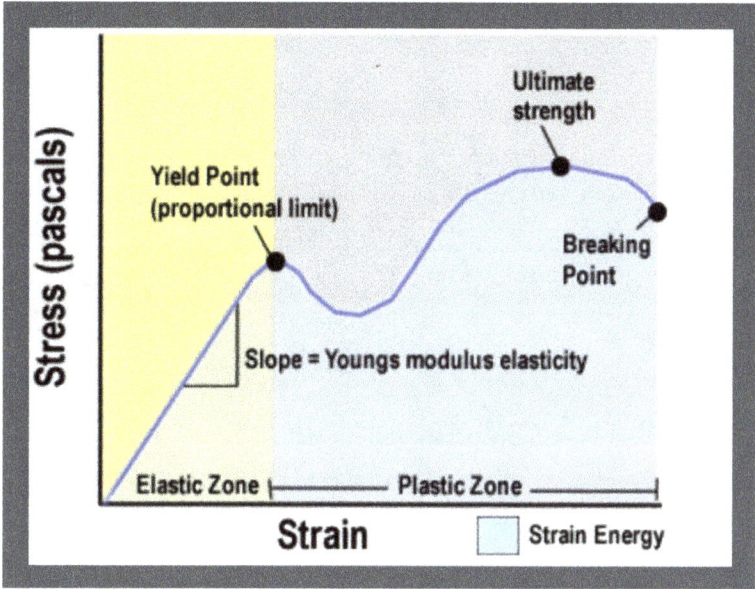

Figure 1: Stress-Strain-Young's modulus, Elastic Zone vs. Plastic Zone

Male Sensor	1/18-2/18	2/18-3/18	3/18-4/18	4/18-5/18	5/18-6/18	6/18-7/18	7/18-8/18	8/18-9/18	9/18-10/18	Average
PPG (peak)	134.90	135.13	140.83	133.37	128.06	134.16	120.46	125.43	119.47	130.20
PPG (Average)	126	122	136	125	117	128	115	119	112	122
FPG (Average)	115.11	97.31	113.58	104.81	96.11	100.55	100.23	99.18	91.08	102.00
Carbs/Sugar (grams)	10.54	13.15	12.73	16.18	12.55	9.79	10.67	12.93	11.81	12.26
Walking (K-steps)	4.519	4.763	4.528	4.268	3.895	4.039	4.009	4.148	4.252	4.269
Female Sensor	1/18-2/18	2/18-3/18	3/18-4/18	4/18-5/18	5/18-6/18	6/18-7/18	7/18-8/18	8/18-9/18	9/18-10/18	Average
PPG (peak)	126.37	124.46	120.11	118.37	115.70	127.68	118.24	119.37	112.58	120.32
PPG (Average)	123	121	115	114	113	118	112	113	110	115
FPG (Average)	111.57	107.24	97.65	102.52	106.90	102.98	97.06	100.77	105.65	103.59
Carbs/Sugar (grams)	8.43	10.52	10.18	12.94	10.04	7.83	8.54	10.34	9.45	9.81
Walking (K-steps)	2.260	2.382	2.264	2.134	1.948	2.020	2.005	2.074	2.126	2.13
Male Predicted PPG	127	118	133	139	119	113	116	122	110	122
Male Prediction Accuracy	101%	97%	98%	111%	101%	88%	100%	102%	98%	100%
Female Predicted PPG	119	119	110	122	120	110	106	114	116	115
Female Prediction Accuracy	97%	99%	95%	108%	107%	93%	95%	101%	106%	100%
Male M2 value (Fixed)										3.6
Female M2 value (Fixed)										2.6
Male X: (Carbs*M2)	37.94	47.34	45.83	58.25	45.18	35.24	38.41	46.55	42.52	44.14
Male Y: (Pred PPG)-(0.97FPG)+(Steps*5)	37.94	47.34	45.83	58.25	45.18	35.24	38.41	46.55	42.52	44.14
Female X: (Carbs*M2)	21.92	27.35	26.48	33.65	26.10	20.36	22.19	26.89	24.56	25.50
Female Y: (Pred PPG)-(0.97FPG)+(Steps*5)	21.92	27.35	26.48	33.65	26.10	20.36	22.19	26.89	24.56	25.50

Figure 2: Raw data and calculations for fixed M2 value (1/18/2020 - 10/18/2020)

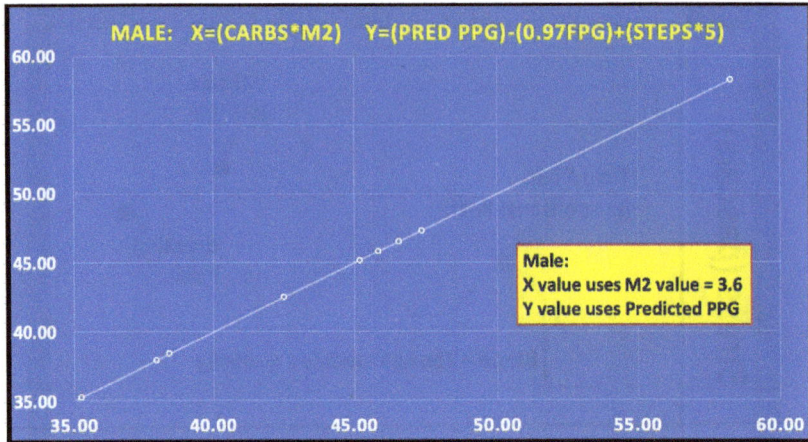

Figure 3: Male case using fixed M2 value of 3.6 (1/18/2020 - 10/18/2020)

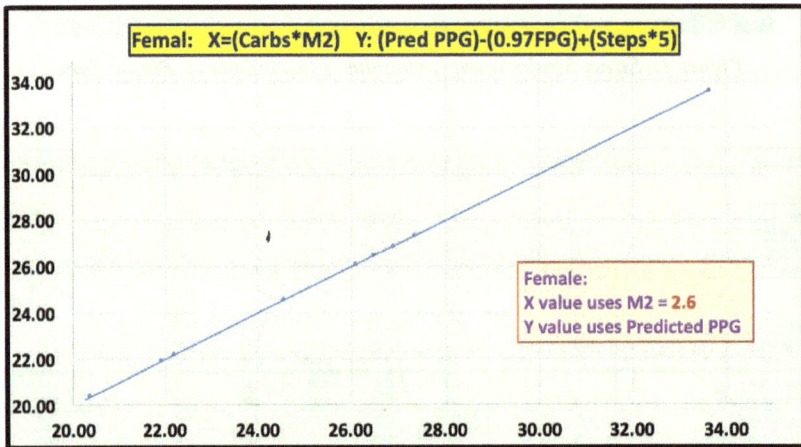

Figure 4: Female case using fixed M2 value of 2.6 (1/18/2020 - 10/18/2020)

Male Sensor	1/18-2/18	2/18-3/18	3/18-4/18	4/18-5/18	5/18-6/18	6/18-7/18	7/18-8/18	8/18-9/18	9/18-10/18	Average
PPG (peak)	134.90	135.13	140.83	133.37	128.06	134.16	120.46	125.43	119.47	130.20
Male Measured PPG (Average)	126	122	136	125	117	128	115	119	112	122
FPG (Average)	115.11	97.31	113.58	104.81	96.11	100.55	100.23	99.18	91.08	102.00
Carbs/Sugar (grams)	10.54	13.15	12.73	16.18	12.55	9.79	10.67	12.93	11.81	12.26
Walking (K-steps)	4.519	4.763	4.528	4.268	3.895	4.039	4.009	4.148	4.252	4.269
Female Sensor	1/18-2/18	2/18-3/18	3/18-4/18	4/18-5/18	5/18-6/18	6/18-7/18	7/18-8/18	8/18-9/18	9/18-10/18	Average
PPG (peak)	126.37	124.46	120.11	118.37	115.70	127.68	118.24	119.37	112.58	120.32
Female MeasuredPPG (Average)	123	121	115	114	113	118	112	113	110	115
FPG (Average)	111.57	107.24	97.65	102.52	106.90	102.98	97.06	100.77	105.65	103.59
Carbs/Sugar (grams)	8.43	10.52	10.18	12.94	10.04	7.83	8.54	10.34	9.45	9.81
Walking (K-steps)	2.260	2.382	2.264	2.134	1.948	2.020	2.005	2.074	2.126	2.13
Male X: (Carbs*M2)	37.07	51.29	48.02	44.94	43.53	50.85	38.14	43.80	45.04	44.74
Male Y: (Meas. PPG)-(0.97FPG)+(Steps*5)	37.07	51.29	48.02	44.94	43.53	50.85	38.14	43.80	45.04	44.74
Female X: (Carbs*M2)	25.69	28.60	31.84	25.02	18.61	28.57	27.48	25.79	18.35	25.55
Female Y: (Meas. PPG)-(0.97FPG)+(Steps*5)	25.69	28.60	31.84	25.02	18.61	28.57	27.48	25.79	18.35	25.55
Male Annual M2 (Variable)	3.5	3.9	3.8	2.8	3.5	5.2	3.6	3.4	3.8	3.7
Female Annual M2 (Variable)	3.0	2.7	3.1	1.9	1.9	3.6	3.2	2.5	1.9	2.7

Figure 5: Raw data and calculations for variable M2 values (1/18/2020 - 10/18/2020)

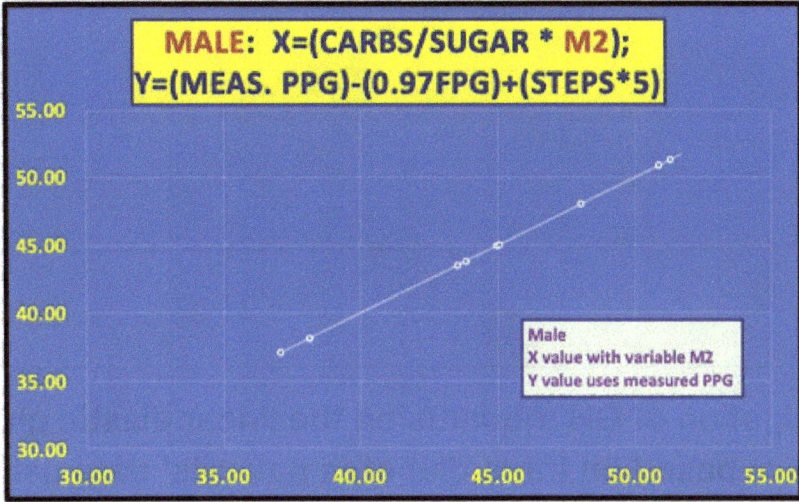

Figure 6: Male case using variable M2 values (1/18/2020 - 10/18/2020)

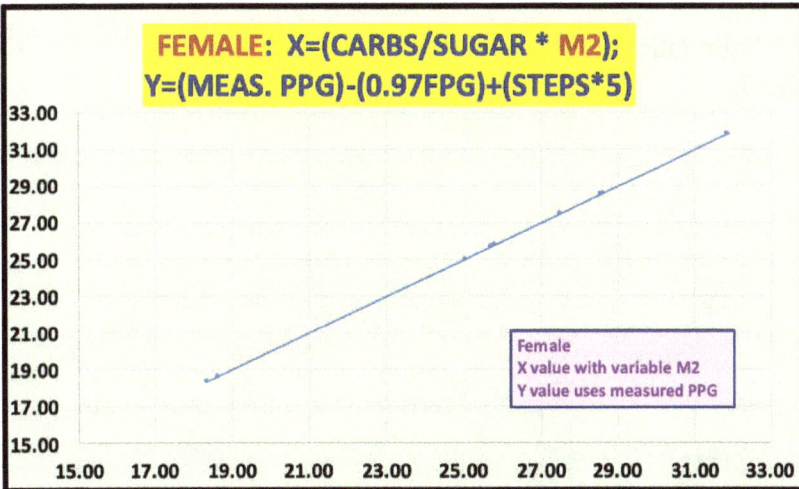

Figure 7: Female case using variable M2 values (1/18/2020 - 10/18/2020)

Investigation of GH modulus on the linear elastic glucose behavior based on three diabetes patients' data using the GH-Method: math-physical medicine, Part 3 (No. 350)

Gerald C. Hsu
eclaireMD Foundation, USA
10/21-23/2020

Abstract:

This article is Part 3 of the linear elastic glucose research work. It is also the continuation of the simple linear equation for predicted PPG (References 2, 3, and 4).

Here is the formula:

Predicted PPG
= (FPG* 0.97) + (carbs/sugar grams * M2) - (post-meal waking K-steps * 5)

The author connected his biomedical equation with a basic concept of linear elasticity which includes stress and strain, along with the Young's modulus of strength of materials in structural & mechanical engineering. By using the collected data of glucose, food, and exercise from three different type 2 diabetes (T2D) patients, he demonstrated once again that a "pseudo-linear" relationship existed in all three clinical cases, between the carbs/sugar intake amount and incremental PPG amount, with a newly defined coefficient of "GH modulus" (same as the M2 multiplier) cited in References 7 and 8. The linear elastic glucose behavior is similar to the Young's modules (E) linking stress and strain of engineering strength of materials.

He selected three T2D patients with different levels of severity. For data consistency purposes, he has chosen data from 7-monthly sub-periods of equal length from 3/18/2020 - 10/18/2020. The main objective of this study is to prove that GH-modulus (M2) indeed vary with the severity of diabetes for these three clinical cases.

The 7-month average value of each monthly M2 variables (i.e, GH-modulus) are 3.7, 2.6, and 1.0, and with an average measured PPG values at 122 mg/dL, 114 md/dL, and 109 mg/dL, for Case A, Case B, and Case C, respectively, which are ranked according to the severity of their diabetes conditions.

In summary, the higher the M2, the higher values of both x (carbs/sugar intake amount) and y (incremental PPG amount) become, and the higher predicted and measured PPG values are. The key conclusion from these three clinical observations is that the M2 values are varying based on patients' body conditions (liver and pancreas), especially their diabetes severity. This is similar to the different inorganic materials having the different Young's modules values, such as nylon ~3 versus steel ~200.

The article represents the author's special interest in using math-physical and engineering modeling methodologies to investigate various biomedical problems. The methodology and approach are a result of his specific academic background and various professional experiences prior to the start of his medical research work in 2010. Therefore, he has been trying to link his newly acquired biomedical knowledge over the past decade with his previously acquired mathematics, physics, computer science, and engineering knowledge over 40 years.

The human body is the most complex system he has dealt with, which includes aerospace, navy defense, nuclear power, computers, and semiconductors. By applying his previous acquired knowledge to his newly found interest of medicine, he can discover many hidden facts or truths inside the biomedical systems. Many basic concepts, theoretical frame of thoughts, and practical modeling techniques from his fundamental disciplines in the past can be applied to his medical research endeavor. After all, science is based on theory via creation and proof via evidence, and as long as we can discover hidden truths, it does not matter which method we use and which option we take. This is the foundation of the GH-Method: math-physics medicine.

The author has spent four decades as a practical engineer and understands the importance of basic concepts, sophisticated theories, and practical equations which serve as the necessary background of all kinds of applications. Therefore, he spent his time and energy to investigate glucose related subjects using variety of methods he studied in the past, including this particular interesting stress-strain approach. On the other hand, he also realize the importance and urgency on helping diabetes patients to control their glucoses. That is why, over the past few years, he has continuously simplified his findings about diabetes and derive more useful formulas or practical tools for meeting the general public's interest on controlling chronic diseases and their complications to reduce their pain and death threat probability.

Introduction:

This article is Part 3 of the linear elastic glucose research work. It is also the continuation of the simple linear equation for predicted PPG (References 2, 3, and 4).

Here is the formula:

Predicted PPG
= (FPG 0.97) + (carbs/sugar grams * M2) - (post-meal waking K-steps * 5)*

The author connected his biomedical equation with a basic concept of linear elasticity which includes stress and strain, along with the Young's modulus of strength of materials in structural & mechanical engineering. By using the collected data of glucose, food, and exercise from three different type 2 diabetes (T2D) patients, he demonstrated once again that a "pseudo-linear" relationship existed in all three clinical cases, between the carbs/sugar intake amount and incremental PPG amount, with a newly defined coefficient of "GH modulus" (same as the M2 multiplier) cited in References 7 and 8. The linear elastic glucose behavior is similar to the Young's modules (E) linking stress and strain of engineering strength of materials.

He selected three T2D patients with different levels of severity. For data consistency purposes, he has chosen data from 7-monthly sub-periods of equal length from 3/18/2020 - 10/18/2020. The main objective of this study is to prove that GH-modulus (M2) indeed vary with the severity of diabetes for these three clinical cases.

Methods:

Background:

To learn more about the author's GH-Method: math-physical medicine (MPM) methodology, readers can refer to his article to understand his developed MPM analysis method in Reference 1.

Highlights of his previous research:

In 2015, the author decomposed the PPG waveforms (data curves) into 19 influential components and identified carbs/sugar intake amount and post-meal walking exercise contributing to approximately 40% of PPG formation, respectively. Therefore, he could safely discount the importance of the remaining ~20% contribution by the 16 other influential components.

In 2016, he utilized optical physics, big data analytics, and artificial intelligence (AI) techniques to develop a computer software to predict PPG based on the patient's food pictures or meal photos. This sophisticated AI approach and iPhone APP software product have reached to a 98.8% prediction accuracy based on ~6,000 meal photos.

In 2017, he also detected that body weight contributes to over 85% to fasting plasma glucose (FPG) formation. Furthermore, in 2019, he identified that FPG could serve as a good indicator of the pancreatic beta cells' health status; therefore, he can apply the FPG value (more precisely, 97% of FPG value) to serve as the baseline PPG value to calculate the PPG incremental amount in order to obtain the predicted PPG.

In 2018, based on his collected ~2,500 meals and associated sensor PPG waveforms, he further applied the perturbation theory from quantum mechanics, using the first bite of his meal as the initial condition to extend and build an entire PPG waveform covering a period of 180 minutes, with a 95% of PPG prediction accuracy.

In 2019, all of his developed PPG prediction mathematical models achieved high percentages of prediction accuracy, but he also realized that his prediction models are too difficult for use by the general public. The above-mentioned sophisticated methods would be difficult for healthcare professionals and diabetes patients to understand, let alone use them in their daily life for diabetes control. Therefore, he supplemented his complex models with a simple linear equation of predicted PPG (see References 2, 3, and 4).

Here is his simple linear formula:

Predicted PPG
= FPG * M1 + (carbs-sugar * M2) - (post-meal walking k-steps * M3)

Where M1, M2, M3 are 3 multipliers.

After lengthy research, trial and error, and data tuning, he finally identified the best multipliers for FPG and exercise as 0.97 for M1 and 5.0 for M3. In comparison with PPG, the FPG is a more stabilized biomarker since it is directly related to body weight. We know that weight reduction is a hard task. However, weight is a calmer and more stabilizing biomarker in comparison to glucose which fluctuates from minute to minute. The influence of exercise (specifically, post-meal walking steps) on PPG (41% contribution and >80% negative correlation with PPG) is almost equal to the influence from the carbs/sugar intake amount on PPG (39% contribution and >80% positive correlation with PPG). In terms of intensity and duration, exercise is a simple and straightforward subject to study. Especially, normal-speed walking is a safe and effective form of exercise for the large portion of diabetes patients, the senior people.

The parameters, FPG and walking, have a lower chance of variation for the author. However, for some diabetes patients, he recommends them to keep the multiplier M3 as a variable if their exercise patterns are different and changing.

The relationship between food nutrition and glucose is a complex and difficult subject to fully understand and effectively manage due to many types of food and their associated carbs/sugar contents. For example, in the author's developed food material and nutrition database, it contains over six million data. As a result, the author decided to implement two multipliers, M1 for FPG and M3 for exercise, as the two "constants" and keep M2 as the only "variable" in his PPG prediction equation and the linear elastic glucose research in this article.

The more simplified linear equation for predicted PPG is listed below:

Predicted PPG
= (0.97*FPG)+(Carbs&sugar * M2) - (post-meal walking k-steps * 5)

Where he created three new terms:

Term 1:
GH modulus = M2

Term 2:
The incremental PPG amount
= Predicted PPG - PPG baseline
 (i.e. 0.97 * FPG) + exercise effect
 (i.e. walking k-steps * 5)

Term 3:
GH modulus
= (Incremental PPG)/(Carbs&sugar)

Stress, Strain, & Young's modulus:
Prior to his medical research work, he was an engineer in the various fields of structural engineering (aerospace, naval defense, and earthquake engineering), mechanical engineering (nuclear power plant equipments, and computer-aided-design), and electronics engineering (computers, semiconductors, and software robot).

The following excerpts comes from internet public domain, including Google and Wikipedia:

"Strain - ε:
Strain is the "deformation of a solid due to stress" - change in dimension divided by the original value of the dimension - and can be expressed as
$\varepsilon = dL / L$
where
$\varepsilon = strain$ *(m/m, in/in)*
$dL = elongation$ *or compression (offset) of object (m, in)*
$L = length$ *of object (m, in)*

Stress - σ:
Stress is force per unit area and can be expressed as
$\sigma = F / A$
where
$\sigma = stress$ *(N/m2, lb/in2, psi)*
$F = applied force$ *(N, lb)*
$A = stress area$ *of object (m2, in2)*

Stress includes tensile stress, compressible stress, shearing stress, etc.

E, Young's modulus:
It can be expressed as:
$E = stress / strain$
$= \sigma / \varepsilon$
$= (F / A) / (dL / L)$
where
$E = \underline{Young's\ Modulus\ of\ Elasticity}$ *(Pa, N/m2, lb/in2, psi) was named after the 18th-century English physicist Thomas Young.*

Elasticity:
Elasticity is a property of an object or material indicating how it will restore it to its original shape after distortion. A spring is an example of an elastic object - when stretched, it exerts a restoring force which tends to bring it back to its original length (Figure 1).

Plasticity:
When the force is going beyond the elastic limit of material, it is into a "plastic' zone which means even when force is removed, the material will not return back to its original state (Figure 1).

Based on various experimental results, the following table lists some Young's modulus associated with different materials:

Nylon: 2.7 GPa

Concrete: 17-30 GPa
Glass fibers: 72 GPa
Copper: 117 GPa
Steel: 190-215 GPa
Diamond: 1220 GPa

Young's modules in the above table are ranked from soft material (low E) to stiff material (higher E)."

Professor James Andrews taught the author linear elasticity at the University of Iowa and Professor Norman Jones taught him nonlinear plasticity at Massachusetts Institute of Technology. These two great academic mentors provided him the foundation knowledge to understand these two important subjects in engineering.

Linear elastic glucose research:
In this particular study, he uses the analogy of relationship among stress, strain, and Young's modulus to illustrate a similar relationship among carbs/sugar intake amount, incremental predicted PPG, and GH modulus (i.e. M2). They are listed below for a closer comparison.

GH modulus (M2)
=(Incremental PPG)/(Carbs&sugar)

Young's modulus E
= stress / strain
= σ / ε

Where Incremental PPG is the incremental amount of predicted PPG (note: the predicted PPG is also replaced by the measured PPG in order to conduct a sensitivity study of glucose behaviors.).

The author visualizes the carbs/sugar intake amount as the stress (the force or stimulator) on his liver and the incremental PPG amount as the strain (the response or stimulation) from the liver. The GH modulus (i.e. M2) is similar to the Young's modulus (i.e. E) which describes the "pseudo-linear" relationship existing between the carbs/sugar intake amount (stress) and the incremental predicted PPG (strain).

In Part 1 of the linear elastic glucose study (Reference 7), he proved the existence of the linear relationship between carbs/sugar intake amount and incremental PPG amount. In Part 2, two T2D patients within the same 9-month period (Reference 8), he proved that the more severe a T2D patient is, then the higher GH-modulus. In Part 3, he uses three clinical cases within the same 7-month period to prove again that the orders of magnitude in the GH-modules are following the severities of diabetes conditions in the patients.

Data collection:
Case A (the author) is a 73-year-old male with a 25-year history of T2D. He

began collecting his carbs/sugar intake amount and post-meal walking steps on 7/1/2015. From 7/15/2015 to 10/18/2020 (1,935 days), he has collected 6 data per day, 1 FPG, 3 PPG, carb/sugar, and post-meal walking steps. He utilized these 11,610 data of 1,935 days to conduct his prior research work on the subject of linear elastic glucose study (Reference 7). In addition, on 5/5/2018, he started to use a continuous glucose monitoring (CGM) sensor device to collect 96 glucose data each day.

The period of 7/1/2015 to 10/18/2020 is his "best-controlled" diabetes period, where his average daily glucoses is maintained at 116 mg/dL (<120 mg/dL). He named this as his "linear elastic zone" of diabetes health. It should also be noted that in 2010, his average glucose was 280 mg/dL and HbA1C was 10%, while taking three diabetes medications. Please note that the strong chemical interventions from various diabetes medications would seriously alter glucose physical behaviors. He called the period prior to 2015 as his "nonlinear plastic zone" of diabetes health.

The second set of data comes from his wife (Case B) with a 22-year history of T2D. She began to collect her glucose data via finger-piercing method (finger glucose) since 1/1/2014. However, she does not keep a detailed record of her diet and exercise. Both patients eat almost the same meals prepared by the author, except that she consumes more meat which partially affects her hyperlipidemia and hypertension conditions. From the diabetes research viewpoint, he decided to use 80% of the Case A's carbs/sugar amount for her and use 50% of the Case A's post-meal walking steps for her. On 1/1/2020, she began using the same brand of CGM device to collect her sensor glucose data at the same rate of 96 data per day since 1/1/2020.

Case C is 47-year-old male with a 4-year history of T2D. He started to collect his glucose data using the same model of CGM sensor on 3/18/2020. Through a telephone interview, the author discovered that over the past 7-month period, his average carbs/ sugar intake amount is about the same amount as Case A, and his average post-meal walking steps is at ~25% level compared to Case A.

It should be mentioned here, other than the male case who has collected a complete dataset of diet and exercise, both female and young cases are using the best guess-estimated percentages of male case amount of diet and exercise. Therefore, these data differences would definitely create some degree of result deviation.

In order to maintain data consistency for a fair and accurate comparison, the author took the CGM sensor glucose data from Cases A, B, and C from 3/18/2020 through 10/18/2020 and subdivided them into 7-monthly sub-periods of equal length to study their glucose fluctuation patterns and data. The reason for using sensor glucose data over finger glucose is because they are 13% to 18% higher. Therefore, the sensor data would be more conservative in terms of diabetes severity. Finally, the author calculated the three GH-modulus values via the approach of matching the predicted PPG values with the yardstick of measured PPG values.

Results:

Figure 2 shows the raw data collected from the three cases and their respective predicted PPG values of each sub-period.

Figure 3 lists a data table of calculated x- and y- components, where
x is (carbs&sugar * M2)
and
y is (measured PPG -(FPG * 0.97) + (walking k-steps * 5).

This table provides the most suitable GH-modulus (i.e. M2) values for each month which allows the predicted PPG to match the measured PPG via trial-and-error.

The 7-month average value of each monthly M2 variables (i.e, GH-modulus) are 3.7, 2.6, and 1.0, and with an average measured PPG values at 122 mg/dL, 114 md/dL, and 109 mg/dL, for Case A, Case B, and Case C, respectively, which are ranked according to the severity of their diabetes conditions.

Listed below are the values of the individual M2 multiplier (i.e. GH-modulus) for each of the 7 months in 2020 which are listed in the order of (Case A, Case B, Case C):

3/18 - 4/18: (3.8, 3.1, 1.3)
4/18 - 5/18: (2.8, 1.9, 0.6)
5/18 - 6/18: (3.5, 1.9, 0.7)
6/18 - 7/18: (5.2, 3.6, 0.7)
7/18 - 8/18: (3.6, 3.2, 1.4)
8/18 - 9/18: (3.4, 2.5, 1.2)
9/18 - 10/18: (3.8, 1.9, 1.4)
Variable M2: (3.7, 2.6, 1.0)
Fixed M2: (3.6, 2.6, 1.0)

Case A with the fixed M2 as 3.6, both x and y are within the range of 38 to 48 with an average value of 45 are observed in Figure 4. Case B with the fixed M2 as 2.6, both x and y are within the range of 18 to 32 with an average value of 25 are observed in Figure 5. Case C with the fixed M2 as 1.0, both x and y are within the range of 11 to 17 with an average value of 13 are observed in Figure 6.

In summary, the higher the M2, the higher values of both x (carbs/sugar intake amount) and y (incremental PPG amount) become, and the higher predicted and measured PPG values are. The key conclusion from these three clinical observations is that the M2 values are varying based on patients' body conditions (blood, liver, pancreas), especially their diabetes severity. This is similar to the different inorganic materials having the different Young's modules values, such as nylon ~3 versus steel ~200.

Discussion:

In the table of raw data shown in Figure 2 and the calculation of x, y, variable M2 shown in Figure 3, plus the three graphic figures of 4, 5 and 6, the author utilized **variable** M2 values for each month in order to make the calculated x-component values to match with the calculated y-components values during each monthly sub-period; therefore, to "force" the predicted PPG value to match with the measured PPG value in each month. As a result, a linear or "pseudo-linear" relationship between x-component and y-component could be created and observed.

This forced "pseudo-linear" relationship makes sense in the biomedical field since red blood cells and liver cells are organic materials which are different from those inorganic materials in the engineering systems, such as rubber or steel. The human organ cells are not only organic but also have different lifespans, where they can mutate, change, repair, or die. For example, the lifespan of the red blood cells is 115 to 120 days, the lifespan of liver cells is 300 to 500 days, and the lifespan of pancreatic beta cells is unknown with a slightly adaptive change. As indicated in his previous research, the pancreatic beta cells' self-repair process is very slow, taking approximately 2.7% per year for the author. Not all of the body cells die at the same moment. At any given instance, an organ would have different combination of new cells, sick cells, dying cells, and mutated cells that can mix together. It is an overly complex and extraordinarily situation; therefore, the author has chosen variable M2 values for different months in order to achieve his prediction accuracies for all sub-periods. This would be a reasonable approach for this particular biomedical research. These data have demonstrated that the variable M2 values of different months resulted from the T2D conditions varying month to month for each patient, precisely the combined situation of liver, blood, and pancreas. This means that glucose is a very "dynamic" function instead of being a "static" function. The above discussions are the major differences between the linear elasticity organic glucoses and the traditional linear elasticity of strength of inorganic engineering materials.

Conclusions:

The article represents the author's special interest in using math-physical and engineering modeling methodologies to investigate various biomedical problems. The methodology and approach are a result of his specific academic background and various professional experiences prior to the start of his medical research work in 2010. Therefore, he has been trying to link his newly acquired biomedical knowledge over the past decade with his previously acquired mathematics, physics, computer science, and engineering knowledge over 40 years.

The human body is the most complex system he has dealt with, which includes aerospace, navy defense, nuclear power, computers, and semiconductors. By applying his previous acquired knowledge to his newly found interest of medicine, he can discover many hidden facts or truths inside the biomedical systems. Many basic concepts, theoretical frame of thoughts, and practical modeling techniques from his fundamental disciplines in the past can be applied to his medical research endeavor.

After all, science is based on theory via creation and proof via evidence, and as long as we can discover hidden truths, it does not matter which method we use and which option we take. This is the foundation of the GH-Method: math-physics medicine.

The author has spent four decades as a practical engineer and understands the importance of basic concepts, sophisticated theories, and practical equations which serve as the necessary background of all kinds of applications. Therefore, he spent his time and energy to investigate glucose related subjects using variety of methods he studied in the past, including this particular interesting stress-strain approach. On the other hand, he also realize the importance and urgency on helping diabetes patients to control their glucoses. That is why, over the past few years, he has continuously simplified his findings about diabetes and derive more useful formulas or practical tools for meeting the general public's interest on controlling chronic diseases and their complications to reduce their pain and death threat probability.

References:

1. Hsu, Gerald C., eclaireMD Foundation, USA, No. 310: "Biomedical research methodology based on GH-Method: math-physical medicine"

2. Hsu, Gerald C., eclaireMD Foundation, USA, No. 345: "Application of linear equations to predict sensor and finger based postprandial plasma glucoses and daily glucoses for pre-virus, virus, and total periods using GH-Method: math-physical medicine"

3. Hsu, Gerald C., eclaireMD Foundation, USA, No. 97: "A simplified yet accurate linear equation of PPG prediction model for T2D patients (GH-Method: math-physical medicine)"

4. Hsu, Gerald C., eclaireMD Foundation, USA, No. 99: "Application of linear equation-based PPG prediction model for four T2D clinic cases (GH-Method: math-physical medicine)"

5. Hsu, Gerald C., eclaireMD Foundation, USA, No. 339: "Self-recovery of pancreatic beta cell's insulin secretion based on 10+ years annualized data of food, exercise, weight, and glucose using GH-Method: math-physical medicine)

6. Hsu, Gerald C., eclaireMD Foundation, USA, No. 340: "A neural communication model between brain and internal organs, specifically stomach, liver, and pancreatic beta cells based on PPG waveforms of 131 liquid egg meals and 124 solid egg meals)

7. Hsu, Gerald C., eclaireMD Foundation, USA, No. 346: "Linear relationship between carbohydrates & sugar intake amount and incremental PPG amount via engineering strength of materials using GH-Method: math-physical medicine, Part 1"

8. Hsu, Gerald C., eclaireMD Foundation, USA, No. 349: "Investigation on GH modulus of linear elastic glucose with two diabetes patients data using GH-Method: math-physical medicine, Part 2"

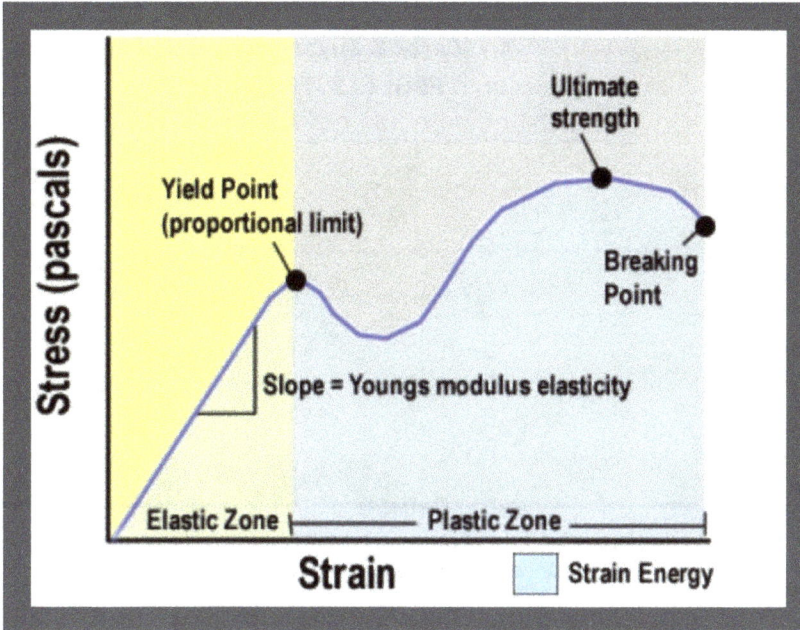

Figure 1: Stress-Strain-Young's modulus, Elastic Zone vs. Plastic Zone

Male Sensor	3/18-4/18	4/18-5/18	5/18-6/18	6/18-7/18	7/18-8/18	8/18-9/18	9/18-10/18	Average
PPG (peak)	141	133	128	134	120	125	119	129
Male Measured PPG	136	125	117	128	115	119	112	122
FPG (Average)	114	105	96	101	100	99	91	101
Carbs/Sugar (grams)	12.73	16.18	12.55	9.79	10.67	12.93	11.81	12.38
Walking (K-steps)	4.528	4.268	3.895	4.039	4.009	4.148	4.252	4.163
Male predicted PPG	133	139	119	113	116	122	116	122
Female Sensor	3/18-4/18	4/18-5/18	5/18-6/18	6/18-7/18	7/18-8/18	8/18-9/18	9/18-10/18	Average
PPG (peak)	120	118	116	128	118	119	113	119
Female Measured PPG	115	114	113	118	112	113	110	114
FPG (Average)	98	103	107	103	97	101	106	102
Carbs/Sugar (grams)	10.18	12.94	10.04	7.83	8.54	10.34	9.45	9.90
Walking (K-steps)	2.264	2.134	1.948	2.020	2.005	2.074	2.126	2.08
Female predicted PPG	110	122	120	110	106	114	116	114
Young Sensor	3/18-4/18	4/18-5/18	5/18-6/18	6/18-7/18	7/18-8/18	8/18-9/18	9/18-10/18	Average
PPG (peak)	132	102	108	105	123	106	107	112
Young Measured PPG	125	101	108	105	121	102	104	109
FPG (Average)	117	100	107	106	115	94	95	105
Carbs/Sugar (grams)	12.73	16.18	12.55	9.79	10.67	12.93	11.81	12.38
Walking (K-steps)	1.132	1.067	0.974	1.010	1.002	1.037	1.063	1.041
Young Predicted PPG with Fixed M2 of 1.0323	121	108	112	108	118	100	99	109
Young Predicted PPG with variable M2	125	101	108	105	121	102	104	109

Figure 2: Raw data and predicted PPG for the 7-months period of three patients

Male X: (Carbs*M2)	48	45	44	51	38	44	45	45
Male Y: (Meas PPG)-(0.97FPG)+(Steps*5)	48	45	44	51	38	44	45	45
Female X: (Carbs*M2)	32	25	19	29	27	26	18	25
Female Y: (Meas. PPG)-(0.97FPG)+(Steps*5)	32	25	19	29	27	26	18	25
Young X: (Carbs*M2)	13	17	13	10	11	13	12	13
Young Y: (Meas. PPG)-(0.97FPG)+(Steps*5)	13	17	13	10	11	13	12	13
Male M2 (Variable)	3.8	2.8	3.5	5.2	3.6	3.4	3.8	3.7
Female M2 (Variable)	3.1	1.9	1.9	3.6	3.2	2.5	1.9	2.6
Young M2 (Variable)	1.3	0.6	0.7	0.7	1.4	1.2	1.4	1.0

Figure 3: Calculated x and y components using variable M2 values for the 7-months period of three patients

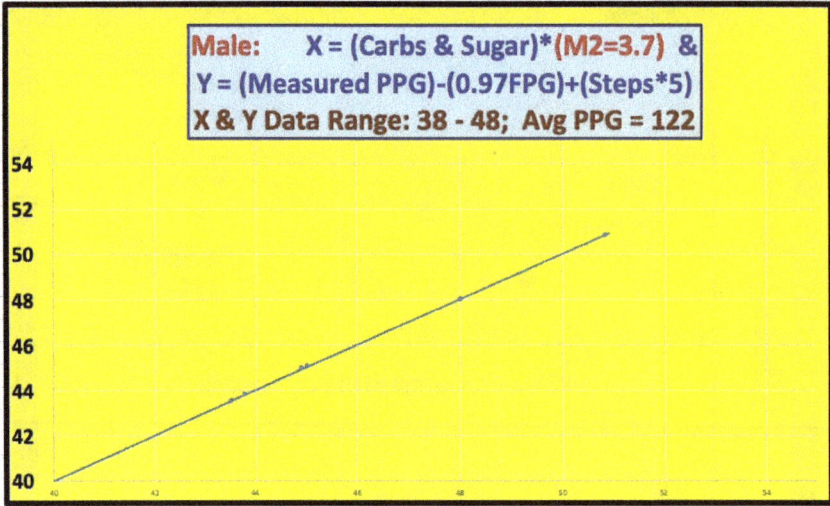

Male: X = (Carbs & Sugar)*(M2=3.7) &
Y = (Measured PPG)-(0.97FPG)+(Steps*5)
X & Y Data Range: 38 - 48; Avg PPG = 122

Figure 4: Linear elastic glucose behavior between cars/sugar input and incremental PPG output for male case during the 7-months period

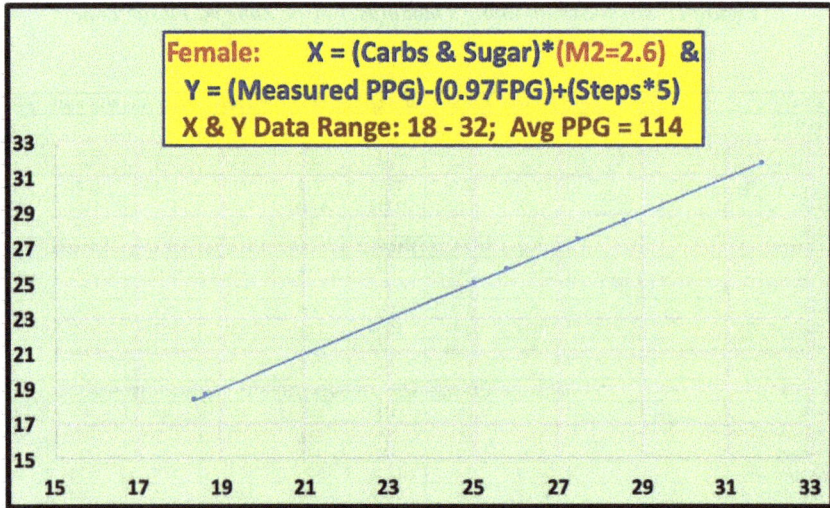

Female: X = (Carbs & Sugar)*(M2=2.6) &
Y = (Measured PPG)-(0.97FPG)+(Steps*5)
X & Y Data Range: 18 - 32; Avg PPG = 114

Figure 5: Linear elastic glucose behavior between cars/sugar input and incremental PPG output for female case during the 7-months period

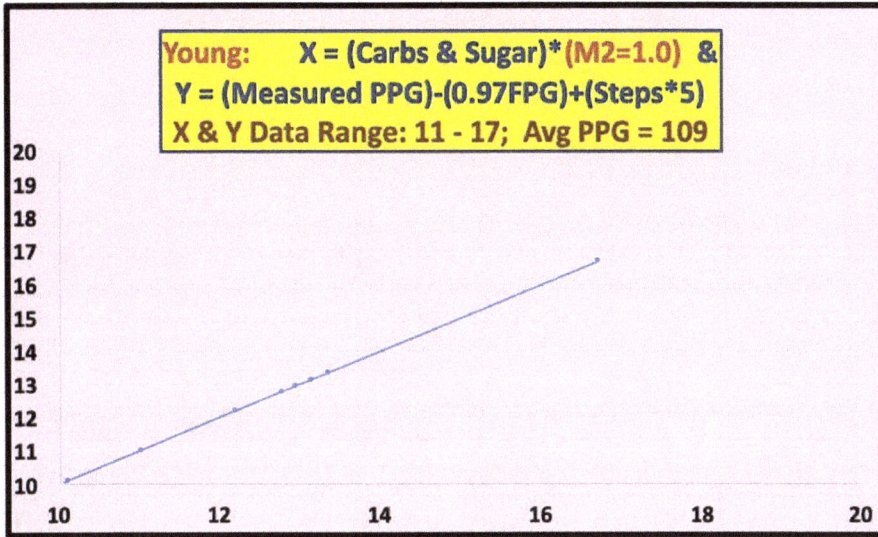

Figure 6: Linear elastic glucose behavior between cars/sugar input and incremental PPG output for young case during the 7-months period

Investigation of linear elastic glucose behavior with GH-modulus linking carbohydrates/sugar intake and incremental PPG via an analogy of Young's modulus from theory of elasticity and engineering strength of materials using GH-Method: math-physical medicine, Parts 1, 2, and 3 (No. 352)

Gerald C. Hsu
eclaireMD Foundation, USA
10/14-25/2020

Abstract:

This article is an extension work of his previous research result of a "simple linear equation of predicted postprandial plasma glucose (PPG)" as shown below:

Predicted PPG
= (FPG * 0.97) + (carbs/sugar grams * M2) - (post-meal waking K-steps * 5)

This article contains special research on the linear elasticity of glucose behaviors with his newly defined GH-modulus (M2) cited in References 7, 8, and 9. The author makes an analogy of stress, strain, and Young's models from engineering strength of materials and theory of elasticity with carbs/sugar (carbs) intake amounts, incremental PPG (PPG delta) and GH-modulus of endocrinology and biomedical science. There are three parts to the study.

In the first part, by using the 6 years of collected data, he attempts to prove a "linear elastic relationship" existing between carbs and PPG delta via the existence of GH-modulus as the "slope" of their straight-line linear relationship.

For the second part, through 9-months data of two diabetes clinical cases, he discovered that the magnitude for the GH-modulus is proportional to the diabetes severity of the patients. This means that the GH-modulus is clearly "material" dependent on the patient's conditions.

In the third part, by examining 7- months data of three diabetes clinical cases, he uncovered the magnitude of GH-modulus varying month to month for all of these three patients. As a result, the GH-modulus is evidently "time" dependent as well.

Part 1 summary: It is obvious that the six-annual data "almost" form a straight line with a slope of 45% between carbs and PPG delta. The author describes the linear phenomenon and data points having small deviations from the straight-line, as a"pseudo-linear" relationship. This is similar to the "elastic zone" of the stress-strain-Young's modulus diagram in theory of elasticity and strength of materials of structural and mechanical engineering (Figure 1). This linear relationship makes the task of incremental PPG prediction through diabetes control via diet much easier.

Part 2 summary: For most of the 9 months, the higher the variable M2, the higher x and y values become, and the higher predicted and measured PPG values are. The key point is that the monthly M2 values (i.e., GH-modulus) are dependent on the patient's body conditions (a combination of blood, liver, and pancreas) of that particular month.

Part 3 summary: *The 7-month averaged values of each monthly M2 variables (i.e., GH-modulus) are 3.7, 2.6, and 1.0, and with an average measured PPG values at 122 mg/dL, 114 md/dL, and 109 mg/dL, for Case A, Case B, and Case C, respectively. They are ranked according to the severity of their diabetes conditions. The higher the M2, the higher values of both x (carbs/sugar intake amount) and y (incremental PPG amount) become, and the higher predicted and measured PPG values are. The key* *conclusion from these three clinical observations is that the M2 values are varying based on patients' body conditions, especially their diabetes severity (i.e. blood, liver, and pancreas). It also indicates that GH-modulus are varying on the time scale because of our body organ cells are "organic" materials.*

Here are the main conclusions of this article:

First, by using an analogy from the theory of elasticity and engineering strength of material, the author has identified a linear relationship existing between carbs and PPG delta with a newly defined GH-modulus, similar to a linear relationship between stress and strain with Young's modulus.

Second, based on two diabetes patients' 9-month data, he has proven that the magnitude of GH-modulus is directly proportional to the *diabetes severity* of the patients.

Third, by utilizing three diabetes patients' 7-month data, he has confirmed that the magnitude of the monthly GH-modulus is directly proportional to the diabetes severity of *that particular month* for each patient.

Fourth, these linear elastic glucose behavior findings are probably *applicable to a glucose range from 70 mg/dL to 180 mg/dL* which covers most situations for a diabetes patient. For glucose values falling outside the range, a nonlinear plastic glucose behavior study is needed.

Introduction:

This article is an extension work of his previous research result of a "simple linear equation of predicted postprandial plasma glucose (PPG)" as shown below:

Predicted PPG
= (FPG * 0.97) + (carbs/sugar grams * M2) - (post-meal waking K-steps * 5)

This article contains special research on the linear elasticity of glucose behaviors with his newly defined GH-modulus (M2) cited in References 7, 8, and 9. The author makes an analogy of stress, strain, and Young's models from engineering strength of materials and theory of elasticity with carbs/sugar (carbs) intake amounts, incremental PPG (PPG delta) and GH-modulus of endocrinology and biomedical science. There are three parts to the study.

In the first part, by using the 6 years of collected data, he attempts to prove a *"linear elastic relationship" existing* between carbs and PPG delta via the existence of GH-modulus as the "slope" of their straight-line linear relationship.

For the second part, through two 9 months of diabetes clinical cases, he discovered that the magnitude for the GH-modulus is proportional to the diabetes severity of the patients. This means that the GH-modulus is clearly "material" dependent on the patient's conditions.

In the third part, by examining 7 months of data from three diabetes clinical cases, he uncovered the magnitude of GH-modulus varying month to month for the three patients. As a result, the GH-modulus is evidently "time" dependent as well.

Methods:
Background:
To learn more about the author's GH-Method: math-physical medicine (MPM) methodology, readers can refer to his article to understand the developed MPM analysis method in Reference 1.

Highlights of his previous research:
In 2015, the author decomposed the PPG waveforms (data curves) into 19 influential components and identified carbs/sugar intake amount and post-meal walking exercise contributing to approximately 40% of PPG formation, respectively. Therefore, he could safely discount the importance of the remaining ~20% contribution by the 16 other influential components.

In 2016, he utilized optical physics, big data analytics, and artificial intelligence (AI) techniques to develop a computer software to predict PPG based on the patient's food pictures or meal photos. This sophisticated AI approach and iPhone APP software product have reached to a 98.8% prediction accuracy based on ~6,000 meal photos.

In 2017, he also detected that body weight contributes to over 85% to fasting plasma glucose (FPG) formation. Furthermore, in 2019, he identified that FPG could serve as a good indicator of the pancreatic beta cells' health status; therefore, he can apply the FPG value (more precisely, 97% of FPG value) to serve as the baseline PPG value to calculate the PPG incremental amount in order to obtain the predicted PPG.

In 2018, based on his collected ~2,500 meals and associated sensor PPG waveforms, he further applied the perturbation theory (a simplified single variable with first-order polynomial function) from quantum mechanics, using the first-bite of his meal as the initial condition and then extend to build the entire predicted PPG waveform covering a period of 180 minutes, with a 95% of PPG prediction accuracy.

In 2019, all of his developed PPG prediction mathematical models have achieved high percentages of prediction accuracy, but he also realized that his prediction models are too difficult to use by the general public. The above-mentioned sophisticated methods would be difficult for healthcare professionals and diabetes patients to understand, let alone use them in their daily life for diabetes control. Therefore, he tried to supplement his complex models with a simple linear equation of predicted PPG (see References 2, 3, and 4).

Here is his simple linear formula:
Predicted PPG
= FPG * M1 + (carbs-sugar * M2) - (post-meal walking k-steps * M3)

Where M1, M2, M3 are 3 multipliers.

After lengthy research, trial and error, and data tuning, he finally identified the best multipliers for FPG and exercise as 0.97 for M1 and 5.0 for M3. In comparison with PPG, the FPG is a more stabilized biomarker since it is directly related to body weight. We know that weight reduction is a hard undertaking. But the weight is a far calmer and more stabilizing biomarker in comparison to glucose which fluctuates from minute to minute. The influence of exercise (specifically, post-meal walking steps) on PPG (41% contribution and >80% negative correlation with PPG) is almost equal to the influence from the carbs/sugar intake amount on PPG (39% contribution and >80% positive correlation with PPG). In terms of intensity and duration, exercise is a much simpler and straightforward subject to study and deal with.

Therefore, for the author, these two parameters, FPG and walking, have a lower chance of variation. However, for other diabetes patients, the author recommends for them to keep the multiplier M3 as a variable if their exercise patterns are complex, different, and fluctuating.

On the other hand, the relationship between food nutrition and glucose is an exceedingly complex and difficult subject or task to fully understand and effectively manage, since there are many types of food and their associated carbs/sugar contents. For example, the author's food nutritional database contains over six million data. As a result, the author decided to implement two multipliers, M1 for FPG and M3 for exercise, as two "constants" and keep M2 as the only "variable" in his PPG prediction equation and the linear elastic glucose study in this particular article.

Here is the simplified linear equation for predicted PPG as follows:

Predicted PPG
= (0.97*FPG)+(Carbs&sugar * M2) - (post-meal walking k-steps * 5)

He also defines the following three new terms in terms 1, 2, and 3:

Term 1:
GH modulus = M2

Term 2:
The incremental PPG amount
= Predicted PPG - baseline PPG
_ (i.e. 0.97 * FPG) + exercise effect_
_ (i.e. walking k-steps * 5)_

Term 3:
GH modulus
= (Incremental PPG)/(Carbs&sugar)

Stress, Strain, & Young's modulus:
Prior to the past decade in his self-study and medical research work, he was an engineer in the fields of structural (aerospace and naval defense), mechanical

(nuclear power plants and computer-aided-design), and electronics (computers and semiconductors).

The following excerpts come from Google and Wikipedia:

"Strain - ε:
Strain is the "deformation of a solid due to stress" - change in dimension divided by the original value of the dimension - and can be expressed as
$$\varepsilon = dL / L$$
where
ε = strain (m/m, in/in)
dL = elongation or compression (offset) of object (m, in)
L = length of object (m, in)

Stress - σ:
Stress is force per unit area and can be expressed as
$$\sigma = F / A$$
where
σ = stress (N/m2, lb/in2, psi)
F = applied force (N, lb)
A = stress area of object (m2, in2)

Stress includes tensile stress, compressible stress, shearing stress, etc.

E, Young's modulus:
It can be expressed as:
$$E = stress / strain$$
$$= \sigma / \varepsilon$$
$$= (F / A) / (dL / L)$$
where
E = Young's Modulus of Elasticity (Pa, N/m2, lb/in2, psi) was named after the 18th-century English physicist Thomas Young.

Elasticity:
Elasticity is a property of an object or material indicating how it will restore it to its original shape after distortion. A spring is an example of an elastic object - when stretched, it exerts a restoring force which tends to bring it back to its original length (Figure 1).

Plasticity:
When the force is going beyond the elastic limit of material, it is into a "plastic' zone which means even when force is removed, the material will not return back to its original state (Figure 1).

Based on various experimental results, the following table lists some of the Young's modulus associated with different materials:

Nylon: 2.7 GPa
Concrete: 17-30 GPa
Glass fibers: 72 GPa
Copper: 117 GPa
Steel: 190-215 GPa
Diamond: 1220 GPa

The Young's modules in the above table are ranked from soft material (low E) to stiff material (higher E)."

Professor James Andrews taught him linear elasticity at the University of Iowa and Professor Norman Jones taught him nonlinear plasticity at Massachusetts Institute of Technology. These two great academic mentors have trained him with the foundation knowledge of these two important subjects.

In this particular study, the above-mentioned Term 4 is *remarkably similar, in concept and format,* to the stress-strain equation as shown below *except that the GH modules and Young's modulus are reciprocal to each other due to their switched abscissa and ordinate.*

GH modulus (i.e. M2)
=(Incremental PPG)/(Carbs&sugar)

Young's modulus E
= stress / strain
$$= \sigma / \varepsilon$$

Where the Incremental PPG is the incremental amount of **predicted** PPG, i.e. PPG delta. (Note: at times, he may also replace the predicted PPG by the measured PPG in order to conduct a sensitivity study of the glucose behaviors.)

The author visualizes the carbs as the stress (the force, cause, or stimulator) on his liver and the PPG delta as the strain (the response, consequence, or stimulation) from the liver. The GH modulus (i.e. M2) is similar to the Young's modulus (i.e. E) which describes the "pseudo-linear" relationship existing between the carbs (stress) and PPG delta (strain).

Conceptually, he is now able to connect the subject of liver glucose production in endocrinology with the subject of strength of materials and theory of elasticity in structural & mechanical engineering.

Data collection:
The author (Case A) is a 73-year-old male with a 25-year history of type 2 diabetes (T2D) history. He began collecting his carbs/sugar intake amount and post-meal walking steps on 7/1/2015. From 7/15/2015 to 10/18/2020 (1,935 days), he has collected 6 data per day, 1 FPG, 3 PPG, carb/sugar, and post-meal walking steps. He utilized these 11,610 data of 1,935 days to conduct his prior research work on the

subject in Part 1 of his linear elastic glucose study (Reference 7).

In addition, on 5/5/2018, he started to use a continuous glucose monitoring (CGM) sensor device to collect 96 glucose data each day.

From 7/1/2015 to 10/18/2020 is his "best-controlled" diabetes period, where his average daily glucoses is maintained at 116 mg/dL (<120 mg/dL). He named this as his "linear elastic zone" of diabetes health. In 2010, his average glucose was 280 mg/dL and HbA1C was 10%, while taking three different diabetes medications (i.e. under very severe type 2 diabetes conditions). Please note that strong chemical interventions from various diabetes medications would seriously alter the physical behaviors of glucose. Prior to 2015, he called that period as his "nonlinear plastic zone" of diabetes health.

The second set of data comes from his wife (Case B) with a 22-year history of T2D. She began to collect her glucose data via finger-piercing method (finger glucose) since 1/1/2014. However, she does not keep a detailed record of her diet and exercise. Since both patients are almost eating the same meals prepared by the author, except that she consumes more meat which partially affects her hyperlipidemia and hypertension conditions. From the diabetes research viewpoint, the author decided to use 80% of Case A's carbs/sugar amount for her and use 50% of Case A's post-meal walking steps for her. She also started to use the same brand of CGM device to collect her sensor glucose data at the same rate of 96 data per day on 1/1/2020.

In order to maintain data consistency for a fair and accurate comparison, the author took both male data and female data from 1/18/2020 through 10/18/2020 and subdivided them into 9 monthly sub-periods of equal length to study their glucose fluctuation patterns and data (Part 2 study).

The third case, Case C, is a 47-year-old male patient with a 4-year history of T2D. He has started to collect his glucose data via the same brand of CGM sensor device on 3/18/2020. Through telephone interviews, the author discovered that during the past 7-month period, his average carbs/sugar intake amount is about the same as Case A and his average post-meal walking steps is at ~25% level of Case A.

In order to maintain data consistency for a fair and accurate comparison, the author took the CGM sensor glucose data from Cases A, B, and C from 3/18/2020 through 10/18/2020 and subdivided them into 7 monthly sub-periods of equal lengths to study their glucose fluctuation patterns and data (Part 3 study).

One of the reasons for using the sensor glucose data is that they are 12.4% (daily glucose) to 16.3% (PPG) higher than finger glucoses on average. Therefore, using the sensor data would be more conservative in terms analyzing diabetes severity. As a result, the author could compare these three sets of GH-modulus values and data patterns from the viewpoint of diabetes severity.

Results:

Part 1:
Fixed & variable M2 of 1 patient

The data calculations in this part use two different sets of M2 values. In Case A, the calculation is based on variable M2 values annually in order to obtain 100% of the PPG prediction accuracy for every year in this period. The 100% accuracy indicates that the annual predicted PPG is identical to the annual measured PPG. In Case B, the calculation is based on a constant value of 1.82 for M2 (using the 6-year average) to obtain six different annual PPG prediction accuracies ranging from 93% to 103%.

Figure 1 and Figure 2 show the graphic results of Case A (variable M2) and Case B (constant M2).

Figure 1 depicts the results from using variable M2 values to achieve a 100% match between the predicted PPG and measured PPG of each year.

Listed below are the values for the variable M2 multiplier (i.e. GH-modulus) for each year:

Year 2015 - 1.56
Year 2016 - 1.76
Year 2017 - 1.59
Year 2018 - 1.87
Year 2019 - 1.75
Year 2020 - 2.41
Averaged - 1.82

In Figure 2, it reflects the results from using a constant GH-modulus (M2) of 1.82 to achieve different predicted PPG values from the measured PPG values, with different prediction accuracy for each year (from 93% to 103%).

Listed below are the values of the prediction accuracy for each year:

Year 2015 - 103%
Year 2016 - 101%
Year 2017 - 103%
Year 2018 - 99%
Year 2019 - 101%
Year 2020 - 93%
Averaged - 100%

In fact, the prediction accuracies varying between 93% to 103% with a 6-year average accuracy of 100% are acceptable for the purpose of practical glucose control for diabetes patients. This is similar to a diabetes patient's situation of glucose prediction accuracy ranging from 112 mg/dL (93%) to 124 mg/dL (103%) using a normal dividing line of 120 mg/dL (100%).

Figure 3 illustrates an x-y data diagram with a "pseudo-linear" relationship between x-values of carbs/sugar multiplied by M2, and y-values of the incremental PPG due to FPG and exercise as defined in the following Equation:

The incremental PPG amount
= Predicted PPG - baseline PPG
* (i.e. FPG * 0.97) + exercise effect*
* (i.e. post-meal walking k-steps * 5)*

The data ranges of x-axis and y-axis are from 20 to 32.

From Figure 4, it is obvious that the six-annual data "almost" form a straight line with a slope of 45% between carbs and PPG delta. The author calls the linear phenomenon and data points having small deviations from the line as a "pseudo-linear" relationship. This is similar to the "elastic zone" of the stress-strain-Young's modulus diagram in theory of elasticity and strength of materials of structural and mechanical engineering (Figure 1). This linear relationship makes the task of incremental PPG prediction through diabetes control via diet much easier.

Part 2:
Fixed & variable M2 of two patients

Fixed M2 Case:
In Part 2, the author utilized two different fixed values of M2 for Case A and Case B, respectively to calculate both x- and y- components of his "linear elastic glucose" equation. *The comparison between Case A's M2 value of 3.6 and Case B's M2 of 2.6 revealed the individual severity of their respective T2D conditions.* Case A indicates a more severe diabetes patient who requires higher M2 (or GH modulus) value to increase his predicted PPG in order to match his higher measured PPG value.

Again, the linear elastic glucose equation using **predicted** PPG is listed below:

Predicted *PPG = (FPG * 0.97) + (carbs&sugar * M2) - (post-meal walking k-steps * 5)*

The *"x-component"* of the linear elastic glucose equation is:
*(carbs&sugar * M2);*
While the *"y-component"* of the linear elastic glucose equation is:
*(**Predicted** PPG - (FPG * 0.97) + (post-meal walking k-steps * 5)*

Due to the linearity characteristics of this equation, the relationship between the x-component and y-component is always guaranteed to be "linear". However, these two different fixed M2 values would result into different data ranges of x and y components. Figures 5 and 6 demonstrate two different fixed M2 values and corresponding data ranges for Case A and Case B, respectively.

Case A with the fixed M2 of 3.6, both x and y are within the range of 35 to 58 with an average value of 44 is shown in Figure 5. Case B with the fixed M2 of 2.6, both x and y are within the range of 22 to 34 with an average value of 26 is observed in Figure 6.

In summary, the higher the M2, the higher x and y values become, and the higher predicted and measured PPG values are. The key point is that the monthly M2 values (i.e. GH-modulus) are dependent on the patient's body conditions (a combination of blood, liver, and pancreas) of that particular month.

Listed below are the values of the prediction accuracy for Case A and Case B for each month. Please note that the prediction accuracy percentage varies with the fixed M2 input; however, their prediction accuracies are 100% for the total period of 9 months for both cases which is the purpose of selecting these two fixed M2 values. However, this approach will cause some degree of sacrifice on monthly PPG prediction's accuracy for each month. It should be noted that the prediction accuracy range are 88%-111% and 93%-108% for Case A and Case B, respectively.

1/18 - 2/18: 101% & 97%
2/18 - 3/18: 97% & 99%
3/18 - 4/18: 98% & 95%
4/18 - 5/18: 111% & 108%
5/18 - 6/18: 101% & 107%
6/18 - 7/18: 88% & 93%
7/18 - 8/18: 100% & 95%
8/18 - 9/18: 102% & 101%
9/18 - 10/18: 98% & 106%
2020 Average: 100% & 100%

Variable M2 Case:
In this section, the author utilized variable value of M2 for each month in order to make the calculated x-component values to match with the calculated y-components values during each monthly sub-period; therefore, to "force" the predicted PPG value to match with the measured PPG value in each month. As a result, a "pseudo-linear" relationship between x-component and y-component could be created and observed.

This forced "pseudo-linear" relationship makes sense in the biomedical field since red blood cells and liver cells are organic materials which are different from those inorganic materials in the engineering systems, such as rubber, concrete, or steel. The human organ cells are not only organic but also have different lifespans, where they can mutate, change, repair, or die. For example, the lifespan of the red blood cells is 115 to 120 days, the lifespan of liver cells is 300 to 500 days, and the lifespan of pancreatic beta cells is unknown with slightly adaptive change. (This is why the pancreatic beta cells' self-repair process is very slow, about 2.7% per year for the author.) Not all of the body cells die at the same moment. At any given instance, an organ would have different combinations of new cells, sick cells, dying cells, and mutated cells, mixing together. It is complex and an extraordinarily situation; therefore, the author has chosen different M2 values for different months in order to achieve his prediction accuracies for all monthly sub-periods. This would be a reasonable approach in proceeding with this biomedical research.

In the previous paragraph, the fixed M2 difference between Case A of 3.6 versus Case B of 2.6 is based on the severity of their T2D between patients. Furthermore, in this paragraph, it has demonstrated that the variable M2 differences of different months are resulted from the T2D conditions varying month to month for each patient. This means that glucose is a "dynamic" function instead of being a "static" function. The above discussions are the major differences between the linear elasticity organic glucoses and the traditional linear elasticity of strength of inorganic engineering materials.

For conducting a further sensitivity analysis, he used the **measured** PPG to replace the predicted PPG in the linear elastic glucose equation as show below:

Measured PPG = (FPG * 0.97) + (carbs&sugar * M2) - (post-meal walking k-steps * 5)

The "*x-component*" of the linear elastic glucose equation is:
*(carbs&sugar * M2);*
While the "*y-component*" of the linear elastic glucose equation is:
*(**Measured** PPG - (FPG * 0.97) + (post-meal walking k-steps * 5)*

By examining the variable M2 values, over 9 monthly sub-periods, Case A has M2 range from 2.8 to 5.2 with an average of 3.7 value (Figure 5), and Case B has M2 range from 1.9 to 3.6 with an average of 2.7 value (Figure 6). Please note the minor difference between fixed M2 of 3.6 versus 2.6 and variable M2 of 3.7 versus 2.7 which are caused by rounding off in the numerical analysis.

For Case A with variable M2, both x and y components are within the range of 37 to 51 with an average value of 45. For Case B with variable M2, both x and y components are within the range of 18 to 32 with an average value of 26.

In summary, similar to the fixed M2 case, for most of the months, the higher the variable M2, the higher x and y values become, and the higher predicted and measured PPG values are. The key point from these two figures is that the monthly M2 values are dependent on the patient's body conditions (combination of blood, liver, and pancreas) for that particular month.

Figures 7 and 8 have graphically demonstrated the linear elastic glucoses data for Case A and Case B, respectively.

Listed below are the values of the individual M2 multiplier (i.e. variable GH-modulus) for each month in 2020, in the order of (Case A vs. Case B).

1/18 - 2/18: 3.5 vs. 3.0
2/18 - 3/18: 3.9 vs. 2.7

3/18 - 4/18: 3.8 vs. 3.1
4/18 - 5/18: 2.8 vs. 1.9
5/18 - 6/18: 3.5 vs. 1.9
6/18 - 7/18: 5.2 vs. 3.6
7/18 - 8/18: 3.6 vs. 3.2
8/18 - 9/18: 3.4 vs. 2.5
9/18 - 10/18: 3.8 vs. 1.9
2020 Average: 3.7 vs. 2.7

The purpose in selecting variable M2 values for each of the 9 monthly sub-periods is to achieve 100% match between x- component and y-component for both cases.

Part 3:
Variable M2 of three patients

Due to the high accuracy of predicted PPG, as mentioned above, there are some insignificant rounding-off errors between the predicted PPG values and measured PPG values. Therefore, he decided to use the measured PPG values in these three cases.

Here is the calculated x- and y- components as follows:

x = (carbs&sugar * M2)
y = (**measured** PPG -(FPG * 0.97) + (walking k-steps * 5)

Listed below are the values of the individual M2 multiplier (i.e. GH-modulus) for each of the 7 months in 2020 which are listed in the order of Case A, Case B, and Case C:

3/18 - 4/18: (3.8, 3.1, 1.3)
4/18 - 5/18: (2.8, 1.9, 0.6)
5/18 - 6/18: (3.5, 1.9, 0.7)
6/18 - 7/18: (5.2, 3.6, 0.7)
7/18 - 8/18: (3.6, 3.2, 1.4)
8/18 - 9/18: (3.4, 2.5, 1.2)
9/18 - 10/18: (3.8, 1.9, 1.4)
Variable M2: (3.7, 2.6, 1.0)
Fixed M2: (3.6, 2.6, 1.0)

Case A with the fixed M2 as 3.6, both x and y are within the range of 38 to 48 with an average value of 45 are observed in Figure 9. Case B with the fixed M2 as 2.6, both x and y are within the range of 18 to 32 with an average value of 25 are observed in Figure 10. Case C with the fixed M2 as 1.0, both x and y are within the range of 11 to 17 with an average value of 13 are observed in Figure 11.

In summary, the 7-month average values of each monthly M2 variables (i.e., GH-modulus) are 3.7, 2.6, and 1.0, and with an average measured PPG values at 122 mg/dL, 114 md/dL, and 109 mg/dL, for Case A, Case B, and Case C, respectively, which are ranked according to the severity of their diabetes conditions. The higher the M2, the higher values of both x (carbs/sugar intake amount) and y (incremental PPG amount) become, and the higher predicted and measured PPG values are. The key conclusion from these three clinical observations is that the M2 values are varying based on patients' body conditions, especially their diabetes severity (i.e. blood, liver, and pancreas). This is similar to the different inorganic engineering materials with the different Young's modules values, such as nylon ~3 versus steel ~200.

Discussion:

Part 1:

One patient

The author was a severe type 2 diabetes patient since 1995. He suffered many life-threatening diabetic complications during the period of Y2000 to Y2012. After experiencing five cardiovascular episodes, with an average glucose value of 280 mg/dL and HbA1C of 10%, he started to self-study and research diabetes and food nutrition in 2010. He collected his diet and exercise data since 6/1/2015. After 2015, his diabetes conditions have been under control via a stringent lifestyle program; therefore, in this study, he used his collected big data of lifestyle details and glucoses to conduct his rather completed numerical analysis. From 7/1/2015 to 10/13/2020, his diabetes conditions have fallen into a linear "elastic" zone (average glucose 116 mg/dL with some peaks). This also suggests that his PPG would land in a reasonable range (around 120 mg/dL or below) when he consumes lesser amounts of carbs/sugar and exercising adequately.

On the other hand, during the period of 2000-2010 (it could even extend to 2013), when his diabetes was totally out of control, he believes that his case should be belonging to a "nonlinear plastic" zone, or at least a "bi-linear plastic" zone, meaning his PPG would remain at a certain elevated level even if he reduced or stopped the intake of carbs/sugar. Worse than having "elevated glucoses" (hyperglycemia i.e. >180 mg/dL), he could suffer from hypoglycemia (glucose <70 mg/dL) leading to insulin shock and eventually sudden death. However, due to the lack of sufficient data collection, he cannot conduct a similar detailed and completed numerical analysis to prove his suspicion of "nonlinear plastic" zone. He can only try to use his scattered data collection from 2010 to 2013 to obtain a guesstimated observation and some partial conclusions.

As shown in Figure 7, he displayed an x-y diagram of predicted PPG versus measured PPG over both periods, the smaller area of linear elastic period of 2015-2020 and the larger area of nonlinear plastic period of 2010-2013. The comparison between these two zones are interesting, but yet he needs to find other ways to collect data and prove his suspicion on the linkage between his glucose spikes and fluctuations (i.e. nonlinearity) of glucoses in the plastic zone and carbs/sugar intake amount in order to compare against his controlled glucoses situations of the pseudo-linear elastic zone.

In his published research papers starting in 2019, he has proven that his pancreatic beta cells' insulin capability of production and quality have been self-repairing at an annual rate of 2.7% (References 5 and 6). It means that 16% of his insulin production and quality problems have been repaired since 2015 which is in the elastic zone, whereas 27% have been repaired since 2011 which covers both partial plastic zone and elastic zone. This type of "organic" cells' regeneration capability and biomedical phenomena was unknown to him when he was an engineer dealing only with variety of "inorganic" materials, such as metal, concrete, and silicon. As a result, since 2010, he has been fascinated in working with the various stimulators and complex stimulations of the biomedical system. The more research work he performs, the more unknown phenomena occur, and the more questions enter his mind, causing him to search for more and better solutions.

Part 2:
Two patients
This "linear elastic glucose" study has started from the verification and improvement for the predicted PPG through his previously defined simple formula of PPG prediction. The author has learned from his engineering background that a linear system approach would be the easiest way to study a relationship between causes and consequences. Therefore, he started to investigate the similarity between elastic glucose system and elastic engineering system using Young's modulus and GH-modulus as his pair of analogy models. Nevertheless, he has never forgotten his ultimate objective is to identify an easier application model with a higher PPG prediction accuracy in order to help other diabetes patients, while maintaining the basic requirement of science that is to seek for truth with high precision.

By either using a fixed M2 value to achieve a high accuracy over a total period of 9 months or using monthly variable M2 values to achieve high accuracies for every monthly sub-period, he has observed a linear relationship existing between carbs/sugar intake amount and incremental PPG amount (including predicted or measured PPG, FPG, and exercise). More importantly, he still maintains an extremely high PPG prediction accuracy in using both approaches.

One important viewpoint is that glucose is an organic biomedical material which consists of both nonlinear and dynamic functional behaviors in its nature. Therefore, in order to fully understand and be able to describe its behavior accurately, a research using a nonlinear plastic model is needed. However, at present time, he lacks of needed and sufficient data to conduct his research. But, similar to linear elasticity engineering applications, this linear elastic glucose behavior study already covers a sufficient scope of biomedical applications which remains to be useful. As a counterpart example, many T2D patients are either in the pre-diabetes range (PPG value at 120 to 140 mg/dL) or their glucose levels fall below the hyperglycemic range (i.e., glucose at 180 mg/dL or lower). This simpler "linear glucose model" can be extremely useful for many diabetes patients worldwide. Depending on the approach, either the overall period's fixed M2 or sub-period's variable M2, it would be easier for diabetes patient to use this linear elastic glucose behavior for their glucose control. The author prefers the fixed M2 model since traditional internal medicine utilizes the HbA1C model. The HbA1C value is remarkably close to the average glucose over a 90-day period (conventionally) or over 120-day period (the author's defined model based on red blood cells life span). Besides, calculating or guess-estimating a single M2 value is much easier and acceptable by patients than using multiple M2 values for every sub-period calculations.

Part 3:
Three patients
In this part, the author has utilized **variable** M2 values for each month in order to make the calculated x-component values to match with the calculated y-components values during each monthly sub-period; therefore, to "force" the predicted PPG value to match with the measured PPG value in each month. As a result, a linear or "pseudo-linear" relationship between x-component and y-component could be created and observed.

This forced "pseudo-linear" relationship makes sense in the biomedical field since red blood cells and liver cells are organic materials which are different from those inorganic materials in the engineering systems, such as rubber or steel. The organic cells system is a complex and extraordinarily situation; therefore, the author has chosen variable M2 values for different months in order to achieve his prediction accuracies for all sub-periods. These data have demonstrated that the variable M2 values of different months resulted from the T2D conditions varying month to month *for each patient, precisely the combined situation of liver, blood, and pancreas.* This means that glucose is a very "dynamic" function instead of being a "static" function. The above discussions are the major differences between the linear elasticity *organic* glucoses and the traditional linear elasticity of strength of *inorganic* engineering materials.

Conclusions:
Here are the main conclusions of this article:

First, by using an analogy from the theory of elasticity and engineering strength of material, the author has identified a linear relationship existing between carbs and PPG delta with a newly defined GH-modulus, similar to a linear relationship between stress and strain with Young's modulus.

Second, based on two diabetes patients' 9-month data, he has proven that the magnitude of GH-modulus is directly proportional to the diabetes severity of the patients.

Third, by utilizing three diabetes patients' 7-month data, he has confirmed that the magnitude of the monthly GH-modulus is directly proportional to the diabetes severity of that particular month for each patient.

Fourth, these linear elastic glucose behavior findings are probably applicable to a glucose range from 70 mg/dL to 180 mg/dL which covers most situations for a diabetes patient. For glucose values falling outside the range, a nonlinear plastic glucose behavior study is needed.

References:

1. Hsu, Gerald C., eclaireMD Foundation, USA, No. 310: "Biomedical research methodology based on GH-Method: math-physical medicine"

2. Hsu, Gerald C., eclaireMD Foundation, USA, No. 345: "Application of linear equations to predict sensor and finger based postprandial plasma glucoses and daily glucoses for pre-virus, virus, and total periods using GH-Method: math-physical medicine"

3. Hsu, Gerald C., eclaireMD Foundation, USA, No. 97: "A simplified yet accurate linear equation of PPG prediction model for T2D patients (GH-Method: math-physical medicine)"

4. Hsu, Gerald C., eclaireMD Foundation, USA, No. 99: "Application of linear equation-based PPG prediction model for four T2D clinic cases (GH-Method: math-physical medicine)"

5. Hsu, Gerald C., eclaireMD Foundation, USA, No. 339: "Self-recovery of pancreatic beta cell's insulin secretion based on 10+ years annualized data of food, exercise, weight, and glucose using GH-Method: math-physical medicine)

6. Hsu, Gerald C., eclaireMD Foundation, USA, No. 340: "A neural communication model between brain and internal organs, specifically stomach, liver, and pancreatic beta cells based on PPG waveforms of 131 liquid egg meals and 124 solid egg meals)

7. Hsu, Gerald C., eclaireMD Foundation, USA, No. 346: "Linear relationship between carbohydrates & sugar intake amount and incremental PPG amount via engineering strength of materials using GH-Method: math-physical medicine, Part 1"

8. Hsu, Gerald C., eclaireMD Foundation, USA, No. 349: "Investigation on GH modulus of linear elastic glucose with two diabetes patients data using GH-Method: math-physical medicine, Part 2"

9. Hsu, Gerald C., eclaireMD Foundation, USA, No. 350: "Investigation of GH modulus (or M2) of linear elastic glucose based on three diabetes patients data using GH-Method: math-physical medicine, Parts 3"

List of Figures:

Figure 2-1: male line with fixed M2
Figure 2-2: female line with fixed M2
Figure 2-3: male line with variable M2
Figure 2-4: female line with variable M2

Part 3: three patients:
Figure 3-1: male line with variable M2
Figure 3-2: female line with variable M2
Figure 3-3: young line with variable M2

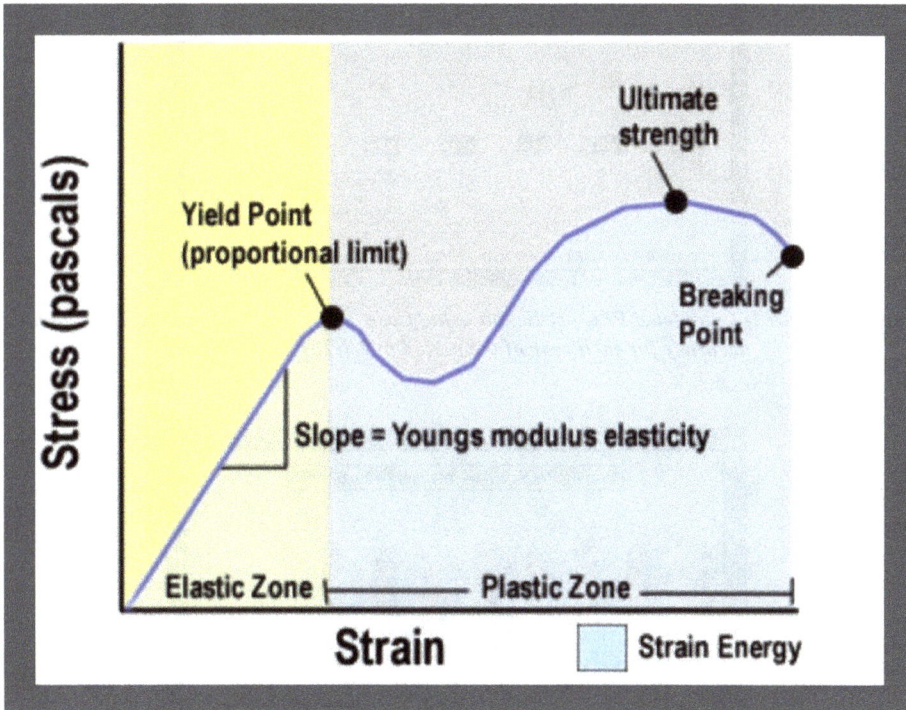

Figure 1: Stress-Strain-Young's modulus, Elastic Zone vs. Plastic Zone

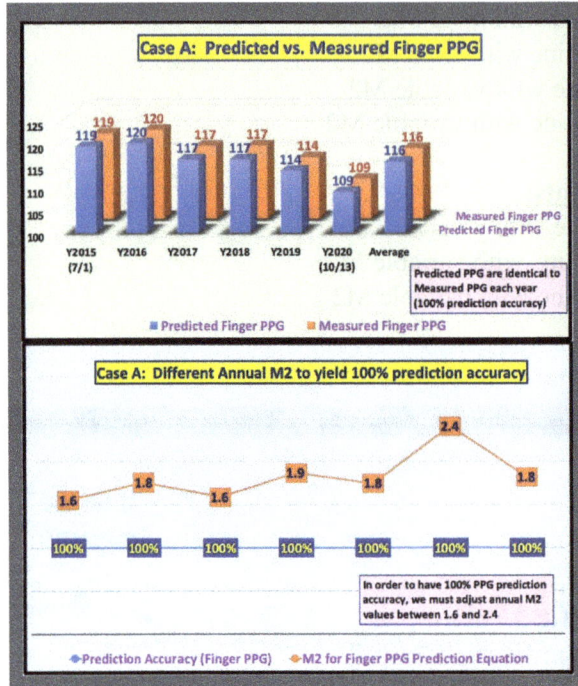

Figure 1-1: (Part 1) Calculated PPG prediction using Case A (variable M2) to have 100% prediction accuracy for each year of the period of 7/1/2015 - 10/13/2020

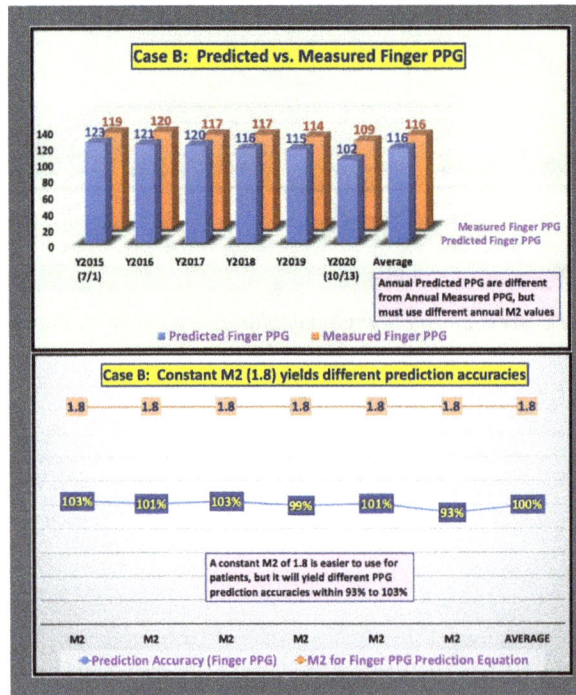

Figure 1-2: (Part 1) Calculated PPG prediction using Case A (constant M2) to have different prediction accuracy for each year (between 93% and 103%) of the period of 7/1/2015 - 10/13/2020

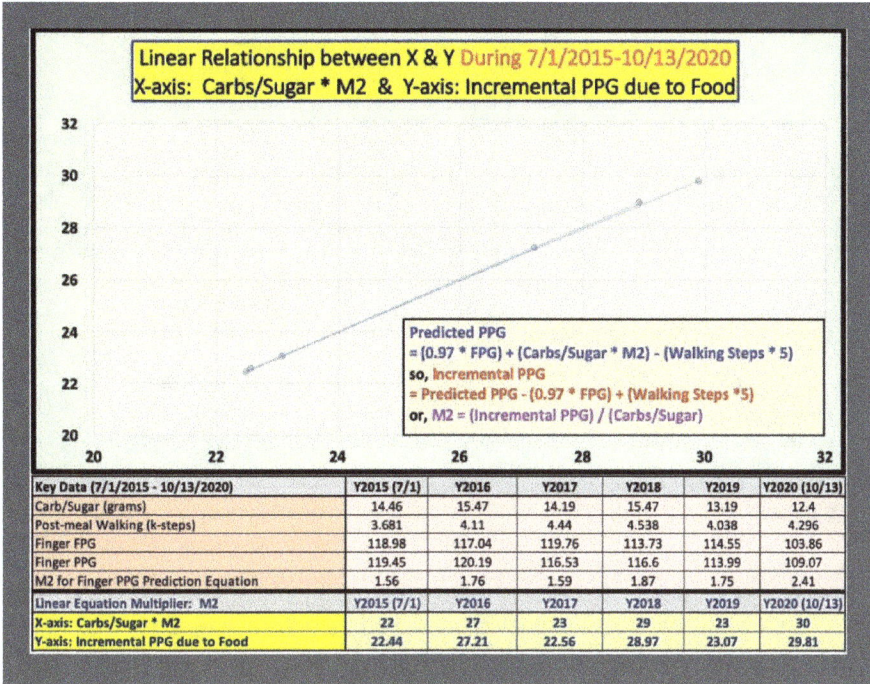

Linear Relationship between X & Y During 7/1/2015-10/13/2020
X-axis: Carbs/Sugar * M2 & Y-axis: Incremental PPG due to Food

Predicted PPG
= (0.97 * FPG) + (Carbs/Sugar * M2) - (Walking Steps * 5)
so, Incremental PPG
= Predicted PPG - (0.97 * FPG) + (Walking Steps *5)
or, M2 = (Incremental PPG) / (Carbs/Sugar)

Key Data (7/1/2015 - 10/13/2020)	Y2015 (7/1)	Y2016	Y2017	Y2018	Y2019	Y2020 (10/13)
Carb/Sugar (grams)	14.46	15.47	14.19	15.47	13.19	12.4
Post-meal Walking (k-steps)	3.681	4.11	4.44	4.538	4.038	4.296
Finger FPG	118.98	117.04	119.76	113.73	114.55	103.86
Finger PPG	119.45	120.19	116.53	116.6	113.99	109.07
M2 for Finger PPG Prediction Equation	1.56	1.76	1.59	1.87	1.75	2.41
Linear Equation Multiplier: M2	Y2015 (7/1)	Y2016	Y2017	Y2018	Y2019	Y2020 (10/13)
X-axis: Carbs/Sugar * M2	22	27	23	29	23	30
Y-axis: Incremental PPG due to Food	22.44	27.21	22.56	28.97	23.07	29.81

Figure 1-3: (Part 1) A "pseudo-linear" relationship between x-values and y-values during the "linear elastic" zone of 2015-2020

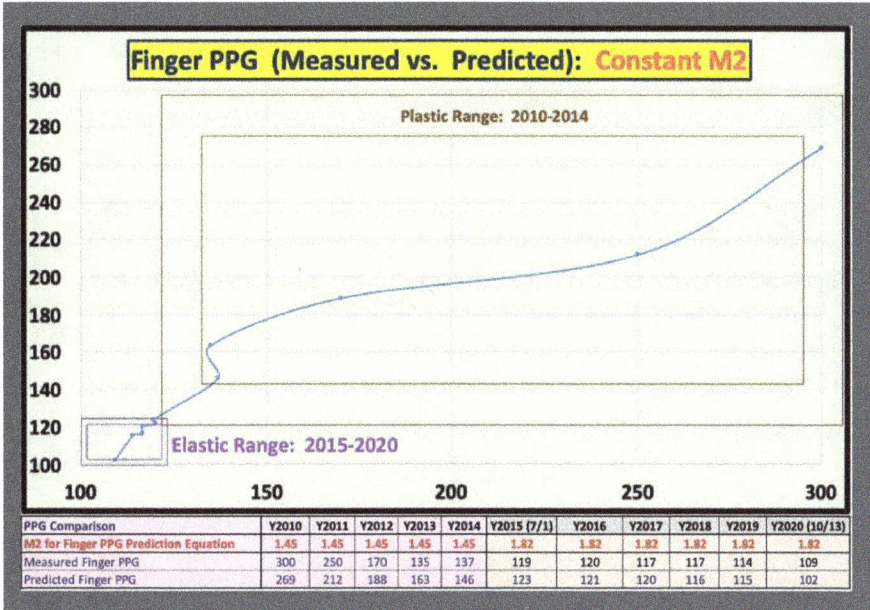

Finger PPG (Measured vs. Predicted): Constant M2

Plastic Range: 2010-2014

Elastic Range: 2015-2020

PPG Comparison	Y2010	Y2011	Y2012	Y2013	Y2014	Y2015 (7/1)	Y2016	Y2017	Y2018	Y2019	Y2020 (10/13)
M2 for Finger PPG Prediction Equation	1.45	1.45	1.45	1.45	1.45	1.82	1.82	1.82	1.82	1.82	1.82
Measured Finger PPG	300	250	170	135	137	119	120	117	117	114	109
Predicted Finger PPG	269	212	188	163	146	123	121	120	116	115	102

Figure 1-4: (Part 1) Discussion of variety relationship between predicted PPG and measured PPG during 2010-2020 (both "pseudo-linear elastic" zone and "nonlinear plastic" zone

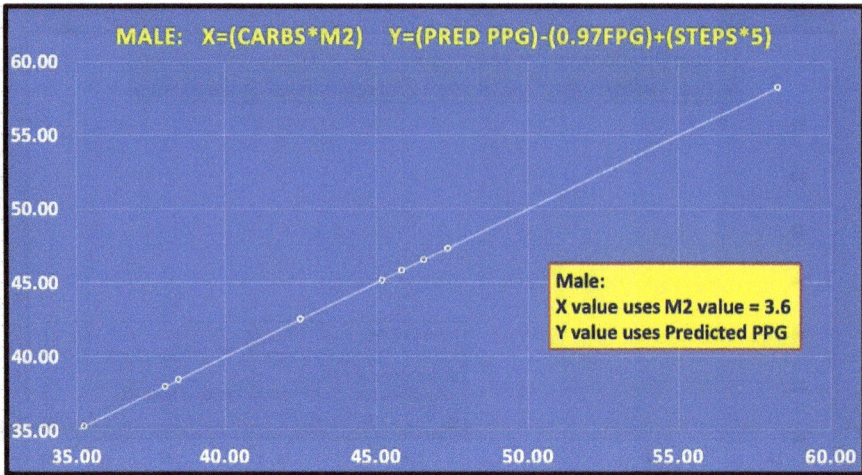

Figure 2-1: (Part 2) Male case using fixed M2 value of 3.6 (1/18/2020 - 10/18/2020)

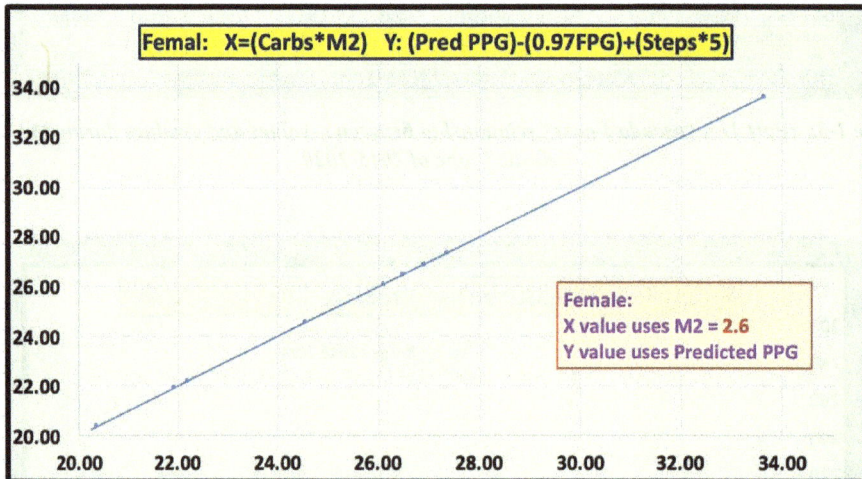

Figure 2-2: (Part 2) Female case using fixed M2 value of 2.6 (1/18/2020 - 10/18/2020)

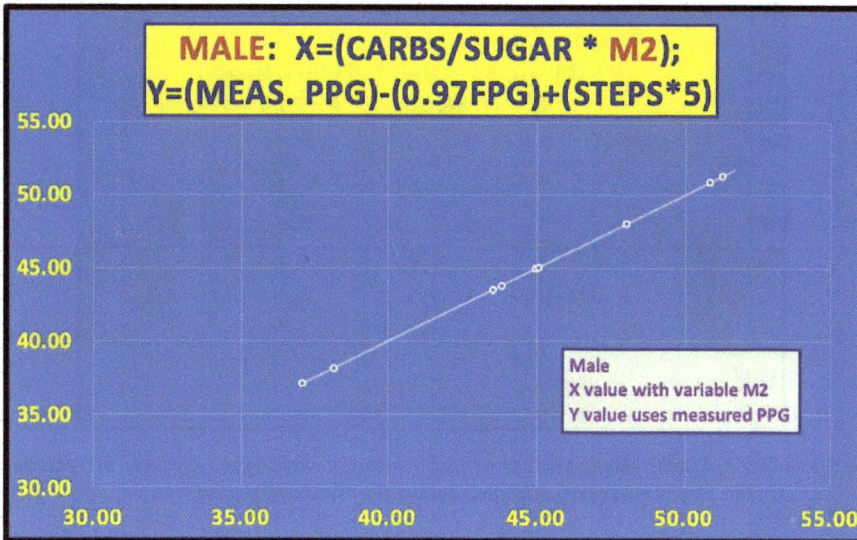

Figure 2-3: (Part 2) Male case using variable M2 values (1/18/2020 - 10/18/2020)

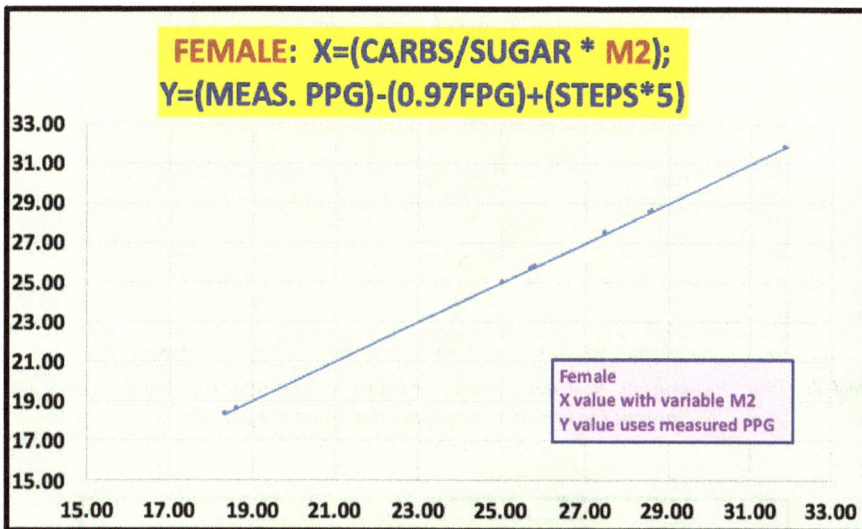

Figure 2-4: (Part 2) Female case using variable M2 values (1/18/2020 - 10/18/2020)

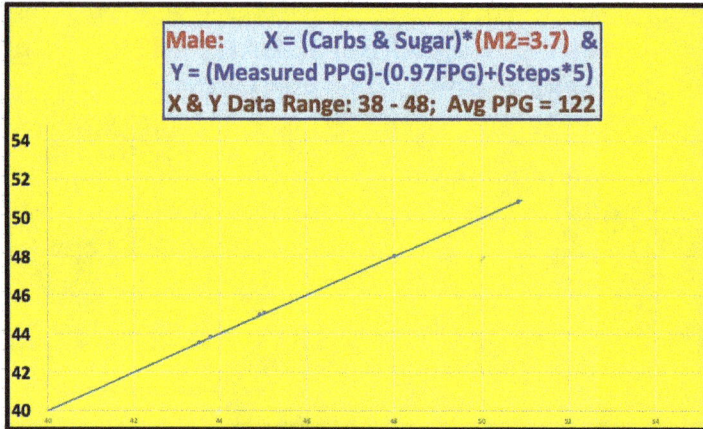

Figure 3-1: (Part 3) Linear elastic glucose behavior between cars/sugar input and incremental PPG output for male case during the 7-months period

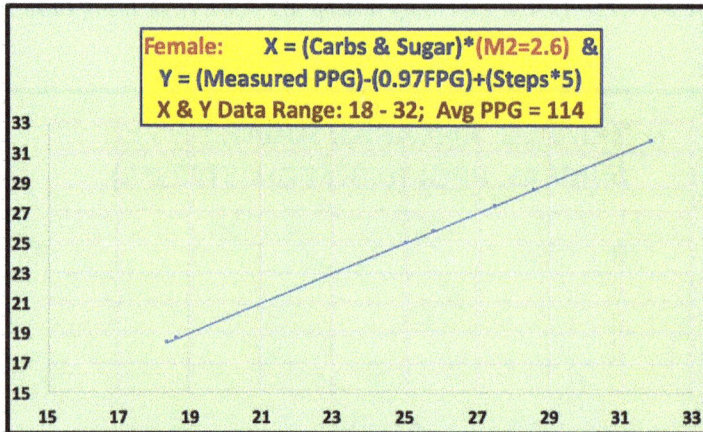

Figure 3-2: (Part 3) Linear elastic glucose behavior between cars/sugar input and incremental PPG output for female case during the 7-months period

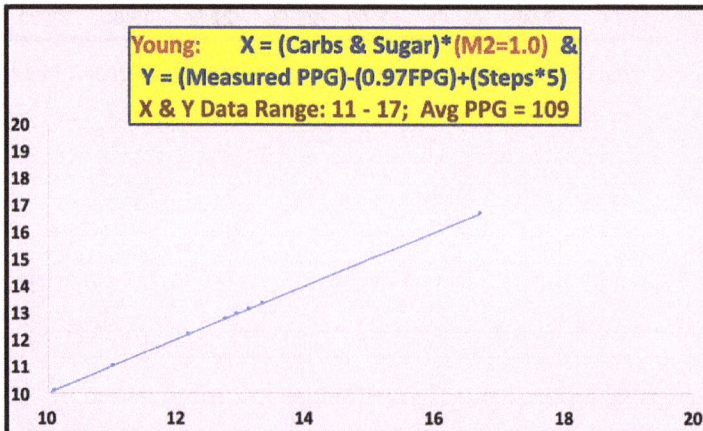

Figure 3-3: (Part 3) Linear elastic glucose behavior between cars/sugar input and incremental PPG output for young case during the 7-months period

Lifestyle medicine practice to diagnose the relationship between sleep patterns and glucoses of three type 2 diabetes patients using GH-Method: math-physical medicine (No. 353)

Gerald C. Hsu
eclaireMD Foundation, USA
10/25-26/2020

Abstract:

The author applies his GH-method: math-physical medicine research methodology and lifestyle medicine practice to diagnose the relationship between sleep patterns and glucoses of three type 2 diabetes (T2D) patients in particular the female case referred to as Case A, who has an irregular sleep pattern.

The key method is to analyze the patient's collected big glucose data and their associated glucose waveforms (glucose curves) to check for curve shapes, changing patterns, rising and dropping speeds, life habits, and consequence interpretation from lifestyle behaviors.

Glucoses are the direct outcomes of lifestyle details, such as diet, exercise, medication, and certain lifetime habits. Instead of delving into the carbs/sugar intake amounts, the intensity and duration of walking exercise, and the effectiveness of different medications, the author can quickly assess a patients' overall health or specific problem areas by examining their lifestyle details hidden behind the glucose data and curves. It should be noted that the three T2D patients are not taking any diabetes medications during this examination period; therefore, this case study excludes the biomedical effects from the medication intervention.

The author has named this method *lifestyle medicine*, which does not rely on the traditional practice of using medications exclusively.

Case A, with a 22-year history of diabetes, has an irregular sleep pattern where she wakes up approximately 4am and then goes back to sleep at 6am. She then wakes up again at around 7am to eat breakfast which continuously pushes up her glucose waveform to reach to a higher breakfast postprandial plasma glucose (PPG) peak about 9am. She has a moderate level of diabetes condition among the three cases. Her irregular sleep pattern has not only raised her fasting plasma glucose (FPG) in the middle of night, but also increases her glucose to connect with her breakfast PPG waveform.

With an irregular sleep pattern, Case A has an unwanted "elevated glucose" between 4am to 6am. Although this 2-hour elevated FPG only occupies a small percentage of her daily average glucose value, its continuous influence of glucose pushing power from FPG to connect with her breakfast PPG cannot be ignored.

This article provides another clinical case study in practicing the lifestyle medicine along with the traditional endocrinology practices.

The author believes that lifestyle medicine should be considered as a branch of general internal medicine. He dedicated the past decade and ~30,000 hours to self-study and research chronic diseases and their complications. To date, he has written 353 articles or research notes over the past 10.3 years. Through presenting ~120 papers at ~65 international medical conferences and publishing ~300 papers on ~100 medical journals, he continuously promote his developed GH-Method: math-physical medicine research methodology, and his learned knowledge through his research of lifestyle, metabolism, and immunity to the healthcare community. In addition, his discoveries from various clinical case studies can inspire other healthcare professionals to join him in saving more lives by using similar methods.

Introduction:

The author applies his GH-method: math-physical medicine research methodology and lifestyle medicine practice to diagnose the relationship between sleep patterns and glucoses of three type 2 diabetes (T2D) patients in particular the female case referred to as Case A, who has an irregular sleep pattern.

The key method is to analyze the patient's collected big glucose data and their associated glucose waveforms (glucose curves) to check for curve shapes, changing patterns, rising and dropping speeds, life habits, and consequence interpretation from lifestyle behaviors.

Glucoses are the direct outcomes of lifestyle details, such as diet, exercise, medication, and certain lifetime habits. Instead of delving into the carbs/sugar intake amounts, the intensity and duration of walking exercise, and the effectiveness of different medications, the author can quickly assess a patients' overall health or specific problem areas by examining their lifestyle details hidden behind the glucose data and curves. It should be noted that the three T2D patients are not taking any diabetes medications during this examination period; therefore, this case study excludes the biomedical effects from the medication intervention.

The author has named this method lifestyle medicine, which does not rely on the traditional practice of using medications exclusively.

Methods:

Background:
To learn more about the author's developed GH-Method: math-physical medicine (MPM) methodology, readers can refer to his article to understand this MPM analysis method in Reference 1.

Highlights of his related research:
In his published medical papers, he has outlined the following key research findings:

(1) FPG and body weight have a high correlation (>77% based on 7-years data) between them. Furthermore, FPG has 5 influential components with weight contributing >85% of FPG formation.
(2) PPG has 19 influential components. Both carbs/sugar intake amount and post-meal walking exercise contribute ~40% of PPG formation, individually.
(3) He has identified that FPG could serve as the baseline level of PPG. Furthermore, FPG is a good indicator for pancreatic beta cells' health status in a diabetes patient.
(4) He proved that his pancreatic beta cells have been self-repairing at an annual rate of 2.7% during the last 6 to 10 years.

(5) Sensor PPG are ~14% to 18% higher than finger PPG, However, average sensor FPG is almost identical to finger FPG (see Figure 1).

(6) For some severe T2D patients, incremental glucose amounts between wake-up moment and first-bite moment of breakfast are around 10 mg/dL to 20 mg/dL.

(7) He has collected more than10 detailed elements regarding daily sleep conditions which can be used for some different and detailed analysis.

Three T2D patients' information:

Case A is a 72-year-old female with a 22-year history of T2D. Her average glucose was 183 mg/dL and HbA1C 8% in 2010. Since 1/1/2019, She has followed some parts of the author's lifestyle management program, especially on diet. She has stopped taking her diabetes medication since 1/1/2019.

Case B is the author himself. He is 73-year-old male with a 25-year history of T2D. His average glucose was 280 mg/dL and HbA1C 10% in 2010 and has suffered from many chronic diseases induced complications between 2000 to 2014. Since 2014, he has started his stringent lifestyle management program on all fronts. He stopped taking three types of prescribed diabetes medications as of 12/8/2015.

Case C is a 47-year-old male with a 4-year history of T2D. His average glucose was 150 mg/dL and HbA1C 6.9% in 2017. He did not follow the author's lifestyle management program. His BMI was 44 in early 2020 and since 4/1/2020, he has started a weight reduction program to reduce ~40 lbs. of his weight to date. He has never taken any diabetes medication.

Data in this case study:

All three patients are using the same brand of a continuous glucose monitoring (CGM) device to collect their glucoses at 15-minute time intervals (Sensor glucoses). Therefore, each patient collects 96 glucose data each day which are stored on a cloud server to be processed and managed via an iPhone APP. For consistency, all the patients' glucoses are sensor glucose data. The starting date for Cases A and B is 1/1/2020 and for Case C is 4/1/2020. The ending date of glucose data for this study is 10/25/2020.

Results:

Figure 2 shows the collected glucose data and curves of the three patients. This figure depicts their hourly glucoses from 00:00 through 09:00.

The author designed his iPhone APP software to include FPG data during the 7 hours of sleep time (from 00:00 throughout 07:00), eating breakfast at one hour after wake-up moment (around 08:00), and reaching to breakfast PPG at one hour after the first bite moment (around 09:00). The software uses a built-in artificial intelligence (AI) feature to automatically correct and re-adjust the timing scale according to the individual patient's life patterns and real time moments.

From Figure 2, Case B has the biggest FPG waveform fluctuation (i.e., up and down with the relative magnitude of peak and valley) which indicates he has the most severe T2D condition. In contrast, Case A has the moderate level of diabetes condition while Case C has the least severe condition. However, when we examine the three waveforms closer, we will find that both Case B and Case C have a similar "salad bowl" shape of waveform, i.e. two extreme peaks located at 00:00 and 09:00, and the valley located in the middle of the bowl around 03:00-04:00. Case A has a completely different shape of waveform which starts at 00:00 trending to its valley around 02:00-03:00, and then rises to its first peak at 06:00, then drops again at 07:00, finally rising again to reach to its second peak at 09:00.

Later, we will examine and discuss Case A's "peculiar" waveform from Figures 3 and 4.

Figure 3 illustrates Case A's monthly glucose waveforms from January through September 2020. It is obvious that almost every single month's glucose waveform over this 9-month period have quite similar patterns.

Figure 4 reveals Case A's synthesized glucose waveform from her glucose data from the period of 1/1/2020 through 10/25/2020.

Let us examine this exclusive diagram closely. Her FPG waveform valleys are 02:00-03:00 then reaches to 102 mg/dL at the same moment of 00:00. After 04:00, her FPG starts to rise from 102 mg/dL to 112 mg/dL at 06:00, with an increased amount of 10 mg/dL. The author has observed this physical from his own FPG waveforms, as indicated in his paper "Hypothesis on the neuroscience communication model existing between the brain and liver regarding glucose secretion in the early morning" (see Reference 7).

Case A's irregular sleep pattern is that she wakes up around 4am and then goes back to sleep again at 6am. She then wakes up again about 7am to eat her breakfast which continuously pushes up her glucose waveform to reach to a higher breakfast PPG peak at approximately 9am.

The author's interpretation about her sleep and glucose situation is described as follows. Her brain receives the "wake-up signal" from her eyes and then issues a "marching order" to the liver to start producing more glucose until 6am when she goes back to sleep. Between 6am to 7am, her FPG drops again down to 107 mg/dL. From her second wake-up moment at 7am with 107 mg/dL to her first bite moment of breakfast at 8am with 120 mg/dL, with her glucose increasing 13 mg/dL. This amount is identical to Case B's increased glucose amount of 13 mg/dL from 106 mg/dL at 7am to 119 mg/dL at 8am. On the other hand, Case C's glucose increased amount is only 1 mg/dL from 107 mg/dL at 7am to 108 mg/dL at 8am due to his non-severe T2D conditions. Case C's situation is still quite similar to a normal person. That is why his FPG waveform is calmer and relatively flat without large fluctuations due to his relative healthy and unharmed pancreatic beta cells.

Summary:

Case A, with a 22-year history, has a moderate level of diabetes condition among the three cases. Her irregular sleep pattern of wakening up around 4am and then going back to sleep at 6am. Not only has this raised her FPG in the middle of night, but it also continuously pushes her glucose to connect with her breakfast PPG waveform.

Case B, with a 25-year history, has the worst diabetes condition. His regular lifestyle routines and good quality of sleep with his 9 lbs. weight reduction in 2020 have directly contributed to his low average sensor FPG.

Case C has the least severe diabetes condition due to his 4-year history of T2D. However, he is an extremely obese patient (BMI 44 on 1/1/2020 and BMI 39 on 10/25/2020). This extreme obesity has caused severe sleep apnea for more than 10 years, where he must depend on a CPAP machine to assist and maintain his sleep. His weight reduction of ~40 lbs. and BMI reduction of 5 in 2020 have already helped his overall glucose control.

Conclusions:

With an irregular sleep pattern, Case A has an unwanted "elevated glucose" between 4am to 6am. Although this 2-hour elevated FPG only occupies a small percentage of her daily average glucose value, its continuous influence of glucose pushing power from FPG to connect with her breakfast PPG cannot be ignored.

This article provides another clinical case study in practicing the lifestyle medicine along with the traditional endocrinology practices.

The author believes that lifestyle medicine should be considered as a branch of general internal medicine. He dedicated the past decade and ~30,000 hours to self-study and research chronic diseases and their complications. To date, he has written 353 articles or research notes over the past 10.3 years. Through presenting ~120 papers at ~65 international medical conferences and publishing ~300 papers on ~100 medical journals, he continuously promote his developed GH-Method: math-physical medicine research methodology, and his learned knowledge through his research of lifestyle, metabolism, and immunity to the healthcare community. In addition, his discoveries from various clinical case studies can inspire other healthcare professionals to join him in saving more lives by using similar methods.

References:

1. Hsu, Gerald C. eclaireMD Foundation, USA. "Biomedical research methodology based on GH-Method: math-physical medicine (No. 310)."

2. Hsu, Gerald C. eclaireMD Foundation, USA. "Application of linear equations to predict sensor and finger based postprandial plasma glucoses and daily glucoses for pre-virus, virus, and total periods using GH-Method: math-physical medicine (No. 345)."

3. Hsu, Gerald C. eclaireMD Foundation, USA. "A simplified yet accurate linear equation of PPG prediction model for T2D patients (GH-Method: math-physical medicine (No. 97)."

4. Hsu, Gerald C., eclaireMD Foundation, USA. "Application of linear equation-based PPG prediction model for four T2D clinic cases (GH-Method: math-physical medicine (No. 99)."

5. Hsu, Gerald C. eclaireMD Foundation, USA. "Self-recovery of pancreatic beta cell's insulin secretion based on 10+ years annualized data of food, exercise, weight, and glucose using GH-Method: math-physical medicine (No. 339).

6. Hsu, Gerald C. eclaireMD Foundation, USA. "A neural communication model between brain and internal organs, specifically stomach, liver, and pancreatic beta cells based on PPG waveforms of 131 liquid egg meals and 124 solid egg meals (No. 340).

7. Hsu, Gerald C. eclaireMD Foundation, USA. "A neuro-communication model between the brain and liver regarding glucose production and secretion in early morning using GH-Method: math-physical medicine (No. 324)."

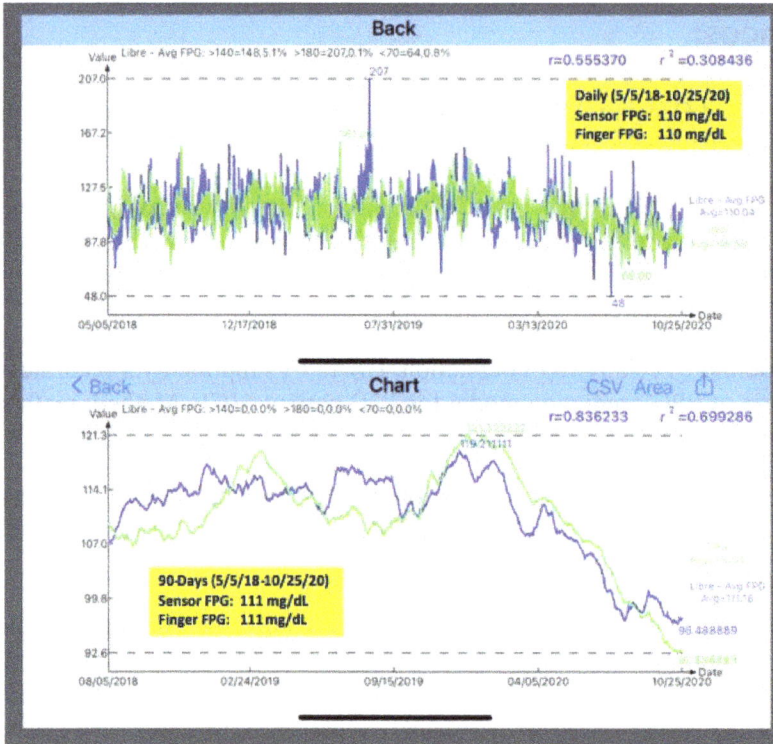

Figure 1: Case B's Sensor FPG versus Finger FPG (5/5/2018 - 10/25/2020)

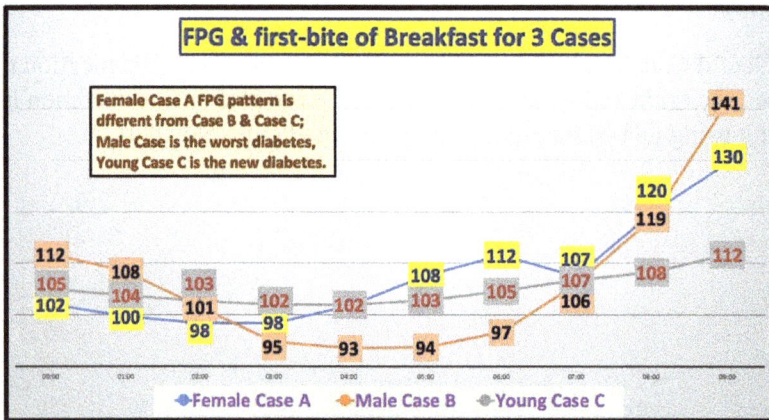

Figure 2: Glucose data and curve of 3 cases (9-hour duration)

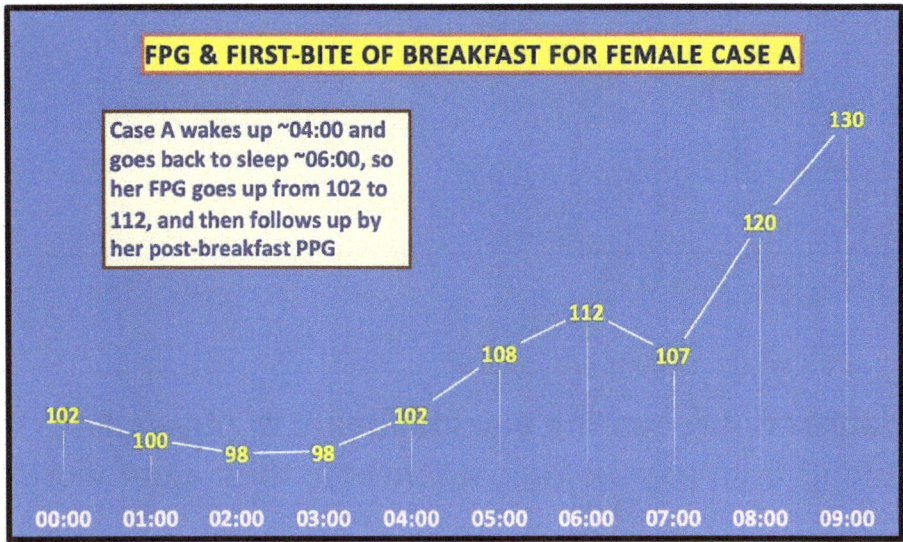

Figure 3: Monthly daily FPG waveforms of Case A (7-hour duration over 9 months)

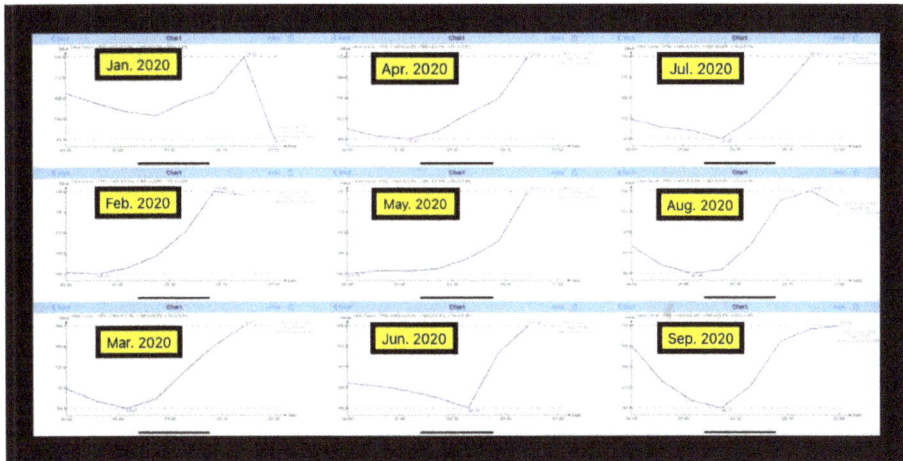

Figure 4: Case A's 9-hour duration covering FPG and her breakfast PPG until peak at 09:00

A manuscript regarding suicidal death of physicians resulting from psychological stress in their inner world (No. 355)

By: Gerald C. Hsu
eclaireMD Foundation, USA
10/31/2020

Abstract:

The author is a 73-year-old medical research scientist who recently read an article regarding *physician health and death* (Reference 1). Inspired by the story and his own past experiences, he decided to write a special manuscript to be shared with medical doctors. This article has a different writing style compared to his previous 354 math-physical medicine research papers, based on a quantitative method to derive analysis results with high precision, aimed at helping patients.

The goal of helping patients must go through the delivery channel of physicians and surgeons, while being concerned about the psychological health of medical doctors. This is the reason why he wrote this article with a qualitative style with an aim at medical physicians.

Being a physician is an enviable profession, where they greatly invested and sacrificed to reach to where they are today. In terms of financial rewards, that is money, even though they are not generously rewarded, at least they are handsomely compensated. With their added knowledge advancement, skill improvement, and society contribution, they may even earn their deserved fame. Their ultimate goal should come from *saving people's life*, not the same as people with political power or financial power. In the author's opinion, saving lives is the outmost power to achieve; therefore, it is a desirable profession indeed.

By having pride and feeling prestige at commencement by getting their MD degree, the physicians should not allow their accomplishments between the ages from 20 to 30 years of age become the only internal strength and emotional support. They should continuously improve themselves to expand into different areas in exploring new findings, learning additional skills and knowledge. This life-long learning will make a broader and more capable person, even for a physician. These newly gained inner strengths will aid physicians to face new challenges in their post-graduate school life.

However, there is a price to pay from having a decent, enviable, and well-compensated profession. In terms of reducing and controlling stress, burdens, and psychological pressure that comes along with their job, life, and relationships, the author believes that they must go deeper into their own inner world, i.e. their mind and heart, to search for strength. When different types of stress overwhelms them, they must return to their original motivation when they decided to become a physician which is helping their patients. Only this type of compassion in their heart, similar to having faith in a religion, can then help them survive many types of tests and challenges they encountered in their profession and private life. For those medical doctors who chose medicine for other reasons, with material or superficial motivations, they should search their heart again to see whether another career is better for them. For example, if their initial motivation was monetary, they better shift their career early enough to be an entrepreneur who takes big risks for larger financial returns.

When physicians face various stressful situations, they should not fight this battle alone. There are plenty of people who would support them as long as they speak up and seek assistance, such as from a mental health professional, like the author did.

The author is an educated individual, knowledgeable scientist, and experienced engineer, but more importantly, he had many rich life experiences that were long, colorful, striving, and challenging. Through his brief self-introduction, the reader can see many similarities and also identify some connections. He cares about his medical colleagues as much as he cares about patients with chronic diseases. This is his motivation of writing this manuscript aiming at physicians, even though he knows that it is a unique article with a qualitative style instead of his previously published quantitative research papers.

If anyone has interest on this subject and would like to provide feedback, please contact the author at g.hsu@eclairemd.com. You will remain anonymous and any information provided will be confidential.

Introduction:

The author is a 73-year-old medical research scientist who recently read an article regarding *physician health and death* (Reference 1). Inspired by the story and his own past experiences, he decided to write a special manuscript to be shared with medical doctors. This article has a different writing style compared to his previous 354 math-physical medicine research papers, based on a quantitative method to derive analysis results with high precision, aimed at helping patients.

The goal of helping patients must go through the delivery channel of physicians and surgeons, while being concerned about the psychological health of medical doctors. This is the reason why he wrote this article with a qualitative style with an aim at medical physicians.

Background:

Author's brief background:
Every person is allowed to express his or her personal thoughts and opinions. Why should physicians read this manuscript?

The author's father was a medical doctor, who started as a surgeon and ended up as an internal medicine physician. When the author was admitted into a medical school, he chose mathematics as his undergraduate major due to the following two reasons. First, he was afraid of the sight of blood (now, he studies hematology, blood, and glucoses). Second, he told his father that he did not want to interface with unhealthy and unhappy patients all day long.

He spent 17 years to study at seven different colleges, where he graduated from one of the top ranked engineering universities. He pursued his career in the fields of aerospace, naval defense, nuclear power, computer hardware and software, and semiconductor chips. After suffering seven business failures over 20 years during his entrepreneur days, he finally became one of the top CEOs in Silicon Valley, where he was generously compensated for his business success.

After achieving business success, he has engaged in many charitable and volunteer opportunities. He spent 9 years to self-study psychology, especially abnormal psychology involving traumatized children who developed a variety of personality disorders. He also established four psychotherapy centers and hired four full-time psychiatrists to take care of over 200 patients for four years until he was physically suffering from long-term health problems in 2010.

The stressful business life caused the collapse of his health. He suffered various complications from his metabolic disorder diseases of obesity and diabetes, including five cardiac episodes, kidney problems, diabetic retinopathy, and others. In order to save his life, in July of 2010, he has initiated his decade-long self-study and medical research in the area of endocrinology, diabetes, metabolism, nutrition, and lifestyle. To date, he has written 354 medical papers, attended over 65 international medical conferences, made more than 120 oral presentations, and published over 300 papers in 100+ medical journals, including nine papers of personal traits and psychological behaviors of patients with chronic diseases (References 2 through 10).

Approximately 40 years ago, when he was in his mid-30s and his son was around 7 years old, he took his son to visit a pediatrician in Northern California. At the clinic, a nurse informed him that his son's female pediatrician (around mid-30s as well) had committed suicide with a pistol in her office a few days earlier. That news shocked him tremendously. At that time, he could not understand why such a young physician with a very promising future would kill herself.

The reason for the brief introduction of the author is to connect himself with physicians who went through similar experiences, who have high degrees of education with difficult disciplines, long and challenging internships, competitive professional struggles, plus financial reward combined with fame, and power, but associated with stress, burnout, depression, and various psychological pressures. Therefore, he understands to some degree, how, why, and what physicians are thinking and doing.

Cited Article:
The article he read recently is "Top causes of death among doctors" in Physician Health & Behavior, by Charlie Williams, published on October 23, 2020 (Reference 1).

Here is an excerpt:

"First, the good news
Being a doctor comes with some serious rewards. Helping people overcome sickness and injury is fulfilling. The opportunity to learn and grow never ceases. And the pay isn't too shabby, either.

Of course, the career is not without risks. Burnout remains pervasive. Exposure to harmful pathogens, radiation, and chemicals is an everyday possibility. Even though hazards and stress are parts of every job, life as a physician brings its own blend of harms—some of which can be deadly (The author's note: such as COVID-19).

Our finding that physicians die older than do others is not unexpected, given the healthy work effect, high socioeconomic status, and prior data showing that physicians tend to make healthy choices. (The author's note: US physicians do have 3% to 5% longer expected life than other professionals.)

The top 10 causes of death for white male physicians in 1990 (heart disease, cancer, cerebrovascular disease, accidents, COPD, pneumonia/influenza, diabetes mellitus, suicide, liver disease, and HIV/AIDS) were essentially the same as those of the general population in the same year.

On the other hand, these doctors were significantly less likely to die from alcoholism, colorectal cancer, bacterial diseases, respiratory diseases (including lung cancer), digestive system diseases, acute myocardial infarction, and non-ischemic heart disease.

Now, the bad news
In a few stand-out areas, doctors appear to be at greater risk of dying than the general population: accidents, suicide, and cerebrovascular disease.

First, *white male physicians were more likely to die from e****xternal causes of injury****— like transport accidents, accidental poisoning, and self-inflicted injury—as well as hepatitis, malignant melanoma, Alzheimer disease, and pancreatic cancer.*

Second, suicide *as the cause of death in physicians between 0% and 4% of the time which is a significantly higher average than the 0.001% rate in the general population* (The author's note: more than several thousand times of probability) *cited by the American Foundation for Suicide Prevention in 2018. Another article, published in The Journal of the Missouri State Medical Association, cited studies that found suicide rates as much as 40% higher in male doctors and 130% higher in female doctors than the general population.*

Third, Cerebrovascular diseases, *like aneurysms, stroke, and arteriovenous malformations, were 9% more likely to be the cause of death for physicians."*

Body of this article:

Key points:
Of course, the author has his personal viewpoints regarding both accidental death (i.e. professional hazards) and death from cerebrovascular diseases. But he would like to focus on one specific subject, **suicidal death**, in this article. The main discussion point is achieving a peaceful and calmer inner world, i.e. heart and mind.

Three Desired targets in life:
Most educated people seek three common targets in their lives, money, fame, and power, in addition to their self-satisfaction (pride) and self-value (esteem). There is nothing wrong to pursue money, fame, or power; however, two important points should be mentioned here. First, driving for anything should have a limit, unlike the phrase, "greed is good, greed works" from the 1987 movie Wall Street played by

Michael Douglas. Second, for most people, you should choose only one target of the three to focus on. When you try to achieve two or more targets at the same time in your life, disaster usually comes along with it. If you want money, then try to be a businessperson or a professional athlete; if you want fame, then try be a scholar or a movie star; if you want power, then try to be a politician or a financial giant. However, for example, if you want power, fame, and money at the same time, most likely you will end up like a corrupted politician and disaster would come along eventually.

Never forget your original heart:
I always ask myself why I wanted to be "someone" when I was young. Similarly, please ask yourself why you wanted to be a medical doctor when you were young. Medicine is a business sector of giving help and providing service. The most noble and correct answer should be: "I truly want to help relieve the patients from their miserable pain, disease, suffering, and death". Of course, probably some young and smart medical school students might be driven by prestige, image, social-economic status, and attractive financial compensation. Those things are equally attractive to most people. Therefore, there is nothing wrong about wanting to get those things; however, please never forget the unique and ultimate objective of choosing medical career is to help patients. Otherwise, you will never achieve your inner peace, self-fulfilling, and true self-pride. The author was a successful high-tech entrepreneur, but he is not proud of his achievements in that sector. Technology itself has no internal evil, but the real-life applications by human society create a 50-50 split which depends on whether you use semiconductor, computer, and AI technology to conduct evil-purpose or good-will actions. On the contrary, his past 10-years of medical research is his most proud and fulfilling period in his lifetime, as long as he does not associate with any money-driven organizations or profit-oriented activities. His medical research work and its ending results are "pure good, nothing evil at all". Therefore, whenever you are having a doubt about your profession and work, please always go back to your original heart and think about the root of your profession which is "helping patients".

Continuous improvements in life:
When individuals receive the highest degree from the finest educational institute between the ages of 20 to 30, this self-pride feeling stays with them for the rest of their lives. However, we should not allow our initial accomplishments at a young age become a hinderance to our continuous improvement and future achievements. The author has met more than 1,000 clinical doctors over the past decades. He has noticed some of them lost their interest on continuous improvement by gaining new knowledge. Of course, they can continuously accumulate their empirical knowledge and work experiences through seeing and treating more patients, though this is a longer and slower process in comparison with learning from deep and thorough medical research results. The author spent 36 years of his 73 years of life (~50% of his life) on learning and studying 10 different academic disciplines. In the past 10 years, he finally realized that all of these 10 different disciplines are actually interconnected with each other and can be applied through medicine. During this decade, he spent more than 30,000 hour studying and researching medicine. He feels the biomedical system is the most complicated system he has ever touched or studied. As a result,

some of his friends laughed at him because he was not enjoying his retirement instead, he was working hard on his research. Helping patients through medical research became his post-retirement hobby. What is more enjoyable than spending your time on your hobby? In summary, life is a long journey which is filled with many surprising turns and interesting explorations. Therefore, do not allow the initial accomplishments to become the hinderance of your continuous success in your future. Learning and growing are a true and long-lasting characteristics of maturity.

Stress, burnout, depression:

Every type of job has its good side, bad side, ups and downs. Stress, burnout, and depression are often inevitable and they go along with any profession you choose. The author has gone through many life hardships, at least he has had more shares than a normal person, such as shorting money to pay for food, washing 1,000 toilets to pay for school tuition, working three years without any income, driving a truck within the US continent to demonstrate his developed product, being chased by industrial enemy with 27 lawsuits, spending $1.4 billion dollars to defend himself legally, being physically arrested from not violating any laws, being forced to sell his established enterprise due to his poor health, etc.

After having to sell his well-established semiconductor company, a deep and sad inner feeling emerged which is remarkably similar to killing one's own baby, he went through a difficult 3-year depression which required continuous psychological counseling. That was why he began to self-study psychology for 9 years after his business career ended. He heard once from a medical doctor who describes the psychiatrist as a "voodoo doctor". We should not hold any biased opinion against any professional field. Each field has its own strengths and weaknesses, and medicine is no exception. Bias and discrimination against other academic or professional fields only limit our own feasibility of further exploration and continuous growth. When we realize that our stress level from our work, our private life, or our inter-personal relationships become unbearable, we should seek immediate help. We may start seeking help from our family members or trusted friends, but do not stop seeking help from other professionals, such as psychiatrists. Depression, stress, burnout are not shameful, and they should not be hidden. We should speak out and seek help. The act of suicide is a sad and shameful ending that shows a true sign of a failure. No medical doctor should be a failure in life. In particular, physicians should not commit suicide after going through the huge investments of family expectation and support, medical educational tuition and expenses. and internship physical struggles. It is important to be a positive example for others to admire and learn from, along with their own additional rewards in their lifetime.

No matter what kind of problems or challenges you are facing now, it may feel unbearable, but it is not the end of the world. Fight against those problems hard with your inner strength and you will succeed eventually. The author has faced many similar or harder challenges in his life and has always survived, even becoming stronger after these difficulties.

Conclusion:

Being a physician is an enviable profession, where they greatly invested and sacrificed to reach to where they are today. In terms of financial rewards, that is *money*, even though they are not generously rewarded, at least they are *handsomely compensated*. With their added knowledge advancement, skill improvement, and society contribution, they may even earn their deserved fame. Their ultimate goal should come from *saving people's life*, not the same as people with political power or financial power. In the author's opinion, saving lives is the outmost power to achieve; therefore, it is a desirable profession indeed.

By having pride and feeling prestige at commencement by getting their MD degree, the physicians should not allow their accomplishments between the ages from 20 to 30 years of age become the only internal strength and emotional support. They should continuously improve themselves to expand into different areas in exploring new findings, learning additional skills and knowledge. This life-long learning will make a broader and more capable person, even for a physician. These newly gained inner strengths will aid physicians to face new challenges in their post-graduate school life.

However, there is a price to pay from having a decent, enviable, and well-compensated profession. In terms of reducing and controlling stress, burdens, and psychological pressure that comes along with their job, life, and relationships, the author believes that they must go deeper into their own inner world, i.e. their mind and heart, to search for strength. When different types of stress overwhelms them, they must return to their original motivation when they decided to become a physician which is *helping their patients*. Only this type of compassion in their heart, similar to having faith, can then help them survive many types of tests and challenges they encountered in their profession and private life. For those medical doctors who chose medicine for other reasons, with material or superficial motivations, they should search their heart again to see whether another career is better for them. For example, if their initial motivation was monetary, they better shift their career early enough to be an entrepreneur who takes big risks for larger financial returns.

When physicians face various stressful situations, they should not fight this battle alone. There are plenty of people who would support them as long as they speak up and seek assistance, such as from a mental health professional, like the author did.

The author is an educated individual, knowledgeable scientist, and experienced engineer, but more importantly, he had many rich life experiences that were long, colorful, striving, and challenging. Through his brief self-introduction, the reader can see many similarities and also identify some connections. He cares about his medical colleagues as much as he cares about patients with chronic diseases. This is his motivation of writing this unique manuscript aiming at physicians, even though he knows that it is a unique article with a qualitative style instead of his previously published quantitative research papers.

If anyone has interest on this subject and would like to provide feedback, please

contact the author at g.hsu@eclairemd.com. **You will remain anonymous and any information provided will be confidential.**

References:

1. William, Charlie, on Physician Health & Behavior, October 23, 2020, "Top causes of death among doctors."

2. Hsu, Gerald C. eclaireMD Foundation, USA. "Behavior psychology and body weight reduction of a T2D patient using GH-Method: math-physical medicine or mentality-personality modeling (No. 308)."

3. Hsu, Gerald C. eclaireMD Foundation, USA. "Glucose control and behavior psychology of a T2D patient using GH-Method: mentality-personality modeling via math-physical medicine (N0. 306)."

4. Hsu, Gerald C. eclaireMD Foundation, USA. "Quantitative measurements of stressors and symptoms for people with Borderline Personality Disorder before and during COVID-19 quarantine period using GH-Method: math-physical medicine (No. 296)."

5. Hsu, Gerald C. eclaireMD Foundation, USA. "Using artificial intelligence technology to overcome some behavioral psychological resistance for diabetes patients on controlling their glucose level using GH-Method: math-physical medicine & mentality-personality modeling (No. 93)."

6. Hsu, Gerald C. eclaireMD Foundation, USA. "Using GH-Method: math-physical medicine, mentality-personality modeling, and segmentation pattern analysis to compare two clinic cases about linkage between T2D patient's psychological behavior and physiological characteristics (No. 72)."

7. Hsu, Gerald C. eclaireMD Foundation, USA. "Trending pattern analysis and progressive behavior modification of two clinic cases of correlation between patient psychological behavior and physiological characteristics of T2D Using GH-Method: math-physical medicine & mentality-personality modeling (No. 53)."

8. Hsu, Gerald C. eclaireMD Foundation, USA. "Using wave characteristic analysis to study T2D patient's personality traits and psychological behavior using GH-Method: math-physical medicine (No. 52)."

9. Hsu, Gerald C. eclaireMD Foundation, USA. "Using wave characteristic analysis to study a diabetic patient's personality traits and psychological behavior via math-physical medicine (No. 49)."

10. Hsu, Gerald C. eclaireMD Foundation, USA. "Using a quantitative wave characteristic analysis to provide an initial look of type 2 diabetes patient's personality traits and psychological behavior on glucose control via math-physical medicine (No. 48)."

Coefficient of GH.f-modulus in the linear elastic fasting plasma glucose behavior study based on health data of three diabetes patients using the GH-Method: math-physical medicine, Part 4 (No. 356)

Gerald C. Hsu
eclaireMD Foundation, USA
11/4-5/2020

Abstract:

This article is Part 4 of the author's linear elastic glucose behavior study, which focuses on fasting plasma glucose (FPG) component. It is the continuation of his previous three studies, Parts 1, 2, and 3, on linear elastic postprandial plasma glucose (PPG) behaviors.

Here is his defined linear elastic FPG equation:

*FPG = GH.f-modulus * Weight*

Where Weight is the input component (similar to stress) and FPG is the output component (similar to strain). The close relationship between Weight and FPG can also be found in his previous published medical papers (Reference 10).

GH.f-modulus is a newly defined coefficient to connect both weight and FPG, similar to the theory of elasticity in engineering:

*Stress = Young's modulus * Strain*

Where Young's modulus connects both stress and strain except Young's modulus and GH.f-modulus are reciprocal to each other.

The author is able to connect this biomedical FPG equation with the basic concept of linear elasticity which involves stress and strain, along with the Young's modulus of strength of materials in structural & mechanical engineering. He uses the collected data of daily body weight and daily FPG data from three type 2 diabetes (T2D) patients with separate severity levels of obesity and diabetes within three *different* time ranges. In addition, he uses an identical 8-month period of collected data for the three patients to conduct his analysis. He demonstrated once again that using GH.f-modulus, a "pseudo-linear" relationship connecting both weight and FPG exists in all three clinical cases, except the value of this coefficient depends on the individual patient's severity level of chronic diseases, specifically obesity and diabetes.

The main objectives of this study is threefold. First, it is to offer a simpler FPG prediction equation to the patients. Second, it is to prove that similar to GH.p-modulus for PPG, the coefficient of GH.f-modulus indeed varies with the severity of chronic diseases in these clinical cases. Third, this constant coefficient of GH.f-modulus also differs from one-time range to another due to dynamic behavior, because blood is a living organic material.

The 7-month average value of each monthly M2 variables (i.e., GH-modulus) are 3.7, 2.6, and 1.0, and with an average measured PPG values at 122 mg/dL, 114 md/dL, and 109 mg/dL, for Case A, Case B, and Case C, respectively, which are ranked according to the severity of their diabetes conditions.

In summary, the higher the M2, the higher values of both x (carbs/sugar intake amount) and y (incremental PPG amount) become, and the higher predicted and measured PPG values are. The key conclusion from these three clinical observations is that the M2 values are varying based on the patients' body conditions (liver and pancreas), especially their diabetes severity. This is similar to the different inorganic materials having the different Young's modules values, such as nylon ~3 versus steel ~200.

The article represents the author's special interest in using math-physical and engineering modeling methodologies to investigate various biomedical problems. The methodology and approach are a result of his specific academic background and various professional experiences prior to the start of his medical research work in 2010. Therefore, he has been trying to link his newly acquired biomedical knowledge over the past decade with his previously acquired knowledge of mathematics, physics, computer science, and engineering for over 40 years.

The human body is the most complex system he has dealt with, which includes aerospace, navy defense, nuclear power, computers, and semiconductors. By applying his previous acquired knowledge to his newly found interest of medicine, he can discover many hidden facts or truths inside the biomedical systems. Many basic concepts, theoretical frame of thoughts, and practical modeling techniques from his fundamental disciplines in the past can be applied to his medical research endeavor. After all, science is based on theory from creation and proof via evidence, and as long as we can discover hidden truths, it does not matter which method we use and which option we take. This is the foundation of the GH-Method: math-physics medicine.

The author has spent four decades as a practical engineer and understands the importance of basic concepts, sophisticated theories, and practical equations which serve as the necessary background of all kinds of applications. Therefore, he spent his time and energy to investigate glucose related subjects using variety of methods he studied in the past, including this particular interesting stress-strain approach. On the other hand, he also realizes the importance and urgency on helping diabetes patients to control their glucoses. That is why, over the past few years, he has continuously simplified his findings about diabetes and try to derive more useful formulas and simple tools for meeting the general public's interest on controlling chronic diseases and their complications to reduce their pain and probability of death.

Introduction:

This article is Part 4 of the author's linear elastic glucose behavior study, which focuses on fasting plasma glucose (FPG) component. It is the continuation of his previous three studies, Parts 1, 2, and 3, on linear elastic postprandial plasma glucose (PPG) behaviors.

Here is his defined linear elastic FPG equation:

FPG = GH.f-modulus * Weight

Where Weight is the input component (similar to stress) and FPG is the output component (similar to strain). The close relationship between Weight and FPG can also be found in his previous published medical papers (Reference 10).

GH.f-modulus is a newly defined coefficient to connect both weight and FPG, similar to the theory of elasticity in engineering:

Stress = Young's modulus * Strain

Where Young's modulus connects both stress and strain except **Young's modulus and GH.f-modulus are reciprocal to each other.**

The author is able to connect this biomedical FPG equation with the basic concept of linear elasticity which involves stress and strain, along with the Young's modulus of strength of materials in structural & mechanical engineering. He uses the collected data of daily body weight and daily FPG data from three type 2 diabetes (T2D) patients with separate severity levels of obesity and diabetes within three different time ranges. In addition, he uses an identical 8-month period of collected data for the three patients to conduct his analysis. He demonstrated once again that using GH.f-modulus, a "pseudo-linear" relationship connecting both weight and FPG exists in all three clinical cases, except the value of this coefficient depends on the individual patient's severity level of chronic diseases, specifically obesity and diabetes.

The main objectives of this study is threefold. First, it is to offer a simpler FPG prediction equation to the patients. Second, it is to prove that similar to GH.p-modulus for PPG, the coefficient of GH.f-modulus indeed varies with the severity of chronic diseases in these clinical cases. Third, this constant coefficient of GH.f-modulus also differs from one-time range to another due to dynamic behavior, because blood is a living organic material.

Patients with varying chronic diseases would have different coefficient of GH.f-modulus. Both Case A and Case B are long-term T2D patients; however, their weights are still within the boundary of normal and slightly overweight with BMI around 25. Therefore, using 14 semi-annual periods for Case A and 10 months for Case B, their coefficients are the same at 0.67. However, due to Case A's stringent lifestyle management to control his diabetes, his weight and glucoses, including FPG, have reduced significantly, especially in 2020 where his coefficient became 0.59 in comparison with Case B's 0.66.

Case C is another story. His extreme-obese condition (BMI at 40.7) is much more serious than his diabetes conditions with a 4-year history. In order to compensate for his heavy weight, he must have a lower value of the GH.f-modulus (his coefficient of 0.36 is at 54% level of 0.67 for both Case A and Case B) in order to match with his measured FPG level (almost normal).

At first glance of this coefficient, it appears that it as a variable, rather than a constant. However, by examining their values within a reasonable time span, they do not vary that much. That is why it is called a "pseudo-linear" relationship. Once we have collected sufficient data for a particular time period, we can then easily figure out the suitable coefficients for both FPG and PPG, i.e. GH.f-modulus and GH.p-modulus respectively, to be used in glucose predictions.

Methods:

Background:
To learn more about the author's GH-Method: math-physical medicine (MPM) methodology, readers can refer to his article to understand his developed MPM analysis method in Reference 1.

Highlights of his related research:
In 2015 and 2016, the author decomposed the PPG waveforms (data curves) into 19 influential components and identified carbs/sugar intake amount and post-meal walking exercise contributing to approximately 40% of PPG formation, respectively. Therefore, he could safely discount the importance of the remaining ~20% contribution by the 16 other influential components.

In March of 2017, he also detected that body weight contributes to over 85% to fasting plasma glucose (FPG) formation. Furthermore, he identified the correlation coefficient between weight and FPG are higher than 90% for different diabetes patients. In addition, he has found other 4 secondary contribution factors of FPG formation.

In 2019, all of his developed prediction mathematical models for both FPG and PPG have achieved high percentages of prediction accuracy, but he also realized that his prediction models are too difficult for use by the general public. Their theoretical background and sophisticated methods would be difficult for healthcare professionals and diabetes patients to understand, let alone use them in their daily life for diabetes control. Therefore, he supplemented his complex models with a simple linear equation of predicted FPG and predicted PPG (see References 2, 3, and 4).

Stress, Strain, & Young's modulus:
Prior to his medical research work, he was an engineer in the various fields of structural engineering (aerospace, naval defense, and earthquake engineering), mechanical engineering (nuclear power plant equipments, and computer-aided-design),

and electronics engineering (computers, semiconductors, graphic software, and software robot).

The following excerpts comes from internet public domain, including Google and Wikipedia:

"Strain - ε:
Strain is the "deformation of a solid due to stress" - change in dimension divided by the original value of the dimension - and can be expressed as
$\varepsilon = dL / L$
where
ε *= strain (m/m, in/in)*
dL = elongation or compression (offset) of object (m, in)
L = length of object (m, in)

Stress - σ:
Stress is force per unit area and can be expressed as
$\sigma = F / A$
where
σ *= stress (N/m2, lb/in2, psi)*
F = applied force (N, lb)
A = stress area of object (m2, in2)

Stress includes tensile stress, compressible stress, shearing stress, etc.

E, Young's modulus:
It can be expressed as:

E = stress / strain
   $= \sigma / \varepsilon$
   $= (F / A) / (dL / L)$

where
E = Young's Modulus of Elasticity (Pa, N/m2, lb/in2, psi) was named after the 18th-century English physicist Thomas Young.

Elasticity:
Elasticity is a property of an object or material indicating how it will restore it to its original shape after distortion. A spring is an example of an elastic object - when stretched, it exerts a restoring force which tends to bring it back to its original length (Figure 1).

Plasticity:
When the force is going beyond the elastic limit of material, it is into a plastic zone which means even when force is removed, the material will not return back to its original state (Figure 1).

Based on various experimental results, the following table lists some Young's modulus associated with different materials:

Nylon: 2.7 GPa
Concrete: 17-30 GPa
Glass fibers: 72 GPa
Copper: 117 GPa
Steel: 190-215 GPa
Diamond: 1220 GPa

Young's modules in the above table are ranked from soft material (low E) to stiff material (higher E)."

Professor James Andrews taught the author linear elasticity at the University of Iowa and Professor Norman Jones taught him nonlinear plasticity at Massachusetts Institute of Technology. These two great academic mentors provided him the necessary foundation knowledge to understand these two important subjects in engineering.

Linear elastic FPG behavior:
In this particular study, he uses the analogy of relationship among stress, strain, and Young's modulus to illustrate a similar relationship between body weight and predicted FPG via a newly defined coefficient of GH.f-modulus which is listed below:

GH.f-modulus
= FPG / Weight

Young's modulus E
= stress / strain

Where FPG is the amount of predicted FPG (note: the predicted FPG can also be replaced by the measured FPG in order to conduct a sensitivity study of FPG behaviors).

Data collection:
Case A (the author) is a 73-year-old male with a 25-year history of T2D. From 7/1/2015 to 10/31/2020 (1,962 days), he has collected 2 data per day, weight and FPG. He utilized these data to conduct his linear elastic FPG behavior research.

In addition, on 5/5/2018, he started to use a continuous glucose monitoring (CGM) sensor device to collect 96 glucose data each day. Within this time period, he uses a sensor device to collect 28 FPG data per day from 00:00 to 07:00 at each 15-minutes time interval. Based on his research, this averaged sensor FPG value is within 1% of margin (i.e., 99% accuracy) from his measured FPG at the wake-up moment using finger-piercing and test strip method (Finger FPG).

The period of 7/1/2015 to 10/31/2020 is his "best-controlled" diabetes period, where his average daily glucoses is maintained at 116 mg/dL (<120 mg/dL). He named this as his "linear elastic zone" of diabetes health. Especially, due to his

It should also be noted that in 2010, his average glucose was 280 mg/dL and HbA1C was 10%, while taking three diabetes medications. Please note that the strong chemical interventions from various diabetes medications could seriously alter glucose physical behaviors. He called the period prior to 2015 as his "nonlinear plastic zone" of diabetes health.

The second set of data comes from his wife (Case B) with a 22-year history of T2D. She began to collect her glucose data via finger-piercing method (finger glucose) since 1/1/2014. On 1/1/2020, she began using the same brand of CGM sensor device to collect her sensor FOG data at the same rate of 28 FPG data per day since 1/1/2020. She discontinued her diabetes medication in 2020.

Case C is 47-year-old male with a BMI over 40 (obesity) and a 4-year history of T2D (new and non-severe diabetes). He started to collect his glucose data using the same model of CGM sensor on 3/18/2020. He has never taken any diabetes medications.

The following lists the different time spans of his four analysis:

(1) Case A:
From 1/1/2014 to 10/31/2020, every 6 months (semi-annually)
(2) Case B:
From 1/1/2020 to 10/31/2020, every month (monthly)
(3) Case C:
From 3/1/2020 to 10/31/2020, every month (monthly)
(4) Case A, Case B, and Case C
From 3/1/2020 to 10/31/2020, every month (monthly)

He then calculates the value of GH.f-modules by dividing FPG by Weight for each time period. Using the averaged GH.f-modulus as a constant to plug it into the following equation to obtain the predicted FPG.

Predicted FPG
= Weight * GH.f-modulus

Finally, he compared the predicted FPG with the measured FPG to obtain prediction accuracies for each time period.

Results:

Figure 2 shows the raw data and the combined two charts, Weight versus FPG and the coefficient of GH.f-modulus, into one diagram for Case A (male patient with 14 semi-annual periods). His average weight is 173 lbs. and average FPG is 117 mg/dL. His average GH.f-modulus is a constant of 0.67 with a variance between 0.55 and 0.74. It should be noted that his significantly lower coefficient of 0.55 in the second half of 2020 is the direct result of his COVID-19 quarantined life. The compatible moving trend (i.e., high correlation) between weight and FPG over these periods is quite obvious. His average predicted FPG using the constant of 0.67 (i.e., a constant GH.f-modulus) is also 117 mg/dL, but with a variance range of FPG prediction error margin between -8% to +5%, excluding significantly positive contribution on his overall health conditions from a stabilized 2020 quarantined lifestyle.

Figure 3 depicts the raw data and the combined two charts, Weight versus FPG and the coefficient of GH.f-modulus, into one diagram for Case B (female patient with 10 monthly periods). Her average weight is 155 lbs. and average FPG is 104 mg/dL. Her average GH.f-modulus is a constant of 0.67 as well (same as Case A) with a variance between 0.63 and 0.70. It should be noted that her relatively more evenly distributed GH.f-modulus is due to the relatively smaller changes of her health conditions since 2010 instead of the 7-year-time period for Case A. The compatible moving trend (i.e., high correlation) between Weight and FPG over these 10 months is also quite evident. Her average predicted FPG using the constant of 0.67 (i.e., a constant GH.f-modulus) is also 104 mg/dL, but with a variance range of FPG prediction error margin between -5% to +6%.

Figure 4 illustrates the raw data and the combined two charts, Weight versus FPG and the coefficient of GH.f-modulus, into one diagram for Case C (younger male patient with 8 monthly periods). His average weight is 292 lbs. (extremely obese) and average FPG is 105 mg/dL (similar to Case B). His average GH.f-modulus is a constant of 0.36 due to his obesity, with a variance between 0.34 and 0.40. The compatible moving trend (i.e., high correlation) between Weight and FPG over these 8 months is also quite obvious. It should be highlighted that he has reduced his monthly average weight from 301 lbs. in January 2020 to 273 lbs. in October 2020. This significant weight reduction effort has assisted him with his average FPG reduction from 120 mg/dL in March 2020 to 95 mg/dL in October 2020. His average predicted FPG using the constant of 0.36 (i.e., a constant GH.f-modulus) is also 105 mg/dL, but with a variance range of FPG prediction error margin between -9% to +5%.

Figure 5 reflects the results of a special analysis by using a consistent time period (monthly data from 3/1/2020 to 10/31/2020) for Cases A, B, and C. The key objective of conducting this timeframe analysis is to compare their GH.f-modulus over the same 8-month-time frame.

Listed below are the values of the GH.f-modulus for each patient over the 8-month period in 2020, which are listed in the order of (Case A, Case B, Case C):

March 2020: (0.63, 0.64, 0.40)
April 2020: (0.66, 0.66, 0.36)
May 2020: (0.58, 0.69, 0.35)
June 2020: (0.58, 0.64, 0.35)
July 2020: (0.56, 0.68, 0.36)
August 2020: (0.58, 0.63, 0.38)
September 2020: (0.59, 0.68, 0.34)
October 2020: (0.56, 0.68, 0.35)

Average GH.f: (0.59, 0.66, 0.36)

Although the coefficient changes from month to month, the magnitude of its changes are not significant. The results for Case C is the same as in Figure 4, but the results for Case B is smaller than in Figure 3 due to a shorter 8-month period used. The most significant difference is for Case A. The 14 semi-annual analysis has an average GH.f-modulus of 0.67, while his 8-month analysis has an average GH.f-modulus of 0.59. The 12% difference is a result from the different time spans chosen, which demonstrate the characteristics of organic blood material. There are more sources of influences than blood alone. In reality, weight and glucose are involved with many internal organs and hormones produced by the body.

Discussion:

Patients with varying chronic diseases would have different coefficient of GH.f-modulus. Both Case A and Case B are long-term T2D patients; however, their weights are still within the boundary of normal and slightly overweight with BMI around 25. Therefore, using 14 semi-annual periods for Case A and 10 months for Case B, their coefficients are the same at 0.67. However, due to Case A's stringent lifestyle management to control his diabetes, his weight and glucoses, including FPG, have reduced significantly, especially in 2020 where his coefficient became 0.59 in comparison with Case B's 0.66.

Case C is another story. His extreme-obese condition (BMI at 40.7) is much more serious than his diabetes conditions with a 4 years of short history. In order to compensate for his heavy weight, he must have a much lower value of the GH.f-modulus (his coefficient of 0.36 is at 54% level of 0.67 for both Case A and Case B) in order to match with his measured FPG level at 105 mg/dL (normal glucose level).

At first glance of this coefficient, it appears that it as a variable, rather than a constant. However, by examining their values within a reasonable time span, they do not vary that much. That is why it is called a "pseudo-linear" relationship. Once we have collected sufficient data for a particular time period, we can then easily figure out the suitable coefficients for both FPG and PPG respectively, i.e. GH.f-modulus and GH.p-modulus, to be used in glucose predictions.

Conclusions:

The article represents the author's special interest in using math-physical and engineering modeling methodologies to investigate various biomedical problems. The methodology and approach are a result of his specific academic background and various professional experiences prior to the start of his medical research work in 2010. Therefore, he has been trying to link his newly acquired biomedical knowledge over the past decade with his previously acquired knowledge of mathematics, physics, computer science, and engineering for over 40 years.

The human body is the most complex system he has dealt with, which includes aerospace, navy defense, nuclear power, computers, and semiconductors. By applying his previous acquired knowledge to his newly found interest of medicine, he can discover many hidden facts or truths inside the biomedical systems. Many basic concepts, theoretical frame of thoughts, and practical modeling techniques from his fundamental disciplines in the past can be applied to his medical research endeavor. After all, science is based on theory from creation and proof via evidence, and as long as we can discover hidden truths, it does not matter which method we use and which option we take. This is the foundation of the GH-Method: math-physics medicine.

The author has spent four decades as a practical engineer and understands the importance of basic concepts, sophisticated theories, and practical equations which serve as the necessary background of all kinds of applications. Therefore, he spent his time and energy to investigate glucose related subjects using variety of methods he studied in the past, including this particular interesting stress-strain approach. On the other hand, he also realizes the importance and urgency on helping diabetes patients to control their glucoses. That is why, over the past few years, he has continuously simplified his findings about diabetes and try to derive more useful formulas and simple tools for meeting the general public's interest on controlling chronic diseases and their complications to reduce their pain and probability of death.

°References:

1. Hsu, Gerald C., eclaireMD Foundation, USA, No. 310: "Biomedical research methodology based on GH-Method: math-physical medicine"

2. Hsu, Gerald C., eclaireMD Foundation, USA, No. 345: "Application of linear equations to predict sensor and finger based postprandial plasma glucoses and daily glucoses for pre-virus, virus, and total periods using GH-Method: math-physical medicine"

3. Hsu, Gerald C., eclaireMD Foundation, USA, No. 97: "A simplified yet accurate linear equation of PPG prediction model for T2D patients (GH-Method: math-physical medicine)"

4. Hsu, Gerald C., eclaireMD Foundation, USA, No. 99: "Application of linear equation-based PPG prediction model for four T2D clinic cases (GH-Method: math-physical medicine)"

5. Hsu, Gerald C., eclaireMD Foundation, USA, No. 339: "Self-recovery of pancreatic beta cell's insulin secretion based on 10+ years annualized data of food, exercise, weight, and glucose using GH-Method: math-physical medicine)

6. Hsu, Gerald C., eclaireMD Foundation, USA, No. 340: "A neural communication model between brain and internal organs, specifically stomach, liver, and pancreatic beta cells based on PPG waveforms of 131 liquid egg meals and 124 solid egg meals)

7. Hsu, Gerald C., eclaireMD Foundation, USA, No. 346: "Linear relationship between carbohydrates & sugar intake amount and incremental PPG amount via engineering strength of materials using GH-Method: math-physical medicine, Part 1"

8. Hsu, Gerald C., eclaireMD Foundation, USA, No. 349: "Investigation on GH modulus of linear elastic glucose with two diabetes patients data using GH-Method: math-physical medicine, Part 2"

9. Hsu, Gerald C., eclaireMD Foundation, USA, No. 349: "Investigation of GH modulus on the linear elastic glucose behavior based on three diabetes patients' data using the GH-Method: math-physical medicine, Part 3"

10. Hsu, Gerald C., eclaireMD Foundation, USA, No. 349: "Using Math-Physics Medicine to Predict FPG"

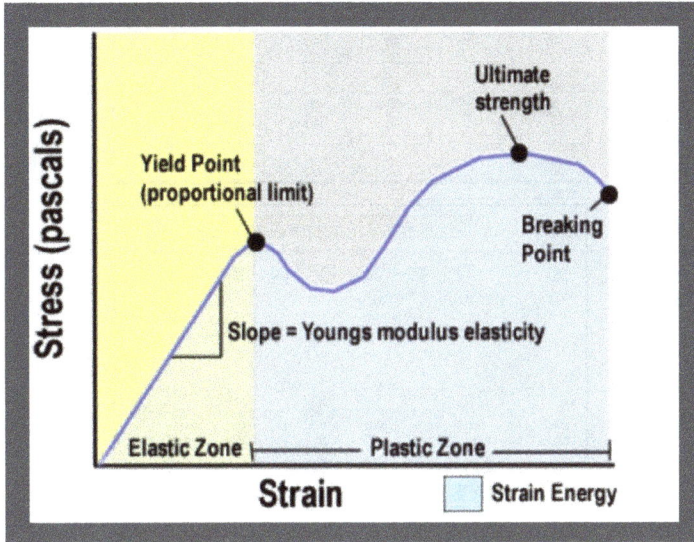

Figure 1: Stress-Strain-Young's modulus, Elastic Zone vs. Plastic Zone

Case A (BMI 25.5)	lbs	mg/dL		FPG / Weight		
Periods	Weight	Measured FPG	Periods	GH.f-modulus	Predicted FPG	Prediction %
2014-1H	177	131	2014-1H	0.74	120	-8%
2014-2H	178	128	2014-2H	0.72	120	-6%
2015-1H	173	125	2015-1H	0.72	117	-6%
2015-2H	172	119	2015-2H	0.69	116	-3%
2016-1H	172	115	2016-1H	0.67	116	1%
2016-2H	174	119	2016-2H	0.68	117	-2%
2017-1H	176	124	2017-1H	0.70	119	-4%
2017-2H	172	116	2017-2H	0.67	116	0%
2018-1H	171	117	2018-1H	0.69	115	-2%
2018-2H	171	110	2018-2H	0.64	115	5%
2019-1H	172	113	2019-1H	0.66	116	2%
2019-2H	173	116	2019-2H	0.67	117	1%
2020-1H	172	110	2020-1H	0.64	116	6%
2020-2H	169	93	2020-2H	0.55	114	23%
Average	173	117	Average	0.67	117	0%

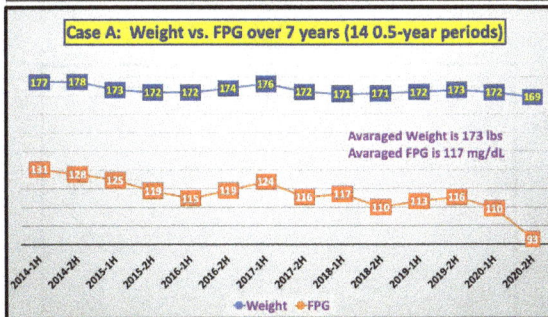

Case A: Weight vs. FPG over 7 years (14 0.5-year periods)

Avaraged Weight is 173 lbs
Avaraged FPG is 117 mg/dL

Weight: 177 178 173 172 172 174 176 172 171 171 172 173 172 169
FPG: 131 128 125 119 115 119 124 116 117 110 113 116 110 93

● Weight ● FPG

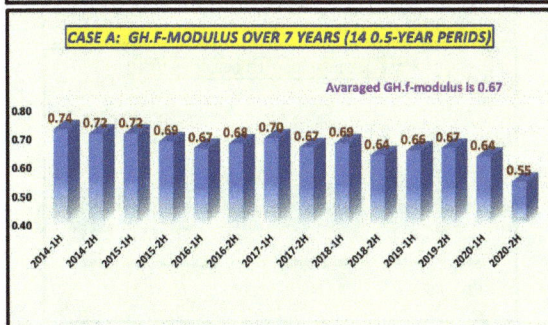

CASE A: GH.F-MODULUS OVER 7 YEARS (14 0.5-YEAR PERIDS)

Avaraged GH.f-modulus is 0.67

0.74 0.72 0.72 0.69 0.67 0.68 0.70 0.67 0.69 0.64 0.66 0.67 0.64 0.55

Figure 2: Case A data & charts

Case B (BMI 25.8)	lbs	mg/dL		FPG / Weight		
Periods	Weight	Measured FPG	Periods	GH.f-modulus	Predicted FPG	Prediction %
Jan, 2020	155	108	Jan, 2020	0.70	104	-4%
Feb, 2020	157	111	Feb, 2020	0.71	105	-5%
Mar, 2020	157	100	Mar, 2020	0.64	105	6%
Apr, 2020	155	103	Apr, 2020	0.66	104	1%
May, 2020	156	108	May, 2020	0.69	105	-3%
Jun, 2020	157	100	Jun, 2020	0.64	105	5%
Jul, 2020	156	106	July, 2020	0.68	104	-2%
Aug, 2020	155	98	Aug, 2020	0.63	104	6%
Sept, 2020	154	105	Sept, 2020	0.68	103	-2%
Oct, 2020	155	105	Oct, 2020	0.68	104	-1%
Average	155	104	Average	0.67	104	0%

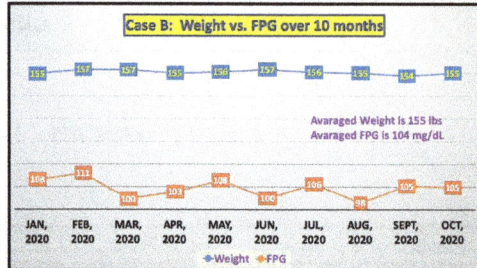

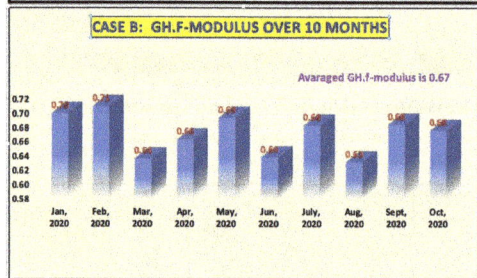

Figure 3: Case B data & charts

Case C (BMI 40.7)	lbs	mg/dL		FPG / Weight		
Periods	Weight	Measured FPG	Periods	GH.f-modulus	Predicted FPG	Prediction %
Mar, 2020	301	120	Mar, 2020	0.40	109	-9%
Apr, 2020	299	107	Apr, 2020	0.36	108	1%
May, 2020	300	105	May, 2020	0.35	108	3%
Jun, 2020	299	105	Jun, 2020	0.35	108	3%
Jul, 2020	296	107	July, 2020	0.36	107	0%
Aug, 2020	288	108	Aug, 2020	0.38	104	-4%
Sept, 2020	281	97	Sept, 2020	0.34	101	5%
Oct, 2020	273	95	Oct, 2020	0.35	99	4%
Average	292	105	Average	0.36	105	0%

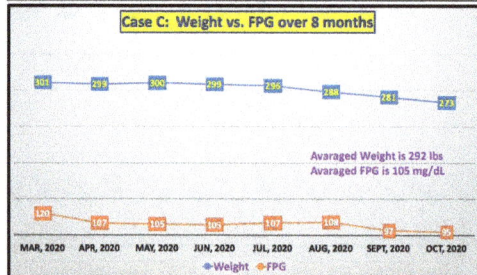

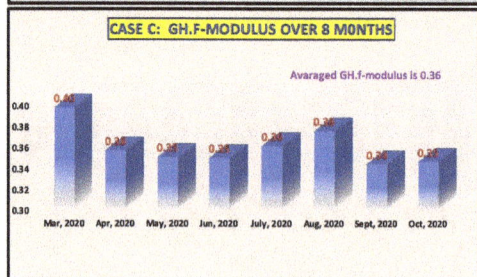

Figure 4: Case C data & charts

BMI 25.5	lbs	mg/dl	BMI 25.5	FPG / Weight	BMI 25.8	lbs	mg/dl	BMI 25.8	FPG / Weight	BMI 40.7	lbs	mg/dl	BMI 40.7	FPG / Weight
Case A:	Weight	FPG	Case A:	GH.f-modulus	Case B:	Weight	FPG	Case B:	GH.f-modulus	Case C:	Weight	FPG	Case C:	GH.f-modulus
Mar, 2020	172	108	Mar, 2020	0.63	Mar, 2020	157	100	Mar, 2020	0.64	Mar, 2020	301	120	Mar, 2020	0.40
Apr, 2020	172	113	Apr, 2020	0.66	Apr, 2020	155	103	Apr, 2020	0.66	Apr, 2020	299	107	Apr, 2020	0.36
May, 2020	173	100	May, 2020	0.58	May, 2020	156	108	May, 2020	0.69	May, 2020	300	105	May, 2020	0.35
Jun, 2020	172	100	Jun, 2020	0.58	Jun, 2020	157	100	Jun, 2020	0.64	Jun, 2020	299	105	Jun, 2020	0.35
Jul, 2020	170	95	July, 2020	0.56	Jul, 2020	156	106	July, 2020	0.68	Jul, 2020	296	107	July, 2020	0.36
Aug, 2020	171	99	Aug, 2020	0.58	Aug, 2020	155	98	Aug, 2020	0.63	Aug, 2020	288	108	Aug, 2020	0.38
Sept, 2020	169	100	Sept, 2020	0.59	Sept, 2020	154	105	Sept, 2020	0.68	Sept, 2020	281	97	Sept, 2020	0.34
Oct, 2020	167	93	Oct, 2020	0.56	Oct, 2020	155	105	Oct, 2020	0.68	Oct, 2020	273	95	Oct, 2020	0.35
Average	171	101	Average	0.59	Average	155	103	Average	0.66	Average	292	105	Average	0.36

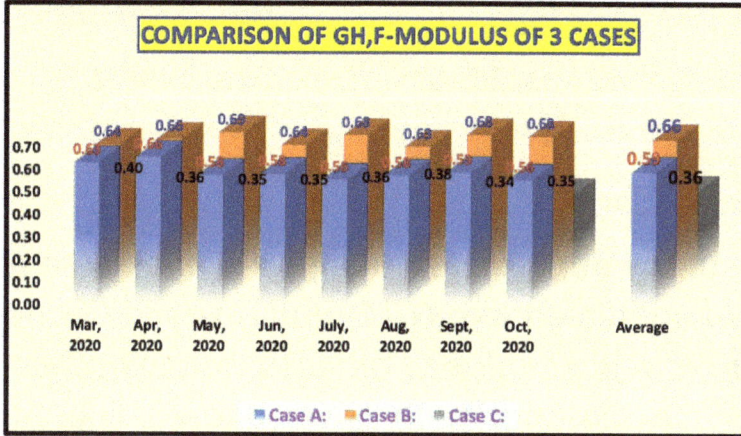

Figure 5: GH.f-modulus during the consistent 8-months time span of Cases A, B, and C

High accuracy of predicted postprandial plasma glucose using two coefficients of GH.f-modulus and GH.p-modulus from linear elastic glucose behavior theory based on GH-Method: math-physical medicine, Part 5 (No. 357)

Gerald C. Hsu
eclaireMD Foundation, USA
11/5-6/2020

Abstract:

This article is Part 5 of the author's linear elastic glucose behavior study, which focuses on the predicted postprandial plasma glucose (PPG). This study is the combination and continuation of his previous four studies, Parts 1, 2, 3, and 4, on linear elastic glucose behaviors

Listed below are his two recently developed linear elastic glucose equations with two defined coefficients of GH-modulus and his third equation for the predicted PPG from combining these two equations together:

*(1) FPG = GH.f-modulus * Weight*

Where Weight is the input component (similar to stress) and FPG is the output component (similar to strain).

(2) Incremental PPG
*= GH.p-modulus * Carbs&sugar*

Where
Incremental PPG
= Predicted PPG - (0.97 * FPG)
+ (post-meal walking k-steps * 5)

When he combines the above two linear elastic equations into one, he has the following new PPG prediction equation:

(3) Predicted PPG
*= (0.97 * GH.f-modulus * Weight) +(GH.p-modulus * Carbs&sugar) - (post-meal walking k-steps * 5)*

The three equations from above were inspired by his prior knowledge in the theory of elasticity in strengths of engineering materials which has the following engineering equation developed in 1807 by a British scientist, Thomas Young:

*Stress = Young's modulus * Strain*

Young's modulus and the two biomedical coefficients (GH.f-modulus and GH.p-modulus) are reciprocal to each other.

The main objective of this study is to offer numerical proof for the PPG prediction accuracy using the above-mentioned equation (3) and based on his own health data collected from 7/1/2015 to 10/31/2020.

Listed below are the annual values of the GH.f-modulus, GH.p-modulus, PPG prediction % for the author's case which reflect his severity levels of both obesity and

diabetes, and PPG prediction accuracy %:

Y2015: (0.71, 1.6,   97%)
Y2016: (0.68, 1.8,   99%)
Y2017: (0.69, 1.6, 100%)
Y2018: (0.66, 1.9, 100%)
Y2019: (0.66, 1.8,   99%)
Y2020: (0.59, 2.4, 103%)

Average: (0.67, 1.9, 100%)

The author applied his linear elastic glucose theory of both FPG and PPG behaviors on the predicted PPG value with high accuracy in order to help other diabetes patients. The five major internal organs involved in glucose production are the brain, stomach, intestines, liver, and pancreas along with three major inter-organ systems including blood, nerves, and hormones. This study has further proved via a quantitative analysis that PPG level has a close connection with FPG, weight (food quantity), carb/sugar intake (food quality), and exercise.

This article represents the author's special interest in using math-physical and engineering modeling methodologies to investigate various biomedical problems. The methodology and approach are the results of his specific academic background and various professional experiences prior to the start of his medical research work in 2010. Therefore, he has attempted to link his newly acquired biomedical knowledge over the past decade with his previously acquired knowledge of mathematics, physics, computer science, and engineering for over 40 years.

The human body is the most complex system he has dealt with, which includes aerospace, navy defense, nuclear power, computers, and semiconductors. By applying his previous acquired knowledge to his newly found interest of medicine, he can discover many hidden facts or truths inside the biomedical systems. Many basic concepts, theoretical frame of thoughts, and practical modeling techniques from his fundamental disciplines in the past can be applied to his medical research endeavor. After all, science is based on theory via creation and proof via evidence, and as long as we can discover hidden truths, it does not matter which method we use and which option we take. This is the foundation of the GH-Method: math-physics medicine.

The author has spent four decades as a practical engineer and understands the importance of basic concepts, sophisticated theories, and practical equations which serve as the necessary background of all kinds of applications. As a result, he spent his time and energy to investigate glucose related subjects using variety of methods he studied in the past, including this particular interesting stress-strain approach. On the other hand, he also realizes the importance and urgency on helping diabetes patients to control their glucoses. That is why, over the past few years, he has continuously simplified his findings about diabetes and to derive more useful formulas and simple tools for meeting the general public's interest on controlling chronic diseases and their complications to reduce their pain and probability of death.

Introduction:

This article is Part 5 of the author's linear elastic glucose behavior study, which focuses on the predicted postprandial plasma glucose (PPG). This study is the combination and continuation of his previous four studies, Parts 1, 2, 3, and 4, on linear elastic glucose behaviors

Listed below are his two recently developed linear elastic glucose equations with two defined coefficients of GH-modulus and his third equation for the predicted PPG from combining these two equations together:

*(2) FPG = GH.f-modulus * Weight*

Where Weight is the input component (similar to stress) and FPG is the output component (similar to strain).

(2) Incremental PPG
*= GH.p-modulus * Carbs&sugar*

Where
Incremental PPG
= Predicted PPG - (0.97 * FPG)
+ (post-meal walking k-steps * 5)

When he combines the above two linear elastic equations into one, he has the following new PPG prediction equation:

(3) Predicted PPG
*= (0.97 * GH.f-modulus * Weight) +(GH.p-modulus * Carbs&sugar) - (post-meal walking k-steps * 5)*

The three equations from above were inspired by his prior knowledge in the theory of elasticity in strengths of engineering materials which has the following engineering equation developed in 1807 by a British scientist, Thomas Young:

*Stress = Young's modulus * Strain*

Young's modulus and the two biomedical coefficients (GH.f-modulus and GH.p-modulus) are reciprocal to each other.

The main objective of this study is to offer numerical proof for the PPG prediction accuracy using the above-mentioned equation (3) and based on his own health data collected from 7/1/2015 to 10/31/2020.

Methods:

Background:

To learn more about the author's GH-Method: math-physical medicine (MPM) methodology, readers can refer to his article to understand his developed MPM analysis method in Reference 1.

Highlights of his related research:

In 2015 and 2016, the author decomposed the PPG waveforms (data curves) into 19 influential components and identified carbs/sugar intake amount and post-meal walking exercise contributing to approximately 40% of PPG formation, respectively. Therefore, he could safely discount the importance of the remaining ~20% contribution by the 16 other influential components.

In 2016, he utilized optical physics, big data analytics, and artificial intelligence (AI) techniques to develop a computer software to predict PPG based on the patient's food pictures or meal photos. This sophisticated AI approach and iPhone APP software product have reached to a 98.8% prediction accuracy based on ~6,000 meal photos.

In March of 2017, he also detected that body weight contributes to over 85% to fasting plasma glucose (FPG) formation. Furthermore, in 2019, he identified that FPG could serve as a good indicator of the pancreatic beta cells' health status; therefore, he can apply the FPG value (more precisely, 97% of FPG value) to serve as the baseline PPG value to calculate the PPG incremental amount in order to obtain the predicted PPG.

In 2018, based on his collected ~2,500 meals and associated sensor PPG waveforms, he further applied the perturbation theory from quantum mechanics, using the first bite of his meal as the initial condition to extend and build an entire PPG waveform covering a period of 180 minutes, with a 95% of PPG prediction accuracy.

In 2019, all of his developed PPG prediction models achieved high percentages of prediction accuracy, but he also realized that his prediction models are too difficult for use by the general public. The above-mentioned sophisticated methods would be difficult for healthcare professionals and diabetes patients to understand, let alone use them in their daily life for diabetes control. As a result, he supplemented his complex models with a simple linear equation of predicted PPG (see References 2, 3, 4, and 12).

Here is his simple linear formula:

Predicted PPG
= FPG * M1 + (carbs-sugar * M2) - (post-meal walking k-steps * M3)

Where M1, M2, M3 are 3 multipliers.

After lengthy research, trial and error, and data tuning, he finally identified the best multipliers for FPG and exercise as 0.97 for M1 and 5.0 for M3. In comparison with PPG, the FPG is a more stabilized biomarker since it is directly related to body weight. We know that weight reduction is a hard task. However, weight is a calmer and more stabilizing biomarker in comparison to glucose which fluctuates from minute to minute. The influence of exercise (specifically, post-meal walking steps) on PPG (41% contribution and >80% negative correlation with PPG) is almost equal to the influence from the carbs/sugar intake amount on PPG (39% contribution and >80% positive correlation with PPG). In terms of intensity and duration, exercise is a simple and straightforward subject to study. Especially, normal-speed walking is a safe and effective form of exercise for the large portion of diabetes patients, particularly senior citizens.

The parameters, FPG and walking, have a lower chance of variation for the author. However, for some diabetes patients, he recommends them to keep the multiplier M3 as a variable if their exercise patterns are different and changing.

The relationship between food nutrition and glucose is a complex and difficult subject to fully understand and effectively manage due to many types of food and their associated carbs/sugar contents. For example, in the author's developed food material and nutritional database, it contains over six million data. As a result, the author decided to implement two multipliers, M1 for FPG and M3 for exercise, as the two "constants" and keep M2 as the only "variable" in his PPG prediction equation and the linear elastic glucose research in this article.

The more simplified linear equation for predicted PPG is listed below:

Predicted PPG
= (0.97*FPG)+(Carbs&sugar * M2) - (post-meal walking k-steps * 5)

He further created two new terms:

Term 1:
GH.p-modulus = M2

Term 2:
The incremental PPG amount
= Predicted PPG - PPG baseline
(i.e. 0.97 * FPG) + exercise effect
(i.e. walking k-steps * 5)

<u>*The linear elastic PPG equation:*</u>
GH.p-modulus
= (Incremental PPG)/(Carbs&sugar)
Recently, he developed his linear elastic FPG equation (Reference 11) as follows:

<u>*The linear elastic FPG equation:*</u>
GH.f-modulus = (FPG) / (Weight)

Stress, Strain, & Young's modulus:

Prior to his medical research work, he was an engineer in the various fields of structural engineering (aerospace, naval defense, and earthquake engineering), mechanical engineering (nuclear power plant equipments, and computer-aided-design), and electronics engineering (computers, semiconductors, graphic software, and software robot).

The following excerpts comes from internet public domain, including Google and Wikipedia:

"Strain - ε:
Strain is the "deformation of a solid due to stress" - change in dimension divided by the original value of the dimension - and can be expressed as
$\varepsilon = dL / L$
where
ε = strain (m/m, in/in)
dL = elongation or compression (offset) of object (m, in)
L = length of object (m, in)

Stress - σ:
Stress is force per unit area and can be expressed as
$\sigma = F / A$
where
σ = stress (N/m2, lb/in2, psi)
F = applied force (N, lb)
A = stress area of object (m2, in2)

Stress includes tensile stress, compressible stress, shearing stress, etc.

E, Young's modulus:
It can be expressed as:

E = stress / strain
  $= \sigma / \varepsilon$
  $= (F / A) / (dL / L)$

where
E = <u>Young's Modulus of Elasticity</u> (Pa, N/m2, lb/in2, psi) was named after the 18th-century English physicist Thomas Young.

Elasticity:
Elasticity is a property of an object or material indicating how it will restore it to its original shape after distortion. A spring is an example of an elastic object - when stretched, it exerts a restoring force which tends to bring it back to its original length (Figure 1).

Plasticity:

When the force is going beyond the elastic limit of material, it is into a plastic zone which means even when force is removed, the material will not return back to its original state (Figure 1).

Based on various experimental results, the following table lists some Young's modulus associated with different materials:

Nylon: 2.7 GPa
Concrete: 17-30 GPa
Glass fibers: 72 GPa
Copper: 117 GPa
Steel: 190-215 GPa
Diamond: 1220 GPa

Young's modules in the above table are ranked from soft material (low E) to stiff material (higher E)."

Professor James Andrews taught the author linear elasticity at the University of Iowa and Professor Norman Jones taught him nonlinear plasticity at Massachusetts Institute of Technology. These two great academic mentors provided him the necessary foundation knowledge to understand these two important subjects in engineering.

Data collection:

The author is a 73-year-old male with a 25-year history of T2D. He began collecting his carbs/sugar intake amount and post-meal walking steps on 7/1/2015. From 7/1/2015 to 10/31/2020 (1,962 days), he has collected 6 data per day, i.e. 1 FPG, 3 PPG, carb/sugar amount, and post-meal walking steps. He utilized these 11,772 data of 1,962 days to conduct his prior research work on the subject of linear elastic PPG study (Reference 7). In addition, on 5/5/2018, he started to use a continuous glucose monitoring (CGM) sensor device to collect 96 glucose data each day. Within this time period, he uses the same sensor device to collect 28 FPG data per day from 00:00 to 07:00 at each 15-minute time interval. Based on his prior research, this averaged sensor FPG value is within 1% of margin of error (i.e. 99% accuracy) from his measured FPG at the wake-up moment using finger-piercing and test strip method (Finger FPG).

The period of 7/1/2015 to 10/31/2020 is his "better-controlled" diabetes period, where his average daily glucoses is maintained at 116 mg/dL (<120 mg/dL). He named this as his "linear elastic zone" of diabetes health. It should also be noted that in 2010, his average glucose was 280 mg/dL and HbA1C was 10%, while taking three diabetes medications. The strong chemical interventions from various diabetes medications would seriously alter glucose physical behaviors. He called the period prior to 2015 as his "nonlinear plastic zone" of diabetes health.

Results:

Listed below are his two recently developed linear elastic glucose equations with two defined coefficients of GH-modulus and his third equation of predicted PPG from combining these two equations:

*(3) FPG = GH.f-modulus * Weight*

Where Weight is the input component (similar to stress) and FPG is the output component (similar to strain).

(2) Incremental PPG
*= GH.p-modulus * Carbs&sugar*

Incremental PPG
= Predicted PPG - (0.97 * FPG)
+ (post-meal walking k-steps * 5)

When he combines above two linear elastic equations into one, he has the following new PPG prediction equation:

(3) Final PPG prediction equation:
Predicted PPG
*= (0.97 * GH.f-modulus * Weight) +(GH.p-modulus * Carbs&sugar) - (post-meal walking k-steps * 5)*

Where *GH.f-modulus* is a coefficient connecting Weight and FPG, and GH.p-modulus is a coefficient connecting Incremental PPG and Carbs&sugar amount. Incremental PPG includes baseline PPG, containing FPG and Weight, and exercise effect. These two coefficients are directly depending on the severity level of patient's two chronic diseases, specifically obesity and diabetes. The suitable values of these two coefficients of GH-modulus can be estimated from a patient's values of Weight and HbA1C with a reasonably high accuracy.

The input data of this final PPG prediction equation would avoid using complicated and troublesome measuring devices, either finger-piercing or CGM sensor. This prediction formula only needs weight, post-meal walking steps, and carbs/sugar intake amount. However, estimation of carbs and sugar amount from food or meal is an overly complicated subject and not easy for most patients. The author utilized optical physics and artificial intelligence to develop a software for estimating carbs and sugar amount from the photos of food and meal which achieved 98.8% prediction accuracy. However, it still requires a smartphone or computer which is difficult for some patients in underdeveloped nations and senior citizens, who are not familiar with technology. Therefore, the author has continued his development effort on simplifying his prediction formula in order to cover a larger group of potential users while still maintaining its prediction accuracy.

Figure 2 shows the raw data and his calculation of predicted PPG with accuracy percentages. He used his annual data from 2015 to 2020, except for Y2015 from 7/1/2015 to 12/31/2015 and Y2020 from 1/1/2020 to 10/31/2020. Listed below are the annual values of the (GH.f-modulus, GH.p-modulus, and PPG prediction %) for the author's case which reflect his severity levels of both obesity and diabetes, and PPG prediction accuracy %:

Y2015: (0.71, 1.6, 97%)
Y2016: (0.68, 1.8, 99%)
Y2017: (0.69, 1.6, 100%)
Y2018: (0.66, 1.9, 100%)
Y2019: (0.66, 1.8, 99%)
Y2020: (0.59, 2.4, 103%)

Average: (0.67, 1.9, 100%)

Figure 3 depicts the direct comparison between his predicted annual PPG and his finger-piercing measured annual PPG. Although there are some small deviations from year to year, those deviations are within the range of +/- 3%. Over the 6- year period, both the predicted PPG and measured PPG are at 116 mg/dL. As mentioned above, this period is his "better-controlled" elastic range which his developed linear elastic glucose behavior theory can be applied. If a patient has remarkably high glucose levels or hyperglycemia condition, for example above 200 mg/dL, then this predicted PPG would start to deviate from the measured PPG. The author needs more reliable collected health data from some severe diabetes patients in order to continue his "nonlinear plastic glucose" research.

Figure 4 reveals the PPG prediction accuracy percentages over these 6 years. The annual PPG prediction accuracy are varying between 97% and 103%, but the overall 6-year average accuracy is 100%.

Conclusions:

The author applied his linear elastic glucose theory of both FPG and PPG behaviors on the predicted PPG value with high accuracy in order to help other diabetes patients. The five major internal organs involved in glucose production are the brain, stomach, intestines, liver, and pancreas along with three major inter-organ systems including blood, nerves, and hormones. This study has further proved via a quantitative analysis that PPG level has a close connection with FPG, weight (food quantity), carb/sugar intake (food quality), and exercise.

This article represents the author's special interest in using math-physical and engineering modeling methodologies to investigate various biomedical problems. The methodology and approach are the results of his specific academic background and various professional experiences prior to the start of his medical research work in 2010. Therefore, he has attempted to link his newly acquired biomedical knowledge over the past decade with his previously acquired knowledge of mathematics, physics, computer science, and engineering for over 40 years.

The human body is the most complex system he has dealt with, which includes aerospace, navy defense, nuclear power, computers, and semiconductors. By applying his previous acquired knowledge to his newly found interest of medicine, he can discover many hidden facts or truths inside the biomedical systems. Many basic concepts, theoretical frame of thoughts, and practical modeling techniques from his fundamental disciplines in the past can be applied to his medical research endeavor. After all, science is based on theory via creation and proof via evidence, and as long as we can discover hidden truths, it does not matter which method we use and which option we take. This is the foundation of the GH-Method: math-physics medicine.

The author has spent four decades as a practical engineer and understands the importance of basic concepts, sophisticated theories, and practical equations which serve as the necessary background of all kinds of applications. As a result, he spent his time and energy to investigate glucose related subjects using variety of methods he studied in the past, including this particular interesting stress-strain approach. On the other hand, he also realizes the importance and urgency on helping diabetes patients to control their glucoses. That is why, over the past few years, he has continuously simplified his findings about diabetes and to derive more useful formulas and simple tools for meeting the general public's interest on controlling chronic diseases and their complications to reduce their pain and probability of death.

References:

1. Hsu, Gerald C., eclaireMD Foundation, USA, No. 310: "Biomedical research methodology based on GH-Method: math-physical medicine"

2. Hsu, Gerald C., eclaireMD Foundation, USA, No. 345: "Application of linear equations to predict sensor and finger based postprandial plasma glucoses and daily glucoses for pre-virus, virus, and total periods using GH-Method: math-physical medicine"

3. Hsu, Gerald C., eclaireMD Foundation, USA, No. 97: "A simplified yet accurate linear equation of PPG prediction model for T2D patients (GH-Method: math-physical medicine)"

4. Hsu, Gerald C., eclaireMD Foundation, USA, No. 99: "Application of linear equation-based PPG prediction model for four T2D clinic cases (GH-Method: math-physical medicine)"

5. Hsu, Gerald C., eclaireMD Foundation, USA, No. 339: "Self-recovery of pancreatic beta cell's insulin secretion based on 10+ years annualized data of food, exercise, weight, and glucose using GH-Method: math-physical medicine)

6. Hsu, Gerald C., eclaireMD Foundation, USA, No. 340: "A neural communication model between brain and internal organs, specifically stomach, liver, and pancreatic beta cells based on PPG waveforms of 131 liquid egg meals and 124 solid egg meals)

7. Hsu, Gerald C., eclaireMD Foundation, USA, No. 346: "Linear relationship between carbohydrates & sugar intake amount and incremental PPG amount via engineering strength of materials using GH-Method: math-physical medicine, Part 1"

8. Hsu, Gerald C., eclaireMD Foundation, USA, No. 349: "Investigation on GH modulus of linear elastic glucose with two diabetes patients data using GH-Method: math-physical medicine, Part 2"

9. Hsu, Gerald C., eclaireMD Foundation, USA, No. 349: "Investigation of GH modulus on the linear elastic glucose behavior based on three diabetes patients' data using the GH-Method: math-physical medicine, Part 3"

10. Hsu, Gerald C., eclaireMD Foundation, USA, No. 349: "Using Math-Physics Medicine to Predict FPG"

11. Hsu, Gerald C., eclaireMD Foundation, USA, No. 356: "Coefficient of GH.f-modulus in the linear elastic fasting plasma glucose behavior study based on health data of three diabetes patients using the GH-Method: math-physical medicine, Part 4 "

12. Hsu, Gerald C., eclaireMD Foundation, USA, No. 264: "Community and Family Medicine via Doctors without distance: Using a simple glucose control card to assist T2D patients in remote rural areas (GH-Method: math-physical medicine)"

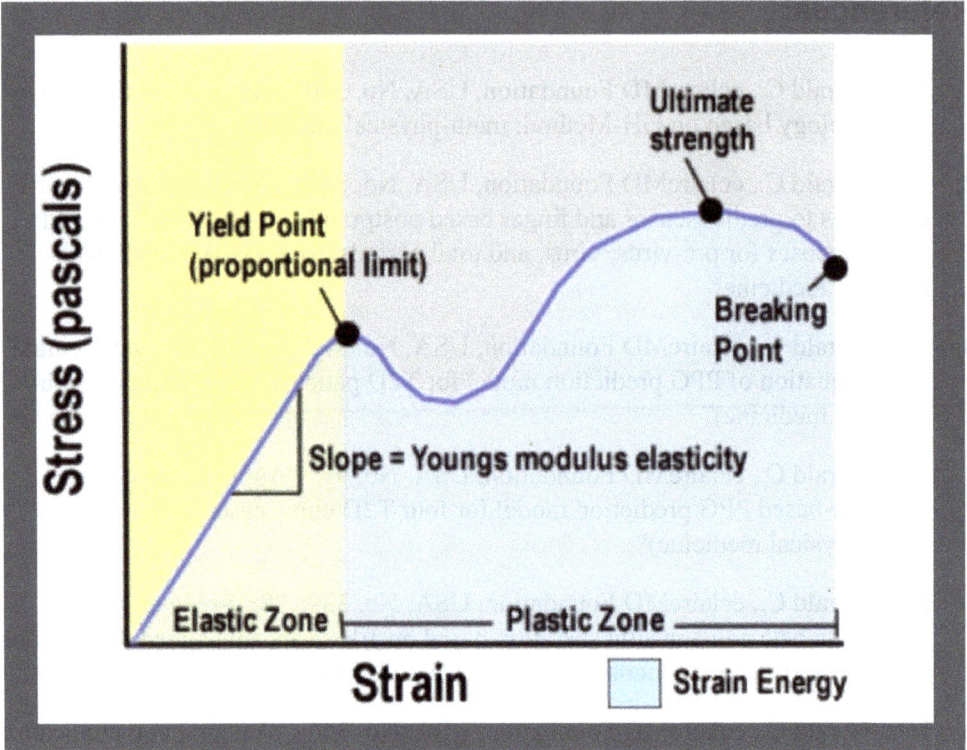

Figure 1: Stress-Strain-Young's modulus, Elastic Zone vs. Plastic Zone

Case A	lbs	FPG / Weight	gram	K-steps	Incremental PPG	Case A	mg/dL	mg/dL	Case A	PPG Prediction
Year	Weight	GH.f-modulus	Carbs/Sugar	Walking	GH.p-modulus	Year	Predicted PPG	Measured PPG	Year	Accuracy %
Y2015	173	0.71	14.46	3.681	1.6	Y2015	123	119	Y2015	97%
Y2016	173	0.68	15.47	4.110	1.8	Y2016	121	120	Y2016	99%
Y2017	174	0.69	14.19	4.440	1.6	Y2017	117	117	Y2017	100%
Y2018	171	0.66	15.47	4.538	1.9	Y2018	117	117	Y2018	100%
Y2019	173	0.66	13.19	4.038	1.8	Y2019	115	114	Y2019	99%
Y2020	171	0.59	12.34	4.345	2.4	Y2020	106	109	Y2020	103%
Average	172	0.67	14.19	4.192	1.9	Average	116	116	Average	100%

Figure 2: Raw data and calculated data

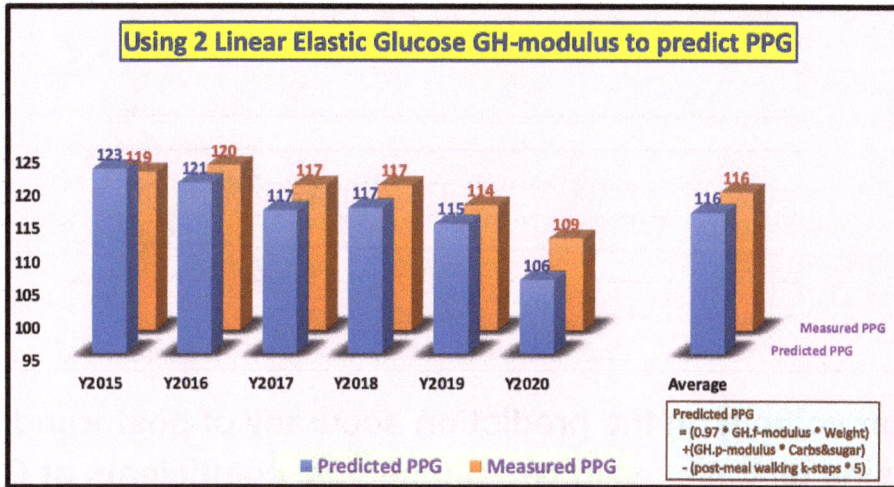

Figure 3: Predicted PPG vs. Measured PPG (2015-2020)

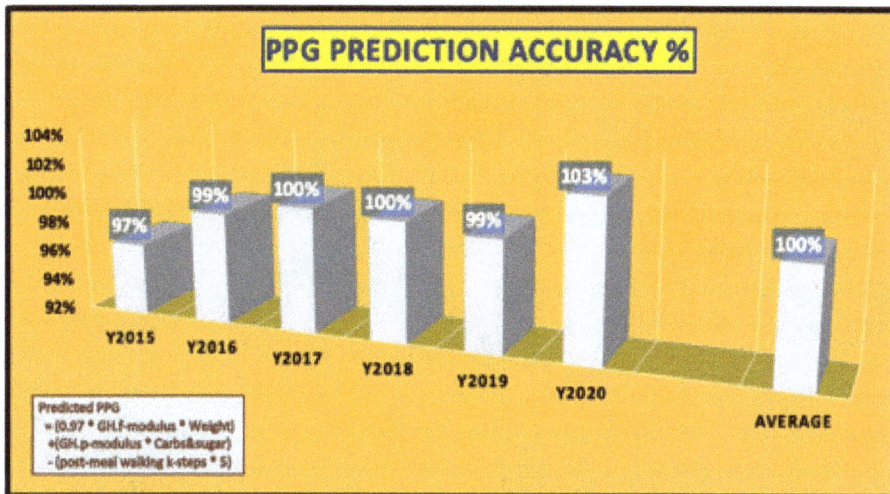

Figure 4: Prediction accuracy % of Predicted PPG vs. Measured PPG (2015-2020

Improvement on the prediction accuracy of postprandial plasma glucose using two biomedical coefficients of GH-modulus from linear elastic glucose theory based on GH-Method: math-physical medicine, Part 6 (No. 358)

Gerald C. Hsu
eclaireMD Foundation, USA
11/7/2020

Abstract:

This article is Part 6 of the author's linear elastic glucose behavior study, which focuses on the prediction accuracy of postprandial plasma glucose (PPG) over the pre-virus period, from 9/1/2015 to 12/31/2019, and the COVID-19 virus period, from 1/1/2020 to 11/6/2020. This research is the continuation of his previous five studies on linear elastic glucose behaviors. As a comparison, this study also utilized his developed artificial intelligence (AI) software to predict his PPG values.

The main objective is to offer numerical proof for the high prediction accuracy of PPG based on linear elastic glucose theory with two biomedical coefficients of GH-modulus and the adjustment of the baseline PPG (i.e. pancreatic beta cells' health conditions) during the COVID-19 virus period.

Based on the author's engineering background, he defines the GH.p-modulus to represent the linear elastic PPG behaviors followed by his defined GH.f-modulus to represent his linear elastic FPG behaviors.

He then discovered that these two unique biomedical coefficients are dependent upon health conditions of a patient, i.e. his/her severity level of obesity and diabetes. Furthermore, he also observed that these two biomedical coefficients behave like a "pseudo-constant" during a period of 3 to 4 months. The average lifespan of red blood cells are approximately 115 to 120 days. Red blood cells carry both oxygen and glucose to circulate the entire body for transporting its needed nutrition and energy to maintain the body's operations, especially for the internal organs.

As the next step, he applied the linear elastic glucose equation on certain selected meals and observed extremely high accuracies of predicted PPG values. He then followed his research by choosing annualized PPG data over a period of 5+ years to do his calculations. He also observed their impressively high prediction accuracies.

In this article, he compares his predicted PPG values against the finger measured PPG values over the pre-virus period (9/1/2015 - 12/31/2019) and virus period (1/1/2020 - 11/6/2020) to see the subtle differences of the prediction accuracy due to different lifestyles using both AI approach and NI approach.

The virus period has achieved 99.98% accuracy with NI and 98.44% accuracy with AI, while the pre-virus period has achieved 99.65% accuracy with NI and 99.30% accuracy with AI. The reason for the virus period in achieving a slightly higher prediction accuracy using NI than the pre-virus period is that the virus period has implemented an adjustment of a lower baseline PPG. **In summary, when a patient implements a stringent lifestyle management program, his/her weight would be reduced, and then lead into a lower glucose level, both FPG and PPG.**

The linear elastic predicted PPG equation cited in this article is simple enough for patients to apply on their weight and diabetes control. The only required input data are body weight, carbs/sugar intake amount, and post-meal walking steps, without the problematic collection in obtaining glucose data.

Introduction:

This article is Part 6 of the author's linear elastic glucose behavior study, which focuses on the prediction accuracy of postprandial plasma glucose (PPG) over the pre-virus period, from 9/1/2015 to 12/31/2019, and the COVID-19 virus period, from 1/1/2020 to 11/6/2020. This research is the continuation of his previous five studies on linear elastic glucose behaviors. As a comparison, this study also utilized his developed artificial intelligence (AI) software to predict his PPG values.

The main objective is to offer numerical proof for the high prediction accuracy of PPG based on linear elastic glucose theory with two biomedical coefficients of GH-modulus and the adjustment of the baseline PPG (i.e. pancreatic beta cells' health conditions) during the COVID-19 virus period.

Methods:

Background:
To learn more about the author's GH-Method: math-physical medicine (MPM) methodology, readers can refer to his article to understand his developed MPM analysis method in Reference 1.

Highlights of his related research:
In 2015 and 2016, the author decomposed the PPG waveforms (data curves) into 19 influential components and identified carbs/sugar intake amount and post-meal walking exercise contributing to approximately 40% of PPG formation, respectively. Therefore, he could safely discount the importance of the remaining ~20% contribution by the 16 other influential components.

In March of 2017, he also detected that body weight contributes to over 85% to fasting plasma glucose (FPG) formation. Furthermore, in 2019, he identified that FPG could serve as a good indicator of the pancreatic beta cells' health status; therefore, he can apply the FPG value (more precisely, 97% of FPG value) to serve as the baseline PPG value to calculate the PPG incremental amount in order to obtain the predicted PPG.

In 2018, based on his collected ~2,500 meals and associated sensor PPG waveforms, he further applied the perturbation theory from quantum mechanics, using the first bite of his meal as the initial condition to extend and build an entire PPG waveform covering a period of 180 minutes, with a 95% of PPG prediction accuracy.

In 2019, all of his developed PPG prediction models achieved high percentages of prediction accuracy, but he also realized that his prediction models are too difficult for use by the general public. The above-mentioned sophisticated methods would be difficult for healthcare professionals and diabetes patients to understand, let alone use them in their daily life for diabetes control. As a result, he supplemented his complex models with a simple linear equation of predicted PPG (see References 2, 3, 4, and 12).

Here is his simple linear formula:

Predicted PPG
= FPG * M1 + (carbs-sugar * M2) - (post-meal walking k-steps * M3)

Where M1, M2, M3 are 3 multipliers.

After lengthy research, trial and error, and data tuning, he finally identified the best multipliers for FPG and exercise as 0.97 for M1 and 5.0 for M3. In comparison with PPG, the FPG is a more stabilized biomarker since it is directly related to body weight, not food or exercise. We know that weight reduction is a hard task. However, weight is a calmer and more stabilized biomarker in comparison to glucose which changes from minute to minute with a bigger magnitude of fluctuation. The influence of exercise (specifically, post-meal walking steps) on PPG (41% contribution and >80% negative correlation with PPG) is almost equal to the influence from the carbs/sugar intake amount on PPG (39% contribution and >80% positive correlation with PPG). In terms of intensity and duration, exercise is a simple and straightforward subject to study. Especially, normal-speed walking is a safe and effective form of exercise for the large portion of diabetes patients, particularly senior citizens.

The parameters, FPG and walking, have a lower chance of variation for the author. However, for some diabetes patients, he recommends them to keep the multiplier M3 as a variable if their exercise patterns are different and changing (i.e. dynamic).

The relationship between food nutrition and glucose is a complex and difficult subject to fully understand and effectively manage due to many types of available food (in terms of both quality and quantity of meals) with different carbs/sugar contents. For example, in the author's developed database of food material and nutritional ingredients, it contains over six million data. As a result, the author decided to implement two multipliers, M1 for FPG and M3 for exercise, as the two "constants", and keep M2 as the only "variable" in his PPG prediction equation.

Therefore, an easier linear equation for predicted PPG is developed and listed below:

Predicted PPG
*= (0.97*FPG)+(Carbs&sugar * M2) - (post-meal walking k-steps * 5)*

He further created two new terms for his developed two linear elastic glucose coefficients:

Term 1:
GH.p-modulus = M2
Term 2:
The incremental PPG from diet
= Predicted PPG - baseline PPG
* (i.e. 0.97 * FPG) + (walking * 5)*
Coefficient 1 for PPG:

GH.p-modulus
= (Incremental PPG)/(Carbs&sugar)

Coefficient 2 for FPG:
GH.f-modulus = (FPG) / (Weight)

After combining the above 2 terms and 2 coefficients, he obtained the following linear equation of predicted PPG:

Predicted PPG =
(0.97 * GH.f-modulus * Weight) +(GH.p-modulus * Carbs&sugar) - (post-meal walking k-steps * 5)

By using this equation, a patient only needs the data of body weight, carbs & sugar intake amount, and post-meal walking steps to calculate the predicted PPG without obtaining any measured glucose data.

AI versus NI:
In 2016, he utilized optical physics, big data analytics, and artificial intelligence (AI) techniques to develop a customized computer software to predict PPG based on the patient's food pictures or meal photos. This sophisticated AI approach and iPhone APP software product have reached to a 98.8% prediction accuracy based on ~6,000 meal photos.

Each photo of food or meal on the iPhone contains ~20 million pixels and each pixel requires 8 unique combination of alpha-numerical digits to represent the uniqueness of a pixel. Therefore, there are ~160 million pixels contained in a picture with many different types and shades of multiple colors. Different color's wavelength is closely related to different molecular structures of the food ingredients. Therefore, through this optical physics approach combined with AI technique, his developed software can quickly figure out the estimated carbohydrates and sugar amount of that particular food or meal. Using this estimated carbs/sugar amount and above predicted PPG equation, a predicted PPG value can be calculated and then compared against the finger-piercing measured PPG value to obtain AI % of prediction accuracy.

The author has spent past 10 years to study endocrinology, metabolism, and food nutrition. Therefore, he has also accumulated vast amount of knowledge of internal medicine and food nutrition in his brain. There are many complicated and deep relationships which cannot be easily programmed into his software program entirely. Besides, the retina can recognize and capture more sophisticated images and is more capable than any advanced camera. After consuming each meal, the author always input two sets of carbs/sugar intake amount data into his software, NI and AI. Here NI stands for natural intelligence which means to use his eyes and brain to make his decision regarding carbs/sugar intake amount. His developed software can quickly provide the results via both AI approach and NI approach.
Stress, Strain, & Young's modulus:
Prior to his medical research work, he was an engineer in the various fields of

structural engineering (aerospace, naval defense, and earthquake engineering), mechanical engineering (nuclear power plant equipments, and computer-aided-design), and electronics engineering (computers, semiconductors, graphic software, and software robot).

The two biomedical coefficients of GH-modulus mentioned above were inspired by his prior knowledge in the theory of elasticity in strengths of engineering materials which has the following engineering equation developed in 1807 by a British scientist, Thomas Young:

Stress = Young's modulus * Strain

(Note: Young's modulus and the two biomedical coefficients, both GH.f-modulus and GH.p-modulus, are reciprocal to each other.)

The following excerpts comes from internet public domain, including Google and Wikipedia:

"Strain - ε:
Strain is the "deformation of a solid due to stress" - change in dimension divided by the original value of the dimension - and can be expressed as
$\varepsilon = dL / L$
where
ε = strain (m/m, in/in)
dL = elongation or compression (offset) of object (m, in)
L = length of object (m, in)

Stress - σ:
Stress is force per unit area and can be expressed as
$\sigma = F / A$
where
σ = stress (N/m2, lb/in2, psi)
F = applied force (N, lb)
A = stress area of object (m2, in2)

Stress includes tensile stress, compressible stress, shearing stress, etc.

E, Young's modulus:
It can be expressed as:

$E = stress / strain$
   $= \sigma / \varepsilon$
   $= (F / A) / (dL / L)$

where
E = Young's Modulus of Elasticity (Pa, N/m2, lb/in2, psi) was named after the 18th-century English physicist Thomas Young.

Elasticity:

Elasticity is a property of an object or material indicating how it will restore it to its original shape after distortion. A spring is an example of an elastic object - when stretched, it exerts a restoring force which tends to bring it back to its original length (Figure 1).

Plasticity:

When the force is going beyond the elastic limit of material, it is into a plastic zone which means even when force is removed, the material will not return back to its original state (Figure 1).

Based on various experimental results, the following table lists some Young's modulus associated with different materials:

Nylon: 2.7 GPa
Concrete: 17-30 GPa
Glass fibers: 72 GPa
Copper: 117 GPa
Steel: 190-215 GPa
Diamond: 1220 GPa

Young's modules in the above table are ranked from soft material (low E) to stiff material (higher E)."

Professor James Andrews taught the author linear elasticity at the University of Iowa and Professor Norman Jones taught him nonlinear dynamic plasticity at Massachusetts Institute of Technology. These two great academic mentors provided him the necessary foundation knowledge to understand these two important subjects in engineering.

Data collection:

The author is a 73-year-old male with a 25-year history of T2D. He began collecting his carbs/sugar intake amount and post-meal walking steps on 6/1/2015. In order to achieve the data integrity and stability in his 90-days moving averaged calculation, he omitted the first three-months data. Therefore, from 9/1/2015 to 11/6/2020 (1,906 days), he has collected 7 data per day, i.e. weight, one FPG, three PPG, carb/sugar intake amount, and post-meal walking steps. He utilized these 13,342 data of 1,906 days to conduct this study.

The period of 9/1/2015 to 12/31/2019 is already his "better-controlled" diabetes period, where his average daily glucoses is maintained at 116 mg/dL (<120 mg/dL, the normal range). He named this period as his "linear elastic zone" of diabetes health. It should also be noted that in 2010, his average glucose was 280 mg/dL and HbA1C was 10%, while taking three diabetes medications. The strong chemical interventions from various diabetes medications would seriously alter glucose physical behaviors. He called the period prior to 2015 as his "nonlinear plastic zone" of diabetes health.

It should be pointed out that, this year of 2020 is his "best-performed" health period due to a stabilized routine and without any traveling lifestyle during the COVID-19 quarantined period. During this special period, his 90-days average daily glucose dropped to 101 mg/dL and his weight went below 170 lbs. (BMI <25). He reduced his weight from above 200 lbs down to around 175 lbs in 2015 and had been maintained at that level for 5 years. This means that his pancreatic beta cells' health condition has reached to his "best state" in the past 25 years of his diabetes history.

Results:

Listed below are his summarized key data of his body weight (lbs.) and baseline PPG (mg/dL) during the non-virus period (9/1/2015 - 12/31/2019) and virus period (1/1/2020 - 11/6/2020). Please note that the baseline PPG is moving in a downward trend from ~100 mg/dL in the pre-virus period toward ~90 mg/dL in the virus period.

Y2017: 178 lbs., 102 mg/dL
Pre-virus: 173 lbs., 99 mg/dL
Virus: 171 lbs., 98 mg/dL
11/2020: 167 lbs., 96 mg/dL

The above example data have used the following formula and coefficient:

baseline PPG
= (GH.f-modulus * 0.97 * FPG)

GH.f-modulus
= 0.59

Figure 2 shows the comparison between NI % (99.65%) and AI % (99.30%) using the "AI predicted" PPG vs. finger-measured PPG during the pre-virus period. The NI prediction is 0.35% higher than the AI prediction which means that the human brain is slightly better than the computer brain (CPU plus data storage).

Figure 3 depicts the comparison between NI % (99.98%) and AI % (98.44%) using the "AI predicted" PPG vs. finger-measured PPG during the virus period. The NI prediction is 1.54% higher than AI prediction which means that the human brain is better than computer brain (CPU plus data storage) again.

Both NI and AI have produced extremely high accuracies of the predicted PPG. However, the human brain still beats the computer with AI by 0.35% to 0.54%. The subtle differences of the phenomena observed by the human eyes and the vast learned knowledge stored and processed by the human brain are always superior to any computer. Theoretically, when and if AI can store all of the people's correct knowledge and high intelligence plus can collect everything from every human brain, then AI system can indeed beat the human's natural intelligence. Of course, this is just the author's personal opinion.

Another observation is that the author's health condition has reached to the best state for the past 25 years of history with obesity and diabetes. In his previous research, he has already identified that his pancreatic beta cells are repairing themselves at a slow rate of 2.7% per year over the last 6 to 8 years (Reference 14). This improvement on his insulin function reflects his downward trend of his baseline PPG value. The above-mentioned phenomenon and necessary system adjustment have already been inserted into his AI software algorithm recently for the time period after 1/1/2010.

Conclusions:

Based on the author's engineering background, he defines the GH.p-modulus to represent the linear elastic PPG behaviors followed by his defined GH.f-modulus to represent his linear elastic FPG behaviors.

He then discovered that these two unique biomedical coefficients are dependent upon health conditions of a patient, i.e. his/her severity level of obesity and diabetes. Furthermore, he also observed that these two biomedical coefficients behave like a "pseudo-constant" during a period of 3 to 4 months. The average lifespan of red blood cells are approximately 115 to 120 days. Red blood cells carry both oxygen and glucose to circulate the entire body for transporting its needed nutrition and energy to maintain the body's operations, especially for the internal organs.

As the next step, he applied the linear elastic glucose equation on certain selected meals and observed extremely high accuracies of predicted PPG values. He then followed his research by choosing annualized PPG data over a period of 5+ years to do his calculations. He also observed their impressively high prediction accuracies.

In this article, he compares his predicted PPG values against the finger measured PPG values over the pre-virus period (9/1/2015 - 12/31/2019) and virus period (1/1/2020 - 11/6/2020) to see the subtle differences of the prediction accuracy due to different lifestyles using both AI approach and NI approach.

The virus period has achieved 99.98% accuracy with NI and 98.44% accuracy with AI, while the pre-virus period has achieved 99.65% accuracy with NI and 99.30% accuracy with AI. The reason for the virus period in achieving a slightly higher prediction accuracy using NI than the pre-virus period is that the virus period has implemented an adjustment of a lower baseline PPG. **In summary, when a patient implements a stringent lifestyle management program, his/her weight would be reduced, and then lead into a lower glucose level, both FPG and PPG.**

The linear elastic predicted PPG equation cited in this article is simple enough for patients to apply on their weight and diabetes control. The only required input data are body weight, carbs/sugar intake amount, and post-meal walking steps, without the problematic collection in obtaining glucose data.

References:

1. Hsu, Gerald C., eclaireMD Foundation, USA, No. 310: "Biomedical research methodology based on GH-Method: math-physical medicine"

2. Hsu, Gerald C., eclaireMD Foundation, USA, No. 345: "Application of linear equations to predict sensor and finger based postprandial plasma glucoses and daily glucoses for pre-virus, virus, and total periods using GH-Method: math-physical medicine"

3. Hsu, Gerald C., eclaireMD Foundation, USA, No. 97: "A simplified yet accurate linear equation of PPG prediction model for T2D patients (GH-Method: math-physical medicine)"

4. Hsu, Gerald C., eclaireMD Foundation, USA, No. 99: "Application of linear equation-based PPG prediction model for four T2D clinic cases (GH-Method: math-physical medicine)"

5. Hsu, Gerald C., eclaireMD Foundation, USA, No. 339: "Self-recovery of pancreatic beta cell's insulin secretion based on 10+ years annualized data of food, exercise, weight, and glucose using GH-Method: math-physical medicine)

6. Hsu, Gerald C., eclaireMD Foundation, USA, No. 340: "A neural communication model between brain and internal organs, specifically stomach, liver, and pancreatic beta cells based on PPG waveforms of 131 liquid egg meals and 124 solid egg meals)

7. Hsu, Gerald C., eclaireMD Foundation, USA, No. 346: "Linear relationship between carbohydrates & sugar intake amount and incremental PPG amount via engineering strength of materials using GH-Method: math-physical medicine, Part 1"

8. Hsu, Gerald C., eclaireMD Foundation, USA, No. 349: "Investigation on GH modulus of linear elastic glucose with two diabetes patients data using GH-Method: math-physical medicine, Part 2"

9. Hsu, Gerald C., eclaireMD Foundation, USA, No. 349: "Investigation of GH modulus on the linear elastic glucose behavior based on three diabetes patients' data using the GH-Method: math-physical medicine, Part 3"

10. Hsu, Gerald C., eclaireMD Foundation, USA, No. 349: "Using Math-Physics Medicine to Predict FPG"

11. Hsu, Gerald C., eclaireMD Foundation, USA, No. 356: "Coefficient of GH.f-modulus in the linear elastic fasting plasma glucose behavior study based on health data of three diabetes patients using the GH-Method: math-physical medicine, Part 4 "

12. Hsu, Gerald C., eclaireMD Foundation, USA, No. 264: "Community and Family Medicine via Doctors without distance: Using a simple glucose control card to assist T2D patients in remote rural areas (GH-Method: math-physical medicine)"

13. Hsu, Gerald C., eclaireMD Foundation, USA, No. 357: "High accuracy of predicted postprandial plasma glucose using two coefficients of GH.f-modulus and GH.p-modulus from linear elastic glucose behavior theory based on GH-Method: math-physical medicine, Part 5"

14. Hsu, Gerald C., eclaireMD Foundation, USA, No. 339: "Self-recovery of pancreatic beta cell's insulin secretion based on 10+ years annualized data of food, exercise, weight, and glucose using GH-Method: math-physical medicine"

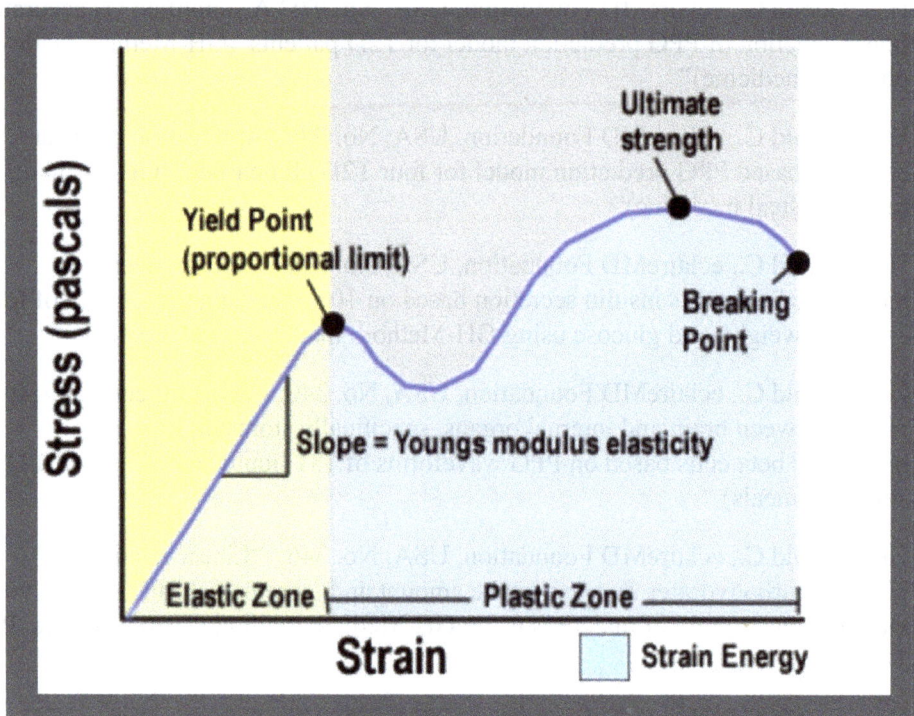

Figure 1: Stress-Strain-Young's modulus, Elastic Zone vs. Plastic Zone

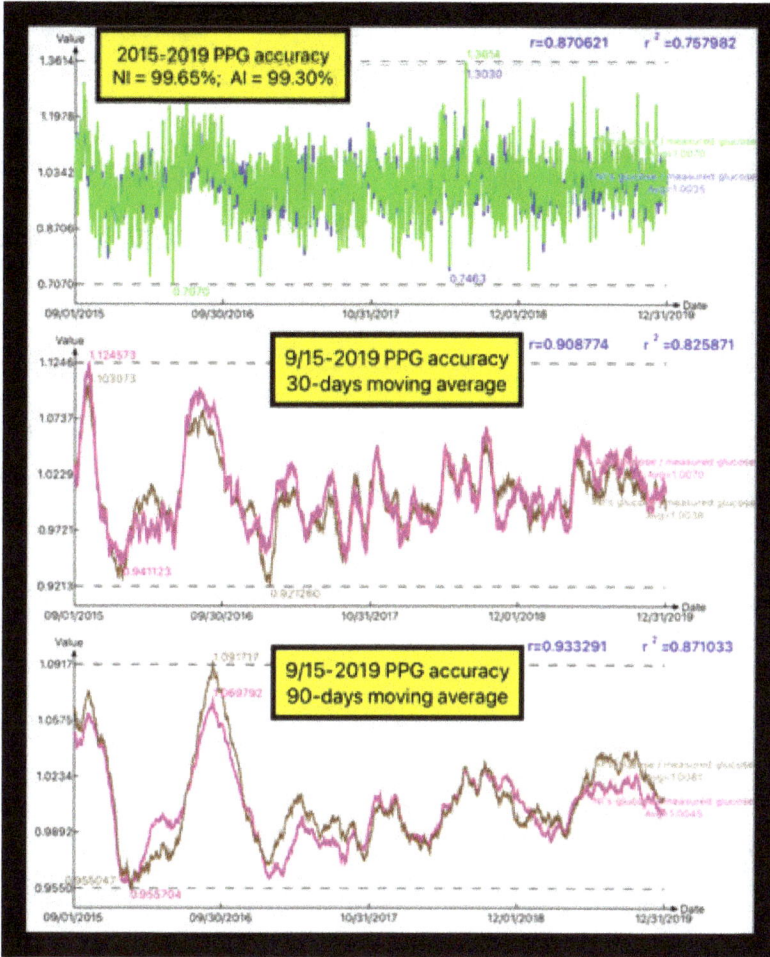

Figure 2: NI 99.65% and AI 99.30% of Pre-virus period (9/1/2015 - 12/31/2019)

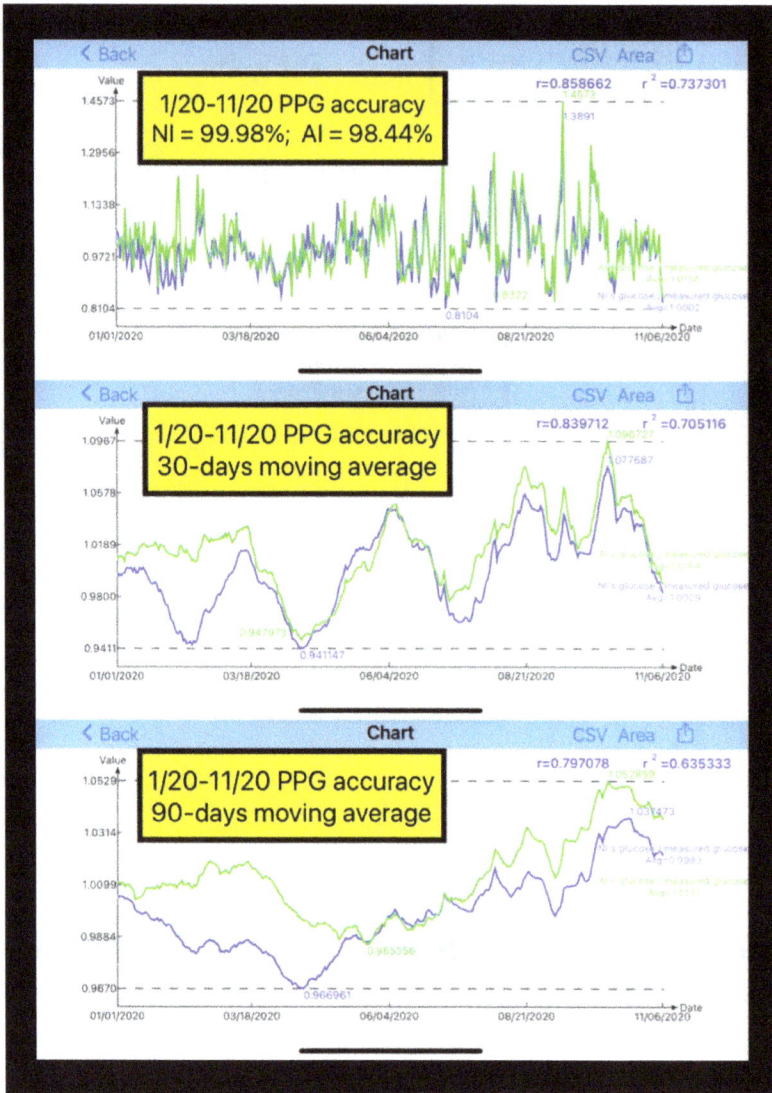

Figure 3: NI 99.98% and AI 98.44% of Virus period (1/1/2020 - 11/6/2020)

High glucose predication accuracy of postprandial plasma glucose and fasting plasma glucose during the COVID-19 period using two glucose coefficients of GH-modulus from linear elastic glucose theory based on GH-Method: math-physical medicine, Part 7 (No. 359)

Gerald C. Hsu
eclaireMD Foundation, USA
11/9/2020

Abstract:

This article is Part 7 of the author's linear elastic glucose behavior study, which focuses on the prediction accuracy of the postprandial plasma glucose (PPG) and fasting plasma glucose (FPG) over the COVID-19 quarantined period, from 1/1/2020 to 11/8/2020. This research is the continuation of his previous six studies on linear elastic glucose behaviors.

The main objective is to offer numerical proof for the high prediction accuracy of both PPG and FPG based on linear elastic glucose theory with two newly defined biomedical coefficients of GH-modulus, during the COVID-19 period when his overall health conditions have reached to the best performed state.

The following lists the average values over this period of 10+ months from 1/1/2020 to 11/8/2020:

Weight: 170 lbs.
Measured FPG: 102 mg/dL
Predicted FPG: 102 mg/dL
Carbs/sugar: 12.19 grams
Post-meal Walking: 4.447 k-steps
Measured PPG: 108.3 mg/dL
Predicted PPG: 109.2 mg/dL
Average GH.f-modulus: 0.60
Average GH.p-modulus: 2.64
Accuracy of predicted FPG: 100.0%
Accuracy of predicted PPG: 99.2%

Where Predicted PPG
= baseline PPG + carbs - walking
= 99.3 + 32.2 - 22.2
= 109.2 mg/dL

The most important finding in this study is ***the extremely high accuracies of predicted glucoses, including FPG with 100.0% accuracy and PPG with 99.2% accuracy.*** The result proves the applicability of his developed linear elastic glucose behaviors models on his glucose predictions efforts during a "better-controlled" COVID-19 quarantined period.

Here is the equation again:

Predicted PPG =
(0.97 * GH.f-modulus * Weight) +(GH.p-modulus * Carbs&sugar) - (post-meal walking k-steps * 5)

In practice, when diabetes patients use the above equation, they only need the input data of weight, carbs/sugar intake amount, and post-meal walking steps, without glucose measurement.

The author will continue his research work to develop corresponding ranges for these two biomedical "glucose coefficients" from GH.p-modulus and GH.f-modulus to match the different groups of health states for patients. He will cover this subject in article No. 360.

The secondary finding for the two "pseudo-linear" or "near-constant" relationship associated with the two glucose coefficients, GH.p-modulus and GH.f-modulus, are also observed in this particular period, which is similar to the cases in his previous research work. The relatively lower values of glucose coefficients have further indicated that his diabetes control during the COVID-19 period has been successful.

Introduction:

This article is Part 7 of the author's linear elastic glucose behavior study, which focuses on the prediction accuracy of the postprandial plasma glucose (PPG) and fasting plasma glucose (FPG) over the COVID-19 quarantined period, from 1/1/2020 to 11/8/2020. This research is the continuation of his previous six studies on linear elastic glucose behaviors.

The main objective is to offer numerical proof for the high prediction accuracy of both PPG and FPG based on linear elastic glucose theory with two newly defined biomedical coefficients of GH-modulus, during the COVID-19 period when his overall health conditions have reached to the best performed state.

Methods:

Background:
To learn more about the author's GH-Method: math-physical medicine (MPM) methodology, readers can refer to his article to understand his developed MPM analysis method in Reference 1.

Highlights of his related research:
In 2015 and 2016, the author decomposed the PPG waveforms (data curves) into 19 influential components and identified carbs/sugar intake amount and post-meal walking exercise contributing to approximately 40% of PPG formation, respectively. Therefore, he could safely discount the importance of the remaining ~20% contribution by the 16 other influential components.

In March of 2017, he also detected that body weight contributes to over 85% to FPG formation. Furthermore, in 2019, he identified that FPG could serve as a good indicator of the pancreatic beta cells' health status; therefore, he can apply the FPG value (more precisely, 97% of FPG value) to serve as the baseline PPG value to calculate the PPG incremental amount in order to obtain the predicted PPG.

In 2019, all of his developed PPG prediction models achieved high percentages of prediction accuracy, but he also realized that his prediction models are too difficult for use by the general public. As a result, he supplemented his complex models with a simple linear equation of predicted PPG (see References 2 and 3).

Here is his simple linear formula (Reference 4):

Predicted PPG
= FPG * M1 + (carbs-sugar * M2) - (post-meal walking k-steps * M3)

Where M1, M2, M3 are 3 multipliers.

After lengthy research, trial and error, and data tuning, he finally identified the best multipliers for FPG and exercise as 0.97 for M1 and 5.0 for M3. In comparison with PPG, the FPG is a more stabilized biomarker since it is directly related to body weight, not food or exercise. We know that weight reduction is a hard task. However, weight is a calmer and more stabilized biomarker in comparison to glucose which changes from minute to minute with a bigger magnitude of fluctuation. The influence of exercise (specifically, post-meal walking steps) on PPG (41% contribution and >80% negative correlation with PPG) is almost equal to the influence from the carbs/sugar intake amount on PPG (39% contribution and >80% positive correlation with PPG). In terms of intensity and duration, exercise is a simple and straightforward subject to study. Especially, normal-speed walking is a safe and effective form of exercise for the large portion of diabetes patients, particularly senior citizens.

The parameters, FPG and walking, have a lower chance of variation for the author since he is stringent on maintaining his body weight and his daily exercise routine.

On the other hand, the relationship between food nutrition and glucose is a quite complex and difficult subject to fully understand and effectively manage due to many types of available food (in terms of both quality and quantity of meals) with different nutritional ingredients, including carbohydrates and sugar contents. For example, in the author's developed database of food material and nutritional ingredients, it contains over six million data. As a result, the author decided to implement two multipliers, M1 for FPG and M3 for exercise, as the two "constants", and keep M2 as the only "variable" in his PPG prediction equation.

Therefore, an easier linear equation for predicted PPG is listed below:

Predicted PPG
*= (0.97*FPG)+(Carbs&sugar * M2) - (post-meal walking k-steps * 5)*

He further created two new terms for his developed two linear elastic glucose coefficients:

Term 1:
GH.p-modulus = M2

Term 2:
The incremental PPG from diet
= Predicted PPG - baseline PPG
 *(i.e. 0.97 * FPG) + (walking * 5)*

Glucose Coefficient for PPG:
GH.p-modulus
= (Incremental PPG)/(Carbs&sugar)

Glucose Coefficient for FPG:
GH.f-modulus = (FPG) / (Weight)

After combining the above 2 terms and 2 glucose coefficients, he has finally obtained the following linear equation of predicted PPG:

Predicted PPG =
(0.97 * GH.f-modulus * Weight) +(GH.p-modulus * Carbs&sugar) - (post-meal walking k-steps * 5)

By using this equation, a patient only needs the data of body weight, carbs & sugar intake amount, and post-meal walking steps to calculate the predicted PPG without obtaining any measured glucose data.

Stress, Strain, & Young's modulus:
Prior to his medical research work, he was an engineer in the various fields of structural engineering (aerospace, naval defense, and earthquake engineering), mechanical engineering (nuclear power plant equipments, and computer-aided-design), and electronics engineering (computers, semiconductors, graphic software, and software robot).

The two biomedical coefficients of GH-modulus mentioned above were inspired by his prior knowledge in the theory of elasticity in strengths of engineering materials which has the following engineering equation developed in 1807 by a British scientist, Thomas Young:

Stress = Young's modulus * Strain

(Note: Young's modulus and the two biomedical coefficients, both GH.f-modulus and GH.p-modulus, are reciprocal to each other.)

The following excerpts comes from internet public domain, including Google and Wikipedia:

"Strain - ε:
Strain is the "deformation of a solid due to stress" - change in dimension divided by the original value of the dimension - and can be expressed as
ε = dL / L
where
ε = strain (m/m, in/in)
dL = elongation or compression (offset) of object (m, in)
L = length of object (m, in)

Stress - σ:
Stress is force per unit area and can be expressed as
$\sigma = F / A$
where
σ = stress (N/m2, lb/in2, psi)
F = applied force (N, lb)
A = stress area of object (m2, in2)

Stress includes tensile stress, compressible stress, shearing stress, etc.

E, Young's modulus:
It can be expressed as:

E = stress / strain
  $= \sigma / \varepsilon$
  $= (F / A) / (dL / L)$

where
E = Young's Modulus of Elasticity (Pa, N/m2, lb/in2, psi) was named after the 18th-century English physicist Thomas Young.

Elasticity:
Elasticity is a property of an object or material indicating how it will restore it to its original shape after distortion. A spring is an example of an elastic object - when stretched, it exerts a restoring force which tends to bring it back to its original length (Figure 1).

Plasticity:
When the force is going beyond the elastic limit of material, it is into a plastic zone which means even when force is removed, the material will not return back to its original state (Figure 1).

Based on various experimental results, the following table lists some Young's modulus associated with different materials:

Nylon: 2.7 GPa
Concrete: 17-30 GPa
Glass fibers: 72 GPa
Copper: 117 GPa
Steel: 190-215 GPa
Diamond: 1220 GPa

Young's modules in the above table are ranked from soft material (low E) to stiff material (higher E)."

Professor James Andrews taught the author linear elasticity at the University of Iowa and Professor Norman Jones taught him nonlinear dynamic plasticity at Massachusetts Institute of Technology. These two great academic mentors provided him the necessary foundation knowledge to understand these two important subjects in engineering.

Data collection:

The author is a 73-year-old male with a 25-year history of T2D. He began collecting his carbs/sugar intake amount and post-meal walking steps on 6/1/2015. Therefore, from 6/1/2015 to 11/6/2020, he has collected 7 data per day, i.e. weight, one FPG, three PPG, carb/sugar intake amount, and post-meal walking steps. He utilized these big data associated to conduct various studies.

The period of 9/1/2015 to 12/31/2019 is already his "better-controlled" diabetes period, where his average daily glucoses is maintained at 116 mg/dL (<120 mg/dL, the normal range). He named this period as his "linear elastic zone" of diabetes health. It should also be noted that in 2010, his average glucose was 280 mg/dL and HbA1C was 10%, while taking three diabetes medications. The strong chemical interventions from various diabetes medications would seriously alter glucose physical behaviors. He called the period prior to 2015 as his "nonlinear plastic zone" of diabetes health.

It should be pointed out that 2020 is his "best-performed" health period due to his stabilized routine without any traveling for the duration of the COVID-19 quarantined timeframe. During this special period, his 90-days average daily glucose dropped to 101 mg/dL and his weight went below 170 lbs. (BMI <25). He reduced his weight from 200+ lbs. to approximately 175 lbs. in 2015, while maintaining the same level for 5 years. This means that his pancreatic beta cells' health condition has reached to his "best state" in the past 25 years of his diabetes history (References 5 and 6).

Recent linear elastic glucose studies:
Utilizing the concept of Young's modulus and stress/strain, during the past 30 days, the author has initiated and engaged in this linear elastic glucose behaviors research. The following highlights have outlined his findings during this process.

First, he discovered that there is a "pseudo-linear" relationship existed between carbs & sugar intake amount and incremental PPG amount. Therefore, he defined a new glucose coefficient of GH.p-modulus for PPG.

Second, similar to Young's modulus relating to stiffness of engineering inorganic materials, he found that the GH.p-modulus is depended upon the patient's severity level of obesity and diabetes.

Third, similar to GH.p-modulus for PPG, he uncovered a similar pseudo-linear relationship existed between weight and FPG. Therefore, he defined another new glucose coefficient of GH.f-modulus for FPG.

Fourth, he inserted the two glucose coefficients, GH.p-modulus and GH.f-modulus, into the PPG prediction equation to remove the responsibility of collecting measured glucoses by patients.

Fifth, by experimenting and calculating many predicted PPG values over a variety of time length of different patients with different health conditions, he finally revealed that GH.p-modulus seems to be "near-constant" or "pseudo-linearized" over a short period of 3 to 4 months. This short period is compatible with the known lifespan of red blood cells. They are living organic materials which is different from engineering materials, such as steel or concrete. The same finding can also be observed in the monthly GH.p-modulus values from this particular study in the COVID-19 period.

Results:

There are only two graphic figures which demonstrate the findings in this study.

Figure 2 shows the data table of the linear elastic glucose behaviors models and their operational calculations of the following key equation:

Predicted PPG =
(0.97 * GH.f-modulus * Weight) +(GH.p-modulus * Carbs&sugar) - (post-meal walking k-steps * 5)

The following lists the average values over this period of 10+ months from 1/1/2020 to 11/8/2020:

Weight: 170 lbs.
Measured FPG: 102 mg/dL
Predicted FPG: 102 mg/dL
Carbs/sugar: 12.19 grams
Post-meal Walking: 4.447 k-steps
Measured PPG: 108.3 mg/dL
Predicted PPG: 109.2 mg/dL
Average GH.f-modulus: 0.60
Average GH.p-modulus: 2.64
Accuracy of predicted FPG: 100.0%
Accuracy of predicted PPG: 99.2%

Where
Predicted PPG
= baseline PPG + carbs - walking
= 99.3 + 32.2 - 22.2
= 109.2 mg/dL

Figure 3 depicts monthly values of GH.f-modulus and GH.p-modulus. There are two noteworthy observations. First, the GH.f-modulus values seem to be more stabilized than the GH.p-modulus values. They are within the range of 0.53 to 0.69, but most of coefficient values are within the range of 0.56 to 0.66. This phenomenon is due to both weight and FPG as being more of a stable biomarker than PPG. Second, the coefficient values of GH.p-modulus has more fluctuations (i.e., amplitude difference) than the GH.f-modulus. However, within a shorter time span of 3 to 4 months, there are several "more-closely clustered" patterns, such as from January through April, June through August, August through October, and September through November. Within these more-closely clustered sub-periods, the coefficients act more like "pseudo-constants".

Conclusions:

The most important finding in this study is the extremely high accuracies of predicted glucoses, including FPG with 100.0% accuracy and PPG with 99.2% accuracy. The result proves the applicability of his developed linear elastic glucose behaviors models on his glucose predictions efforts during a "better-controlled" COVID-19 quarantined period.

Here is the equation again:

Predicted PPG =
(0.97 * GH.f-modulus * Weight) +(GH.p-modulus * Carbs&sugar) - (post-meal walking k-steps * 5)

In practice, when diabetes patients use the above equation, they only need the input data of weight, carbs/sugar intake amount, and post-meal walking steps, without glucose measurement.

The author will continue his research work to develop corresponding ranges for these two biomedical "glucose coefficients" of GH.p-modulus and GH.f-modulus to match the different groups of health states for patients. He will cover this subject in one of his future articles.

The secondary finding for the two "pseudo-linear" or "near-constant" relationship associated with the two glucose coefficients, GH.p-modulus and GH.f-modulus, are also observed in this particular period, which is similar to the cases in his previous research work. The relatively lower values of glucose coefficients have further indicated that his diabetes control during the COVID-19 period has been successful.

References:

1. Hsu, Gerald C., eclaireMD Foundation, USA, No. 310: "Biomedical research methodology based on GH-Method: math-physical medicine"

2. Hsu, Gerald C., eclaireMD Foundation, USA, No. 345: "Application of linear equations to predict sensor and finger based postprandial plasma glucoses and daily glucoses for pre-virus, virus, and total periods using GH-Method: math-physical medicine"

3. Hsu, Gerald C., eclaireMD Foundation, USA, No. 97: "A simplified yet accurate linear equation of PPG prediction model for T2D patients (GH-Method: math-physical medicine)"

4. Hsu, Gerald C., eclaireMD Foundation, USA, No. 99: "Application of linear

equation-based PPG prediction model for four T2D clinic cases (GH-Method: math-physical medicine)"

5. Hsu, Gerald C., eclaireMD Foundation, USA, No. 339: "Self-recovery of pancreatic beta cell's insulin secretion based on 10+ years annualized data of food, exercise, weight, and glucose using GH-Method: math-physical medicine)

6. Hsu, Gerald C., eclaireMD Foundation, USA, No. 340: "A neural communication model between brain and internal organs, specifically stomach, liver, and pancreatic beta cells based on PPG waveforms of 131 liquid egg meals and 124 solid egg meals)

7. Hsu, Gerald C., eclaireMD Foundation, USA, No. 349: "Using Math-Physics Medicine to Predict FPG"

8. Hsu, Gerald C., eclaireMD Foundation, USA, No. 264: "Community and Family Medicine via Doctors without distance: Using a simple glucose control card to assist T2D patients in remote rural areas (GH-Method: math-physical medicine)"

9. Hsu, Gerald C., eclaireMD Foundation, USA, No. 346: "Linear relationship between carbohydrates & sugar intake amount and incremental PPG amount via engineering strength of materials using GH-Method: math-physical medicine, Part 1"

10. Hsu, Gerald C., eclaireMD Foundation, USA, No. 349: "Investigation on GH modulus of linear elastic glucose with two diabetes patients data using GH-Method: math-physical medicine, Part 2"

11. Hsu, Gerald C., eclaireMD Foundation, USA, No. 349: "Investigation of GH modulus on the linear elastic glucose behavior based on three diabetes patients' data using the GH-Method: math-physical medicine, Part 3"

12. Hsu, Gerald C., eclaireMD Foundation, USA, No. 356: "Coefficient of GH.f-modulus in the linear elastic fasting plasma glucose behavior study based on health data of three diabetes patients using the GH-Method: math-physical medicine, Part 4 "

13. Hsu, Gerald C., eclaireMD Foundation, USA, No. 357: "High accuracy of predicted postprandial plasma glucose using two coefficients of GH.f-modulus and GH.p-modulus from linear elastic glucose behavior theory based on GH-Method: math-physical medicine, Part 5"

14. Hsu, Gerald C., eclaireMD Foundation, USA, No. 339: "Self-recovery of pancreatic beta cell's insulin secretion based on 10+ years annualized data of food, exercise, weight, and glucose using GH-Method: math-physical medicine"

15. Hsu, Gerald C., eclaireMD Foundation, USA, No. 358: "Improvement on the prediction accuracy of postprandial plasma glucose using two biomedical coefficients of GH-modulus from linear elastic glucose theory based on GH-Method: math-physical medicine, Part 6"

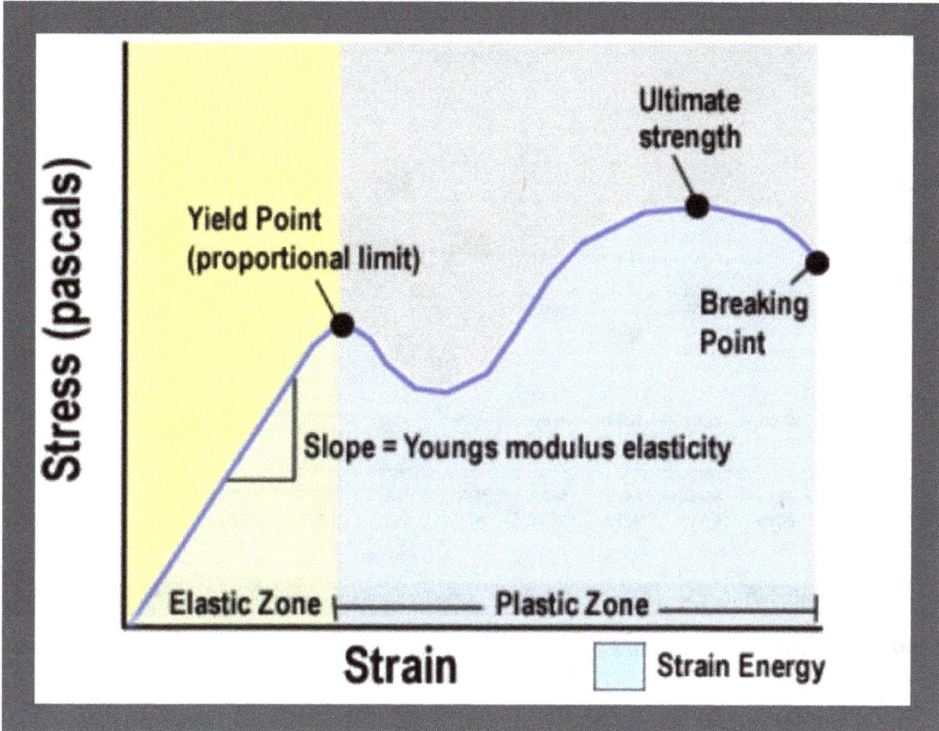

Figure 1: Stress-Strain-Young's modulus, Elastic Zone vs. Plastic Zone

Case A:	lbs Weight	mg/dL Measured FPG	FPG / Weight GH.f-modulus	Case A:	grams Carbs/Sugar	K-steps Walking	Incremental PPG GH.p-modulus	mg/dL Predicted PPG	mg/dL Measured PPG	PPG Prediction Accuracy %
Jan, 2020	170	117	0.69	Jan, 2020	14.38	4.587	1.65	114	114	100%
Feb, 2020	171	112	0.66	Feb, 2020	11.36	4.574	2.13	110	110	100%
Mar, 2020	172	108	0.63	Mar, 2020	12.93	4.869	2.20	109	109	100%
Apr, 2020	172	113	0.66	Apr, 2020	13.49	4.365	1.75	111	111	100%
May, 2020	173	100	0.58	May, 2020	15.41	4.013	2.05	108	108	100%
Jun, 2020	172	100	0.58	Jun, 2020	11.59	3.850	2.95	112	112	100%
Jul, 2020	170	95	0.56	Jul, 2020	10.43	4.250	3.70	109	109	100%
Aug, 2020	171	99	0.58	Aug, 2020	10.79	3.962	2.68	105	105	100%
Sept, 2020	169	100	0.59	Sept, 2020	11.38	4.024	2.45	104	104	100%
Oct, 2020	167	93	0.56	Oct, 2020	11.94	4.807	3.01	102	102	100%
Nov, 2020	167	89	0.53	Nov, 2020	10.42	5.614	4.45	105	105	100%
Case A:	Weight	Measured FPG	GH.f-modulus	Case A:	Carbs/Sugar	Walking	GH.p-modulus	Predicted PPG	Measured PPG	Accuracy %
Calculated	170	102	0.60	Calculated	12.19	4.447	2.64	109.2	108.3	99.2%
Averaged	170	102	0.60	Averaged	12.19	4.447	2.64	108.3	108.3	100.0%
Case A:	Weight	Measured FPG	GH.f-modulus	Case A:				Predicted PPG	Measured PPG	Accuracy %
Averaged	170	102	0.60	Averaged				102.4	102.4	100.0%

Baseline PPG	99.3	= 0.97* (Weight * GH.f-modulus, i.e. FPG)
+ Carbs/sugar	32.2	= Carbs/sugar * GH.p-modulus
- walking	22.2	= Walking k-steps * 5
Predicted PPG	109.2	= baseline PPG + carbs/sugar - walking k-steps

Figure 2: Data table and equation calculations during COVID-19 period (1/1/2020 - 11/8/2020)

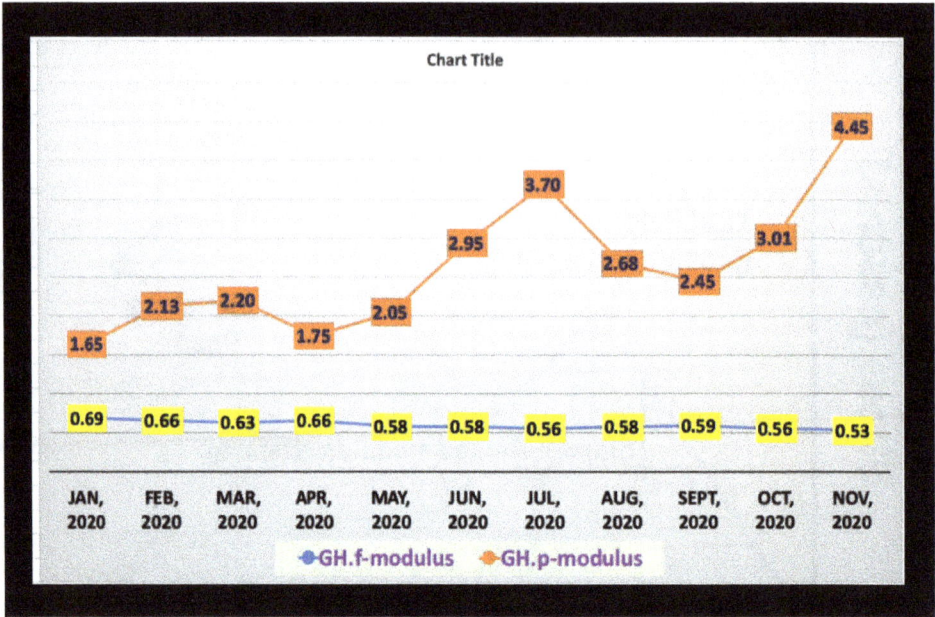

Figure 3: Glucose coefficients of both GH.f-modulus and GH.p-modulus during COVID-19 period (1/1/2020 - 11/8/2020)

Investigation of two glucose coefficients of GH.f-modulus and GH.p-modulus based on the data of three clinical cases during the COVID-19 period using linear elastic glucose theory of GH-Method: math-physical medicine, Part 8 (No. 360)

Gerald C. Hsu
eclaireMD Foundation, USA
11/10-11/2020

Abstract:

This article is Part 8 of the author's linear elastic glucose behavior study which focuses on the deeper understanding of these two newly defined glucose coefficients, GH.f-modulus and GH.p-modulus. Findings have shown the sensitive relationships with health conditions such as obesity and diabetes and certain lifestyle components, e.g. carbs/sugar intake amount and post-meal walking steps. Hopefully in the near future, he will be able to develop a reasonable and applicable numerical ranges of these two glucose coefficients. He used his measured glucose data and predicted glucose models for both fasting plasma glucose (FPG) and postprandial plasma glucose (PPG) for three patients with chronic diseases over the COVID-19 quarantined period, from 3/1/2020 to 11/10/2020.

The consolidated diagram below shows a complicated presentation of multiple components and a variety of results. It is a four-dimensional chart that illustrates the PPG prediction via carbs/sugar and post-meal walking under the influence of the glucose coefficient, GH.p-modulus, for three clinical cases during this timeframe. This single diagram demonstrates the complete results of this study.

The research of the linear elastic glucose behaviors theory summarizes all of his previous findings from Parts 1 through 7. This article utilizes the clinical cases with different severities of obesity and diabetes.

Through different weights along with differing FPG, the author calculates the GH.f-modulus values for each patient which indicates the relative severity between obesity and diabetes.

Furthermore, through the linearity relationship or the linear indication of GH.p-modulus between incremental PPG and carbs/sugar intake amount, he can connect the complicated components of cars/sugar, exercise, weight or FPG into his final predicted PPG equation.

His developed linear elastic glucose theory inspired by his previously acquired knowledge of engineering theory of elasticity which has been proven useful for diabetes control. These research results from the biomedical linearity situations probably are applicable for ~80% of worldwide diabetes patients. However, for a smaller amount of diabetes patients' hyperglycemia situations, ~20% of the total population whose glucose frequently exceed 200 mg/dL level, a nonlinear plastic theory may need to be developed and then applied to these extreme situations.

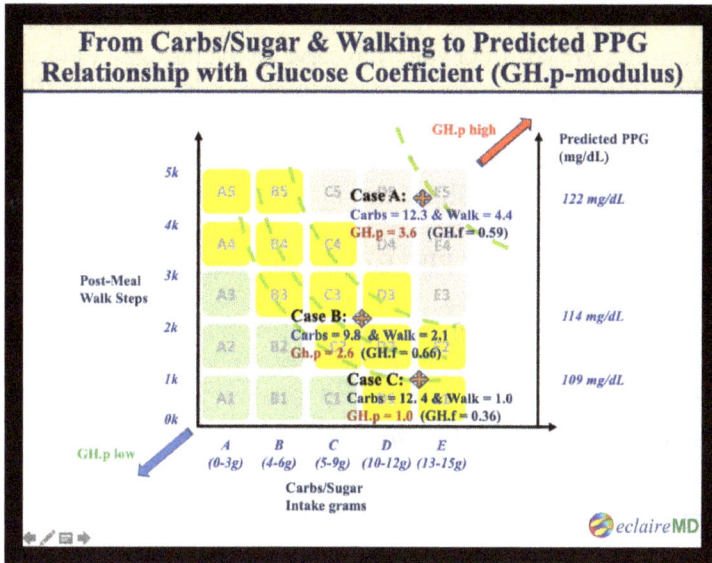

From Carbs/Sugar & Walking to Predicted PPG Relationship with Glucose Coefficient (GH.p-modulus)

Introduction:

This article is Part 8 of the author's linear elastic glucose behavior study which focuses on the deeper understanding of these two newly defined glucose coefficients, GH.f-modulus and GH.p-modulus. Findings have shown the sensitive relationships with health conditions such as obesity and diabetes and certain lifestyle components, e.g. carbs/sugar intake amount and post-meal walking steps. Hopefully in the near future, he will be able to develop a reasonable and applicable numerical ranges of these two glucose coefficients. He used his measured glucose data and predicted glucose models for both fasting plasma glucose (FPG) and postprandial plasma glucose (PPG) for three patients with chronic diseases over the COVID-19 quarantined period, from 3/1/2020 to 11/10/2020.

Methods:

Background:
To learn more about the author's GH-Method: math-physical medicine (MPM) methodology, readers can refer to his article to understand his developed MPM analysis method in Reference 1.

Highlights of his related research:
In 2015 and 2016, the author decomposed the PPG waveforms (data curves) into 19 influential components and identified carbs/sugar intake amount and post-meal walking exercise contributing to approximately 40% of PPG formation, respectively. Therefore, he could safely discount the importance of the remaining ~20% contribution by the 16 other influential components.

In March of 2017, he detected that body weight contributes over 85% to FPG formation. Furthermore, in 2019, he identified that FPG could serve as a good indicator of the pancreatic beta cells' health status; therefore, he can apply the FPG value (more precisely, 97% of FPG value) to serve as the baseline PPG value to calculate the PPG incremental amount in order to obtain the predicted PPG.

In 2019, all of his developed PPG prediction models achieved high percentages of prediction accuracy, but he also realized that his prediction models are too difficult for use by the general public. As a result, he supplemented his complex models with a simple linear equation of predicted PPG (see References 2 and 3).

Here is his simple linear formula (Reference 4):

Predicted PPG
= FPG * M1 + (carbs-sugar * M2) - (post-meal walking k-steps * M3)

Where M1, M2, M3 are 3 multipliers.

After lengthy research, trial and error, and data tuning, he finally identified the best multipliers for FPG and exercise as 0.97 for M1 and 5.0 for M3. In comparison with PPG, the FPG is a more stabilized biomarker since it is directly related to body weight, not food or exercise. Most of us know that weight reduction is a hard task. However, weight is a calmer and more stabilized biomarker in comparison to glucose which changes from minute to minute with a bigger magnitude of fluctuation. The influence of exercise (specifically, post-meal walking steps) on PPG (41% contribution and >80% negative correlation with PPG) is almost equal to the influence from the carbs/sugar intake amount on PPG (39% contribution and >80% positive correlation with PPG). In terms of intensity and duration, exercise is a rather simple and straightforward subject to study. Walking is especially safe and an effective form of exercise for the majority of diabetes patients, particularly senior citizens.

For the author, these two parameters, FPG and walking, have a lower chance of variation since he is stringent on maintaining his body weight and his daily exercise routine.

On the other hand, the relationship between food nutrition and glucose is a quite complex and difficult subject to fully understand and effectively manage due to many types of available food, in terms of quality and quantity of meals, with different nutritional ingredients, including carbohydrates and sugar contents. For example, in the author's developed database of food material and nutritional ingredients, it contains over six million data. As a result, the author decided to implement two multipliers, M1 for FPG and M3 for exercise, as the two fixed "constants", and keep M2 as the only "variable" in his PPG prediction equation.

Therefore, an *easier* linear equation for predicted PPG is listed below:

Predicted PPG
= (0.97*FPG)+(Carbs&sugar * M2) - (post-meal walking k-steps * 5)

He further created two new terms for his developed two linear elastic glucose coefficients:

Term 1:
GH.p-modulus = M2

Term 2:
*The **incremental PPG** from diet*
= Predicted PPG - baseline PPG:
* (i.e. 0.97 * FPG) + (walking * 5)*

Glucose Coefficient for PPG:
GH.p-modulus
= (Incremental PPG)/(Carbs&sugar)

Glucose Coefficient for FPG:
GH.f-modulus *= (FPG) / (Weight)*

After combining the above 2 terms and 2 glucose coefficients, he has finally obtained the following linear equation of predicted PPG:

Predicted PPG =
(0.97 * GH.f-modulus * Weight) +(GH.p-modulus * Carbs&sugar) - (post-meal walking k-steps * 5)

By using this equation, a patient only needs the data of body weight, carbs & sugar intake amount, and post-meal walking steps to calculate the predicted PPG without obtaining any measured glucose data.

Stress, Strain, & Young's modulus:
Prior to his medical research work, he was an engineer in the various fields of structural engineering (aerospace, naval defense, and earthquake engineering), mechanical engineering (nuclear power plant equipments, and computer-aided-design), and electronics engineering (computers, semiconductors, graphic software, and software robot).

The two biomedical coefficients of GH-modulus mentioned above were inspired by his prior knowledge in the theory of elasticity in strengths of engineering materials which has the following engineering equation developed in 1807 by a British scientist, Thomas Young:

Stress = Young's modulus * Strain

(Note: Young's modulus and the two biomedical coefficients, both GH.f-modulus and GH.p-modulus, are reciprocal to each other.)

The following excerpts comes from the internet public domain, including Google and Wikipedia:

"Strain - ε:

Strain is the "deformation of a solid due to stress" - change in dimension divided by the original value of the dimension - and can be expressed as

$\varepsilon = dL / L$

where

ε = strain (m/m, in/in)

dL = elongation or compression (offset) of object (m, in)

L = length of object (m, in)

Stress - σ:

Stress is force per unit area and can be expressed as

$\sigma = F / A$

where

σ = stress (N/m2, lb/in2, psi)

F = applied force (N, lb)

A = stress area of object (m2, in2)

Stress includes tensile stress, compressible stress, shearing stress, etc.

E, Young's modulus:

It can be expressed as:

E = stress / strain

  $= \sigma / \varepsilon$

  $= (F / A) / (dL / L)$

where

E = Young's Modulus of Elasticity (Pa, N/m2, lb/in2, psi) was named after the 18th-century English physicist Thomas Young.

Elasticity:

Elasticity is a property of an object or material indicating how it will restore it to its original shape after distortion. A spring is an example of an elastic object - when stretched, it exerts a restoring force which tends to bring it back to its original length (Figure 1).

Plasticity:

When the force is going beyond the elastic limit of material, it is into a plastic zone which means even when force is removed, the material will not return back to its original state (Figure 1).

Based on various experimental results, the following table lists some Young's modulus associated with different materials:

Nylon: 2.7 GPa

Concrete: 17-30 GPa

Glass fibers: 72 GPa

Copper: 117 GPa
Steel: 190-215 GPa
Diamond: 1220 GPa

Young's modules in the above table are ranked from soft material (low E) to stiff material (higher E)."

Professor James Andrews taught the author linear elasticity at the University of Iowa, and Professor Norman Jones taught him nonlinear dynamic plasticity at Massachusetts Institute of Technology. These two great academic mentors provided him the necessary foundation knowledge to understand these two important subjects in engineering.

Data collection:
Case A (the author) is a 73-year-old male with a 25-year history of T2D. He began collecting his carbs/sugar intake amount and post-meal walking steps on 7/1/2015. Since 7/15/2015, he has collected 6 data per day, 1 FPG, 3 PPG, carb/sugar, and post-meal walking steps. He utilized these data to conduct his prior research work on the subject of linear elastic glucose study (Reference 7).
In addition, on 5/5/2018, he started to use a continuous glucose monitoring (CGM) sensor device to collect 96 glucose data each day.

The timeframe from 7/1/2015 to 11/10/2020 is his "best-controlled" diabetes period, where his average daily glucoses is maintained at 116 mg/dL (<120 mg/dL). He named this as his "linear elastic zone" of diabetes health. It should also be noted that in 2010, his average glucose was 280 mg/dL and HbA1C was 10%, while taking three diabetes medications. Please note that the strong chemical interventions from various diabetes medications would seriously alter glucose physical behaviors. He called the period prior to 2015 as his "nonlinear plastic zone" of diabetes health.

Case B is a 73-year-old female with a 22-year history of T2D. She began to collect her glucose data via finger-piercing method (finger glucose) since 1/1/2014. However, she does not keep a detailed record of her diet and exercise. Both patients eat almost the same meals prepared by the author, except that she consumes more meat which partially affects her hyperlipidemia and hypertension conditions, not her diabetes conditions. From the viewpoint of this diabetes research, he decided to use 80% of the Case A's carbs/sugar amount for her and use 50% of the Case A's post-meal walking steps for her. She also began using the same brand of CGM device to collect her sensor glucose data at the same rate of 96 data per day since 1/1/2020.

Case C is a 47-year-old male with a 4-year history of T2D. He started to collect his glucose data using the same model of CGM sensor on 3/1/2020. Through a telephone interview, the author discovered that over the past 8-month period, his average carbs/ sugar intake amount is about the same amount as Case A, and his average post-meal walking steps is at ~25% level compared to Case A.

It should be mentioned here, other than Case A, who has collected a complete dataset of diet and exercise, Case B and Case C are using the best guess-estimated percentages of Case A's amount of diet and exercise. Therefore, these data differences would definitely create some degree of result deviation.

In order to maintain data consistency for a fair and accurate comparison, the author took the CGM sensor glucose data from Cases A, B, and C from 3/1/2020 through 11/10/2020 to use them in this analysis. The reason for using the sensor glucose data over finger glucose is because they are 13% to 18% higher. Therefore, the sensor data would be more conservative in terms of diabetes severity. Finally, the author calculated the two GH-modulus values via the approach of matching the predicted PPG values with the yardstick of measured PPG values.

It should be mentioned here that, regardless his various models developed and analytical methods used, his predicted glucose values have reached a 98.5% to 99.9% of accuracies in comparison with his measured glucoses.

Recent linear elastic glucose studies:
By utilizing the concept of Young's modulus and stress/strain, over the past 30 days, the author has initiated and engaged in this linear elastic glucose behaviors research. The following highlights outline the findings during this process.

First, he discovered that there is a "pseudo-linear" relationship existing between carbs & sugar intake amount and incremental PPG amount. Therefore, he defined a new glucose coefficient of GH.p-modulus for PPG.

Second, similar to Young's modulus relating to stiffness of engineering inorganic materials, he found that the GH.p-modulus is depended upon the patient's severity level of obesity and diabetes in terms of glucose sensitivity to carbs/sugar intake amount.

Third, comparable to the GH.p-modulus for PPG, he uncovered a similar pseudo-linear relationship existed between weight and FPG. Therefore, he defined another new glucose coefficient of GH.f-modulus for FPG.

Fourth, he inserted these two glucose coefficients, GH.p-modulus and GH.f-modulus, into the PPG prediction equation to remove the burden of collecting measured glucoses by patients.

Fifth, by experimenting and calculating many predicted PPG values over a variety of time length based on three patients with different health conditions, he finally revealed that GH.p-modulus seems to be "near-constant" or "pseudo-linearized" over a short period of 3 to 4 months. This short period is compatible with the known lifespan of red blood cells, which are living organic materials, that are different from engineering materials, such as steel or concrete. The same finding can also be observed in the monthly GH.p-modulus values from this study over the 10-months in the COVID-19 period.

Results:

His defined linear elastic glucose behaviors model is shown below:

Predicted PPG =
(0.97 * GH.f-modulus * Weight) +(GH.p-modulus * Carbs&sugar) - (post-meal walking k-steps * 5)

There are 5 figures in this article which demonstrate the following 4 comparisons over the COVID-19 period from 3/1/2020 to 11/10/2020.

Figure 2 depicts the relationship between weight and FPG via GH.f-modulus among the three cases. It also indicates the severity of obesity and diabetes of each case.

Figure 3 reflects carbs/sugar intake amount (grams) and post-meal walking (k-steps) of the three cases which are major influential factors relating to PPG via GH.p-modulus.

Figure 4 reveals the relationship between GH.p-modules and PPG among the three cases. It indicates that the magnitudes of GH.p-modulus is proportional to PPG values.

Figure 5 demonstrates graphically the comparison between GH.f-modules and GH.p-modules. GH.f-modules indicates the severity of obesity of each patient, where Case C is considered extremely obese, Case B is over-weight, and Case A is normal weight. GH.p-modules indicates the severity of diabetes of each case, Case A (3.6) is the most severe diabetes patient, Case B (2.6) is a moderate diabetes patient, and Case C (1.0) has the least severity of diabetes. More precisely, GH.p-modulus shows the relationship between diabetes severity (i.e. PPG sensitivity) and glucose sensitivity to carbs/sugar intake amount under the assumption of constant level of exercise for one specific patient. A variety of food is more complicated than an assortment of exercises, because it is difficult for people to change their daily routines.

Figure 6 indicates that the values of both (Incremental PPG) and (Carbs * GH.p-modulus) are almost equal, for the three clinical cases, during the COVID-19 period. This has further proved the linearity of elastic glucose behaviors among different patients.

The consolidated diagram of Figure 7 shows a complicated presentation of multiple components and a variety of results. It is a four-dimensional chart that illustrates the PPG prediction via carbs/sugar and post-meal walking under the influence of the glucose coefficient, GH.p-modulus, for three clinical cases during this timeframe. This figure has demonstrated the complicated results of this study in a single diagram.

Conclusions:

The research of the linear elastic glucose behaviors theory summarizes all of his previous findings from Parts 1 through 7. This article utilizes the clinical cases with different severities of obesity and diabetes.

Through different weights along with differing FPG, the author calculates the GH.f-modulus values for each patient which indicates the relative severity between obesity and diabetes.

Furthermore, through the linearity relationship or the linear indication of GH.p-modulus between incremental PPG and carbs/sugar intake amount, he can connect the complicated components of cars/sugar, exercise, weight or FPG into his final predicted PPG equation.

His developed linear elastic glucose theory inspired by his previously acquired knowledge of engineering theory of elasticity which has been proven useful for diabetes control. These research results from the biomedical linearity situations probably are applicable for ~80% of worldwide diabetes patients. However, for a smaller amount of diabetes patients' hyperglycemia situations, ~20% of the total population whose glucose frequently exceed 200 mg/dL level, a nonlinear plastic theory may need to be developed and then applied to these extreme situations.

References:

1. Hsu, Gerald C., eclaireMD Foundation, USA, No. 310: "Biomedical research methodology based on GH-Method: math-physical medicine"

2. Hsu, Gerald C., eclaireMD Foundation, USA, No. 345: "Application of linear equations to predict sensor and finger based postprandial plasma glucoses and daily glucoses for pre-virus, virus, and total periods using GH-Method: math-physical medicine"

3. Hsu, Gerald C., eclaireMD Foundation, USA, No. 97: "A simplified yet accurate linear equation of PPG prediction model for T2D patients (GH-Method: math-physical medicine)"

4. Hsu, Gerald C., eclaireMD Foundation, USA, No. 99: "Application of linear equation-based PPG prediction model for four T2D clinic cases (GH-Method: math-physical medicine)"

5. Hsu, Gerald C., eclaireMD Foundation, USA, No. 339: "Self-recovery of pancreatic beta cell's insulin secretion based on 10+ years annualized data of food, exercise, weight, and glucose using GH-Method: math-physical medicine)

6. Hsu, Gerald C., eclaireMD Foundation, USA, No. 340: "A neural communication model between brain and internal organs, specifically stomach, liver, and pancreatic beta cells based on PPG waveforms of 131 liquid egg meals and 124 solid egg meals)

7. Hsu, Gerald C., eclaireMD Foundation, USA, No. 349: "Using Math-Physics Medicine to Predict FPG"

8. Hsu, Gerald C., eclaireMD Foundation, USA, No. 264: "Community and Family Medicine via Doctors without distance: Using a simple glucose control card to assist T2D patients in remote rural areas (GH-Method: math-physical medicine)"

9. Hsu, Gerald C., eclaireMD Foundation, USA, No. 346: "Linear relationship between carbohydrates & sugar intake amount and incremental PPG amount via engineering strength of materials using GH-Method: math-physical medicine, Part 1"

10. Hsu, Gerald C., eclaireMD Foundation, USA, No. 349: "Investigation on GH modulus of linear elastic glucose with two diabetes patients data using GH-Method: math-physical medicine, Part 2"

11. Hsu, Gerald C., eclaireMD Foundation, USA, No. 349: "Investigation of GH modulus on the linear elastic glucose behavior based on three diabetes patients' data using the GH-Method: math-physical medicine, Part 3"

12. Hsu, Gerald C., eclaireMD Foundation, USA, No. 356: "Coefficient of GH.f-modulus in the linear elastic fasting plasma glucose behavior study based on health data of three diabetes patients using the GH-Method: math-physical medicine, Part 4 "

13. Hsu, Gerald C., eclaireMD Foundation, USA, No. 357: "High accuracy of predicted postprandial plasma glucose using two coefficients of GH.f-modulus and GH.p-modulus from linear elastic glucose behavior theory based on GH-Method: math-physical medicine, Part 5"

14. Hsu, Gerald C., eclaireMD Foundation, USA, No. 339: "Self-recovery of pancreatic beta cell's insulin secretion based on 10+ years annualized data of food, exercise, weight, and glucose using GH-Method: math-physical medicine"

15. Hsu, Gerald C., eclaireMD Foundation, USA, No. 358: "Improvement on the prediction accuracy of postprandial plasma glucose using two biomedical coefficients of GH-modulus from linear elastic glucose theory based on GH-Method: math-physical medicine, Part 6"

16. Hsu, Gerald C., eclaireMD Foundation, USA, No. 359: "High glucose predication accuracy of postprandial plasma glucose and fasting plasma glucose during the COVID-19 period using two glucose coefficients of GH-modulus from linear elastic glucose theory based on GH-Method: math-physical medicine, Part 7"

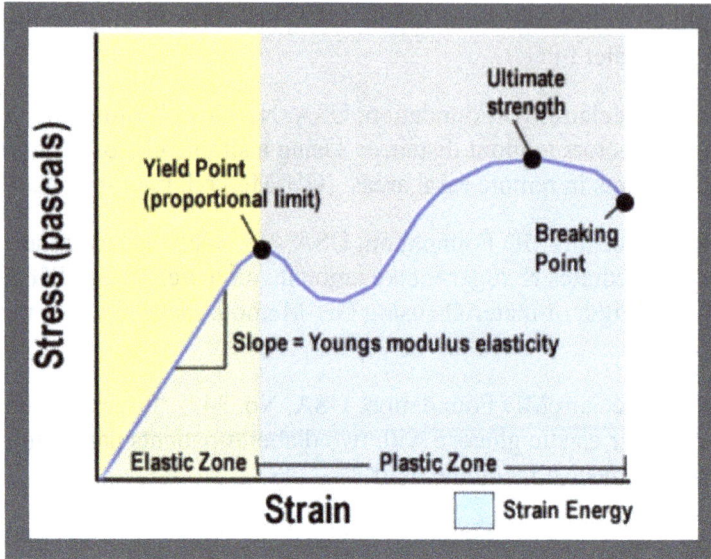

Figure 1: Stress-Strain-Young's modulus, Elastic Zone vs. Plastic Zone

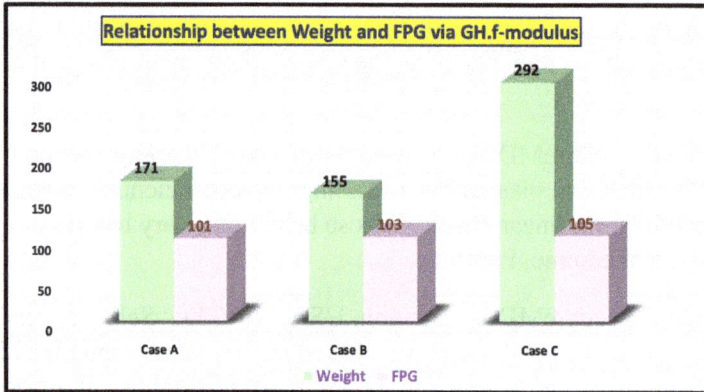

Figure 2: Relationship between weight and FPG via GH.f-modulus during COVID-19 period (3/1/2020 - 11/10/2020)

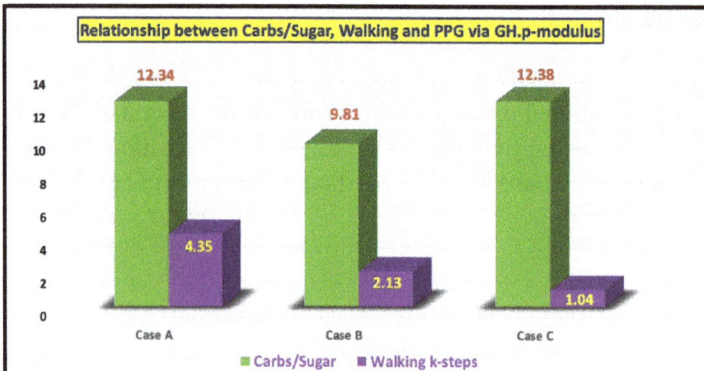

Figure 3: Carbs/sugar and post-meal walking k-steps during COVID-19 period (3/1/2020 - 11/10/2020)

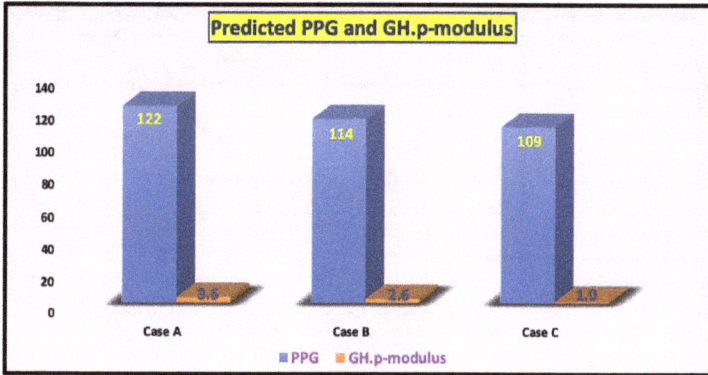

Figure 4: Relationship between Predicted PPG and GH.p-modulus during COVID-19 period (3/1/2020 - 11/10/2020)

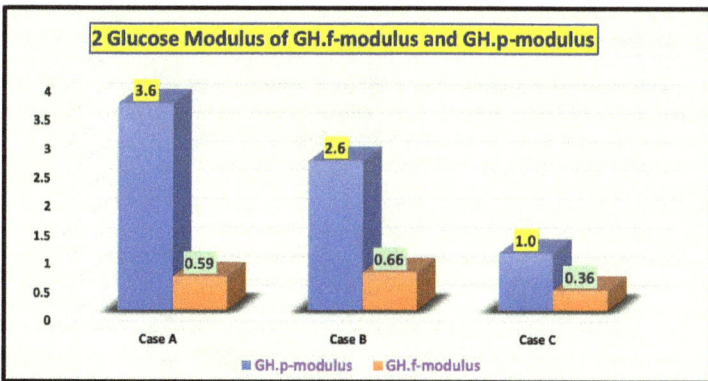

Figure 5: 2 Glucose coefficients of GH.f-modulus and GH.p-modulus during COVID-19 period (3/1/2020 - 11/10/2020)

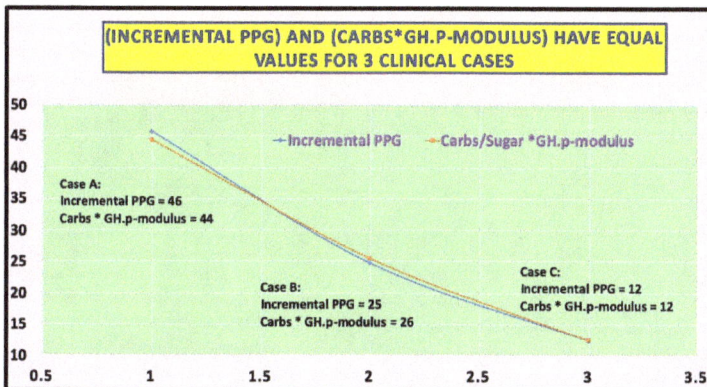

*Figure 6: (Incremental PPG) and (Carbs * GH.p-modulus) have equal values of three clinical cases during COVID-19 period (3/1/2020 - 11/10/2020)*

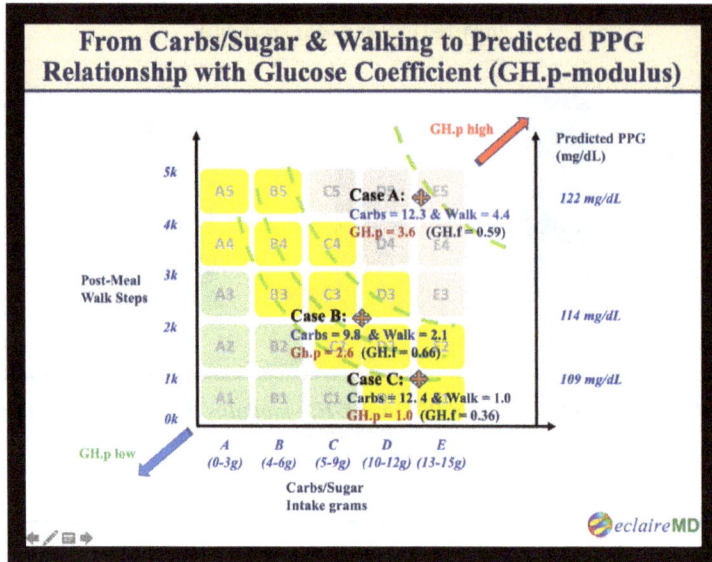

Figure 7: A 4-dimensional chart shows that PPG prediction via carbs/sugar and post-meal walking with Glucose coefficient of GH.p-modulus of 3 clinical cases during COVID-19 period (3/1/2020 - 11/10/2020)

Postprandial plasma glucose lower and upper boundary study using two glucose coefficients of GH-modulus from linear elastic glucose theory based on GH-Method: math-physical medicine, Part 9 (No. 361)

Gerald C. Hsu
eclaireMD Foundation, USA
11/11-13/2020

Abstract:

This article is Part 9 of the author's linear elastic glucose behavior study, which focuses on searching for an applicable data range of two glucose coefficients of both GH.f-modules and GH.p-modules via lower-bound and upper-bounds of predicted postprandial plasma glucose (PPG) values which would be useful to most type 2 diabetes (T2D) patients.

The linear elastic glucose behavior equation is:

Predicted PPG =
(0.97 * GH.f-modulus * Weight) +(GH.p-modulus * Carbs&sugar) - (post-meal walking k-steps * 5)

This equation is useful in predicting PPG values and helping patients with their diabetes control.

Here is the step-by-step PPG boundary analysis of the eight standard cases using linear elastic glucose theory as described in this paper and References 10 through 17:

Baseline PPG has only two values, i.e. using lower bound of FPG 100*0.97 = 97, and upper bound of FPG 150*0.97 =146
plus carbs/sugar intake amount's lower-bound of 10 grams of carbs/sugar intake: 97+10*GH.p 2.0 = 97+20 = 117 mg/dL, and higher bound of 25 grams of carbs/sugar intake: 146 + 25*6.0 = 146+150 = 296 mg/dL
minus post-meal walking k-steps' lower-bound of 4K steps: -5*4 = - 20 = 117-20 =97 mg/dL, and higher bound of 1K steps: -5*1 = -5 = 296-5 = 291 mg/dL
Therefore, the boundary of *predicted PPG* shows data is located within the numerical range of lower bound of 97 mg/dL & upper bound of 291 mg/dL.

Resuts of Boundary Analysis	Lower-Bound	Upper-Bound
BMI	25	35
Height (inch)	64	69
Weight (pound)	146	237
FPG (mg/dL)	100	150
GH.f-modulus	0.42	1.03
Baseline PPG 9mg/dL)	97	146
GH.p-modulus	2.0	6.0
Carbs/Sugar (standard gram)	10	25
Carbs/Sugar (extreme gram)	10	50
Carbs *GH.p (standard gram)	20	150
Carbs *GH.p (extreme gram)	20	300
Walking (standard k-steps)	1	4
Walking (extreme k-steps)	1	5
Predicted PPG (standard case)	97	276
Predicted PPG (extreme case)	92	475

The author has demonstrated the biomedical meaning and data sensitivity of these two glucose coefficients of GH.f-modulus and GH.p-modulus. From clinical viewpoints, the applicable glucose data range using the calculated lower and upper bounds of PPG values for the eight standard cases seems reasonable.

Introduction:

This article is Part 9 of the author's linear elastic glucose behavior study, which focuses on searching for an applicable data range of two glucose coefficients of both GH.f-modules and GH.p-modules via lower-bound and upper-bounds of predicted postprandial plasma glucose (PPG) values which would be useful to most type 2 diabetes (T2D) patients.

Methods:

Background:
To learn more about the author's GH-Method: math-physical medicine (MPM) methodology, readers can refer to his article to understand his developed MPM analysis method in Reference 1.

Highlights of his related research & Engineering theory of elasticity:
The readers can view the details of his previous research work related to this subject in the Reference. He would like to present again the linear elastic equation of the predicted PPG with two glucose coefficients of both GH.f-modules and GH.p-modules:

Predicted PPG =
*(0.97 * GH.f-modulus * Weight) +(GH.p-modulus * Carbs&sugar) - (post-meal walking k-steps * 5)*

Where
fasting plasma glucose (FPG)
= Weight * GH.f-modulus

By using this equation, a patient only needs the input data of body weight, carbs &
sugar intake amount, and post-meal walking steps in order to calculate the predicted
PPG without obtaining any measured glucose data.

Linear elastic glucose behaviors:
By utilizing the concept of Young's modulus with stress and strain, which the author
learned from engineering schools, he has initiated and engaged this linear elastic
glucose behaviors research since 10/14/2020. The following paragraphs describe his
research findings during the past month:

First, he discovered that there is a "pseudo-linear" relationship existed between carbs
& sugar intake amount and incremental PPG amount. Based on this finding, he
defined his first glucose coefficient of GH.p-modulus for PPG.

Second, similar to Young's modulus relating to stiffness of engineering inorganic
materials, he found that the GH.p-modulus is depended upon the patient's severity
level of obesity and diabetes, i.e. health conditions.

Third, comparable to GH.p-modulus for PPG, he uncovered a similar pseudo-linear
relationship existing between weight and FPG in 2017. Therefore, he defined his
second glucose coefficient of GH.f-modulus for FPG.

Fourth, he inserted these two glucose coefficients, GH.p-modulus and GH.f-modulus,
into the PPG prediction equation to remove the burden of collecting measured glucoses
by patients.

Fifth, by experimenting and calculating many predicted PPG values over a variety of
time length from different diabetes patients with different health conditions, he finally
revealed that GH.p-modulus seems to be "near-constant" or "pseudo-linearized"
over a short period of 3 to 4 months. This short period is compatible with the known
lifespan of red blood cells, which are living organic cells, that are different from the
engineering inorganic materials, such as steel or concrete. The same conclusion was
also observed using the monthly GH.p-modulus data from one particular patient during
the 2020 COVID-19 period.

Sixth, he used three clinical cases during the 2020 COVID-19 period to delve
into the hidden characteristics of the physical parameters and their biomedical
relationships. More importantly, through the comparison study in Part 7, he was able
to identify more biomedical interpretations of his two defined glucose coefficients of
GH.p-modulus and GH.f-modulus.

Data processing in this article:
First, he used the average height of a US male (5'9") and US female (5'4") and two

BMI values, 25 for normal weight and 35 for obesity, to separate his hypothetical data into four general groups, i.e. normal male, obese male, normal female, and obese female. He then used two different diabetes levels, normal FPG at 100 mg/dL and diabetic FPG at 150 mg/dL, to further separate them into eight standard cases.

Second, he calculated the first glucose coefficient of GH.f-modulus using the following formula:

GH.f-modulus = FPG / Weight

In this way, he was able to obtain eight different GH.f-modulus values which are corresponding to eight individual standard cases.

Third, he calculated the baseline PPG value using the following formula:

Baseline PPG
= 0.97 * FPG
= 0.97 * Weight * GH.f-modulus

He noticed from his calculated results that due to his specific definition of standard cases, there are only two fixed values of Baseline PPG which are 97 mg/dL for a non-diabetic person, and 146 mg/dL for a diabetic person, regardless of gender and weight.

Fourth, he selected two extreme-end values of the GH.p-modulus, i.e. 2.0 for the case where glucose is quite insensitive to carbs/sugar intake amount (i.e. non-severe diabetes) and 6.0 for the case where glucose is extremely sensitive to carbs/sugar intake amount (i.e. severe diabetes), in calculating the PPG influences from food intake. He believes that, in reality, for most diabetes patients the GH.p-modulus values are within the range between 2.0 to 6.0. Furthermore, he selected four levels of carbs/sugar intake amounts, i.e. 10g, 15g, 20g, and 25g for his calculation using either 2.0 or 6.0 for GH.p-modulus values. He assumed that for most diabetes patients health concerns, their average carbs/sugar intake amount should be under 25 grams per meal. Otherwise, their diabetes conditions would be very difficult to control via a lifestyle management approach unless they are on numerous medications. For any patient who does follow the author's suggestion regarding diet, then this carbs/sugar intake amount recommendation would be very helpful to him or her. From a mathematical viewpoint, in the later part of this article, the author has also conducted an extreme "stress test" of 50 grams per meal of carbs/sugar intake amount which would push this hypothetical patient's PPG level up to 475 mg/dL. This hyperglycemia situation does happen to some severe diabetes patients.

Fifth, he calculated the increased PPG amount due to food by using the following formula:

Increased PPG by food
= Carbs/sugar * GH.p-modulus

Sixth, he selected four exercise levels of post-meal waking steps of 1k, 2k, 3k, and 4k. In his extreme "stress test", he also added in a 5k walking steps of exercise to further reduce his predicted PPG by an additional 5 mg/dL. Over the past 7 years, the author's average post-meal walking is approximately 4,500 steps. Therefore, he does understand how much of an effort is needed to maintain this good habit.

Seventh, he calculated the decreased PPG amount due to exercise by using the following formula:

Decreased PPG by walking
*= Walking k-steps * 5*

Eighth, he could calculate the predicted PPG by using the following formula:

Predicted PPG
= Baseline PPG + PPG by carbs/sugar - PPG by walking
= (0.97 * Weight * GH.f-modulus) + (Carbs/sugar * GH.p-modulus) - (Walking k-steps * 5)

Finally, the ninth step is to use these 256 separated calculation groups (256 = 8*2*4*4) from his detailed calculations to figure out the PPG "boundaries", i.e. the lower-bound and upper-bound of the predicted PPG values. He then checked those boundaries against the realistic biomedical boundary of clinical diabetes conditions.

In this study, he used Excel to conduct his grouping boundary calculations instead of writing a customized software for this task. After obtaining more proof, evidence, and validation, he would consider in transforming the above steps and calculations into an APP program for the mobile phones for use by a larger pool of diabetes patients.

Results:

Figure 1 shows the data table and calculation table of the eight standard cases and three clinical cases based on the above described method.

Figure 2 depicts the bar-chart comparison of 11 different glucose coefficient of GH.f-modulus from eight hypothetical standard cases and three clinical cases.

Figure 3 illustrates the detailed data table of the calculations using food and exercise in obtaining the predicted PPG values of the eight standard cases. The calculation is straightforward but it is also the most tedious part.

Figure 4 reflects the upper and lower bounds of the predicated PPG values of eight standard cases. Each standard case contains 32 (=2 GH.p * 4 carbs/sugar * 4 walking) sets of detailed calculations. Nevertheless, he chose the lowest PPG value of 97 mg/dL as the lower-bound value and the highest PPG value of 291 mg/dL as the upper-bound value for these eight hypothetical standard cases. In this diagram, he also performed an extreme "stress test" by increasing the carbs/sugar intake amount to 50 grams for pushing the PPG value or by increasing the walking steps to 5k steps for reducing the PPG value. This stress test has provided a new lower-bound PPG of 92 mg/dL by walking 5k steps and a new upper-bound PPG of 475 mg/dL by consuming 50 grams of carbs/sugar per meal. Based on the author's personal experience and his collected glucose record regarding his diabetes conditions, these lower bound of 97 mg/dL and upper bound of 271 mg/dL are quite close to his own collected glucose data range. By observing other T2D patients, the lower bound of 92 mg/dL and upper bound of 475 mg/dL for extreme stress test are also feasible. In Figure 5, he shows his past PPG record of post-lunch PPG of 280 mg/dL from consuming a local island food and sweets in Hawaii in May of 2018. This extreme high PPG value must accompany with a higher GH.p-modulus value which also reveals his glucose's super sensitivity to carbs/sugar intake at that time. In other words, this GH.p-modulus reflects the overall health conditions of his liver and pancreatic beta cells at that time.

In Figure 6, he applied a special 4-dimensional presentation diagram developed by him as described in Reference 17 to graphically present these four extreme PPG locations together in terms of their close relationships with carbs/sugar and post-meal walking along with the hidden relationship with GH.f-modulus (weight and FPG) and GH.p-modulus (diet and exercise). This special 4-dimensional diagram can clearly present the four PPG boundary points.

Some results in Figure 7 are recopied from Part 1 through Part 8 of his research work (References 10 through 17). The three clinical cases are different from the eight standard cases since each case has a unique set of input data (weight, FPG, carbs, walking, GH-modulus) and output data (GH-modulus and PPG) instead of the eight standard cases constituting a "numerical range" of input and output data. As a comparison, the three clinical cases data are very well located within the data range (i.e., from lower bound to upper bound) of the eight standard cases. It should be pointed out that the results from the clinical cases are more skewed toward the lower bound side of the eight standard cases, which means that their diabetes condition are quite well under control.

Figure 8 shows the summarized results of lower-bound and upper-bound of predicted PPG boundary analysis.

Conclusions:

The linear elastic glucose behavior equation is:

Predicted PPG =
(0.97 * GH.f-modulus * Weight) +(GH.p-modulus * Carbs&sugar) - (post-meal walking k-steps * 5)

This equation is useful in predicting PPG values and helping patients with their diabetes control.

Here is the step-by-step PPG boundary analysis of the eight standard cases using linear elastic glucose theory as described in this paper and References 10 through 17:

Baseline PPG has only two values, i.e. using lower bound of FPG 100*0.97 = 97, and upper bound of FPG 150*0.97 =146
plus carbs/sugar intake amount's lower-bound of 10 grams of carbs/sugar intake: 97+10*GH.p 2.0 = 97+20 = 117 mg/dL, and higher bound of 25 grams of carbs/sugar intake: 146 + 25*6.0 = 146+150 = 296 mg/dL
minus post-meal walking k-steps' lower-bound of 4K steps: -5*4 = - 20 = 117-20 =97 mg/dL, and higher bound of 1K steps: -5*1 = -5 = 296-5 = 291 mg/dL
Therefore, the boundary of predicted PPG shows data is located within the numerical range of lower bound of 97 mg/dL & upper bound of 291 mg/dL.

The author has demonstrated the biomedical meaning and data sensitivity of these two glucose coefficients of GH.f-modulus and GH.p-modulus. From clinical viewpoints, the applicable glucose data range using the calculated lower and upper bounds of PPG values for the eight standard cases seems reasonable.

References:

1. Hsu, Gerald C., eclaireMD Foundation, USA, No. 310: "Biomedical research methodology based on GH-Method: math-physical medicine"

2. Hsu, Gerald C., eclaireMD Foundation, USA, No. 345: "Application of linear equations to predict sensor and finger based postprandial plasma glucoses and daily glucoses for pre-virus, virus, and total periods using GH-Method: math-physical medicine"

3. Hsu, Gerald C., eclaireMD Foundation, USA, No. 97: "A simplified yet accurate linear equation of PPG prediction model for T2D patients (GH-Method: math-physical medicine)"

4. Hsu, Gerald C., eclaireMD Foundation, USA, No. 99: "Application of linear equation-based PPG prediction model for four T2D clinic cases (GH-Method: math-physical medicine)"

5. Hsu, Gerald C., eclaireMD Foundation, USA, No. 339: "Self-recovery of pancreatic beta cell's insulin secretion based on 10+ years annualized data of food, exercise, weight, and glucose using GH-Method: math-physical medicine)

6. Hsu, Gerald C., eclaireMD Foundation, USA, No. 340: "A neural communication model between brain and internal organs, specifically stomach, liver, and pancreatic beta cells based on PPG waveforms of 131 liquid egg meals and 124 solid egg meals)

7. Hsu, Gerald C., eclaireMD Foundation, USA, No. 349: "Using Math-Physics Medicine to Predict FPG"

8. Hsu, Gerald C., eclaireMD Foundation, USA, No. 264: "Community and Family Medicine via Doctors without distance: Using a simple glucose control card to assist T2D patients in remote rural areas (GH-Method: math-physical medicine)"

9. Hsu, Gerald C., eclaireMD Foundation, USA, No. 339: "Self-recovery of pancreatic beta cell's insulin secretion based on 10+ years annualized data of food, exercise, weight, and glucose using GH-Method: math-physical medicine"

10. Hsu, Gerald C., eclaireMD Foundation, USA, No. 346: "Linear relationship between carbohydrates & sugar intake amount and incremental PPG amount via engineering strength of materials using GH-Method: math-physical medicine, Part 1"

11. Hsu, Gerald C., eclaireMD Foundation, USA, No. 349: "Investigation on GH modulus of linear elastic glucose with two diabetes patients data using GH-Method: math-physical medicine, Part 2"

12. Hsu, Gerald C., eclaireMD Foundation, USA, No. 349: "Investigation of GH modulus on the linear elastic glucose behavior based on three diabetes patients' data using the GH-Method: math-physical medicine, Part 3"

13. Hsu, Gerald C., eclaireMD Foundation, USA, No. 356: "Coefficient of GH.f-modulus in the linear elastic fasting plasma glucose behavior study based on health data of three diabetes patients using the GH-Method: math-physical medicine, Part 4 "

14. Hsu, Gerald C., eclaireMD Foundation, USA, No. 357: "High accuracy of predicted postprandial plasma glucose using two coefficients of GH.f-modulus and GH.p-modulus from linear elastic glucose behavior theory based on GH-Method: math-physical medicine, Part 5"

15. Hsu, Gerald C., eclaireMD Foundation, USA, No. 358: "Improvement on the prediction accuracy of postprandial plasma glucose using two biomedical coefficients of GH-modulus from linear elastic glucose theory based on GH-Method: math-physical medicine, Part 6"

16. Hsu, Gerald C., eclaireMD Foundation, USA, No. 359: "High glucose predication accuracy of postprandial plasma glucose and fasting plasma glucose during the COVID-19 period using two glucose coefficients of GH-modulus from linear elastic glucose theory based on GH-Method: math-physical medicine, Part 7"

17. Hsu, Gerald C., eclaireMD Foundation, USA, No. 360: "Investigation of two glucose coefficients of GH.f-modulus and GH.p-modulus based on data of 3 clinical cases during COVID-19 period using linear elastic glucose theory of GH-Method: math-physical medicine, Part 8"

	Case 1	Case 2	Case 3	Case 4	Case 5	Case 6	Case 7	Case 8	Case A	Case B	Case C
Obesity	Normal Men	Normal Men	Obese Men	Obese Men	Normal Women	Normal Women	Obese Women	Obese Women	Male	Female	Young
Diabetes	No Diabetes	With Diabetes	No Diabetes	With Diabetes	No Diabetes	With Diabetes	No Diabetes	With Diabetes	T2D	T2D	Obesity
Avg. Height (")	69	69	69	69	64	64	64	64	69	64	71
BMI	25	25	35	35	25	25	35	35	25	27	41
Weight (lbs)	169	169	237	237	146	146	204	204	171	155	292
FPG (mg/dL)	100	150	100	150	100	150	100	150	101	103	105
GH.f-modulus	0.59	0.89	0.42	0.61	0.69	1.03	0.49	0.74	0.59	0.66	0.36
Baseline PPG	97	146	97	146	97	146	97	146	98	100	102
GH.p-modulus	2.0	6.0	2.0	6.0	2.0	6.0	2.0	6.0	3.6	2.6	1.0
Carbs/Sugar (g)	10	10	15	15	20	20	25	25	12.34	9.81	12.38
Carbs * GH.p	20	60	30	90	40	120	50	150	44	26	12

	Case 1	Case 2	Case 3	Case 4	Case 5	Case 6	Case 7	Case 8	Case A	Case B	Case C
Carbs/Sugar (g)	10	10	15	15	20	20	25	25	12.34	9.81	12.38
Baseline + Carbs	117	206	127	236	137	266	147	296	142	125	114
PPG from 1K walk	-5	-5	-5	-5	-5	-5	-5	-5	-22	-11	-5
Predicted PPG (1K)	112	201	122	231	132	261	142	291	121	115	109
PPG from 2K walk	-10	-10	-10	-10	-10	-10	-10	-10	-22	-11	-5
Predicted PPG (2K)	107	196	117	226	127	256	137	286	121	115	109
PPG from 4K walk	-20	-20	-20	-20	-20	-20	-20	-20	-22	-11	-5
Predicted PPG (4K)	97	186	107	216	117	246	127	276	121	115	109

	Case 1	Case 2	Case 3	Case 4	Case 5	Case 6	Case 7	Case 8	Case A	Case B	Case C
Gender	Man	Man	Man	Man	Woman	Woman	Woman	Woman	Male	Female	Young
Obesity	No Obesity	No Obesity	Obesity	Obesity	No Obesity	No Obesity	Obesity	Obesity	No Obesity	No Obesity	Obesity
Diabetes	No Diabetes	Diabetes	No Diabetes	Diabetes	No Diabetes	Diabetes	No Diabetes	Diabetes	Pre-Diabetes	Pre-Diabetes	Pre-Diabetes
Weight (lbs)	169	169	237	237	146	146	204	204	171	155	292
FPG (mg/dL)	100	150	100	150	100	150	100	150	101	103	105
Carbs/Sugar (g)	10	10	15	15	20	20	25	25	12.34	9.81	12.38

	Case 1	Case 2	Case 3	Case 4	Case 5	Case 6	Case 7	Case 8	Case A	Case B	Case C
Predicted PPG (1K)	112	201	122	231	132	261	142	291	121	115	109
Predicted PPG (2K)	107	196	117	226	127	256	137	286	121	115	109
Predicted PPG (4K)	97	186	107	216	117	246	127	276	121	115	109

	Case 1	Case 2	Case 3	Case 4	Case 5	Case 6	Case 7	Case 8	Case A	Case B	Case C
Predicted PPG (2.3K)	105	194	115	224	125	254	135	284	121	115	109

	Case 1	Case 2	Case 3	Case 4	Case 5	Case 6	Case 7	Case 8	Case A	Case B	Case C
GH.f-modulus	0.6	0.9	0.4	0.6	0.7	1.0	0.5	0.7	0.59	0.66	0.36
GH.p-modulus	2.0	6.0	2.0	6.0	2.0	6.0	2.0	6.0	3.6		

Stitch It!

Figure 1: Data table and calculation table of 8 standard cases and 3 clinical cases

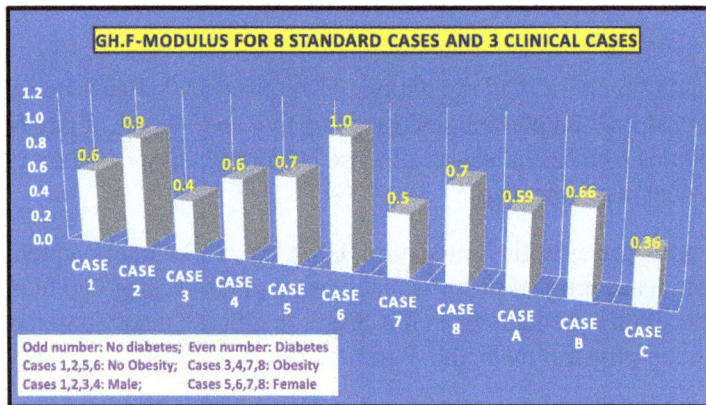

GH.F-MODULUS FOR 8 STANDARD CASES AND 3 CLINICAL CASES

CASE 1: 0.6
CASE 2: 0.9
CASE 3: 0.4
CASE 4: 0.6
CASE 5: 0.7
CASE 6: 1.0
CASE 7: 0.5
CASE 8: 0.7
CASE A: 0.59
CASE B: 0.66
CASE C: 0.36

Odd number: No diabetes; Even number: Diabetes
Cases 1,2,5,6: No Obesity; Cases 3,4,7,8: Obesity
Cases 1,2,3,4: Male; Cases 5,6,7,8: Female

Figure 2: Different Glucose coefficients of GH.f-modulus for 8 standard cases and 3 clinical cases

Figure 3 data table (8 standard cases):

GH.p-modulus	2.0	2.0	2.0	2.0	6.0	6.0	6.0	6.0	Case 1
Carbs/Sugar (g)	10	15	20	25	10	15	20	25	Man Walking
Predicted PPG (1K)	112	122	132	142	152	182	212	242	1.0
Predicted PPG (2K)	107	117	127	137	147	177	207	237	2.0
Predicted PPG (3K)	102	112	122	132	142	172	202	232	3.0
Predicted PPG (4K)	97	107	117	127	137	167	197	227	4.0
GH.p-modulus	2.0	2.0	2.0	2.0	6.0	6.0	6.0	6.0	Case 2
Carbs/Sugar (g)	10	15	20	25	10	15	20	25	Man Walking
Predicted PPG (1K)	161	171	181	191	201	231	261	291	1.0
Predicted PPG (2K)	156	166	176	186	196	226	256	286	2.0
Predicted PPG (3K)	151	161	171	181	191	221	251	281	3.0
Predicted PPG (4K)	146	156	166	176	186	216	246	276	4.0
GH.p-modulus	2.0	2.0	2.0	2.0	6.0	6.0	6.0	6.0	Case 3
Carbs/Sugar (g)	10	15	20	25	10	15	20	25	Man Walking
Predicted PPG (1K)	112	122	132	142	152	182	212	242	1.0
Predicted PPG (2K)	107	117	127	137	147	177	207	237	2.0
Predicted PPG (3K)	102	112	122	132	142	172	202	232	3.0
Predicted PPG (4K)	97	107	117	127	137	167	197	227	4.0
GH.p-modulus	2.0	2.0	2.0	2.0	6.0	6.0	6.0	6.0	Case 4
Carbs/Sugar (g)	10	15	20	25	10	15	20	25	Man Walking
Predicted PPG (1K)	161	171	181	191	201	231	261	291	1.0
Predicted PPG (2K)	156	166	176	186	196	226	256	286	2.0
Predicted PPG (3K)	151	161	171	181	191	221	251	281	3.0
Predicted PPG (4K)	146	156	166	176	186	216	246	276	4.0
GH.p-modulus	2.0	2.0	2.0	2.0	6.0	6.0	6.0	6.0	Case 5
Carbs/Sugar (g)	10	15	30	25	10	15	20	25	Woman Walking
Predicted PPG (1K)	112	122	132	142	152	182	212	242	1.0
Predicted PPG (2K)	107	117	127	137	147	177	207	237	2.0
Predicted PPG (3K)	102	112	122	132	142	172	202	232	3.0
Predicted PPG (4K)	97	107	117	127	137	167	197	227	4.0
GH.p-modulus	2.0	2.0	2.0	2.0	6.0	6.0	6.0	6.0	Case 6
Carbs/Sugar (g)	10	15	20	25	10	15	20	25	Woman Walking
Predicted PPG (1K)	161	171	181	191	201	231	261	291	1.0
Predicted PPG (2K)	156	166	176	186	196	226	256	286	2.0
Predicted PPG (3K)	151	161	171	181	191	221	251	281	3.0
Predicted PPG (4K)	146	156	166	176	186	216	246	276	4.0
GH.p-modulus	2.0	2.0	2.0	2.0	6.0	6.0	6.0	6.0	Case 7
Carbs/Sugar (g)	10	15	20	25	10	15	20	25	Woman Walking
Predicted PPG (1K)	112	122	132	142	152	182	212	242	1.0
Predicted PPG (2K)	107	117	127	137	147	177	207	237	2.0
Predicted PPG (3K)	102	112	122	132	142	172	202	232	3.0
Predicted PPG (4K)	97	107	117	127	137	167	197	227	4.0
GH.p-modulus	2.0	2.0	2.0	2.0	6.0	6.0	6.0	6.0	Case 9
Carbs/Sugar (g)	10	15	20	25	10	15	20	25	Woman Walking
Predicted PPG (1K)	161	171	181	191	201	231	261	391	1.0
Predicted PPG (2K)	156	166	176	186	196	226	256	286	2.0
Predicted PPG (3K)	151	161	171	181	191	221	251	281	3.0
Predicted PPG (4K)	146	156	166	176	186	216	246	276	4.0

Figure 3: Data table of food influences and predicted PPG for 8 standard cases

The Author's Case:	Formula	Lower-Bound	Upper-Bound
FPG	Author choice	100	150
Baseline PPG	= 0.97 * FPG	97	146
Carbs/Sugar	Author choice	10	25
GH.p-modulus	Author choice	2.0	6.0
+ Carbs/Sugar	= Carbs * GH.p	20	150
Walking K-steps	Author choice	1.0	4.0
- Walking	= K-steps * 5	-20	-5
Predicted PPG	=Baseline +Carbs-Walk	97	291
The Extreme Case:	Formula	Lower-Bound	Upper-Bound
FPG	Author choice	100	180
Baseline PPG	= 0.97 * FPG	97	175
Carbs/Sugar	Author choice	10	50
GH.p-modulus	Author choice	2.0	6.0
+ Carbs/Sugar	= Carbs * GH.p	20	300
Walking K-steps	Author choice	0.0	5.0
- Walking	= K-steps * 5	-25	0
Predicted PPG	=Baseline +Carbs-Walk	92	475

Figure 4: Lower-bound and Upper-bound of Predicted PPG values from 8 standard cases and the extreme "stress test" case

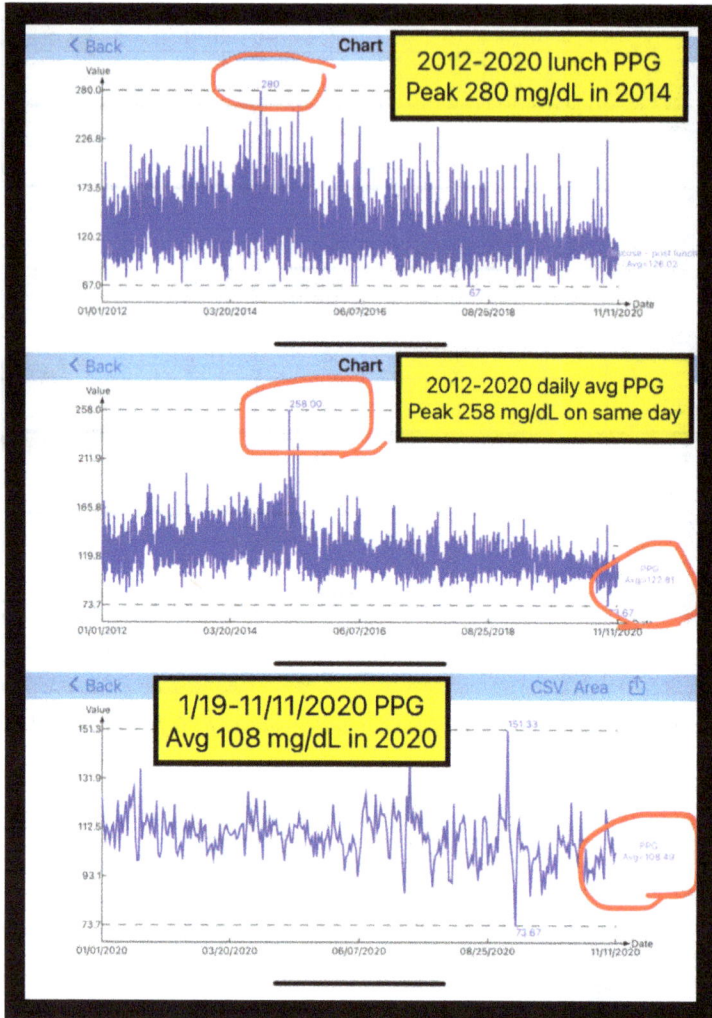

Figure 5: Clinical case A's hyperglycemia data example in May of 2015

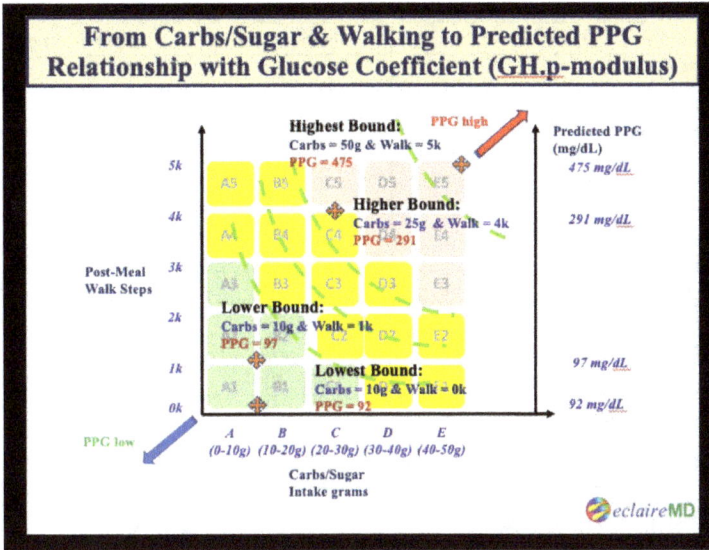

Figure 6: A special 4-dimensional representation of upper-bound and lower-bound of predicted PPG values, including carbs/sugar, walking, PPG, and the "hidden" GH.p-modulus

	Case A	Case B	Case C
Obesity	Male	Female	Young
Diabetes	T2D	T2D	Obesity
Avg. Height (")	69	64	71
BMI	25	27	41
Weight (lbs)	171	155	292
FPG (mg/dL)	101	103	105
GH.f-modulus	0.59	0.66	0.36
Baseline PPG	98	100	102
GH.p-modulus	3.6	2.6	1.0
Carbs/Sugar (g)	12.34	9.81	12.38
Carbs * GH.p	44	26	12
	Case A	Case B	Case C
Carbs/Sugar (g)	12.34	9.81	12.38
Baseline + Carbs	142	125	114
Walking K-steps	4.35	2.13	1.04
- PPG from Walk	-22	-11	-5
Predicted PPG	121	115	109

Figure 7: Predicted Glucose values of 3 clinical cases

Resuts of Boundary Analysis	Lower-Bound	Upper-Bound
BMI	25	35
Height (inch)	64	69
Weight (pound)	146	237
FPG (mg/dL)	100	150
GH.f-modulus	0.42	1.03
Baseline PPG 9mg/dL)	97	146
GH.p-modulus	2.0	6.0
Carbs/Sugar (standard gram)	10	25
Carbs/Sugar (extreme gram)	10	50
Carbs *GH.p (standard gram)	20	150
Carbs *GH.p (extreme gram)	20	300
Walking (standard k-steps)	1	4
Walking (extreme k-steps)	1	5
Predicted PPG (standard case)	97	276
Predicted PPG (extreme case)	92	475

Figure 8: Results of lower-bound and upper-bound of predicted PPG boundary analysis

Six international clinical cases demonstrating prediction accuracies of postprandial plasma glucoses and suggested methods for improvements using linear elastic glucose theory of GH-Method: math-physical medicine, Part 10 (No. 362)

Gerald C. Hsu (1)
eclaireMD Foundation, USA
Professor Than (2)
Myanmar
11/15/2020

Abstract:

This article is Part 10 of the author's linear elastic glucose behavior study. It focuses on validating his recently defined two glucose coefficients of GH.f-modulus and GH.p-modulus, while interpreting their biomedical meaning and correlations with chronic disease conditions, specifically, obesity and diabetes. In addition, this article illustrates the applicability of his developed predicted postprandial plasma glucose (PPG) equation through data from six international clinical cases. Hopefully, this linear elastic glucose model would be useful in real life applications to most of type 2 diabetes (T2D) patients worldwide on controlling their conditions.

Here is the step-by-step explanation of the predicted PPG equation from the six clinical cases using linear elastic glucose theory as described in References 10 through 18:

Baseline PPG equals to 97% of FPG value, or 97% * (weight * GH.f-Modulus).
Baseline PPG *plus* increased amount of PPG due to food, i.e. plus (carbs/sugar intake amount * GH.p-Modulus).
Baseline PPG plus *increased PPG due to food, and then subtracts reduction amount of PPG due to exercise, i.e. minus (post-meal walking k-steps * 5).*
The *Predicted PPG* equals to *Baseline PPG plus the food influences, and then subtracts the exercise influences.*

The linear elastic glucose equation is:

Predicted PPG =
*(0.97 * GH.f-modulus * Weight) +(GH.p-modulus * Carbs&sugar) - (post-meal walking k-steps * 5)*

By using this linear equation, a diabetes patient only needs the input data of body weight, carbs & sugar intake amount, and post-meal walking steps in order to calculate the predicted PPG value without obtaining any measured glucose data.

The biomedical interpretation of these two glucose coefficients are as follows:

When a patient's obesity is worsening (i.e. gaining weight), then the GH.f-Modulus would be lower; however, when the same patient's diabetes is worsening (FPG higher), then the GH.f-Modulus would be higher. Usually, a patient's weight and FPG are closely related to each other with a higher than 90% of correlation. Therefore, the combination in severity of both obesity and diabetes is reflected in the magnitude of GH.f-modules.

On the other hand, the situation of GH.p-Modulus is simpler which mainly shows a patient's glucose sensitivity to carbs/sugar intake amount (the higher the glucose sensitivity depicts worsening diabetes conditions). When a more severe diabetes patient who has a higher GH.p-Modulus consumes the same amount of carbs/sugar, his/her PPG value would be higher than a not-so-severe diabetes patient. This

GH.p-modulus also reflects the health state of pancreatic beta cells of a particular patient. GH.p-modulus (similar to Young's modulus in engineering) indicates the linear relationship between the carbs/sugar intake amount (similar to stress) and the incremental PPG amount (similar to strain) with different slopes for different patients.

The ultimate PPG value is determined by the combination of weight, FPG, carbs/sugar intake amount, post-meal walking steps, with two glucose coefficients of GH.f-Modulus, and GH.p-Modulus.

It should be mentioned here that different from engineering inorganic material which does not change during a long period of time, human blood contains millions organic living red blood cells which have an averaged lifespan of 115 to 120 days. Therefore, the glucose coefficients of GH.f-Modulus and GH.p-Modulus are "pseudo-constants" during a time span of 3 to 4 months, similar to the tested values of HbA1C. Giving his observed personal HbA1C data during the past 10 years with a change rate within 1% to 11%, the author guesses that these two glucose coefficients should have a similar change rate within 1% to 11% as well. The maximum 11% change rate of GH.p-Modulus from 3.6 to 4.0 would increase his predicted PPG value from 121 mg/dL to 127 mg/dL. In addition, both of weight reduction and glucose change are slow processes. A significant change usually takes a reasonable long period of time, such as years.

This study provides a quantitative proof with high precision from six clinical cases of obesity and diabetes conditions, either by adopting or rejecting the lifestyle management program. Linear elastic glucose theory and its associated predicted PPG equation have shown their power and applicability on diabetes control for a wide range of patients.

By adopting this theory and linear equation, the author is capable of providing customized quantitative advice and precise recommendations to three Myanmar patients on how to better control their obesity and T2D conditions. This chronic diseases control via a lifestyle management program using linear elastic glucose theory of GH-Method: math-physical medicine can indeed provide a solid scientific background to support the practical guidance as the branch of "Lifestyle Medicine".

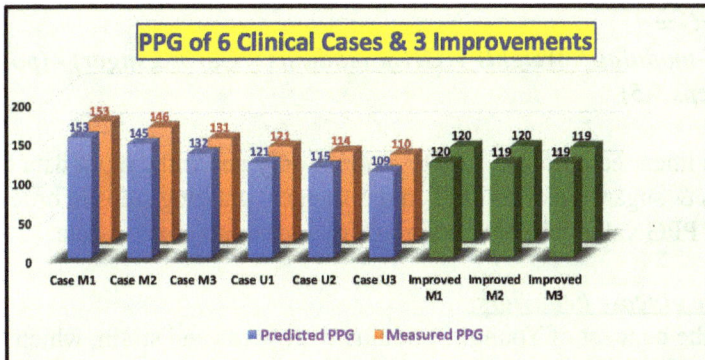

Introduction:

This article is Part 10 of the author's linear elastic glucose behavior study. It focuses on validating his recently defined two glucose coefficients of GH.f-modulus and GH.p-modulus, while interpreting their biomedical meaning and correlations with chronic disease conditions, specifically, obesity and diabetes. In addition, this article illustrates the applicability of his developed predicted postprandial plasma glucose (PPG) equation through data from six international clinical cases. Hopefully, this linear elastic glucose model would be useful in real life applications to most of type 2 diabetes (T2D) patients worldwide on controlling their conditions.

Methods:

Background:
To learn more about the author's GH-Method: math-physical medicine (MPM) methodology, readers can refer to his article to understand his developed MPM analysis method in Reference 1.

Highlights of the related research & Engineering theory of elasticity:
The readers can view the details of his previous research work related to this subject listed in the Reference section.

Here is the step-by-step explanation of the predicted PPG equation from the six clinical cases using linear elastic glucose theory as described in References 10 through 18:

Baseline PPG equals to 97% of FPG value, or 97% * (weight * GH.f-Modulus).
Baseline PPG **plus** increased amount of PPG due to food, i.e. plus (carbs/sugar intake amount * GH.p-Modulus).
Baseline PPG **plus** increased PPG due to food, and then **subtracts** reduction amount of PPG due to exercise, i.e. minus (post-meal walking k-steps * 5).
The **Predicted PPG** equals to **Baseline PPG plus the food influences, and then subtracts the exercise influences.**

The linear elastic glucose equation is:

*Predicted PPG =
(0.97 * GH.f-modulus * Weight) +(GH.p-modulus * Carbs&sugar) - (post-meal walking k-steps * 5)*

By using this linear equation, a diabetes patient only needs the input data of body weight, carbs & sugar intake amount, and post-meal walking steps in order to calculate the predicted PPG value without obtaining any measured glucose data.

Linear elastic glucose behaviors:
By utilizing the concept of Young's modulus with stress and strain, which the author learned from engineering schools, he has initiated and engaged this linear elastic glucose behaviors research since 10/14/2020. The following paragraphs describe his

research findings over the past month:

First, he discovered that there is a "pseudo-linear" relationship existed between carbs & sugar intake amount and incremental PPG amount. Based on this finding, he defined his first glucose coefficient of GH.p-modulus for PPG.

Second, similar to Young's modulus relating to stiffness of engineering inorganic materials, he found that the GH.p-modulus is depended upon the patient's severity level of diabetes, i.e. patient's glucose sensitivity on carbs/sugar intake amount.

Third, comparable to GH.p-modulus for PPG, he uncovered a similar pseudo-linear relationship existing between weight and FPG in 2017. Therefore, he defined his second glucose coefficient of GH.f-modulus as the FPG value divided by the weight value. This GH.f-modulus is related to the severity of both obesity and diabetes.

Fourth, he inserted these two glucose coefficients of GH.p-modulus and GH.f-modulus, into the predicted PPG equation to remove the burden of collecting measured glucoses by patients.

Fifth, by experimenting and calculating many predicted PPG values over a variety of time length from different diabetes patients with different health conditions, he finally revealed that GH.p-modulus seems to be "near-constant" or "pseudo-linearized" over a short period of 3 to 4 months. This short period is compatible with the known lifespan of red blood cells, which are living organic cells, that are different from the engineering inorganic materials, such as steel or concrete. The same conclusion was also observed using the monthly GH.p-modulus data from one particular patient during the 2020 COVID-19 period when his lifestyle became routine and stabilized.

Sixth, he used three US clinical cases during the 2020 COVID-19 period to delve into the hidden characteristics of the physical parameters and their biomedical relationships. More importantly, through the comparison study in Part 7, he found explainable biomedical interpretations of his two defined glucose coefficients of GH.p-modulus and GH.f-modulus.

Seventh, he conducted a PPG boundary analysis by discovering a lower-bound and an upper-bound of predicted PPG values for eight hypothetical standard cases and three US clinical cases. The derived numerical values of these two boundaries make sense from a biomedical viewpoint and also matched with the situations of the three US clinical cases. He even conducted two extreme stress tests, i.e. increasing carbs/ sugar intake amount to 50 grams per meal and boosting post-meal walking steps to 5k after each meal, to examine the impacts on the lower-bound and upper-bound of PPG values.

Clinical cases in this article:
He selected three clinical cases from Myanmar (Cases M1, M2, and M3) and three clinical cases from the US (Cases U1, U2, and U3) in order to cover a broader range of race, gender, food, weather temperature, and environment.

Described below are the key status of each patient's chronic diseases, obesity and diabetes:

- M1 is a male around 40-50 years old, with normal weight, but has severe diabetes conditions.

- M2 is a female around 40-50 years old, who is obese, and has severe diabetes conditions.

- M3 is a female around 40-50 years old, who is obese, and has pre-diabetes conditions.

- U1 is a male over 70 years old, with normal weight, and has a controlled diabetes conditions.

- U2 is a female over 70 years old, who is overweight, but has a controlled diabetes conditions.

- U3 is a male around 40-50 years old, who is extremely obese (BMI over 40), and has pre-diabetes conditions.

It should be mentioned that the three US cases are based on 9-months data in 2020. while the three Myanmar cases are based on around 6-months data in 2019.

Results:

Figure 1 shows the data table of the measured health data and calculated PPG data using the step-by-step-process described in the Method section.

The three clinical cases U1, U2, and U3 have adopted the author's recommended lifestyle management program during the entire year of 2020. Therefore, all of their measured FPG values are between 101 mg/dL to 105 mg/dL and their measured PPG values are between 109 mg/dL to 121 mg/dL.

The three Myanmar cases did not follow the author's advice on lifestyle management providing excuses such as difficulty in reducing weight, unable to reduce food portions, and incapable to exercise in hot weather. As a result, all of their measured FPG values are between 133 mg/dL to 141 mg/dL and their measured PPG values are between 131 mg/dL to 153 mg/dL.

Therefore, the author has different suggestions in improving the PPG values for cases M1, M2, and M3. For M1, he will reduce his carbs/sugar intake amount by 2 grams from 15.42g down to 13.42g, while increasing his post-meal walking from 1k to 3k steps, this will drop his PPG value to 120 mg/dL.

For both M2 and M3, the major problem causing their hyperglycemia is due to their heavy weight, if they could reduce their weight to 200 lbs. by cutting 20% off from their normal meal portion, most of their diabetes problems will go away. For M2, the author also suggested for her to reduce carbs/sugar intake amount by 3 grams, from

15.35g to 12.34g, while increasing the post-meal walking from 2.5k to 4.4K steps. For M3, there is no need to adjust her diet and exercise for diabetes concerns, but to focus on her weight reduction.

If cases M1, M2, and M3 could follow his advice and suggestions, all of their predicted PPG values would be dropped down to ~120 mg/dL.

Figure 2 demonstrated the final comparison of the predicted PPG using linear elastic glucose theory versus measured PPG. It is obviously that they match each other extremely well. Figure 2 is extended into to Figure 3 for the prediction accuracy bars for each case. All of these prediction accuracies are within +/- 1% margin of error which means they have reached 99% to 100% of prediction accuracies.

Conclusions:

The biomedical interpretation of these two glucose coefficients are as follows:

When a patient's obesity is worsening (i.e. gaining weight), then the GH.f-Modulus would be lower; however, when the same patient's diabetes is worsening (FPG higher), then the GH.f-Modulus would be higher. Usually, a patient's weight and FPG are closely related to each other with a higher than 90% of correlation. Therefore, the combination in severity of both obesity and diabetes is reflected in the magnitude of GH.f-modules.

On the other hand, the situation of GH.p-Modulus is simpler which mainly shows a patient's glucose sensitivity to carbs/sugar intake amount (the higher the glucose sensitivity depicts worsening diabetes conditions). When a more severe diabetes patient who has a higher GH.p-Modulus consumes the same amount of carbs/sugar, his/her PPG value would be higher than a not-so-severe diabetes patient. This GH.p-modulus also reflects the health state of pancreatic beta cells of a particular patient. GH.p-modulus (similar to Young's modulus in engineering) indicates the linear relationship between the carbs/sugar intake amount (similar to stress) and the incremental PPG amount (similar to strain) with different slopes for different patients.

The ultimate PPG value is determined by the combination of weight, FPG, carbs/ sugar intake amount, post-meal walking steps, with two glucose coefficients of GH.f- Modulus, and GH.p-Modulus.

It should be mentioned here that different from engineering inorganic material which does not change during a long period of time, human blood contains millions organic living red blood cells which have an averaged lifespan of 115 to 120 days. Therefore, the glucose coefficients of GH.f-Modulus and GH.p-Modulus are "pseudo-constants" during a time span of 3 to 4 months, similar to the tested values of HbA1C. Giving his observed personal HbA1C data during the past 10 years with a change rate within 1% to 11%, the author guesses that these two glucose coefficients should have a similar change rate within 1% to 11% as well. The maximum 11% change rate of GH.p-Modulus from 3.6 to 4.0 would increase his predicted PPG value from 121 mg/

dL to 127 mg/dL. In addition, both of weight reduction and glucose change are slow processes. A significant change usually takes a reasonable long period of time, such as years.

This study provides a quantitative proof with high precision from six clinical cases of obesity and diabetes conditions, either by adopting or rejecting the lifestyle management program. Linear elastic glucose theory and its associated predicted PPG equation have shown their power and applicability on diabetes control for a wide range of patients.

By adopting this theory and linear equation, the author is capable of providing customized quantitative advice and precise recommendations to three Myanmar patients on how to better control their obesity and T2D conditions. This chronic diseases control via a lifestyle management program using linear elastic glucose theory of GH-Method: math-physical medicine can indeed provide a solid scientific background to support the practical guidance as the branch of "Lifestyle Medicine".

References:

1. Hsu, Gerald C., eclaireMD Foundation, USA, No. 310: "Biomedical research methodology based on GH-Method: math-physical medicine"

2. Hsu, Gerald C., eclaireMD Foundation, USA, No. 345: "Application of linear equations to predict sensor and finger based postprandial plasma glucoses and daily glucoses for pre-virus, virus, and total periods using GH-Method: math-physical medicine"

3. Hsu, Gerald C., eclaireMD Foundation, USA, No. 97: "A simplified yet accurate linear equation of PPG prediction model for T2D patients (GH-Method: math-physical medicine)"

4. Hsu, Gerald C., eclaireMD Foundation, USA, No. 99: "Application of linear equation-based PPG prediction model for four T2D clinic cases (GH-Method: math-physical medicine)"

5. Hsu, Gerald C., eclaireMD Foundation, USA, No. 339: "Self-recovery of pancreatic beta cell's insulin secretion based on 10+ years annualized data of food, exercise, weight, and glucose using GH-Method: math-physical medicine)

6. Hsu, Gerald C., eclaireMD Foundation, USA, No. 340: "A neural communication model between brain and internal organs, specifically stomach, liver, and pancreatic beta cells based on PPG waveforms of 131 liquid egg meals and 124 solid egg meals)

7. Hsu, Gerald C., eclaireMD Foundation, USA, No. 349: "Using Math-Physics Medicine to Predict FPG"

8. Hsu, Gerald C., eclaireMD Foundation, USA, No. 264: "Community and Family Medicine via Doctors without distance: Using a simple glucose control card to assist T2D patients in remote rural areas (GH-Method: math-physical medicine)"

9. Hsu, Gerald C., eclaireMD Foundation, USA, No. 339: "Self-recovery of pancreatic beta cell's insulin secretion based on 10+ years annualized data of food, exercise, weight, and glucose using GH-Method: math-physical medicine"

10. Hsu, Gerald C., eclaireMD Foundation, USA, No. 346: "Linear relationship between carbohydrates & sugar intake amount and incremental PPG amount via engineering strength of materials using GH-Method: math-physical medicine, Part 1"

11. Hsu, Gerald C., eclaireMD Foundation, USA, No. 349: "Investigation on GH modulus of linear elastic glucose with two diabetes patients data using GH-Method: math-physical medicine, Part 2"

12. Hsu, Gerald C., eclaireMD Foundation, USA, No. 349: "Investigation of GH modulus on the linear elastic glucose behavior based on three diabetes patients' data using the GH-Method: math-physical medicine, Part 3"

13. Hsu, Gerald C., eclaireMD Foundation, USA, No. 356: "Coefficient of GH.f-modulus in the linear elastic fasting plasma glucose behavior study based on health data of three diabetes patients using the GH-Method: math-physical medicine, Part 4 "

14. Hsu, Gerald C., eclaireMD Foundation, USA, No. 357: "High accuracy of predicted postprandial plasma glucose using two coefficients of GH.f-modulus and GH.p-modulus from linear elastic glucose behavior theory based on GH-Method: math-physical medicine, Part 5"

15. Hsu, Gerald C., eclaireMD Foundation, USA, No. 358: "Improvement on the prediction accuracy of postprandial plasma glucose using two biomedical coefficients of GH-modulus from linear elastic glucose theory based on GH-Method: math-physical medicine, Part 6"

16. Hsu, Gerald C., eclaireMD Foundation, USA, No. 359: "High glucose predication accuracy of postprandial plasma glucose and fasting plasma glucose during the COVID-19 period using two glucose coefficients of GH-modulus from linear elastic glucose theory based on GH-Method: math-physical medicine, Part 7"

17. Hsu, Gerald C., eclaireMD Foundation, USA, No. 360: "Investigation of two glucose coefficients of GH.f-modulus and GH.p-modulus based on data of 3 clinical cases during COVID-19 period using linear elastic glucose theory of GH-Method: math-physical medicine, Part 8"

18. Hsu, Gerald C., eclaireMD Foundation, USA, No. 361: "Postprandial plasma glucose lower and upper boundary study using two glucose coefficients of GH-modulus from linear elastic glucose theory based on GH-Method: math-physical medicine, Part 9"

T2D Patients	Case M1	Case M2	Case M3	Case U1	Case U2	Case U3	Improved M1	Improved M2	Improved M3
Weight (pound)	150	237	228	167	157	273	150	200	200
FPG (mg/dL)	141	137	133	101	103	105	120	125	120
GH.f-modulus	0.94	0.58	0.58	0.60	0.66	0.38	0.80	0.63	0.60
Baseline PPG 9mg/dL)	137	133	129	98	100	102	116	121	116
GH.p-modulus	1.4	1.6	0.5	3.6	2.6	1.0	1.4	1.6	0.5
Carbs/Sugar (standard gram)	15.42	15.35	15.61	12.34	9.81	12.38	13.42	12.34	15.61
Carbs *GH.p-modulus	22	25	8	44	26	12	19	20	8
Walking (standard k-steps)	1.0	2.5	1.0	4.4	2.1	1.0	3.0	4.4	1.0
T2D Patients	Case M1	Case M2	Case M3	Case U1	Case U2	Case U3	Improved M1	Improved M2	Improved M3
Predicted PPG	153	145	132	121	115	109	120	119	119
Measured PPG	153	146	131	121	114	110	120	120	119
T2D Patients	Case M1	Case M2	Case M3	Case U1	Case U2	Case U3	Improved M1	Improved M2	Improved M3
Accuracy of Predicted PPG	100%	100%	101%	100%	101%	99%	100%	99%	100%

Figure 1: Data table and PPG calculations of 6 clinical cases

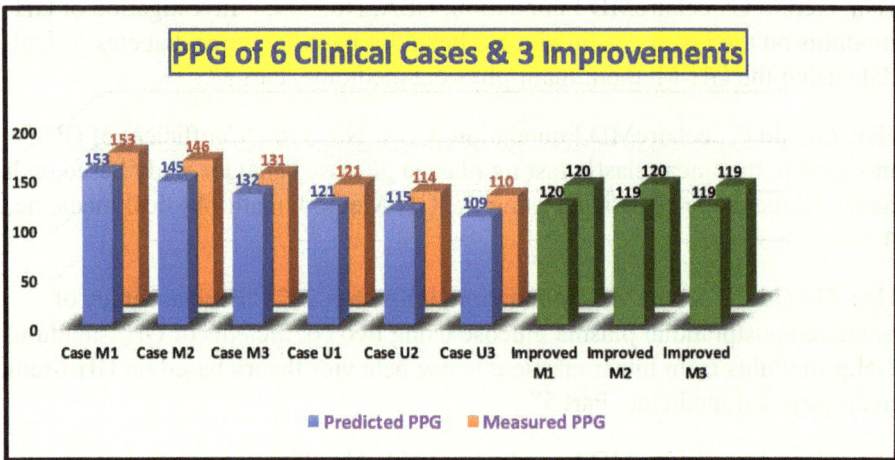

Figure 2: Comparison between predicted PPG and measured PPG for 6 clinical cases with customized recommendations of improvements for 3 Myanmar patients

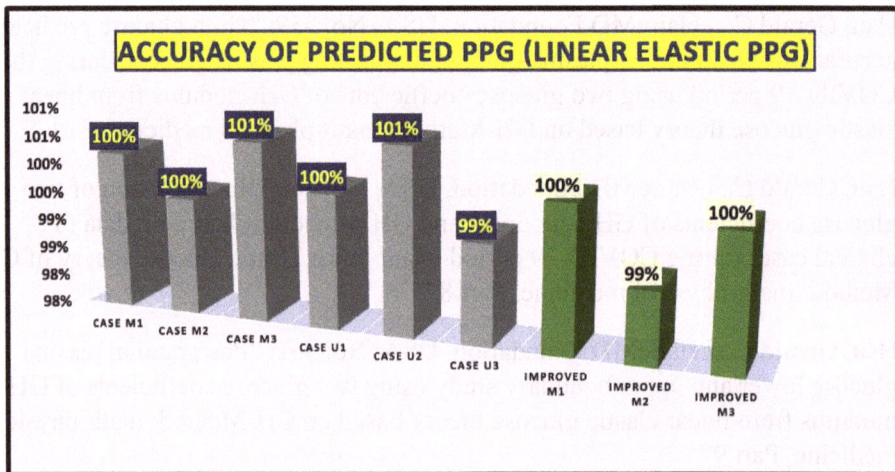

Figure 3: prediction accuracies for 6 clinical cases

A special Neuro-communication influences on GH.p-modulus of linear elastic glucose theory based on data from 159 liquid egg and 126 solid egg meals using GH-Method: math-physical medicine, Part 11 (No. 363)

Gerald C. Hsu
eclaireMD Foundation, USA
11/17-18/2020

Abstract:

This article is Part 11 of the author's linear elastic glucose behavior study. It focuses on a deeper investigation regarding the specific glucose coefficient of GH.p-modulus, which involves the influence of the neuro-communication between the stomach, brain, and liver pertaining to the postprandial plasma glucose (PPG) production amount (see Reference 6). When a person consumes a meal in a liquid state such as egg drop soup, the stomach would "trick" or "trigger" the brain to recognize the arrival of fluids, then it issues a marching order to the liver to produce a lesser amount of PPG. Due to the smaller value of carb intake and the mathematical definition of the incremental PPG, the value of GH.p-modulus must be raised to a higher value in order to achieve a high prediction accuracy for egg meals, especially for solid egg meals with the same small intake amount of carbs/sugar.

This article provides the background data, observed physical phenomena, and mathematical derivations to interpret and prove these higher values of GH.p-modulus for egg meals. By using two different time periods, it also demonstrates the strong linkage between GH.p-modulus and the patient's overall diabetes status, either it is improving (through a dropped GH.p-modulus) or worsening (through a raised GH.p-modulus).

Here is the step-by-step explanation of the predicted PPG equation from the six clinical cases using linear elastic glucose theory as described in References 9 through 18:

*(1) **Baseline PPG** equals to 97% of FPG value, or 97% * (weight * GH.f-Modulus).*
*(2) Baseline PPG **plus** increased amount of PPG due to food, i.e. plus (carbs/sugar intake amount * GH.p-Modulus).*
*(3) Baseline PPG **plus** increased PPG due to food, and then **subtracts** reduction amount of PPG due to exercise, i.e. minus (post-meal walking k-steps * 5).*
*(4) The **Predicted PPG** equals to **Baseline PPG plus the food influences, and then subtracts the exercise influences.***

The linear elastic glucose equation is:

Predicted PPG =
(0.97 * GH.f-modulus * Weight) +(GH.p-modulus * Carbs&sugar) - (post-meal walking k-steps * 5)

Where

Incremental PPG =Predicted PPG - Baseline PPG + Exercise impact

GH.f-modulus = FPG / Weight

GH.p-modulus =

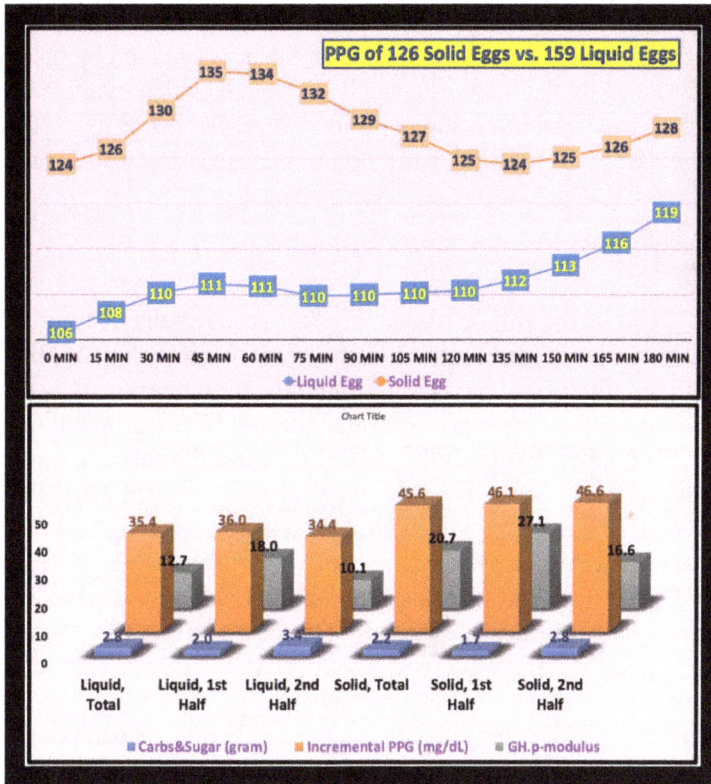

PPG of 126 Solid Eggs vs. 159 Liquid Eggs

Incremental PPG / Carbs intake

This article uses the neuro-scientific experiment results of two physical states of egg meals to further investigate the two glucose coefficients, in particular the GH.p-modulus value and meaning.

The GH.p-modulus is not only the direct result of lifestyle difference (diet and exercise) but also includes the status difference of the chronic diseases (baseline PPG via weight and FPG). It also reflects the general health state of pancreatic beta cells of a particular patient which can be described by the fasting plasma glucose (FPG) level. In addition, it further contains the neuroscience of communication model between the brain and stomach regarding the amount of glucose production or glucose release in response to a specific message of the timing of the food's entry and the physical state of the stomach and intestine. This neurology viewpoint makes the GH.p-modulus even more complex. Nevertheless, the linear elastic glucose theory still applies to the special case of the neuro-scientific egg meals, even though it creates a much higher GH.p-modulus value that can be considered as one of the boundary cases in this linear elasticity study.

With the neuro-scientific case study, it is clear that this linear elastic glucose behaviors are much more complicated than the classical engineering elasticity theory because the engineering inorganic materials do not change for a long period of time. The human body is made from organic living cells. For example, blood contains millions of organic living red blood cells with an average lifespan of 115 to 120 days and liver cells that last about 300 to 500 days. In addition, the glucose production and release are controlled by the brain. The glucose level is further regulated by insulin (a type of hormone) produced by the pancreas which is also controlled by the brain. The communication between the brain and nervous system can throw a curve ball into the glucoses game making this research work not only more complicated but also more interesting.

Introduction:

This article is Part 11 of the author's linear elastic glucose behavior study. It focuses on a deeper investigation regarding the specific glucose coefficient of GH.p-modulus, which involves the influence of the neuro-communication between the stomach, brain, and liver pertaining to the postprandial plasma glucose (PPG) production amount (see Reference 6). When a person consumes a meal in a liquid state such as egg drop soup, the stomach would "trick" or "trigger" the brain to recognize the arrival of fluids, then it issues a marching order to the liver to produce a lesser amount of PPG. Due to the smaller value of carb intake and the mathematical definition of the incremental PPG, the value of GH.p-modulus must be raised to a higher value in order to achieve a high prediction accuracy for egg meals, especially for solid egg meals with the same small intake amount of carbs/sugar.

This article provides the background data, observed physical phenomena, and mathematical derivations to interpret and prove these higher values of GH.p-modulus for egg meals. By using two different time periods, it also demonstrates the strong linkage between GH.p-modulus and the patient's overall diabetes status, either it is improving (through a dropped GH.p-modulus) or worsening (through a raised GH.p-modulus).

Methods:

Background:
To learn more about the author's GH-Method: math-physical medicine (MPM) methodology, readers can refer to his article to understand his developed MPM analysis method in Reference 1.

Highlights of linear elastic glucose theory:
Here is the step-by-step explanation of the predicted PPG equation using linear elastic glucose theory as described in References 9 through 18:

*(5) **Baseline PPG** equals to 97% of FPG value, or 97% * (weight * GH.f-Modulus).*
*(6) Baseline PPG **plus** increased amount of PPG due to food, i.e. plus (carbs/sugar intake amount * GH.p-Modulus).*
*(7) Baseline PPG **plus** increased PPG due to food, and then **subtracts** reduction amount of PPG due to exercise, i.e. minus (post-meal walking k-steps * 5).*
*(8) The **Predicted PPG** equals to **Baseline PPG plus the food influences, and then subtracts the exercise influences.***

The linear elastic glucose equation is:

Predicted PPG =
(0.97 * GH.f-modulus * Weight) +(GH.p-modulus * Carbs&sugar) - (post-meal walking k-steps * 5)

By using this linear equation, a diabetes patient only needs the input data of body weight, carbs & sugar intake amount, and post-meal walking steps in order to calculate the predicted PPG value without obtaining any measured glucose data except for data calibrating purposes.

The readers can view the details of his previous research work related to this subject listed in the Reference section.

In 2014, the author came up with the analogy between theory of elasticity and plasticity and the severity of diabetes when he was developing his mathematical model of metabolism.

On 10/14/2020, by utilizing the concept of Young's modulus with stress and strain, which was taught in engineering schools, he initiated and engaged this linear elastic glucose behaviors research. The following paragraphs describe his research findings at different stages of this research period:

First, he discovered that there is a "pseudo-linear" relationship existed between carbs & sugar intake amount and incremental PPG amount. Based on this finding, he defined his first glucose coefficient of GH.p-modulus for PPG.

Second, similar to Young's modulus relating to stiffness of engineering inorganic materials, he found that the GH.p-modulus is depended upon the patient's severity level of diabetes, i.e. patient's glucose sensitivity on carbs/sugar intake amount.

Third, comparable to GH.p-modulus for PPG, in 2017, he uncovered a similar pseudo-linear relationship existing between weight and FPG with high correlation coefficient of greater than 90%. Therefore, he defined his second glucose coefficient of GH.f-modulus as the FPG value divided by the weight value. This GH.f-modulus is related to the severity of chronic diseases, including both obesity and diabetes.

Fourth, he inserted these two glucose coefficients of GH.p-modulus and GH.f-modulus, into the predicted PPG equation to remove the burden of collecting measured glucoses by patients.

Fifth, by experimenting and calculating many predicted PPG values over a variety of time length from different diabetes patients with varying health conditions, he finally revealed that GH.p-modulus seems to be "near-constant" or "pseudo-linearized" over a short period of 3 to 4 months. This short period is compatible with the known lifespan of red blood cells, which are living organic cells, that are different from the engineering inorganic materials, such as steel or concrete. The same conclusion was observed using his monthly GH.p-modulus data during the COVID-19 period in 2010 when his lifestyle became routine and stabilized.

Sixth, he used three US clinical cases during the 2020 COVID-19 period to delve into the hidden characteristics of the physical parameters and their biomedical relationships. More importantly, through the comparison study in Part 7, he found explainable biomedical interpretations of his two defined glucose coefficients of GH.p-modulus and GH.f-modulus.

Seventh, he conducted a PPG boundary analysis by discovering a lower bound and an upper bound of predicted PPG values for eight hypothetical standard cases and three US clinical cases. The derived numerical values of these two boundaries make sense from a biomedical viewpoint and also matched with the situations of the three US clinical cases. He even conducted two extreme stress tests, i.e. increasing carbs/sugar intake amount to 50 grams per meal and boosting post-meal walking steps to 5k after each meal, to examine the impacts on the lower bound and upper bound of PPG values.

Eighth, based on six international clinical cases, he further explored the influences from the combination of obesity and diabetes. Using a lifestyle medicine approach, he offered suggestions to reduce their PPG from 130-150 mg/dL down to below 120 mg/dL via reducing carbs/sugar intake and increasing exercise such as walking steps.

Egg meal cases in this article:
In multiple published articles from his previous neuroscience research work, he separated his egg meals into two distinctive physical states, liquid state (159 egg drop soup) and solid state (126 pan-fried egg or hard broiled egg), during the period from 5/5/2018 to 11/17/2020. The majority of his egg meals data are concentrated in 2020; therefore, he further established two sub-periods, the first half from 5/5/2018 to 6/30/2020 (pre-virus period) and the second half from 7/1/2020 to 11/17/2020 (virus period). It happens that the second half sub-period matches with his COVID-19 quarantined period. Due to a special quiet and routine lifestyle without any traveling, his overall health conditions, including both weights and glucoses, have reached to his "best-performed" status over the past 25 years. This special characteristic also contributed to the values of GH-modulus.

He then segregated his collected data according to the categories of weight, FPG, carbs, walking, and PPG. By using the average data within each sub-period and the total period, he then calculated his corresponding glucose coefficients of GH.f-modulus and GH.f-modulus.

Finally, he compared his calculated coefficients of three periods to study their biomedical meaning and interpretation.

Results:

Figure 1 shows the comparison of PPG waveforms between solid egg meals and liquid egg meals. It is obvious that the solid egg PPG values are higher than the liquid egg PPG values, with a difference of 18 mg/dL higher at 0-minute (open moment), 24 mg/dL higher at 45-minutes (maximum moment), and 15 mg/dL higher at 120-minutes (moment of finger-piercing PPG measurement). In paper No. 340 (Reference 6), the author explained his hypothesis and offered the neuroscientific interpretation and proof regarding the communication model among the stomach, brain, and liver to determine the glucose level based on the incoming food's physical state, i.e. liquid vs. solid. It should be noted that both solid egg meals and liquid egg meals are based on one large egg which has a minimal amount of carbohydrates around 2 grams. Furthermore, his post-meal walking exercises are usually around 4,500 steps.

Figure 2 depicts the background data for calculations of predicted PPG and derivations of 2 glucose coefficients, both GH.f-modulus and GH.p-modulus.

Figure 3 reveals the GH.f-modulus linking Weight and Sensor FPG to indicate a patient's (with chronic diseases) relative health state in terms of both obesity and diabetes. These two meals associated with the GH.f-modulus value, 59 for liquid eggs and 64 for solid eggs, are within the general range of his recorded weight and FPG from 5/5/2018 to 11/17/2020. It should be pointed out that the GH.f-modulus has no "direct" relationship with diet and exercise, however, they do have some "indirect" relationships with food and exercise through body weight.

Figures 4 illustrates the GH.p-modulus linking Carbs/Sugar amount and Incremental PPG value to indicate a patient's glucose sensitivity to carbs & sugar amount related to the two types of egg meals. The linear elastic glucose behavior can be expressed via the following linear equation:

Incremental PPG =
*Carbs/Sugar intake * GH.p-modulus*

The two GH.p-modulus values are 12.7 for liquid eggs and 20.7 for solid eggs which are much higher than the author's previously acquired research knowledge and learned PPG prediction experience regarding the GH.p-modulus values. The author guesses that the general GH.p-modulus range of 1.0 to 5.0 is probably suitable for the majority of clinical cases (the author's GH.p-modulus range is between 2.1 and 3.4). For a period of 5 years, the author has maintained an average carbs/sugar intake amount approximately less than 15 grams per meal in order to control his severe diabetes conditions without taking any medication. However, in order to conduct his own neuroscience experiments, he chose only one egg per meal which contains a mere ~2 grams of carbs/sugar. This extremely low carb amount must accompany with a much higher GH.p-modulus value in order to accomplish his desired health maintenance goal via his predicted PPG level matching with his measured PPG.

Here is a summary:

Liquid eggs:
2g * *12.7* = 25.4
Solid eggs:
2g * *20.7* = 41.4
Normal meals:
15g * *1.7* = 25.5
15g * *2.75* = 41.3

Figure 5 shows GH.f-modulus, Weight, Sensor FPG for both liquid egg meals and solid egg meals for three different periods, including the total period, first half period (non-virus), and second half period (virus period).

Figure 6 represents the GH.p-modulus, Carbs amount, incremental FPG for both liquid egg meals and solid egg meals for three different periods, periods, including the total period, first half period (pre-virus), and second half period (virus period).

Figure 5 and Figure 6 provide a comparison of the two glucose coefficients, GH.f-modulus and GH.p-modulus between two sub-periods, the first half and second half. There is not much difference between the first-half period and second-half period on the GH.f-modulus values due to both weight and FPG not changing significantly.

However, the difference of the GH.p-modulus value between the first-half period versus second-half period are more obvious, i.e. 18 vs. 10 and 27 vs. 17. The bigger differences are caused by the combined effect of value reduction on weight, FPG, Baseline PPG, and measured PPG from the pre-virus period to virus period. In other words, the patient's overall diabetes conditions have been improving in the second half of the virus sub-period.

Conclusions:

This article uses the neuro-scientific experiment results of two physical states of egg meals to further investigate the two glucose coefficients, in particular the GH.p-modulus value and meaning.

The GH.p-modulus is not only the direct result of lifestyle difference (diet and exercise) but also includes the status difference of the chronic diseases (baseline PPG via weight and FPG). It also reflects the general health state of pancreatic beta cells of a particular patient which can be described by the fasting plasma glucose (FPG) level. In addition, it further contains the neuroscience of communication model between the brain and stomach regarding the amount of glucose production or glucose release in response to a specific message of the timing of the food's entry and the physical state of the stomach and intestine. This neurology viewpoint makes the GH.p-modulus even more complex. Nevertheless, the linear elastic glucose theory still applies to the special case of the neuro-scientific egg meals, even though it creates a much higher GH.p-modulus value that can be considered as one of the boundary cases in this linear elasticity study.

With the neuro-scientific case study, it is clear that this linear elastic glucose behaviors are much more complicated than the classical engineering theory of elasticity because the engineering inorganic materials do not change for a long period of time. The human body is made from organic living cells. For example, blood contains millions of organic living red blood cells with an average lifespan of 115 to 120 days and liver cells that last about 300 to 500 days. In addition, the glucose production and release are controlled by the brain. The glucose level is further regulated by insulin (a type of hormone) produced by the pancreas which is also controlled by the brain. The communication between the brain and nervous system can throw a curve ball into the glucoses game making this research work not only more complicated but also more interesting.

References:

1. Hsu, Gerald C., eclaireMD Foundation, USA, No. 310: "Biomedical research methodology based on GH-Method: math-physical medicine"

2. Hsu, Gerald C., eclaireMD Foundation, USA, No. 345: "Application of linear equations to predict sensor and finger based postprandial plasma glucoses and daily glucoses for pre-virus, virus, and total periods using GH-Method: math-physical medicine"

3. Hsu, Gerald C., eclaireMD Foundation, USA, No. 97: "A simplified yet accurate linear equation of PPG prediction model for T2D patients (GH-Method: math-physical medicine)"

4. Hsu, Gerald C., eclaireMD Foundation, USA, No. 99: "Application of linear equation-based PPG prediction model for four T2D clinic cases (GH-Method: math-physical medicine)"

5. Hsu, Gerald C., eclaireMD Foundation, USA, No. 339: "Self-recovery of pancreatic beta cell's insulin secretion based on 10+ years annualized data of food, exercise, weight, and glucose using GH-Method: math-physical medicine)

6. Hsu, Gerald C., eclaireMD Foundation, USA, No. 340: "A neural communication model between brain and internal organs, specifically stomach, liver, and pancreatic beta cells based on PPG waveforms of 131 liquid egg meals and 124 solid egg meals)

7. Hsu, Gerald C., eclaireMD Foundation, USA, No. 349: "Using Math-Physics Medicine to Predict FPG"

8. Hsu, Gerald C., eclaireMD Foundation, USA, No. 264: "Community and Family Medicine via Doctors without distance: Using a simple glucose control card to assist T2D patients in remote rural areas (GH-Method: math-physical medicine)"

9. Hsu, Gerald C., eclaireMD Foundation, USA, No. 346: "Linear relationship between carbohydrates & sugar intake amount and incremental PPG amount via engineering strength of materials using GH-Method: math-physical medicine, Part 1"

10. Hsu, Gerald C., eclaireMD Foundation, USA, No. 349: "Investigation on GH modulus of linear elastic glucose with two diabetes patients data using GH-Method: math-physical medicine, Part 2"

11. Hsu, Gerald C., eclaireMD Foundation, USA, No. 349: "Investigation of GH modulus on the linear elastic glucose behavior based on three diabetes patients' data using the GH-Method: math-physical medicine, Part 3"

12. Hsu, Gerald C., eclaireMD Foundation, USA, No. 356: "Coefficient of GH.f-modulus in the linear elastic fasting plasma glucose behavior study based on health data of three diabetes patients using the GH-Method: math-physical medicine, Part 4 "

13. Hsu, Gerald C., eclaireMD Foundation, USA, No. 357: "High accuracy of predicted postprandial plasma glucose using two coefficients of GH.f-modulus and GH.p-modulus from linear elastic glucose behavior theory based on GH-Method: math-physical medicine, Part 5"

14. Hsu, Gerald C., eclaireMD Foundation, USA, No. 358: "Improvement on the prediction accuracy of postprandial plasma glucose using two biomedical coefficients of GH-modulus from linear elastic glucose theory based on GH-Method: math-physical medicine, Part 6"

15. Hsu, Gerald C., eclaireMD Foundation, USA, No. 359: "High glucose predication accuracy of postprandial plasma glucose and fasting plasma glucose during the COVID-19 period using two glucose coefficients of GH-modulus from linear elastic glucose theory based on GH-Method: math-physical medicine, Part 7"

16. Hsu, Gerald C., eclaireMD Foundation, USA, No. 360: "Investigation of two glucose coefficients of GH.f-modulus and GH.p-modulus based on data of 3 clinical cases during COVID-19 period using linear elastic glucose theory of GH-Method: math-physical medicine, Part 8"

17. Hsu, Gerald C., eclaireMD Foundation, USA, No. 361: "Postprandial plasma glucose lower and upper boundary study using two glucose coefficients of GH-modulus from linear elastic glucose theory based on GH-Method: math-physical medicine, Part 9"

18. Hsu, Gerald C., eclaireMD Foundation, USA, No. 362: "Six international clinical cases demonstrating prediction accuracies of postprandial plasma glucoses and suggested methods for improvements using linear elastic glucose theory of GH-Method: math-physical medicine, Part 10"

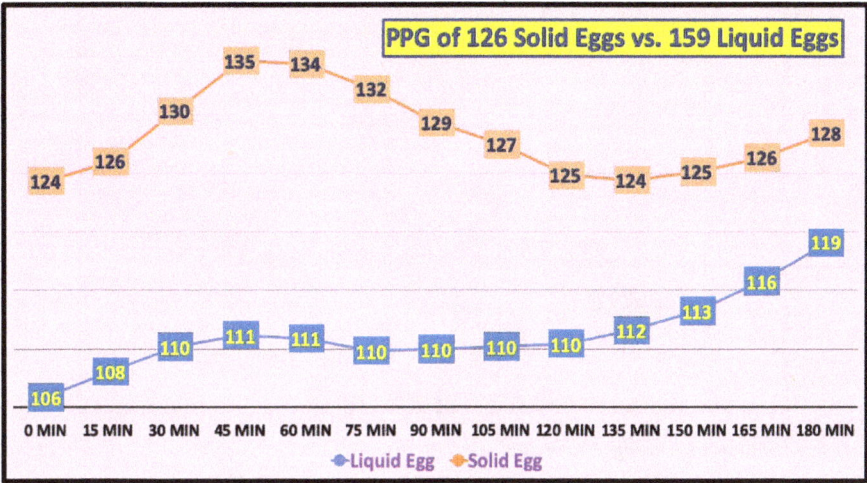

Figure 1: PPG waveform comparison between 159 egg drop soups vs. 126 solid eggs (pan-fried egg, hard broiled egg)

Figure 2: Definition of GH.f-modulus, GH.p-modulus, Baseline PPG, Incremental PPG and calculation of Predicted PPG with comparison against Measured PPG during various time periods

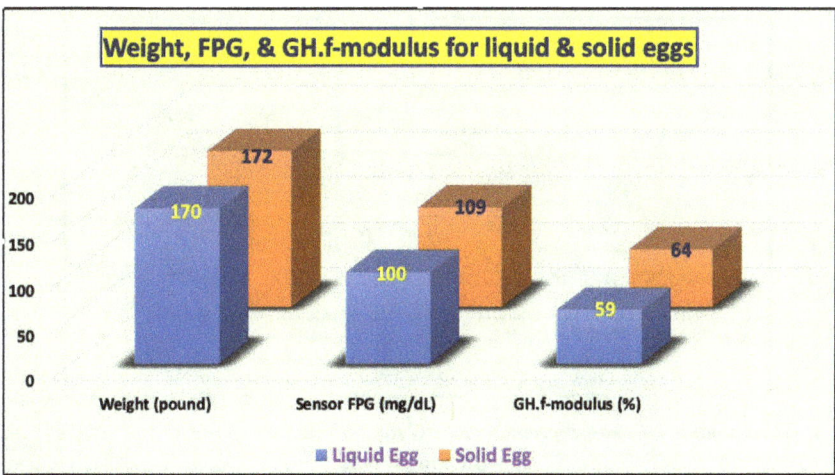

Figure 3: GH.f-modulus linking Weight and Sensor FPG to show a patient's relative health state in terms of both obesity and diabetes

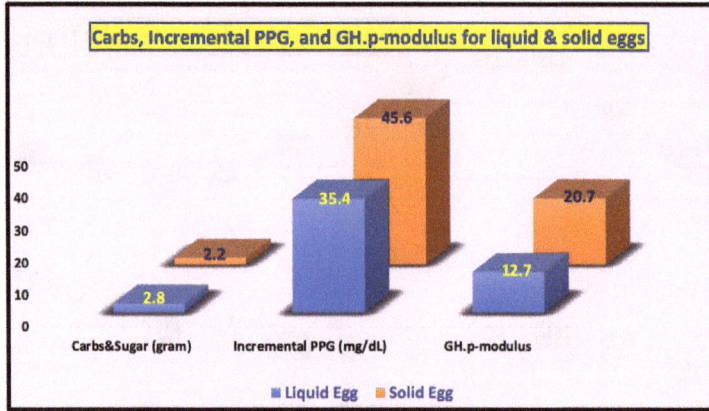

Figure 4: GH.p-modulus linking Carbs and Incremental PPG to show a patient's glucose sensitivity to carbs & sugar intake amount relative to egg meals

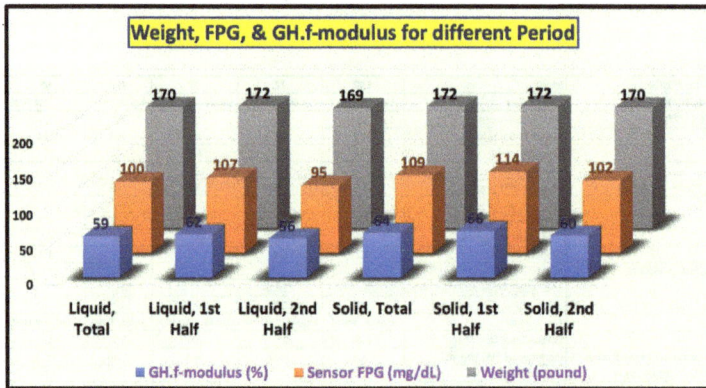

Figure 5: GH.f-modulus, Weight, Sensor FPG for both liquid egg meals and solid egg meals for different periods

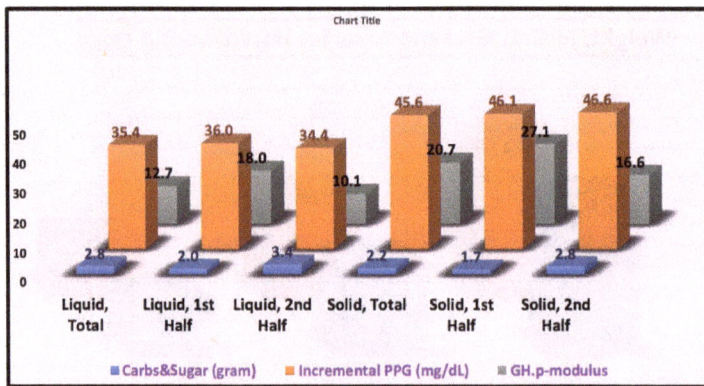

Figure 6: GH.p-modulus, Carbs, incremental FPG for both liquid egg meals and solid egg meals for different periods.

The difference of GH.p-modulus between first half period and second half periods are also shown.

GH.p-modulus study of linear elastic glucose theory based on data from 159 liquid egg meals, 126 solid egg meals, and 2,843 total meals using GH-Method: math-physical medicine, Part 12 (No. 364)

Gerald C. Hsu
eclaireMD Foundation, USA
11/17-18/2020

Abstract:

This article is Part 12 of the author's linear elastic glucose behavior study. It focuses on a deeper investigation of GH.p-modulus through the comparison of the results from his neuroscience study of egg meals against his 2,843 total meals during the period of 5/5/2018 to 11/17/2020. In the comparison study, he can explore the potential range (variance) of GH.p-modulus values with special cases of 285 egg meals and general case of 2,843 total meals. As a result, it extends to connect the study of his eight hypothetical standard cases presented in paper No. 361 (Reference 17).

Here is the step-by-step explanation of the predicted postprandial plasma glucose (PPG) equation using linear elastic glucose theory as described in References 9 through 19:

(1) **Baseline PPG** equals to 97% of FPG value, or 97% * (weight * GH.f-Modulus).
(2) Baseline PPG **plus** increased amount of PPG due to food, i.e. plus (carbs/sugar intake amount * GH.p-Modulus).
(3) Baseline PPG **plus** increased PPG due to food, and then **subtracts** reduction amount of PPG due to exercise, i.e. minus (post-meal walking k-steps * 5).
(4) The **Predicted PPG** equals to **Baseline PPG plus the food influences, and then subtracts the exercise influences.**

The linear elastic glucose equation is:

Predicted PPG =
(0.97 * GH.f-modulus * Weight) +(GH.p-modulus * Carbs&sugar) - (post-meal walking k-steps * 5)

Where
(1) ***Incremental PPG = Predicted PPG - Baseline PPG + Exercise impact***
(2) ***GH.f-modulus = FPG / Weight***
(3) ***GH.p-modulus = Incremental PPG / Carbs intake***

It is quite interesting to put the author's 285 special egg meals experimental data side by side with his 2,843 total meals data together. The differences of the carb amount and GH.p-modulus values between the egg meals and total meals are vast and obvious.

The neuroscience egg meals are offered as extreme cases for the GH.p-modulus boundary situations by having an extremely low carb intake amount per meal with an associated much higher GH.p-modulus value. However, the conclusions from the case of 2,843 total meals could offer general guidelines for type 2 diabetes patients who want to control their diabetic conditions via lifestyle management program. The author thinks that a general GH.p-modulus range of 1.0 to 5.0 is probably suitable for the majority of clinical cases (the author's own range is 2.1 to 3.4). From a practical angle, a patient can use this GH.p-modulus value as a multiplier of his carbs/sugar amount and use a number of 5 as his multiplier to the post-meal walking k-steps and then plug them into the following "quick but not so dirty" formula in order to obtain the predicted PPG.

Predicted PPG =
FPG + (GH.p * Carbs) - (k-steps *5)

Where the patient can attempt to use different numbers between 1 through 5 as the GH.p input value to determine the suitable GH.p-modulus.

By using the above estimated PPG formula, diabetes patients can find their PPG level very quickly and accurately without delving into the details of the linear elastic glucose theory.

Introduction:

This article is Part 12 of the author's linear elastic glucose behavior study. It focuses on a deeper investigation of GH.p-modulus through the comparison of the results from his neuroscience study of egg meals against his 2,843 total meals during the period of 5/5/2018 to 11/17/2020. In the comparison study, he can explore the potential range (variance) of GH.p-modulus values with special cases of 285 egg meals and general case of 2,843 total meals. As a result, it extends to connect the study of his eight hypothetical standard cases presented in paper No. 361 (Reference 17).

Methods:

Background:
To learn more about the author's GH-Method: math-physical medicine (MPM) methodology, readers can refer to his article to understand his developed MPM analysis method in Reference 1.

Highlights of linear elastic glucose theory:
Here is the step-by-step explanation of the predicted PPG equation using linear elastic glucose theory as described in References 9 through 19:

*(1) **Baseline PPG** equals to 97% of FPG value, or 97% * (weight * GH.f-Modulus).*
*(2) Baseline PPG **plus** increased amount of PPG due to food, i.e. plus (carbs/sugar intake amount * GH.p-Modulus).*
*(3) Baseline PPG **plus** increased PPG due to food, and then subtracts reduction amount of PPG due to exercise, i.e. minus (post-meal walking k-steps * 5).*
*(4) The **Predicted PPG** equals to **Baseline PPG plus the food influences, and then subtracts the exercise influences.***

The linear elastic glucose equation is:

Predicted PPG =
(0.97 * GH.f-modulus * Weight) +(GH.p-modulus * Carbs&sugar) - (post-meal walking k-steps * 5)

Where
(1) Incremental PPG = Predicted PPG - Baseline PPG + Exercise impact
(2) GH.f-modulus = FPG / Weight
(3) GH.p-modulus = Incremental PPG / Carbs intake

By using this linear equation, a diabetes patient only needs the input data of body weight, carbs & sugar intake amount, and post-meal walking steps in order to calculate the predicted PPG value without obtaining any measured glucose data.

In 2014, the author came up with the analogy between theory of elasticity and plasticity and the severity of diabetes when he was developing his mathematical model of metabolism.

On 10/14/2020, by utilizing the concept of Young's modulus with stress and strain, which was taught in engineering schools, he initiated and engaged this linear elastic glucose behaviors research. The following paragraphs describe his research findings at different stages of this research period:

First, he discovered that there is a "pseudo-linear" relationship existing between carbs & sugar intake amount and incremental PPG amount. Based on this finding, he defined the first glucose coefficient of GH.p-modulus for PPG.

Second, similar to Young's modulus relating to stiffness of engineering inorganic materials, he found that the GH.p-modulus is dependent upon the patient's severity level of diabetes, i.e. patient's glucose sensitivity on carbs/sugar intake amount.

Third, comparable to GH.p-modulus for PPG, in 2017, he uncovered a similar pseudo-linear relationship existing between weight and FPG with high correlation coefficient of above 90%. Therefore, he defined the second glucose coefficient of GH.f-modulus as the FPG value divided by the weight value. This GH.f-modulus is related to the severity of combined chronic diseases, including both obesity and diabetes.

Fourth, he inserted these two glucose coefficients of GH.p-modulus and GH.f-modulus, into the predicted PPG equation to remove the burden of collecting measured glucoses by patients.

Fifth, by experimenting and calculating many predicted PPG values over a variety of time length from different diabetes patients with different health conditions, he finally revealed that GH.p-modulus seems to be "near-constant" or "pseudo-linearized" over a short period of 3 to 4 months. This short period is compatible with the known lifespan of human red blood cells, which are living organic cells. This is quite different from the engineering inorganic materials, such as steel or concrete which can last for an exceptionally long period of time. The same conclusion was observed using his monthly GH.p-modulus data during the COVID-19 period in 2010 when his lifestyle became routine and stabilized.

Sixth, he used three US clinical cases during the 2020 COVID-19 period to delve into the hidden characteristics of the physical parameters and their biomedical relationships. More importantly, through the comparison study in Part 7, he found explainable biomedical interpretations of his two defined glucose coefficients of GH.p-modulus and GH.f-modulus.

Seventh, he conducted a PPG boundary analysis by discovering a lower bound and an upper bound of predicted PPG values for eight hypothetical standard cases and three US specific clinical cases. The derived numerical values of these two boundaries make sense from a biomedical viewpoint and also matched with the situations of the three US clinical cases. He even conducted two extreme stress tests, i.e. increasing carbs/sugar intake amount to 50 grams per meal and boosting post-meal walking steps to 5k after each meal, to examine the impacts on the lower bound and upper bound of PPG values.

Eighth, based on six international clinical cases, he further explored the influences from the combination of obesity and diabetes. Using a "lifestyle medicine" approach, he offered recommendations to reduce their PPG from 130-150 mg/dL down to below 120 mg/dL via reducing carbs/sugar intake and increasing exercise level in walking.

Ninth, based on his neuroscience research work using both 126 solid eggs and 159 liquid eggs with a very low carbs/sugar intake amount of ~2.5 grams producing two totally different sets of PPG values and waveforms, he identified a different set of much higher values of GH.p-modules for these egg meals. Even though this research served as a special boundary case in the study, nevertheless, it has further proven that the GH.p-modules is also influenced directly by the human brain.

Meal cases in this article:
In multiple published articles from his previous neuroscience research work, he separated his egg meals into two distinctive physical states, liquid state (159 egg drop soup) and solid state (126 pan-fried egg or hard broiled egg), during the period from 5/5/2018 to 11/17/2020. This period is selected due to the same glucose measuring period via a continuous glucose monitoring (CGM) sensor device on his arm. His 285 egg meals have an average carb intake amount around 2.5 grams and his average post-meal walking approximately 4.5 k-step. His sensor measured PPG levels are 111 mg/dL for liquid eggs PPG and 128 mg/dL for solid eggs PPG.

During the same time period, he has consumed a total of 2,843 meals with an average carb intake amount of 13.8 grams and his post-meal walking is 4.3 k-step. It should be mentioned that he also continued to measure his PPG using the traditional finger-piercing method at 120-minutes after the first bite of his meal. For this total meal's group, his measured PPG levels are 131 mg/dL for sensor PPG and 113 mg/dL for finger PPG.

He then segregated his collected data according to the categories of weight, FPG, carbs, walking, and PPG. By using the average data within each type of meals and the total period using both sensor and finger methods, he then calculated the four sets of corresponding glucose coefficients of GH.f-modulus and GH.f-modulus.

Finally, he compared his calculated glucose coefficients of these four groups to study their relationships, specific meaning, and identify the proper biomedical interpretations.

Results:

Figure 1 shows the comparison of PPG waveforms between 126 solid egg meals, 159 liquid egg meals, and 2,843 total meals. It is obvious that the **total meals PPG waveform (average PPG 131 g/dL and carbs 13.8 grams)** is the highest one. The solid egg PPG waveform (average PPG 128 g/dL and carbs 2.2 grams) is slightly lower than the total meals. However, the **liquid egg PPG waveform (average PPG 111 g/dL and carbs 2.8 grams)** is the lowest one among these three groups. The finger total meals is not included because they contain only one glucose number per meal instead of 13 PPG data points per meal for a sensor waveform. The Finger PPG value's measuring time (120 minutes after the first bite of meal) usually occurs around the lowest levels of sensor PPG waveform and the average finger PPG is about 16% lower than the average sensor PPG.

Figure 2 depicts the background data for the calculations of predicted PPG and derivations of two glucose coefficients, both GH.f-modulus and GH.p-modulus.

Here again is the step-by-step explanation of the predicted PPG equation:

*(1) **Baseline PPG** equals to 97% of FPG value, or 97% * (weight * GH.f-Modulus).*
*(2) Baseline PPG **plus** increased amount of PPG due to food, i.e. plus (carbs/sugar intake amount * GH.p-Modulus).*
*(3) Baseline PPG **plus** increased PPG due to food, and then **subtracts** reduction amount of PPG due to exercise, i.e. minus (post-meal walking k-steps * 5).*
*(4) The **Predicted PPG** equals to **Baseline PPG plus the food influences, and then subtracts the exercise influences.***

The linear elastic glucose equation is:

Predicted PPG =
*(0.97 * GH.f-modulus * Weight) +(GH.p-modulus * Carbs&sugar) - (post-meal walking k-steps * 5)*

Where
*(1) **Incremental PPG = Predicted PPG - Baseline PPG + Exercise impact***
*(2) **GH.f-modulus = FPG / Weight***
*(3) **GH.p-modulus = Incremental PPG / Carbs intake***

It is interesting to list his calculated results of GH.f-modulus elbow:

Liquid eggs: 0.59
Solid eggs: 0.64
Total meals: 0.64

Regardless of the variety of his meal contents, his overall weight and FPG values are highly consistent. Therefore, this "near-constant" GH.f-modulus values indicate that the conditions of his chronic diseases are under well controlled during the past 2.5-years period.

Figures 3 reflects the GH.p-modulus values link together with Carbs/Sugar amounts and Incremental PPG values for these four groups: liquid eggs, solid eggs, total meals sensor, and total meals finger. As a result, this indicates his glucose sensitivity to carbs & sugar intake amounts of these three groups of meals, excluding total meals finger.

The GH.p-modulus and Incremental PPG relationship can be expressed in the following linear equation:

Incremental PPG =
Carbs intake * GH.p-modulus

The two **GH.p-modulus values are 12.7 for liquid eggs and 20.7 for solid eggs** which are much higher than his two **total meals GH.p-modulus values of 3.4 for total sensor PPG and 2.1 for total finger PPG.** The large differences are due to the extremely low carb intake amount of ~2.5 grams which produces 111 mg/dL for liquid eggs PPG, but a much higher 128 mg/dL for solid eggs PPG resulting from the neuro-communication between the brain and internal organs. Although the total meals finger PPG of 113 mg/dL is quite close to the liquid eggs PPG of 111 mg/dL, but their significant difference of carbs amount (13.8g vs. 2.8g) produces two vastly different GH.p-modulus values (2.1 vs. 12.7).

Here are the key numbers put together in the form of carbs, GH.p:

Liquid eggs: (2.8g, 12.7)
Solid eggs: (2.2g, 20.7)
Total sensor: (13.8g, 3.4)
Total finger: (13.8g, 2.1)

Based on the above findings, during the last 2.5 years, *the author has applied one multiplier of 2.1 for his predicted finger PPG and another multiplier of 3.4 for his predicted sensor PPG to achieve highly accurate PPG prediction.*

Another sanity check to conduct the following calculation in the formula: "Incremental PPG = carbs * GH.p"

Liquid eggs:
2.8g * 12.7 = 35.6 mg/dL
Solid eggs:
2.2g * 20.7 = 45.5 mg/dL
Total meals sensor:
13.8g * 3.4 = 46.9 mg/dL

Total meals finger:
13.8g * 2.1 = 29.0 mg/dL

When he adds the corresponding baseline PPG values of the above calculated incremental PPG values, he accurately obtained the four sets of predicted PPG values which are identical to his measured PPG values.

Conclusions:

It is quite interesting to put the author's 285 special egg meals experimental data side by side with his 2,843 total meals data together. The differences of the carb amount and GH.p-modulus values between the egg meals and total meals are vast and obvious.

The neuroscience egg meals are offered as extreme cases for the GH.p-modulus boundary situations by having an extremely low carb intake amount per meal with an associated much higher GH.p-modulus value. However, the conclusions from the case of 2,843 total meals could offer general guidelines for type 2 diabetes patients who want to control their diabetic conditions via lifestyle management program. The author thinks that a general GH.p-modulus range of 1.0 to 5.0 is probably suitable for the majority of clinical cases (the author's own range is 2.1 to 3.4). From a practical angle, a patient can use this GH.p-modulus value as a multiplier of his carbs/sugar amount and use a number of 5 as his multiplier to the post-meal walking k-steps and then plug them into the following "quick but not so dirty" formula in order to obtain the predicted PPG.

Predicted PPG =
FPG + (GH.p * Carbs) - (k-steps *5)

Where the patient can attempt to use different numbers between 1 through 5 as the GH.p input value to determine the suitable GH.p-modulus.

By using the above estimated PPG formula, diabetes patients can find their PPG level very quickly and accurately without delving into the details of the linear elastic glucose theory.

References:

1. Hsu, Gerald C., eclaireMD Foundation, USA, No. 310: "Biomedical research methodology based on GH-Method: math-physical medicine"

2. Hsu, Gerald C., eclaireMD Foundation, USA, No. 345: "Application of linear equations to predict sensor and finger based postprandial plasma glucoses and daily glucoses for pre-virus, virus, and total periods using GH-Method: math-physical medicine"

3. Hsu, Gerald C., eclaireMD Foundation, USA, No. 97: "A simplified yet accurate linear equation of PPG prediction model for T2D patients (GH-Method: math-physical medicine)"

4. Hsu, Gerald C., eclaireMD Foundation, USA, No. 99: "Application of linear equation-based PPG prediction model for four T2D clinic cases (GH-Method: math-physical medicine)"

5. Hsu, Gerald C., eclaireMD Foundation, USA, No. 339: "Self-recovery of pancreatic beta cell's insulin secretion based on 10+ years annualized data of food, exercise, weight, and glucose using GH-Method: math-physical medicine)

6. Hsu, Gerald C., eclaireMD Foundation, USA, No. 340: "A neural communication model between brain and internal organs, specifically stomach, liver, and pancreatic beta cells based on PPG waveforms of 131 liquid egg meals and 124 solid egg meals)

7. Hsu, Gerald C., eclaireMD Foundation, USA, No. 349: "Using Math-Physics Medicine to Predict FPG"

8. Hsu, Gerald C., eclaireMD Foundation, USA, No. 264: "Community and Family Medicine via Doctors without distance: Using a simple glucose control card to assist T2D patients in remote rural areas (GH-Method: math-physical medicine)"

9. Hsu, Gerald C., eclaireMD Foundation, USA, No. 346: "Linear relationship between carbohydrates & sugar intake amount and incremental PPG amount via engineering strength of materials using GH-Method: math-physical medicine, Part 1"

10. Hsu, Gerald C., eclaireMD Foundation, USA, No. 349: "Investigation on GH modulus of linear elastic glucose with two diabetes patients data using GH-Method: math-physical medicine, Part 2"

11. Hsu, Gerald C., eclaireMD Foundation, USA, No. 349: "Investigation of GH modulus on the linear elastic glucose behavior based on three diabetes patients' data using the GH-Method: math-physical medicine, Part 3"

12. Hsu, Gerald C., eclaireMD Foundation, USA, No. 356: "Coefficient of GH.f-modulus in the linear elastic fasting plasma glucose behavior study based on health data of three diabetes patients using the GH-Method: math-physical medicine, Part 4 "

13. Hsu, Gerald C., eclaireMD Foundation, USA, No. 357: "High accuracy of predicted postprandial plasma glucose using two coefficients of GH.f-modulus and GH.p-modulus from linear elastic glucose behavior theory based on GH-Method: math-physical medicine, Part 5"

14. Hsu, Gerald C., eclaireMD Foundation, USA, No. 358: "Improvement on the prediction accuracy of postprandial plasma glucose using two biomedical coefficients of GH-modulus from linear elastic glucose theory based on GH-Method: math-physical medicine, Part 6"

15. Hsu, Gerald C., eclaireMD Foundation, USA, No. 359: "High glucose predication accuracy of postprandial plasma glucose and fasting plasma glucose during the

COVID-19 period using two glucose coefficients of GH-modulus from linear elastic glucose theory based on GH-Method: math-physical medicine, Part 7"

16. Hsu, Gerald C., eclaireMD Foundation, USA, No. 360: "Investigation of two glucose coefficients of GH.f-modulus and GH.p-modulus based on data of 3 clinical cases during COVID-19 period using linear elastic glucose theory of GH-Method: math-physical medicine, Part 8"

17. Hsu, Gerald C., eclaireMD Foundation, USA, No. 361: "Postprandial plasma glucose lower and upper boundary study using two glucose coefficients of GH-modulus from linear elastic glucose theory based on GH-Method: math-physical medicine, Part 9"

18. Hsu, Gerald C., eclaireMD Foundation, USA, No. 362: "Six international clinical cases demonstrating prediction accuracies of postprandial plasma glucoses and suggested methods for improvements using linear elastic glucose theory of GH-Method: math-physical medicine, Part 10"

19. Hsu, Gerald C., eclaireMD Foundation, USA, No. 362: "A special Neuro-communication influences on GH.p-modulus of linear elastic glucose theory based on data from 159 liquid egg and 126 solid egg meals using GH-Method: math-physical medicine, Part 11"

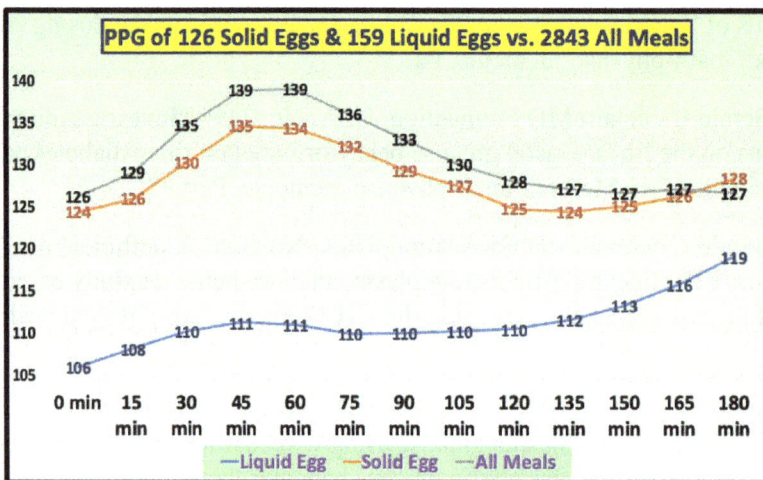

Figure 1: Three PPG waveforms comparison between 159 liquid eggs (egg drop soup), 126 solid eggs (pan-fried egg and hard broiled egg), and 2,843 total meals using sensor device for measuring PPG

Total: 5/5/2018-11/7/2020	Meals:	159	126	2843	2843
	The Author	Liquid Eggs	Solid Eggs	All Meals - Sensor	All Meals -Finger
	GH.f-modulus (%)	59	64	64	64
	Sensor FPG (mg/dL)	100	109	110	110
Formula	Weight (pound)	170	172	171	171
= FPG / Weight	GH.f-modulus	0.59	0.64	0.64	0.64
= 0.97 * Weight * GH.f-modulus	Baseline PPG (mg/dL)	97	106	106	106
	GH.p-modulus	12.7	20.7	3.4	2.1
	Carbs&Sugar (gram)	2.8	2.2	13.8	13.8
	Carbs *GH.p-modulus	35	46	46	28
	Walking (k-steps)	4.2	4.7	4.3	4.3
= Baseline+Carbs*GH.p-Walk*5	Predicted PPG	111.3	128.3	131.0	113.0
	Measured PPG (mg/dL)	111.3	128.3	131.0	113.0
= Predicted PPG / Measured PPG	Accuracy of Predicted PPG	100%	100%	100%	100%
	The Author	Liquid Eggs	Solid Eggs	All Meals - Sensor	All Meals -Finger
	Carbs&Sugar (gram)	2.8	2.2	13.8	13.8
= predcted PPG - Baseline PPG + K-steps*5	Incremental PPG (mg/dL)	35.4	45.6	46.3	28.3
= Incremental PPG / Carbs&Sugar	GH.p-modulus	12.7	20.7	3.4	2.1

Figure 2: Data, definition, and formula using GH.f-modulus, GH.p-modulus, Baseline PPG, Incremental PPG and calculation of Predicted PPG for liquid eggs, solid eggs, and total meals

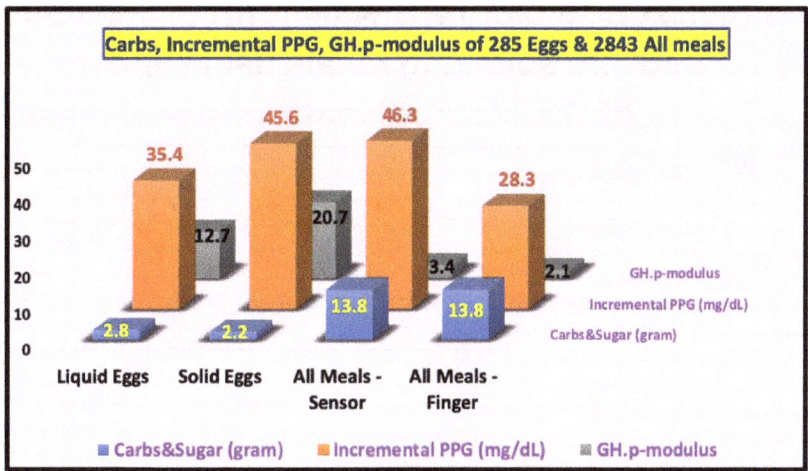

Figure 3: GH.p-modulus linking Carbs and Incremental PPG for liquid eggs, solid eggs, and total meals

Detailed GH.p-modulus values at 15-minute time intervals for a synthesized sensor PPG waveform of 159 liquid egg meals, and 126 solid egg meals using linear elastic glucose theory of GH-Method: math-physical medicine, Part 13 (No. 365)

Gerald C. Hsu
eclaireMD Foundation, USA
11/19-20/2020

Abstract:

This article is Part 13 of the author's linear elastic glucose behavior study. It focuses on a deeper investigation of GH.p-modulus at 15-minute time intervals for a synthesized PPG waveform based on the comparison of the results from his neuroscience study on two types of egg meals during the period from 5/5/2018 to 11/17/2020.

Here is the step by step explanation for the predicted postprandial plasma glucose (PPG) equation using linear elastic glucose theory as described in References 9 through 20:

*(1) **Baseline PPG** equals to 97% of fasting plasma glucose (FPG) value, or 97% * (weight * GH.f-Modulus).*
*(2) Baseline PPG **plus** increased amount of PPG due to food, i.e. plus (carbs/sugar intake amount * GH.p-Modulus).*
*(3) Baseline PPG **plus** increased PPG due to food, and then **subtracts** reduction . amount of PPG due to exercise, i.e. minus (post-meal walking k-steps * 5).*
*(4) The **Predicted PPG** equals to **Baseline PPG plus the food influences, and then subtracts the exercise influences.***

The linear elastic glucose equation is:

Predicted PPG =
(0.97 * GH.f-modulus * Weight) +(GH.p-modulus * Carbs&sugar) - (post-meal walking k-steps * 5)

Where
*(1) **Incremental PPG = Predicted PPG - Baseline PPG + Exercise impact***
*(2) **GH.f-modulus = FPG / Weight***
*(3) **GH.p-modulus = Incremental PPG / Carbs intake***

This study analyzes the glucose coefficient of GH.p-modulus at 15-minute intervals for two synthesized PPG waveforms associated with liquid eggs and solid eggs. The variation range of GH.p-modulus are between 15 and 22 with an average of 18.9 for solid eggs and between 10 and 14 with an average of 11.6 for liquid eggs.

The average GH.p-modulus values of 18.9 for solid eggs and 11.6 for liquid eggs using every 15-minute intervals of the PPG values are comparable with the average GH.p-modulus values of 20.7 for solid eggs and 12.7 for liquid eggs using the average glucose values of 285 egg meals (Reference 19 of paper no. 363).

However, a vast difference can be observed by comparing the 285 egg meals, where the *GH.p-modulus are in double digits*, against his 2,843 total meals (see Reference 19). His GH.p-modulus values of 2,483 total meals are 2.1 using finger PPG and 3.4 using sensor PPG, where the *GH.p-modulus are in a single digit*.

The differences are caused by the neural communication model between the brain and internal organs. This neuroscience contribution factor has caused the higher solid egg meals PPG magnitudes in comparison with the lower liquid egg meals PPG values. Actually, the different peak PPG values of the two different physical states of egg meals, resulting from varying cooking methods, have the same carbs/sugar intake amount of ~2 grams and comparable exercise amount of ~4,500 steps.

Although this paper does not focus on the neuroscience studies of egg meals, it is investigating the possible variance of GH.p-modulus. The study utilizes a step by step illustration of moving from (1) the difference between PPG and FPG, going through (2) Incremental PPG, then finally arriving at (3) Predicted PPG. By moving along with this calculation process, we can observe three waveform variances between liquid egg meals versus solid egg meals.

As a result, the author has gained a great deal of inside knowledge and a clear picture of the characteristics and behaviors of the most difficult glucose coefficient, GH.p-modulus, as presented in his research work on linear elastic glucose behaviors for Part 13.

Introduction:

This article is Part 13 of the author's linear elastic glucose behavior study. It focuses on a deeper investigation of GH.p-modulus at 15-minute time intervals for a synthesized PPG waveform based on the comparison of the results from his neuroscience study on two types of egg meals during the period from 5/5/2018 to 11/17/2020.

Methods:

Background:

To learn more about the author's GH-Method: math-physical medicine (MPM) methodology, readers can refer to his article to understand his developed MPM analysis method in Reference 1.

Highlights of linear elastic glucose theory:

Here is the step by step explanation for the predicted PPG equation using linear elastic glucose theory as described in References 9 through 20:

*(1) **Baseline PPG** equals to 97% of FPG value, or 97% * (weight * GH.f-Modulus).*
*(2) Baseline PPG **plus** increased amount of PPG due to food, i.e. plus (carbs/sugar intake amount * GH.p-Modulus).*
*(3) Baseline PPG **plus** increased PPG due to food, and then **subtracts** reduction amount of PPG due to exercise, i.e. minus (post-meal walking k-steps * 5).*
*(4) The **Predicted PPG** equals to **Baseline PPG plus the food influences, and then subtracts the exercise influences.***

The linear elastic glucose equation is:

Predicted PPG =
(0.97 * GH.f-modulus * Weight) +(GH.p-modulus * Carbs&sugar) - (post-meal
walking k-steps * 5)

Where
(1) Incremental PPG = Predicted PPG - Baseline PPG + Exercise impact
(2) GH.f-modulus = FPG / Weight
(3) GH.p-modulus = Incremental PPG / Carbs intake

By using this linear equation, a diabetes patient only needs the input data of body weight, carbs & sugar intake amount, and post-meal walking steps in order to calculate the predicted PPG value without obtaining any measured glucose data.

In 2014, the author came up with the analogy between theory of elasticity and plasticity and the severity of diabetes when he was developing his mathematical model of metabolism.

On 10/14/2020, by utilizing the concept of Young's modulus with stress and strain, which was taught in engineering schools, he initiated and engaged this linear elastic glucose behaviors research. The following paragraphs describe his research findings at different stages of this research period:

First, he discovered that there is a "pseudo-linear" relationship existing between carbs & sugar intake amount and incremental PPG amount. Based on this finding, he defined the first glucose coefficient of GH.p-modulus for PPG.

Second, similar to Young's modulus relating to stiffness of engineering inorganic materials, he found that the GH.p-modulus is dependent upon the patient's severity level of diabetes, i.e. the patient's glucose sensitivity on carbs/sugar intake amount.

Third, comparable to GH.p-modulus for PPG, in 2017, he uncovered a similar pseudo-linear relationship existing between weight and FPG with high correlation coefficient of above 90%. Therefore, he defined the second glucose coefficient of GH.f-modulus as the FPG value divided by the weight value. This GH.f-modulus is related to the severity of combined chronic diseases, including both obesity and diabetes.

Fourth, he inserted these two glucose coefficients of GH.p-modulus and GH.f-modulus, into the predicted PPG equation to remove the burden of collecting measured glucoses by patients.

Fifth, by experimenting and calculating many predicted PPG values over a variety of time length from different diabetes patients with different health conditions, he finally revealed that GH.p-modulus seems to be "near-constant" or "pseudo-linearized" over a short period of 3 to 4 months. This short period is compatible with the known lifespan of human red blood cells, which are living organic cells. This is quite different from the engineering inorganic materials, such as steel or concrete which can last for an exceptionally long period of time. The same conclusion was observed using his monthly GH.p-modulus data during the COVID-19 period in 2010 when his lifestyle became routine and stabilized.

Sixth, he used three US clinical cases during the 2020 COVID-19 period to delve into the hidden characteristics of the physical parameters and their biomedical relationships. More importantly, through the comparison study in Part 7, he found explainable biomedical interpretations of his two defined glucose coefficients of GH.p-modulus and GH.f-modulus.

Seventh, he conducted a PPG boundary analysis by discovering a lower bound and an upper bound of predicted PPG values for eight hypothetical standard cases and three US specific clinical cases. The derived numerical values of these two boundaries make sense from a biomedical viewpoint and also matched with the situations of the three US clinical cases. He even conducted two extreme stress tests, i.e. increasing carbs/sugar intake amount to 50 grams per meal and boosting post-meal walking steps to 5k after each meal, to examine the impacts on the lower bound and upper bound of PPG values.

Eighth, based on six international clinical cases, he further explored the influences from the combination of obesity and diabetes. Using a "lifestyle medicine" approach, he offered recommendations to reduce their PPG from 130-150 mg/dL down to below 120 mg/dL via reducing carbs/sugar intake and increasing exercise level in walking.

Ninth, based on his neuroscience research work using both 126 solid eggs and 159 liquid eggs with a very low carbs/sugar intake amount of ~2.5 grams producing two totally different sets of PPG values and waveforms, he identified a different set of much higher values of GH.p-modules for these egg meals. Even though this research served as a special boundary case in the study, nevertheless, it has further proven that the GH.p-modules is also influenced directly by the human brain.

Tenth, he compared the above two egg meals results, including PPG values and glucose coefficients, in particular the GH.p-modules, against the total results of his 2,843. He discovered the vast differences of GH.p-modulus magnitudes and also learned the tight relationship between GH.p-modulus value and carbs/sugar intake amount. By distinguishing these GH.p-modulus results from the special boundary cases of 12.7 for liquid egg meals and 20.7 for solid egg meals, his general GH.p-modulus values from his 2,843 total meals are 2.1 using finger PPG and 3.4 using sensor PPG.

Meal cases in this article:
In multiple published articles from his neuroscience research work, he separated his egg meals into two distinctive physical states, liquid state (159 egg drop soup) and solid state (126 pan-fried egg or hard broiled egg), during the period from 5/5/2018 to 11/17/2020. This period is selected due to the same glucose measuring period via a continuous glucose monitoring (CGM) sensor device on his arm. His 285 egg meals have an average carb intake amount around 2.5 grams and his average post-meal walking approximately 4.5 k-steps. His sensor measured PPG levels are 111 mg/dL

for liquid eggs PPG and 128 mg/dL for solid eggs PPG.

During the same time period, he has consumed a total of 2,843 meals with an average carb intake amount of 13.8 grams and his post-meal walking is 4.3 k-step. It should be mentioned that he also continued to measure his PPG using the traditional finger-piercing method at 120-minutes after the first bite of his meal. For this total meal's group, his measured PPG levels are 131 mg/dL for sensor PPG and 113 mg/dL for finger PPG.

At first, he calculates the estimated baseline PPG for these two types of egg meals and then uses the following two equations to calculate the incremental PPG and GH.p-modulus.

Incremental PPG =
baseline PPG (i.e. 0.97*FPG or FPG) + exercise impact (walking ksteps*5)

GH.p-modulus =
(Incremental PPG) / (Carbs amount)

Above two equations are based on his developed "linear elastic glucose theory" which can be described as follows:

FPG = (Weight) * (GH.f-modulus)

and

(Incremental PPG) =
(Carbs amount) * (GH.p-modulus)

Results:

Figure 1 shows the comparison of PPG waveforms between 126 solid egg meals and 159 liquid egg meals. It is obvious that the **solid egg PPG waveform (peak PPG 135 mg/dL at 45-minutes, average PPG 128 g/dL, and carbs 2.2 grams) is higher than the liquid egg PPG waveform (peak PPG 111 mg/dL at 45-minutes, average PPG 111 g/dL and carbs 2.8 grams).** The reason for the PPG differences with the same inputs of both carbs/sugar amount and exercise steps is due to the neural communication between the brain and internal organs regarding the physical states of the food, which is not the main focus in this article.

Of course, in this two-years period of diabetes research and food nutrition experiment, he did not consume both liquid eggs and solid eggs in the same meal. He also knows that different days would have different FPG values which can be served as the baseline PPG for one particular meal. Therefore, the author has modified his software program such that he could extract the FPG values corresponding to the days with one particular type of meals of the same day.

Figure 2 depicts the waveforms of the difference between PPG and FPG. These curves (i.e. waveforms) indicate the amount of PPG minus FPG is the final results from the inputs of both food and exercise. It is interesting to find that solid egg meals curve (peak at 25 mg/dL) is still higher than the liquid egg meals curve (peak at 11 mg/dL). At the peak PPG time (45-min to 60-min), solid egg meal is 14 mg/dL higher than liquid egg meal where both have almost identical carbs/sugar intake amount and post-meal walking steps. Of course, from a neuroscience viewpoint, a reasonable explanation could be offered to explain this strange physical phenomenon.

Figure 3 reflects the waveforms of Incremental PPG for these two egg meals. These 2 Incremental PPG waveform patterns are very similar to those 2 waveforms of (PPG-FPG) in Figure 2, except for the solid egg meals have a peak incremental PPG of 49 mg/dL around 45-60 minutes, while the liquid egg meals have a peak incremental PPG of 32 mg/dL around 45-60 minutes. Again, at the peak PPG time (45-min to 60-min), the solid egg meal is 17 mg/dL higher than liquid egg meal where both have almost identical carbs/sugar intake amount and post-meal walking steps. Once again, from a neuroscience viewpoint, a reasonable explanation could be offered to explain this strange physical phenomenon.

After conducting his calculations for both (PPG-FPG) and incremental PPG, he was able to figure out the different GH.p-modulus values at each 15-minute time interval of the synthesized PPG waveforms for both liquid egg meals and solid egg meals (Figure 4).

Here again is the step by step explanation for the predicted PPG equation:

*(1) **Baseline PPG** equals to 97% of FPG value, or 97% * (weight * GH.f-Modulus).*
*(2) Baseline PPG **plus** increased amount of PPG due to food, i.e. plus (carbs/sugar intake amount * GH.p-Modulus).*
*(3) Baseline PPG **plus** increased PPG due to food, and then **subtracts** reduction amount of PPG due to exercise, i.e. minus (post-meal walking k-steps * 5).*
*(4) The **Predicted PPG** equals to **Baseline PPG plus the food influences, and then subtracts the exercise influences.***

The linear elastic glucose equation is:

Predicted PPG =
(0.97 * GH.f-modulus * Weight) +(GH.p-modulus * Carbs&sugar) - (post-meal walking k-steps * 5)

Where
(1) Incremental PPG = Predicted PPG - Baseline PPG + Exercise impact
(2) GH.f-modulus = FPG / Weight
(3) GH.p-modulus = Incremental PPG / Carbs intake

Here is the list of his final calculated GH.f-modulus values in the form of liquid egg, solid egg at each 15-minute time intervals.

0-min: *(10, 17)*
15-min: *(10, 18)*
30-min: *(11, 20)*
45-min: *(12, 22)*
60-min: *(11, 22)*
75-min: *(11, 21)*
90-min: *(11, 20)*
105-min: (11, 19)
120-min: (11, 18)
135-min: (12, 17)
150-min: (12, 18)
165-min: (13, 18)
180-min: (14, 15)

Average:(11.6, 18.9)

The average GH.p-modulus values of 11.6 for liquid eggs and 18.9 for solid eggs using every 15-minute intervals of the glucose values *are quite comparable with the average GH.p-modulus values of 12.7 for liquid eggs and 20.7 for solid eggs* using the average glucose values for the two types of egg meals (Reference 19).

Conclusions:

This study analyzes the glucose coefficient of GH.p-modulus at 15-minute intervals for two synthesized PPG waveforms associated with liquid eggs and solid eggs. The variation range of GH.p-modulus are between 15 and 22 with an average of 18.9 for solid eggs and between 10 and 14 with an average of 11.6 for liquid eggs.

The average GH.p-modulus values of 18.9 for solid eggs and 11.6 for liquid eggs using every 15-minute intervals of the PPG values are comparable with the average GH.p-modulus values of 20.7 for solid eggs and 12.7 for liquid eggs using the average glucose values of 285 egg meals (Reference 19 of paper no. 363).

However, a vast difference can be observed by comparing the 285 egg meals, where the GH.p-modulus are in double digits, against his 2,843 total meals (see Reference 19). His GH.p-modulus values of 2,483 total meals are 2.1 using finger PPG and 3.4 using sensor PPG, where the GH.p-modulus are in a single digit.

The differences are caused by the neural communication model between the brain and internal organs. This neuroscience contribution factor has caused the higher solid egg meals PPG magnitudes in comparison with the lower liquid egg meals PPG values. Actually, the different peak PPG values of the two different physical states of egg meals, resulting from varying cooking methods, have the same carbs/sugar intake amount of ~2 grams and comparable exercise amount of ~4,500 steps.

Although this paper does not focus on the neuroscience studies of egg meals, it is investigating the possible variance of GH.p-modulus. The study utilizes a step by step illustration of moving from (1) the difference between PPG and FPG, going through (2) Incremental PPG, then finally arriving at (3) Predicted PPG. By moving along with this calculation process, we can observe three waveform variances between liquid egg meals versus solid egg meals.

As a result, the author has gained a great deal of inside knowledge and a clear picture of the characteristics and behaviors of the most difficult glucose coefficient, GH.p-modulus, as presented in his research work on linear elastic glucose behaviors for Part 13.

References:

1. Hsu, Gerald C., eclaireMD Foundation, USA, No. 310: "Biomedical research methodology based on GH-Method: math-physical medicine"

2. Hsu, Gerald C., eclaireMD Foundation, USA, No. 345: "Application of linear equations to predict sensor and finger based postprandial plasma glucoses and daily glucoses for pre-virus, virus, and total periods using GH-Method: math-physical medicine"

3. Hsu, Gerald C., eclaireMD Foundation, USA, No. 97: "A simplified yet accurate linear equation of PPG prediction model for T2D patients (GH-Method: math-physical medicine)"

4. Hsu, Gerald C., eclaireMD Foundation, USA, No. 99: "Application of linear equation-based PPG prediction model for four T2D clinic cases (GH-Method: math-physical medicine)"

5. Hsu, Gerald C., eclaireMD Foundation, USA, No. 339: "Self-recovery of pancreatic beta cell's insulin secretion based on 10+ years annualized data of food, exercise, weight, and glucose using GH-Method: math-physical medicine)

6. Hsu, Gerald C., eclaireMD Foundation, USA, No. 340: "A neural communication model between brain and internal organs, specifically stomach, liver, and pancreatic beta cells based on PPG waveforms of 131 liquid egg meals and 124 solid egg meals)

7. Hsu, Gerald C., eclaireMD Foundation, USA, No. 349: "Using Math-Physics Medicine to Predict FPG"

8. Hsu, Gerald C., eclaireMD Foundation, USA, No. 264: "Community and Family Medicine via Doctors without distance: Using a simple glucose control card to assist T2D patients in remote rural areas (GH-Method: math-physical medicine)"

9. Hsu, Gerald C., eclaireMD Foundation, USA, No. 346: "Linear relationship between carbohydrates & sugar intake amount and incremental PPG amount via engineering strength of materials using GH-Method: math-physical medicine, Part 1"

10. Hsu, Gerald C., eclaireMD Foundation, USA, No. 349: "Investigation on GH

modulus of linear elastic glucose with two diabetes patients data using GH-Method: math-physical medicine, Part 2"

11. Hsu, Gerald C., eclaireMD Foundation, USA, No. 349: "Investigation of GH modulus on the linear elastic glucose behavior based on three diabetes patients' data using the GH-Method: math-physical medicine, Part 3"

12. Hsu, Gerald C., eclaireMD Foundation, USA, No. 356: "Coefficient of GH.f-modulus in the linear elastic fasting plasma glucose behavior study based on health data of three diabetes patients using the GH-Method: math-physical medicine, Part 4 "

13. Hsu, Gerald C., eclaireMD Foundation, USA, No. 357: "High accuracy of predicted postprandial plasma glucose using two coefficients of GH.f-modulus and GH.p-modulus from linear elastic glucose behavior theory based on GH-Method: math-physical medicine, Part 5"

14. Hsu, Gerald C., eclaireMD Foundation, USA, No. 358: "Improvement on the prediction accuracy of postprandial plasma glucose using two biomedical coefficients of GH-modulus from linear elastic glucose theory based on GH-Method: math-physical medicine, Part 6"

15. Hsu, Gerald C., eclaireMD Foundation, USA, No. 359: "High glucose predication accuracy of postprandial plasma glucose and fasting plasma glucose during the COVID-19 period using two glucose coefficients of GH-modulus from linear elastic glucose theory based on GH-Method: math-physical medicine, Part 7"

16. Hsu, Gerald C., eclaireMD Foundation, USA, No. 360: "Investigation of two glucose coefficients of GH.f-modulus and GH.p-modulus based on data of 3 clinical cases during COVID-19 period using linear elastic glucose theory of GH-Method: math-physical medicine, Part 8"

17. Hsu, Gerald C., eclaireMD Foundation, USA, No. 361: "Postprandial plasma glucose lower and upper boundary study using two glucose coefficients of GH-modulus from linear elastic glucose theory based on GH-Method: math-physical medicine, Part 9"

18. Hsu, Gerald C., eclaireMD Foundation, USA, No. 362: "Six international clinical cases demonstrating prediction accuracies of postprandial plasma glucoses and suggested methods for improvements using linear elastic glucose theory of GH-Method: math-physical medicine, Part 10"

19. Hsu, Gerald C., eclaireMD Foundation, USA, No. 363: "A special Neuro-communication influences on GH.p-modulus of linear elastic glucose theory based on data from 159 liquid egg and 126 solid egg meals using GH-Method: math-physical medicine, Part 11"

20. Hsu, Gerald C., eclaireMD Foundation, USA, No. 364: "GH.p-modulus study of linear elastic glucose theory based on data from 159 liquid egg meals, 126 solid egg meals, and 2,843 total meals using GH-Method: math-physical medicine, Part

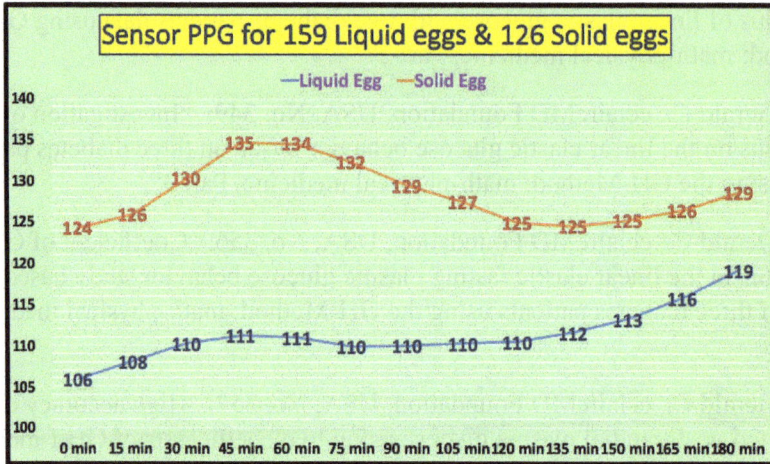

Figure 1: Two PPG waveforms comparison between 159 liquid eggs (egg drop soup) and 126 solid eggs (pan-fried egg and hard broiled egg) using CGM sensor device for measuring PPG values

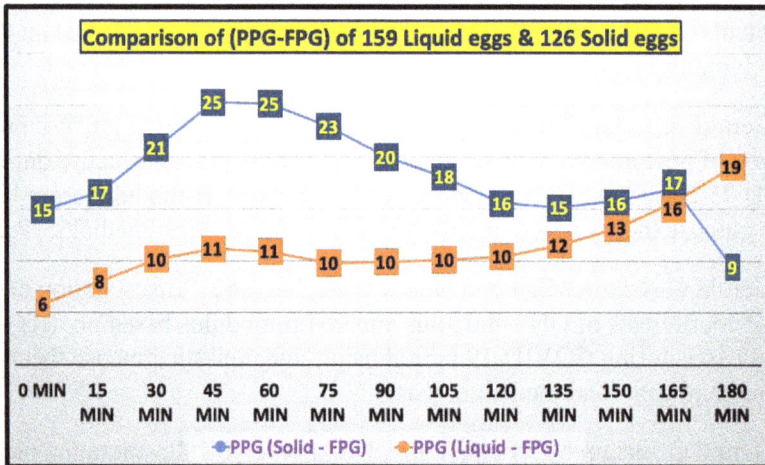

Figure 2: Comparison of values of (PPG minus FPG) between 159 liquid eggs (egg drop soup) and 126 solid eggs (pan-fried egg and hard broiled egg)

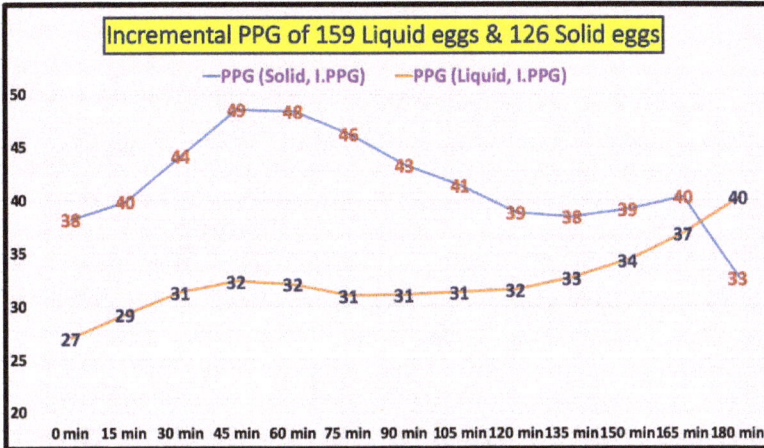

*Figure 3: Comparison of Incremental PPG values (= predicted PPG - 0.97 * FPG + Walking's 1000 steps *5) between 159 liquid eggs (egg drop soup) and 126 solid eggs (pan-fried egg and hard broiled egg)*

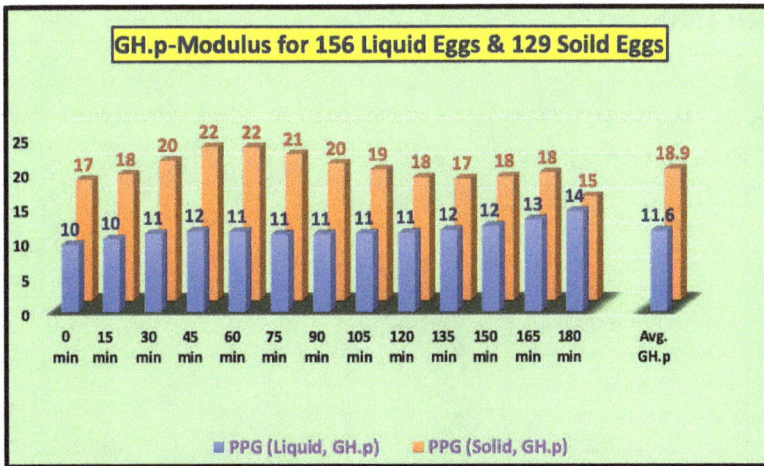

Figure 4: Comparison of GH.p-modulus values (= Incremental PPG divided by Carbs amount) at every 15-minutes time intervals of a synthesized PPG waveform between 159 liquid eggs (egg drop soup) and 126 solid eggs (pan-fried egg and hard broiled egg)

A lifestyle medicine model for family medical practices based on 9-years of clinical data including food, weight, glucose, carbs/sugar, and walking using linear elastic glucose theory (Part 14) and GH-Method: math-physical medicine (No. 367)

By: Gerald C. Hsu
eclaireMD Foundation, USA
11/22-25/2020

Abstract:

This article is aimed at assisting family medical practices for obesity and type 2 diabetes (T2D) control using the lifestyle medicine model, which is also the Part 14 of his recently developed linear elastic glucose theory (LEGT).

More than 33 million Americans, about 1 in 10, have diabetes, and approximately **90% to 95%** of them have type 2 diabetes (T2D), where **86%** also have problems with being overweight or obese. In other words, 7.7% to 8.2 % of the US population or 25 to 27 million Americans have issues with weight, T2D conditions and multiple complications.

The author is a patient who suffered with being overweight/obesity and T2D for over 25 years. He faced many complications from 2002 to 2010. Over the past 11 years, he dedicated himself to research diabetes and its complications. In this article, he describes the simple and straightforward yet highly precise method to control his chronic disease conditions, including weight and glucose. The results of his research provide proof through a big data analytics of his collected input data through the continuous research and implementation efforts during the past 9 years. His findings have finally achieved satisfactory health results with high mathematical precision on his various biomarker predictions.

He named this the "lifestyle medicine" approach. The purpose of writing this article is to offer a simple but practical approach to patients with chronic diseases like himself.

In summary, the author describes his straightforward implementation model in the following four steps:

By reducing his weight from 189 lb. to 170 lb. (-19 lb. or -10% in total weight), cutting off about 50% of his original over-eating food portion size (from 130% in 2012 down to 66% in 2020, which is -7% of his annual food portion reduction from original amount, or -6% averaged annual reduction continuously). This food portion reduction will automatically reduce the intake amount of fat and carbohydrates. But he strictly control his sugar, and sodium amounts. And he maintains a sufficient intake amount of high-quality protein.
When his weight dropped from 189 lbs. to 170 lbs. (-10% or -1.1% per year), his FPG then decreased from 140 mg/dL to 102 mg/dL (-38 mg/dL or -27%, or -3% per year) accordingly. Weight and FPG are highly correlated (93%).
When his FPG dropped, his PPG also reduced from 128 mg/dL to 108 mg/dL (-20 mg/dL or -16%, or -1.7% per year), providing he limits his carb/sugar intake amount below 15 grams per meal and walking at least 30 minutes after each meal. He also increased his post-meal walking from 500 steps to 4,400 steps (+433 post-meal steps per year or +87% per year in comparison with his walking steps in 2012).
He wants to re-emphasize the importance of diet and exercise. Normally, reduction on food and meal portion will automatically assist on limiting the carbs/sugar intake amount. However, patients should always watch out for the overall nutritional balance. For the author, his carbs/sugar intake amount has been cut down from 20

grams to 12.5 grams per meal (-7.5 grams or -38%, or -4% per year) as a result of his food portion reduction from 130% to 66% (-64% of food portion or -7% per year).

This article merely provides a clinical proof using a quantitative and precision approach. These mathematical and biomedical accomplishments are based on careful physical phenomena observations and related biomedical interpretation and proof process. This particular research project of food nutrition and biomedicine has utilized his developed GH-Method: math-physical medicine in which 366 medical papers have been published. The above four statements are simple to understand. Therefore, there is no need to learn fancy theories, complex formulas or equations. No need to take special seminars or attend college courses, take high dosages of medications or supplements, or go through any unnecessary surgeries. There are straight-line relationships existing among food, exercise, weight, and glucose that follow a simple and straight-line route of *"from food portion control to weight reduction and arrive at glucose stability for both FPG and PPG"*.

Introduction:

This article is aimed at assisting family medical practices for obesity and type 2 diabetes (T2D) control using the lifestyle medicine model, which is also the Part 14 of his recently developed linear elastic glucose theory (LEGT).

More than 33 million Americans, about 1 in 10, have diabetes, and approximately **90% to 95%** of them have type 2 diabetes (T2D), where **86%** also have problems with being overweight or obese. In other words, 7.7% to 8.2 % of the US population or 25 to 27 million Americans have issues with weight, T2D conditions and multiple complications.

The author is a patient who suffered with being overweight/obesity and T2D for over 25 years. He faced many complications from 2002 to 2010. Over the past 11 years, he dedicated himself to research diabetes and its complications. In this article, he describes the simple and straightforward yet highly precise method to control his chronic disease conditions, including weight and glucose. The results of his research provide proof through a big data analytics of his collected input data through the continuous research and implementation efforts during the past 9 years. His findings have finally achieved satisfactory health results with high mathematical precision on his various biomarker predictions.

He named this the "lifestyle medicine" approach. The purpose of writing this article is to offer a simple but practical approach to patients with chronic diseases like himself.

Methods:

Background:
To learn more about the author's GH-Method: math-physical medicine (MPM) methodology, readers can refer to his article to understand his developed MPM analysis method in Reference 1.

Case description:
The author has had T2D for over 25-years, while being obese and overweight. In 2010, his weight was 220 lbs. (BMI 32.5), with a daily average glucose over 200 mg/dL. He has also suffered many diabetes complications, including five cardiac episodes, severe kidney complications, foot ulcer, diabetic retinopathy, bladder infections, hypothyroidism, and others. After receiving warnings from three individual physicians regarding his serious conditions and death threats, he decided to self-study those chronic diseases and tried to make a serious change on his overall lifestyle.

After 9 years of his continuous efforts, over the past 6 months in 2020, his average weight is 169.5 lbs. (BMI 24.9) and his average daily glucose is 103 mg/dL (FPG 94, PPG 106) without taking any medications or insulin injections.

Data collection:
Since 1/1/2012, the author developed a research-oriented software on his iPhone to collect all of his diabetes-related medical data and lifestyle details. He also spend the entire year of 2014 to develop a mathematical model of metabolism which has been served as the cornerstone of his follow-up research work. He started to keep a complete daily record of his weight (morning and bedtime) since 4/11/2015, and his glucoses since 6/1/2015. Prior to mid-2015, he had sparse data that were not as complete compared to the period after mid-2015.

In addition, he started to collect his glucose data using a continuous glucose monitor (CGM) sensor device from 5/5/2018. He has accumulated approximately 91 glucose data per day with 13 glucose data per meal over a 3-hour time span. However, he discovered that his average sensor-collected glucoses is about 16% higher than his finger-pierced glucoses, where his postprandial plasma glucose (PPG) data are measured at 2-hours after the first bite of meal. They are usually located at the lowest position on his 3-hour long sensor PPG waveforms.
In order to keep the data consistency and data integrity of his analysis, he decided to use finger glucose values in this particular study since it covers a long time period of 9-years .

Mathematics of data processing:
In this article, he mainly used average annual values from time-series domain and then conducted correlation coefficient calculations, in addition to pattern and trend analysis via observations of moving-average waveforms.

Other than utilizing the two GH-modules based on his recently developed linear elastic glucose theory (LEGT) to verify the existing relationships among weight, PPG, FPG, Carbs/sugar intake amount and post-meal walking k-steps, there are no other elaborate mathematical tools used in this analysis and article.

Factors affect body weight:
There are many factors that can affect body weight. Some of these key factors are:

- Age

- Gender

- Frequency and number of fastings

- Dietary fat vs. burning of body fat

- Exercise persistence

- Stress situations

- Sleep quality

- Calories influence on hormones

- Existing health conditions

- Thyroid conditions

- Insulin resistance

- Metabolic rate

Weight reduction or control is a complex issue and task. To benefit most patients, the author will skip the detailed academic discussions regarding above-mentioned weight influential factors and concentrate on the discovery and identification of a simpler and more straightforward route to accomplish the goal of weight control.

Results:
Figure 1 shows three curves of weight, FPG, and PPG during the period of 2012 to 2020. Figure 2 depicts three curves of Food portion, Carbs/Sugar intake, and Post-meal Walking during the period of 2012 to 2020. In these two diagrams, all of the 5 curves trend downward year after year, except for the exercise curve of post-meal walking steps that trends upward.

Figures 3, 4, and 5 reveal correlation coefficients (R) of two curves in a pair since R can only be calculated between two curves (two sets of data). These three diagrams reflect a total of 9 pairs of results for R with a total of 6 variables: weight, FPG, PPG, food portion percentage, carbs/sugar amount, and post-meal walking k-steps. In statistics, any R greater than 50% means these two variables are closely inter-related with each other. Therefore, from these 9 sets of R percentages, only PPG vs. carbs/sugar has 53% R and weight vs. PPG has 65% (53% and 65% are already high enough), all other R values are greater than 70%. This proves that the 6 variables in this article are highly correlated with one another.

Figure 6 summarizes 9 correlation coefficients into one table. By observing this table, readers will have a clear picture regarding the "tight relationships" among weight, glucoses (both FPG and PPG), food portion percentage, Carbs/sugar intake amount, and post-meal walking steps.

Figure 7 recaps the annual reduction rates of weight, food portion, FPG, PPG, and carbs/sugar amount.

Finally, Figure 8 displays all of the numerical numbers for data used in this analysis and report.

Figure 9 shows the two calculated GH-modulus values based on the linear elastic glucose theory (LEGT). Here are the definitions of the two GH-modulus:

GH.f-modulus = FPG / Weight

Predicted PPG =
(0.97 * FPG) + (carbs/sugar * GH.p-modulus) - (walking k-steps * 5)

Due to his incomplete collected data for both health and lifestyle from 2012-2015, his calculation of GH.p only starts from 2015. There are two key observations of the following conclusive phenomena.

First, GH.f-modulus is continuously moving downward, from 0.74 in 2012 to 0.60 in 2020 which means that his health conditions of being overweight and diabetes are getting better year after year. Second, his GH.p-modulus values are between 1.6 and 2.5 which are expected values based on his prior research. The special and highest GH.p-modulus value of 2.5 in 2020 is due to his excellent control on low carbs/sugar intake and glucose values resulting from no travel and routine lifestyle during the 2020 COVID-19 quarantine period.

The following table lists the reduction amount of each key variable from 2012 to 2020. They are listed in a form of (2012 amount, 2020 amount, **change amount).** The only exceptional variable is the post-meal walking k-steps which is an "increased" amount.

Weight: *(189, 170, **-19**)*
FPG: *(140, 102, -38)*
PPG: *(128, 108. **-20**)*
Food portion: *(130%, 66%, **-64%**)*
Carbs/Sugar: *(20.0, 12.48, **-7.52**)*
Walking steps: *(0.5, 4.404, **+3.904**)*

In other words, for his case, he has reduced ~50% of his annual average meal portion from 130% to 66% with a 19 lb. reduction in his weight (-10%), then his FPG would be decreased by 38 mg/dL (-27%) and his PPG would be reduced by 20 mg/dL (-16%). This proves the existence of a "straight-line route" of ***"from food portion control to weight and glucose control".***

Most T2D patients, who do not possess sufficient knowledge of food nutrition and have bad habits of overeating, their intake of carbohydrates, sugar, proteins, and fat would exceed the recommended amounts. As a result, this would cause problems with controlling both their weight and glucose. Of course, theoretically, when you get too much input energy via food, you must burn off the energy through physical activities and exercise. Unfortunately, most T2D patients are senior citizens. Generally speaking, most of them have a sedentary lifestyle; therefore, their choice and level of activity of exercise are generally limited. So, the author's advice to elderly diabetes patients is to focus on "post-meal walking". They just need to walk with a normal speed for approximately 30 minutes after each meal, which should be sufficient enough for them. In this way, they will easily achieve their target of walking 10,000 steps per day by burning off ~400 calories per day.

The best food choice is limiting the amount of carbs/sugar and sodium with very minimal fat and having sufficient high-quality proteins and vitamins. If T2D patients pay attention to their food and meal portion along with carbs/sugar intake amount, combined with exercise as mentioned above, then their weight and glucose will simultaneously improve.

Conclusions:

In summary, the author describes his straightforward implementation model in the following four steps:

By reducing his weight from 189 lb. to 170 lb. (-19 lb. or -10% in total weight), cutting off about 50% of his original over-eating food portion size (from 130% in 2012 down to 66% in 2020, which is -7% of his annual food portion reduction from original amount, or -6% averaged annual reduction continuously). This food portion reduction will automatically reduce the intake amount of fat and carbohydrates. But he strictly control his sugar, and sodium amounts. And he maintains a sufficient intake amount of high-quality protein.
When his weight dropped from 189 lbs. to 170 lbs. (-10% or -1.1% per year), his FPG then decreased from 140 mg/dL to 102 mg/dL (-38 mg/dL or -27%, or -3% per year) accordingly. Weight and FPG are highly correlated (93%).
When his FPG dropped, his PPG also reduced from 128 mg/dL to 108 mg/dL (-20 mg/dL or -16%, or -1.7% per year), providing he limits his carb/sugar intake amount below 15 grams per meal and walking at least 30 minutes after each meal. He also increased his post-meal walking from 500 steps to 4,400 steps (+433 post-meal steps per year or +87% per year in comparison with his walking steps in 2012).
He wants to re-emphasize the importance of diet and exercise. Normally, reduction on food and meal portion will automatically assist on limiting the carbs/sugar intake amount. However, patients should always watch out for the overall nutritional balance. For the author, his carbs/sugar intake amount has been cut down from 20 grams to 12.5 grams per meal (-7.5 grams or -38%, or -4% per year) as a result of his food portion reduction from 130% to 66% (-64% of food portion or -7% per year).
 This article merely provides a clinical proof using a quantitative and precision

approach. These mathematical and biomedical accomplishments are based on careful physical phenomena observations and related biomedical interpretation and proof process. This particular research project of food nutrition and biomedicine has utilized his developed GH-Method: math-physical medicine in which 366 medical papers have been published. The above four statements are simple to understand. Therefore, there is no need to learn fancy theories, complex formulas or equations. No need to take special seminars or attend college courses, take high dosages of medications or supplements, or go through any unnecessary surgeries. There are straight-line relationships existing among food, exercise, weight, and glucose that follow a simple and straight-line route of *"from food portion control to weight reduction and arrive at glucose stability for both FPG and PPG"*.

References:

1. Hsu, Gerald C., eclaireMD Foundation, USA, No. 310: "Biomedical research methodology based on GH-Method: math-physical medicine"

2. Hsu, Gerald C., eclaireMD Foundation, USA, No. 328: "Investigating the relationship between annualized weight and annualized food portion percentage along with a segmentation analysis on lowering weight less than 170 pounds using GH-Method: math-physical medicine"

3. Hsu, Gerald C., eclaireMD Foundation, USA, No. 327: "Investigating the influential factors on body weight and its impact on glucoses using GH-Method: math-physical medicine"

4. Hsu, Gerald C., eclaireMD Foundation, USA, No. 308: "Behavior psychology and body weight reduction of a T2D patient using GH-Method: math-physical medicine or mentality-personality modeling"

5. Hsu, Gerald C., eclaireMD Foundation, USA, No. 307: "Weight control trend analysis and progressive behavior modification of a T2D patient using GH-Method: math-physical medicine"

6. Hsu, Gerald C., eclaireMD Foundation, USA, No. 27: "From Weight Management via Diabetes Control to Cardiovascular Risk Reduction"

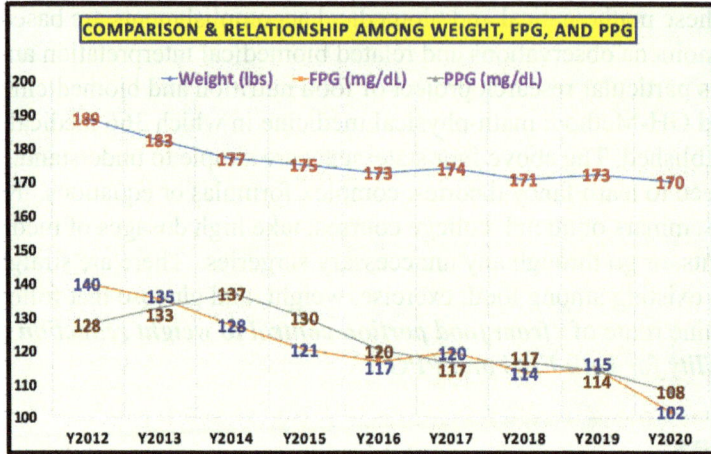

Figure 1: Comparison among Weight, FPG, PPG

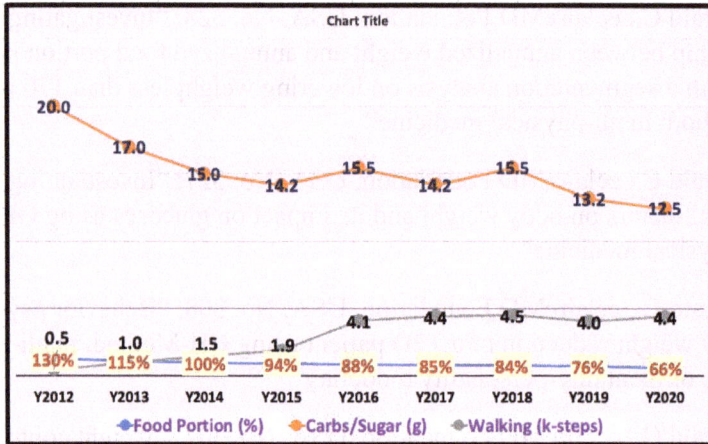

Figure 2: Comparison among Food portion, Carbs/Sugar intake, Post-meal Walking

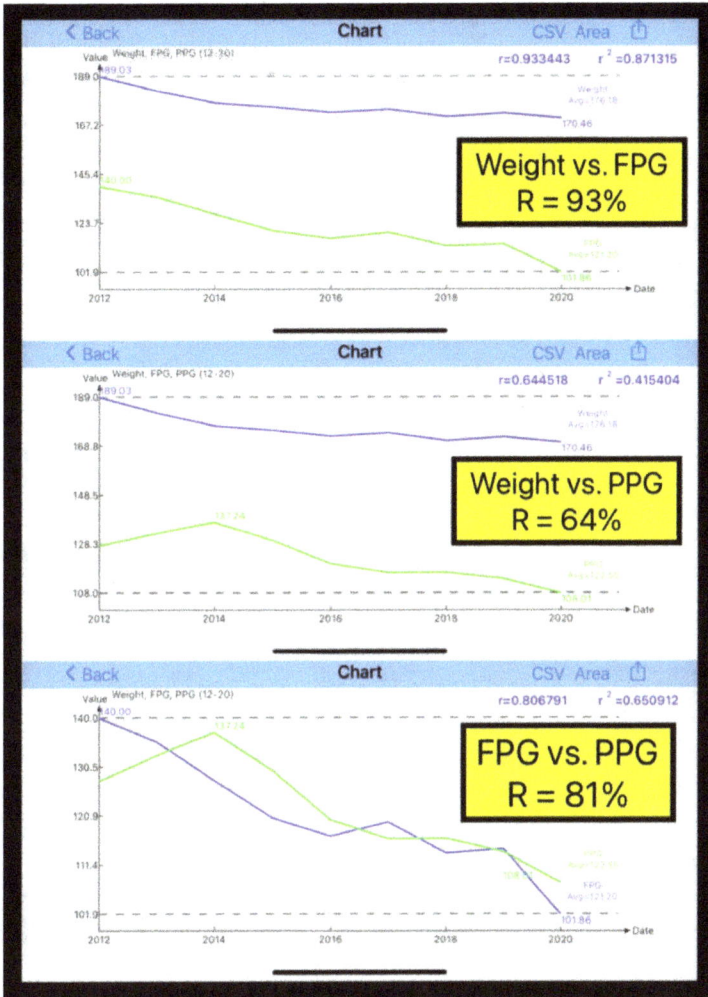

Figure 3: Three correlation coefficients (R) among Weight, FPG, PPG

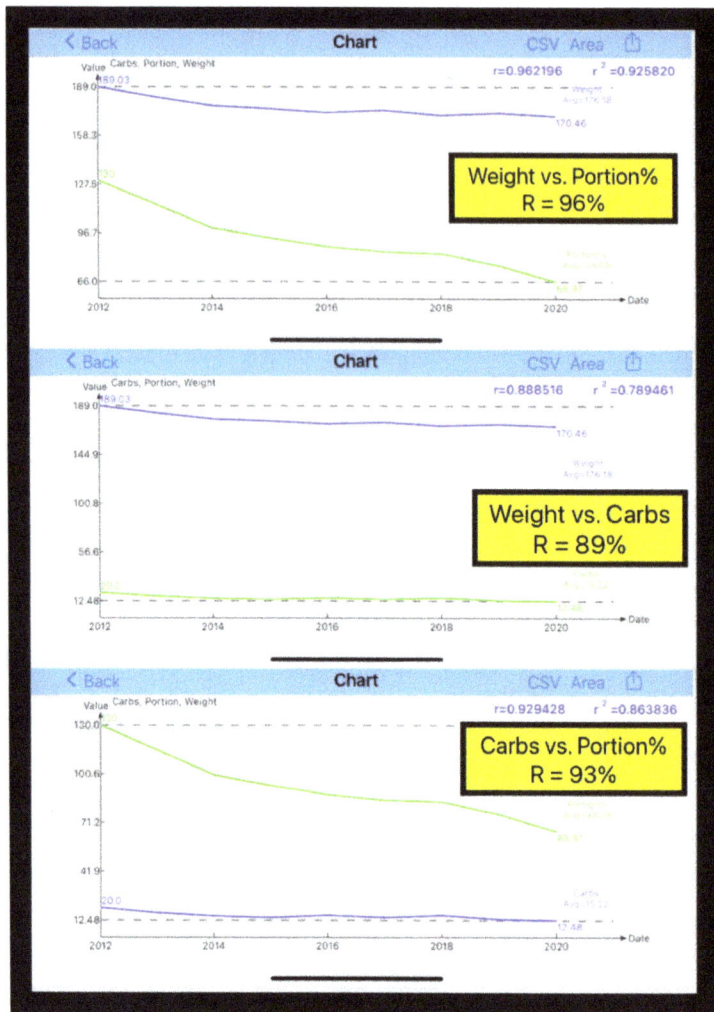

Figure 4: Three correlation (R) among Weight, Food portion, Carbs/Sugar

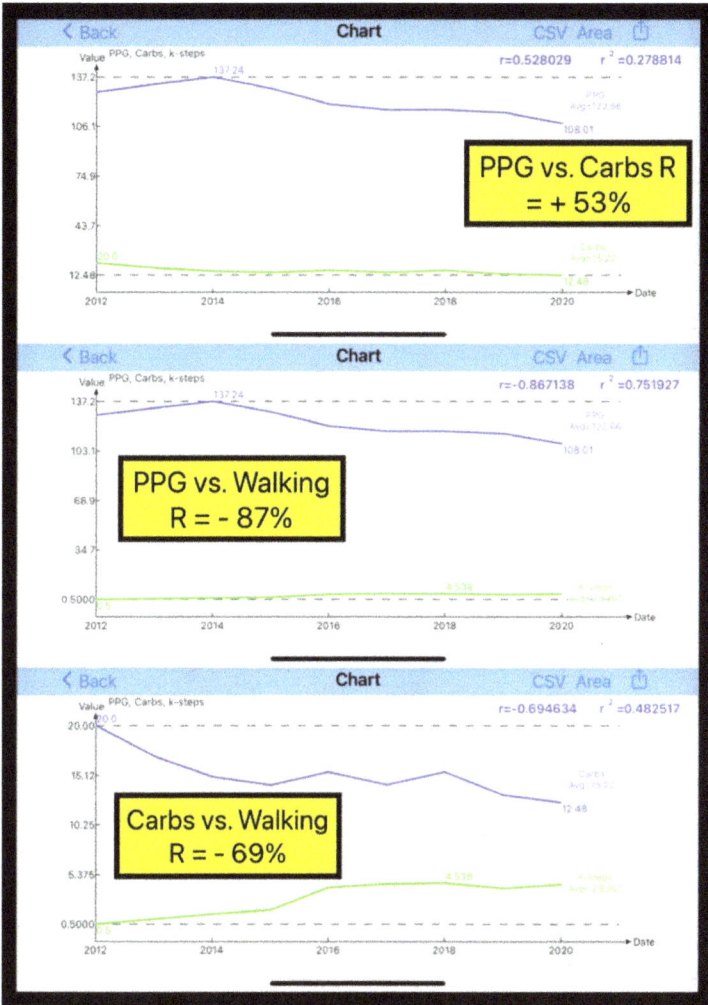

Figure 5: Three correlation coefficients (R) among PPG, Carbs/Sugar, Post-meal walking

Figure 6: Summary table of 9 correlation coefficients

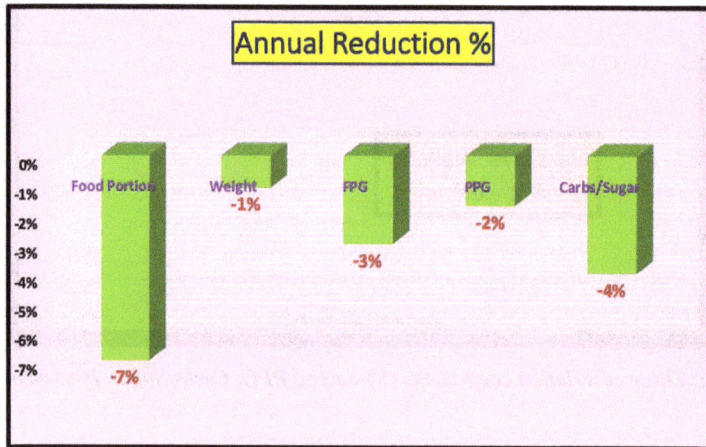

Figure 7: Annual reduction rates

1/1/12	Height (inches)			
11/22/20	69.5			
	Weight (lbs)	FPG (mg/dL)	PPG (mg/dL)	BMI
Y2012	189	140	128	27.5
Y2013	183	135	133	26.6
Y2014	177	128	137	25.8
Y2015	175	121	130	25.5
Y2016	173	117	120	25.2
Y2017	174	120	117	25.4
Y2018	171	114	117	24.9
Y2019	173	115	114	25.1
Y2020	170	102	108	24.8
	Food Portion (%)	Carbs/Sugar (g)	Walking (k-steps)	Glucose (mg/dL)
Y2012	130%	20.0	0.5	131
Y2013	115%	17.0	1.0	133
Y2014	100%	15.0	1.5	135
Y2015	94%	14.2	1.9	128
Y2016	88%	15.5	4.1	119
Y2017	85%	14.2	4.4	117
Y2018	84%	15.5	4.5	116
Y2019	76%	13.2	4.0	114
Y2020	66%	12.5	4.4	106

Figure 8: Data table

	GH.f-modulus	GH.p-modulus	Predicted PPG
Y2012	0.74		
Y2013	0.74		
Y2014	0.72		
Y2015	0.69	1.6	130
Y2016	0.68	1.8	120
Y2017	0.69	1.6	117
Y2018	0.66	1.9	117
Y2019	0.66	1.8	114
Y2020	0.60	2.5	108

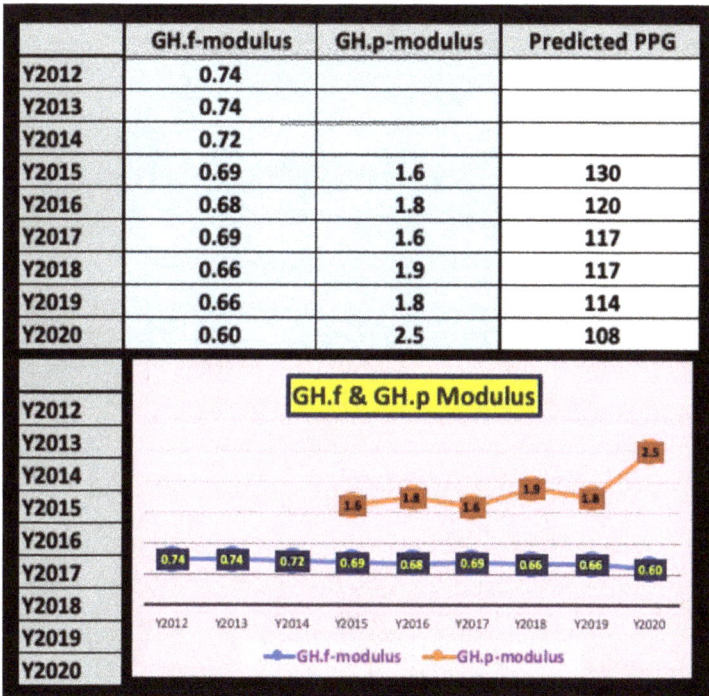

Figure 9: Linear elastic glucose (GH.f-modulus & GH.p-modulus)

GH.p-modulus study during three periods using finger-piercing glucoses and linear elastic glucose theory of GH-Method: math-physical medicine, Part 15 (No. 369)

Gerald C. Hsu
eclaireMD Foundation, USA
11/27-28/2020

Abstract:

This article is Part 15 of the author's linear elastic glucose behavior study. It focuses on a deeper investigation of GH.p-modulus over three periods: 2017-2019, 2020, and 2017-2020.

The author plans to conduct additional studies on linear elastic glucose behavior theory in order to obtain a solid and better understanding on the glucose coefficient of GH.p-modulus.

Here is the step-by-step explanation for the predicted postprandial plasma glucose (PPG) equation using linear elastic glucose theory as described in References 9 through 22:

(1) Baseline PPG equals to 97% of fasting plasma glucose (FPG) value, or 97% * (weight * GH.f-Modulus).
(2) Baseline PPG plus increased amount of PPG due to food, i.e., plus (carbs/sugar intake amount * GH.p-Modulus).
(3) Baseline PPG plus increased PPG due to food, and then subtracts reduction amount of PPG due to exercise, i.e., minus (post-meal walking k-steps * 5).
(4) The Predicted PPG equals to Baseline PPG plus the food influences, and then subtracts the exercise influences.

The linear elastic glucose equation is:

Predicted PPG =
(0.97 * GH.f-modulus * Weight) +(GH.p-modulus * Carbs&sugar) - (post-meal walking k-steps * 5)

Where,

(1) Incremental PPG = Predicted PPG - Baseline PPG + Exercise impact
(2) GH.f-modulus = FPG / Weight
(3) GH.p-modulus = Incremental PPG / Carbs intake

Therefore,

GH.p-modulus = (PPG - (0.97 * FPG) + (post-meal walking k-steps * 5)) / (Carbs&Sugar intake)

The study in this article calculates and analyzes the glucose coefficient of GH.p-modulus values for three periods. The variation range of GH.p-modulus values are between 1.8 for 2017-2019, and 2.2 for 2020 with an average of 1.8 for 2017-2020.

The average GH.p-modulus value of 1.8 for the 2017-2019 (pre-virus) period is quite close to his overall biomarker indicators for health and lifestyle. The average GH.p-modulus value of 2.2 for the 2020 (COVID-19) period is higher than the pre-virus sub-period due to the combination of his lower FPG (-10 mg/dL or -9%), lower PPG (-7 mg/dL or -6%), along with lower carbs/sugar intake amount (-1.6 grams or -11%). However, the average GH.p-modulus value of 1.8 for the total period of 2017-2020 (both pre-virus and COVID-19) reflects his overall and normal situations for health and lifestyle.

This paper investigates the likely situations of the author's health conditions and lifestyle details. The GH.p-modulus values have a small variance between 1.8 to 2.2, where the differences are insignificant. Any number located between the range of 1.8 to 2.2, which skews toward the lower side of the scale, can be used as the application value for the GH.p-modulus in order to predict PPG.

The study utilizes a step-by-step illustration, moving from the difference between PPG and FPG, going through the Incremental PPG, then arriving at the Predicted PPG. In the described steps, the most important variable is the GH.p-modulus. That is why the author has conducted many parts of this research of linear elastic glucose theory in order to acquire a good and solid understanding for the GH.p-modulus.

Introduction:

This article is Part 15 of the author's linear elastic glucose behavior study. It focuses on a deeper investigation of GH.p-modulus over three periods: 2017-2019, 2020, and 2017-2020.

The author plans to conduct additional studies on linear elastic glucose behavior theory in order to obtain a solid and better understanding on the glucose coefficient of GH.p-modulus.

Methods:

Background:
To learn more about the author's GH-Method: math-physical medicine (MPM) methodology, readers can refer to his article to understand his developed MPM analysis method in Reference 1.

Stress, Strain, & Young's modulus:
Prior to his medical research work, he was an engineer in the various fields of structural engineering (aerospace, naval defense, and earthquake engineering), mechanical engineering (nuclear power plant equipments, and computer-aided-design), and electronics engineering (computers, semiconductors, and software robot).

The following excerpts comes from internet public domain, including Google and Wikipedia:

"Strain - ε:
Strain is the "deformation of a solid due to stress" - change in dimension divided by the original value of the dimension - and can be expressed as
$\varepsilon = dL / L$

where
ε = strain (m/m, in/in)
dL = elongation or compression (offset) of object (m, in)
L = length of object (m, in)

*Stress - **σ**:*
Stress is force per unit area and can be expressed as
σ = F / A
where
σ = stress (N/m2, lb./in2, psi)
F = applied force (N, lb.)
A = stress area of object (m2, in2)

Stress includes tensile stress, compressible stress, shearing stress, etc.

<u>*E, Young's modulus:*</u>
It can be expressed as:
E = stress / strain
  = σ / ε
  = (F / A) / (dL / L)
where
E = <u>Young's Modulus of Elasticity</u> (Pa, N/m2, lb./in2, psi) was named after the 18th-century English physicist Thomas Young.

Elasticity:
Elasticity is a property of an object or material indicating how it will restore it to its original shape after distortion. A spring is an example of an elastic object - when stretched, it exerts a restoring force which tends to bring it back to its original length (Figure 1).

Plasticity:
When the force is going beyond the elastic limit of material, it is into a "plastic" zone which means even when force is removed, the material will not return back to its original state.

Based on various experimental results, the following table lists some of Young's modulus associated with different materials:

Nylon: 2.7 GPa
Concrete: 17-30 GPa
Glass fibers: 72 GPa
Copper: 117 GPa
Steel: 190-215 GPa
Diamond: 1220 GPa

Young's modules in the above table are ranked from soft material (low E) to stiff material (higher E)."

Professor James Andrews taught the author strength of materials and linear elasticity at the University of Iowa and Professor Norman Jones taught him nonlinear and dynamic plastic behaviors of structures at Massachusetts Institute of Technology. These two great academic mentors provided him with the foundational knowledge to understand these two important subjects in engineering.

Highlights of linear elastic glucose theory:

Here is the step-by-step explanation for the predicted PPG equation using linear elastic glucose theory as described in References 9 through 22:

(1) Baseline PPG equals to 97% of FPG value, or 97% * (weight * GH.f-Modulus).
(2) Baseline PPG plus increased amount of PPG due to food, i.e., plus (carbs/sugar intake amount * GH.p-Modulus).
(3) Baseline PPG plus increased PPG due to food, and then subtracts reduction amount of PPG due to exercise, i.e., minus (post-meal walking k-steps * 5).
(4) The Predicted PPG equals to Baseline PPG plus the food influences, and then subtracts the exercise influences.

The linear elastic glucose equation is:

Predicted PPG =
*(0.97 * GH.f-modulus * Weight) +(GH.p-modulus * Carbs&sugar) - (post-meal walking k-steps * 5)*

Where
(1) Incremental PPG = Predicted PPG - Baseline PPG + Exercise impact
(2) GH.f-modulus = FPG / Weight
(3) GH.p-modulus = Incremental PPG / Carbs intake

Therefore,

*GH.p-modulus = (PPG - (0.97 * FPG) + (post-meal walking k-steps * 5)) / (Carbs&Sugar intake)*

By using this linear equation, a diabetes patient only needs the input data of body weight, carbs & sugar intake amount, and post-meal walking steps in order to calculate the predicted PPG value without obtaining any measured glucose data.

In 2014, the author came up with the analogy between theory of elasticity and plasticity and the severity of his diabetes conditions when he was developing his mathematical model of metabolism using topology concept and finite element method.

On 10/14/2020, by utilizing the concept of Young's modulus with stress and strain, which was taught in engineering schools, he initiated and engaged this linear elastic glucose behaviors research. The following paragraphs describe his research findings at different stages:
1) He discovered that there is a "pseudo-linear" relationship existing between carbs &

sugar intake amount and incremental PPG amount. Based on this finding, he defined the first glucose coefficient of GH.p-modulus for PPG.

2) Similar to Young's modulus relating to stiffness of engineering inorganic materials, he found that the GH.p-modulus is dependent upon the patient's severity level of diabetes, i.e., the patient's glucose sensitivity on carbs/sugar intake amount, which reflects this patient's health state of liver cells and pancreatic beta cells.

3) Comparable to GH.p-modulus for PPG, in 2017, he uncovered a similar pseudo-linear relationship existing between weight and FPG with high correlation coefficient of above 90%. Therefore, he defined the second glucose coefficient of GH.f-modulus as the FPG value divided by the weight value. This GH.f-modulus is related to the severity of combined chronic diseases, including both obesity and diabetes. More than 33 million Americans, about 1 in 10, have diabetes, and approximately 90% to 95% of them have type 2 diabetes (T2D), where 86% also have problems with being overweight or obese. In other words, 7.7% to 8.2 % of the US population or 25 to 27 million Americans have issues with both obesity and diabetes.

4) He inserted these two glucose coefficients of GH.p-modulus and GH.f-modulus, into the predicted PPG equation to remove the burden of collecting measured glucoses by patients.

5) By experimenting and calculating many predicted PPG values over a variety of time length from different diabetes patients with different health conditions, he finally revealed that GH.p-modulus seems to be "near-constant" or "pseudo-linearized" over a short period of 3 to 4 months. This short period is compatible with the known lifespan of human red blood cells, which are living organic cells. This is quite different from the engineering inorganic materials, such as steel or concrete which can last for an exceptionally long period of time. The same conclusion was observed using his monthly GH.p-modulus data during the COVID-19 period in 2020 when his lifestyle became routine and stabilized.

6) He used three US clinical cases during the 2020 COVID-19 period to delve into the hidden characteristics of the physical parameters and their biomedical relationships. More importantly, through the comparison study in Part 7, he found explainable biomedical interpretations of his two defined glucose coefficients of GH.p-modulus and GH.f-modulus.

7) He conducted a PPG boundary analysis by discovering a lower bound and an upper bound of predicted PPG values for eight hypothetical standard cases and three US specific clinical cases. The derived numerical values of these two boundaries make sense from a biomedical viewpoint and also matched the situations of the three US clinical cases. He conducted two extreme stress tests, i.e., increasing carbs/sugar intake amount to 50 grams per meal and boosting post-meal walking steps to 5k after each meal, to examine the impacts on the lower bound and upper bound of PPG values.

8) Based on six international clinical cases, he further explored the influences from the combination of obesity and diabetes. Using a "lifestyle medicine" approach, he offered recommendations to reduce their PPG from 130-150 mg/dL down to below 120 mg/dL via reducing carbs/sugar intake and increasing exercise level in walking.

9) Based on his neuroscience research work using both 126 solid eggs and 159 liquid eggs with an extremely low carbs/sugar intake amount of ~2.5 grams, producing two totally different sets of PPG data and waveforms based on neurosciences viewpoint. He has also identified a different set of much higher values for GH.p-modules from the exceptionally low carbs/sugar intake of egg meals. Even though this egg neuroscience research results can be served as a special boundary case, it has also further proven that the GH.p-modules is influenced directly by the human brain and nervous system.

10) He compared the above two egg meals results, including PPG values and glucose coefficients, in particular the GH.p-modules, against the total results of his 2,843 meals. He discovered the vast differences of GH.p-modulus magnitudes and also learned the tight relationship between GH.p-modulus value and carbs/sugar intake amount. By distinguishing the GH.p-modulus results from the special boundary cases of 12.7 for liquid egg meals and 20.7 for solid egg meals, his general GH.p-modulus values from his 2,843 total meals are 2.1 using finger PPG and 3.4 using sensor PPG.

11) He used his 365 egg meal data from his neurosciences research papers to further calculate detailed variations of their associated GH.p-modulus.

12) He applied the linear elastic glucose theory to formulate certain guidelines as a part of his practical "lifestyle medicine" approach for family medicine.

Results:

Figures 1, 2, and 3 show the 90-days moving average value of FPG, PPG, Carbs/sugar intake amount, and post-meal walking steps for periods of 2017-2019, 2020, and 2017-2020 respectively.

Here again is the step-by-step explanation for the predicted PPG equation:

(1) Baseline PPG equals to 97% of FPG value, or 97% * (weight * GH.f-Modulus).
(2) Baseline PPG plus increased amount of PPG due to food, i.e., plus (carbs/sugar intake amount * GH.p-Modulus).
(3) Baseline PPG plus increased PPG due to food, and then subtracts reduction amount of PPG due to exercise, i.e., minus (post-meal walking k-steps * 5).
(4) The Predicted PPG equals to Baseline PPG plus the food influences, and then subtracts the exercise influences.

The linear elastic glucose equation is:

Predicted PPG =
*(0.97 * GH.f-modulus * Weight) +(GH.p-modulus * Carbs&sugar) - (post-meal*

walking k-steps * 5)

Where
(1) Incremental PPG = Predicted PPG - Baseline PPG + Exercise impact
(2) GH.f-modulus = FPG / Weight
(3) GH.p-modulus = Incremental PPG / Carbs intake
Therefore,

GH.p-modulus = (PPG - (0.97 * FPG) + (post-meal walking k-steps * 5)) /
(Carbs&Sugar intake)

Here is the list of his average values in the form of FPG, PPG, Carbs&sugar intake grams, Walking k-steps during the three periods.

2017-2019:   (116, 116, 14.3, 4.32)
2020 virus: (106, 109, 12.7, 4.37)
2017-2020:   (114, 114, 13.9, 4.33)

Figure 4 is a data and calculation table that applies above equations. The final results reflect the calculated GH.p-modulus results for these three periods using the 90-days moving averaged input data. The average GH.p-modulus value for the pre-virus period of 2017-2019 is 1.8, while the average GH.p-modulus value for the COVID-19 period of 2020 is 2.2. This higher GH.p-modulus value for the COVID period in 2020 is resulted from the combination of his lower FPG (-10 mg/dL or -9%), lower PPG (-7 mg/dL or -6%), along with the lower carbs/sugar intake amount (-1.6 grams or -11%).

However, the average GH.p-modulus value of 1.8, for the total period of 2017-2020 (both pre-virus and COVID-19) is reflecting his overall and normal situations for health and lifestyle. This GH.p-modulus value of 1.8 also matches his personal experiences of watching and researching his past glucose data and lifestyle details over the past 9 years (2012-2020).

In summary, the GH.p-modulus value coordinates with a patient's weight, FPG, PPG, carbs/sugar intake, and post-meal exercise that fluctuates within a reasonable numerical range. In this study, the GH.p-modulus actually reflects the general health conditions of the author.

Conclusions:

The study in this article calculates and analyzes the glucose coefficient of GH.p-modulus values for three periods. The variation range of GH.p-modulus values are between 1.8 for 2017-2019, and 2.2 for 2020 with an average of 1.8 for 2017-2020.

The average GH.p-modulus value of 1.8 for the 2017-2019 (pre-virus) period is quite close to his overall biomarker indicators for health and lifestyle. The average GH.p-modulus value of 2.2 for the 2020 (COVID-19) period is higher than the pre-virus sub-period due to the combination of his lower FPG (-10 mg/dL or -9%), lower PPG (-7 mg/

dL or -6%), along with lower carbs/sugar intake amount (-1.6 grams or -11%). However, the average GH.p-modulus value of 1.8 for the total period of 2017-2020 (both pre-virus and COVID-19) reflects his overall and normal situations for health and lifestyle.

This paper investigates the likely situations of the author's health conditions and lifestyle details. The GH.p-modulus values have a small variance between 1.8 to 2.2, where the differences are insignificant. Any number located between the range of 1.8 to 2.2, which skews toward the lower side of the scale, can be used as the application value for the GH.p-modulus in order to predict PPG.

The study utilizes a step-by-step illustration, moving from the difference between PPG and FPG, going through the Incremental PPG, then arriving at the Predicted PPG. In the described steps, the most important variable is the GH.p-modulus. That is why the author has conducted many parts of this research of linear elastic glucose theory in order to acquire a good and solid understanding for the GH.p-modulus.

References:

1. Hsu, Gerald C., eclaireMD Foundation, USA, No. 310: "Biomedical research methodology based on GH-Method: math-physical medicine."

2. Hsu, Gerald C., eclaireMD Foundation, USA, No. 345: "Application of linear equations to predict sensor and finger based postprandial plasma glucoses and daily glucoses for pre-virus, virus, and total periods using GH-Method: math-physical medicine."

3. Hsu, Gerald C., eclaireMD Foundation, USA, No. 97: "A simplified yet accurate linear equation of PPG prediction model for T2D patients using GH-Method: math-physical medicine."

4. Hsu, Gerald C., eclaireMD Foundation, USA, No. 99: "Application of linear equation-based PPG prediction model for four T2D clinic cases using GH-Method: math-physical medicine."

5. Hsu, Gerald C., eclaireMD Foundation, USA, No. 339: "Self-recovery of pancreatic beta cell's insulin secretion based on 10+ years annualized data of food, exercise, weight, and glucose using GH-Method: math-physical medicine."

6. Hsu, Gerald C., eclaireMD Foundation, USA, No. 340: "A neural communication model between brain and internal organs, specifically stomach, liver, and pancreatic beta cells based on PPG waveforms of 131 liquid egg meals and 124 solid egg meals."

7. Hsu, Gerald C., eclaireMD Foundation, USA, No. 349: "Using Math-Physics Medicine to Predict FPG."

8. Hsu, Gerald C., eclaireMD Foundation, USA, No. 264: "Community and Family Medicine via Doctors without distance: Using a simple glucose control card to assist T2D patients in remote rural areas via GH-Method: math-physical medicine."

9. Hsu, Gerald C., eclaireMD Foundation, USA, No. 346: "Linear relationship between carbohydrates & sugar intake amount and incremental PPG amount via engineering strength of materials using GH-Method: math-physical medicine, Part 1."

10. Hsu, Gerald C., eclaireMD Foundation, USA, No. 349: "Investigation on GH modulus of linear elastic glucose with two diabetes' patients data using GH-Method: math-physical medicine, Part 2."

11. Hsu, Gerald C., eclaireMD Foundation, USA, No. 349: "Investigation of GH modulus on the linear elastic glucose behavior based on three diabetes patients' data using the GH-Method: math-physical medicine, Part 3."

12. Hsu, Gerald C., eclaireMD Foundation, USA, No. 356: "Coefficient of GH.f-modulus in the linear elastic fasting plasma glucose behavior study based on health data of three diabetes patients using the GH-Method: math-physical medicine, Part 4. "

13. Hsu, Gerald C., eclaireMD Foundation, USA, No. 357: "High accuracy of predicted postprandial plasma glucose using two coefficients of GH.f-modulus and GH.p-modulus from linear elastic glucose behavior theory based on GH-Method: math-physical medicine, Part 5."

14. Hsu, Gerald C., eclaireMD Foundation, USA, No. 358: "Improvement on the prediction accuracy of postprandial plasma glucose using two biomedical coefficients of GH-modulus from linear elastic glucose theory based on GH-Method: math-physical medicine, Part 6."

15. Hsu, Gerald C., eclaireMD Foundation, USA, No. 359: "High glucose predication accuracy of postprandial plasma glucose and fasting plasma glucose during the COVID-19 period using two glucose coefficients of GH-modulus from linear elastic glucose theory based on GH-Method: math-physical medicine, Part 7."

16. Hsu, Gerald C., eclaireMD Foundation, USA, No. 360: "Investigation of two glucose coefficients of GH.f-modulus and GH.p-modulus based on data of 3 clinical cases during COVID-19 period using linear elastic glucose theory of GH-Method: math-physical medicine, Part 8."

17. Hsu, Gerald C., eclaireMD Foundation, USA, No. 361: "Postprandial plasma glucose lower and upper boundary study using two glucose coefficients of GH-modulus from linear elastic glucose theory based on GH-Method: math-physical medicine, Part 9."

18. Hsu, Gerald C., eclaireMD Foundation, USA, No. 362: "Six international clinical cases demonstrating prediction accuracies of postprandial plasma glucoses and suggested methods for improvements using linear elastic glucose theory of GH-Method: math-physical medicine, Part 10."

19. Hsu, Gerald C., eclaireMD Foundation, USA, No. 363: "A special Neuro-communication influences on GH.p-modulus of linear elastic glucose theory based on data from 159 liquid egg and 126 solid egg meals using GH-Method: math-physical medicine, Part 11."

20. Hsu, Gerald C., eclaireMD Foundation, USA, No. 364: "GH.p-modulus study of linear elastic glucose theory based on data from 159 liquid egg meals, 126 solid egg meals, and 2,843 total meals using GH-Method: math-physical medicine, Part 12."

21. Hsu, Gerald C., eclaireMD Foundation, USA, No. 365: "Detailed GH.p-modulus values at 15-minute time intervals for a synthesized sensor PPG waveform of 159 liquid egg meals, and 126 solid egg meals using linear elastic glucose theory of GH-Method: math-physical medicine, Part 13."

22. Hsu, Gerald C., eclaireMD Foundation, USA, No. 367: "A lifestyle medicine model for family medical practices based on 9-years of clinical data including food, weight, glucose, carbs/sugar, and walking using linear elastic glucose theory and GH-Method: math-physical medicine, Part 14."

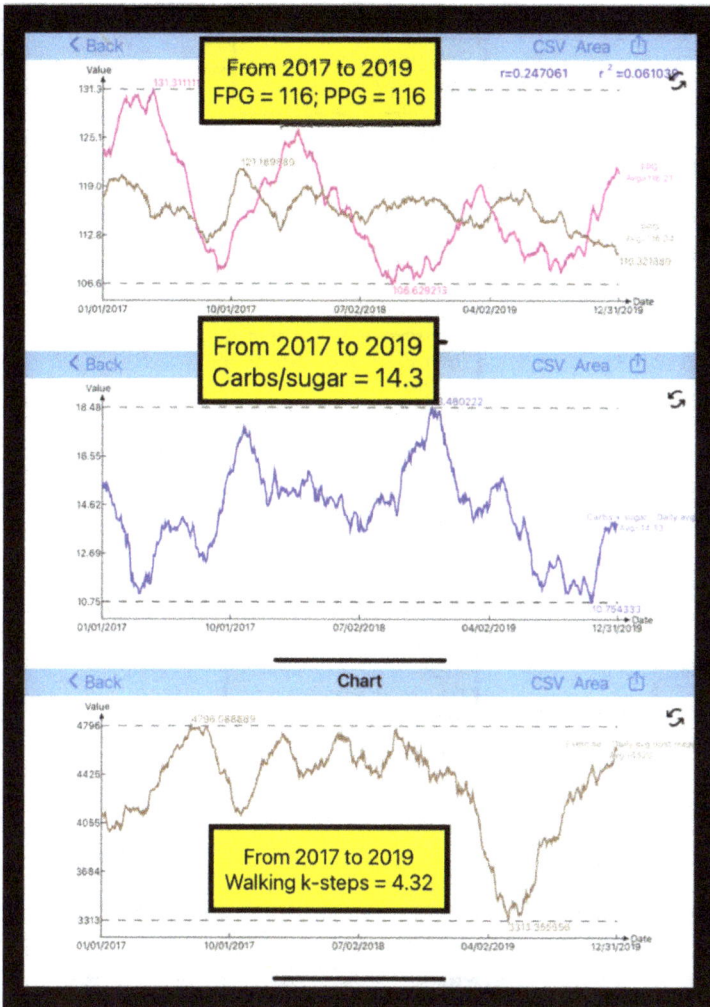

Figure 1: FPG, PPG, Carbs, Walking during 2017-2019

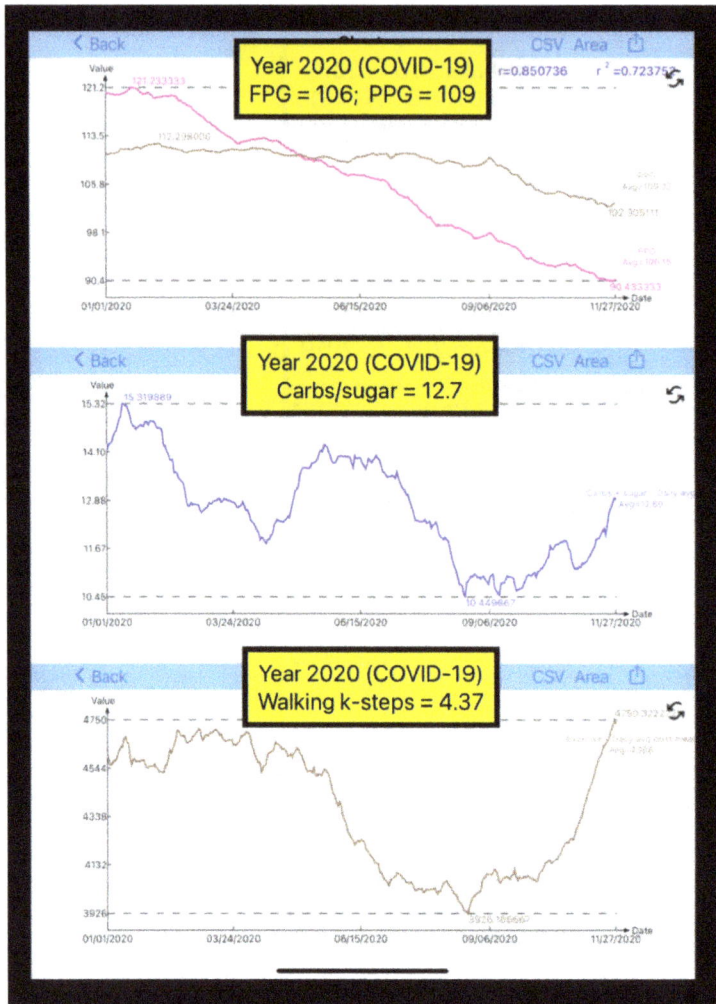

Figure 2: FPG, PPG, Carbs, Walking during 2020 COVID-19

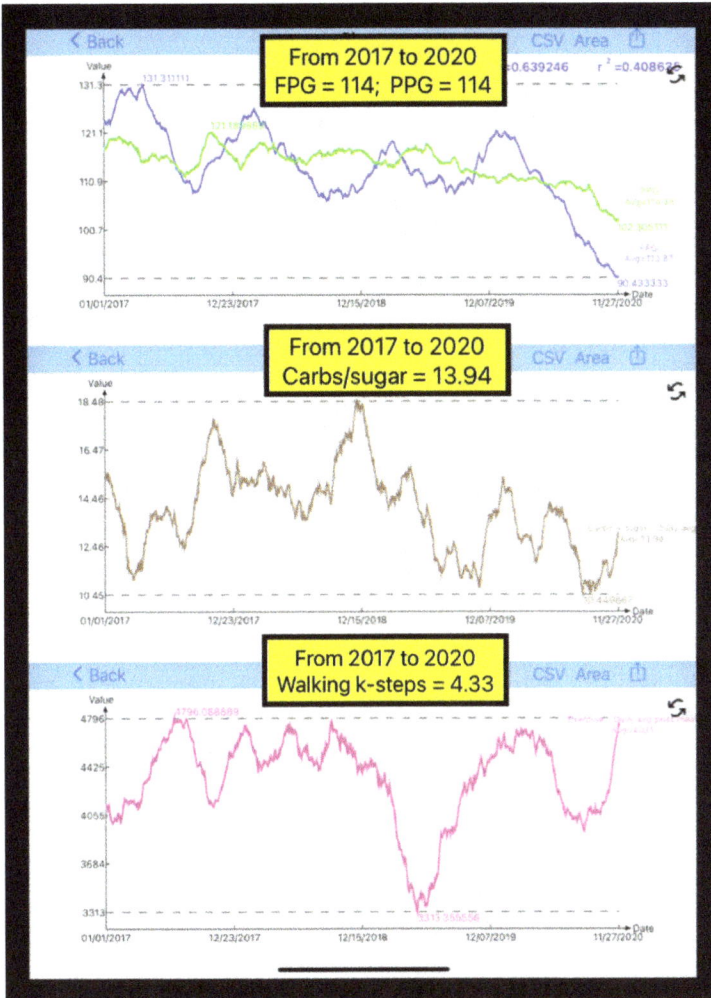

Figure 3: FPG, PPG, Carbs, Walking during 2017-2020

Finger	Y2017-2019	Y2020	Y2017-2020
PPG	116	109	114
FPG	116	106	114
Carbs gram	14.3	12.7	13.9
Walking k-steps	4.32	4.37	4.33
Finger	Y2017-2019	Y2020	Y2017-2020
GH.p (avg. data)	1.8	2.2	1.8

Figure 4: GH.p-modulus during three periods

GH.p-modulus study using both finger and sensor glucoses and linear elastic glucose theory of GH-Method: math-physical medicine, Part 16 (No. 370)

Gerald C. Hsu
eclaireMD Foundation, USA
11/28-29/2020

Abstract:

This article is Part 16 of the author's linear elastic glucose behavior study. It focuses on a deeper investigation of GH.p-modulus over the period from 8/5/2018 through 11/27/2020 using both finger-piercing measured glucoses (finger) and continuous glucose monitor (CGM) sensor collected glucoses (sensor).

The author plans to conduct additional studies on linear elastic glucose behavior theory in order to obtain a solid and better understanding on the glucose coefficient of GH.p-modulus.

Here is the step by step explanation for the predicted postprandial plasma glucose (PPG) equation using linear elastic glucose theory as described in References 9 through 22:

*(1) Baseline PPG equals to 97% of fasting plasma glucose (FPG) value, or 97% * (weight * GH.f-Modulus).*
*(2) Baseline PPG plus increased amount of PPG due to food, i.e. plus (carbs/sugar intake amount * GH.p-Modulus).*
*(3) Baseline PPG plus increased PPG due to food, and then subtracts reduction amount of PPG due to exercise, i.e. minus (post-meal walking k-steps * 5).*
(4) The Predicted PPG equals to Baseline PPG plus the food influences, and then subtracts the exercise influences.

The linear elastic glucose equation is:

Predicted PPG =
*(0.97 * GH.f-modulus * Weight) +(GH.p-modulus * Carbs&sugar) - (post-meal walking k-steps * 5)*

Where,

(1) Incremental PPG = Predicted PPG - Baseline PPG + Exercise impact
(2) GH.f-modulus = FPG / Weight
(3) GH.p-modulus = Incremental PPG / Carbs intake

Therefore,

GH.p-modulus = (PPG - (0.97 * FPG) + (post-meal walking k-steps * 5)) / (Carbs&Sugar intake)

The study in this article calculates and analyzes the glucose coefficient of GH.p-modulus values over the period from 8/5/2018 through 11/27/2020 using both finger glucoses and sensor glucoses. The calculated GH.p-modulus values are 2.0 for finger glucoses, and 3.3 for sensor glucoses.

This paper investigates the likely situations of the author's health conditions and lifestyle details based on two different glucose measuring methods. These two GH.p-modulus values have a relatively small and insignificant variance of 1.2, which is between 2.0 and 3.2. Actually, any number located between the range of 1.8 to 3.3, even if it skews toward the higher side of this scale, can be used as an application to the GH.p-modulus for PPG prediction.

This study utilizes a step by step illustration, moving from the difference between PPG and FPG, going through the Incremental PPG, and then arriving at the Predicted PPG. In the described steps, the most important variable of the linear elastic glucose behaviors is the coefficient of GH.p-modulus (similar to Young's modules in theory of engineering elasticity). That is why the author has conducted a massive amount of research on linear elastic glucose behaviors theory in order to acquire a good and solid understanding for the GH.p-modulus.

Introduction:

This article is Part 16 of the author's linear elastic glucose behavior study. It focuses on a deeper investigation of GH.p-modulus over the period from 8/5/2018 through 11/27/2020 using both finger-piercing measured glucoses (finger) and continuous glucose monitor (CGM) sensor collected glucoses (sensor).

The author plans to conduct additional studies on linear elastic glucose behavior theory in order to obtain a solid and better understanding on the glucose coefficient of GH.p-modulus.

Methods:

Background:
To learn more about the author's GH-Method: math-physical medicine (MPM) methodology, readers can refer to his article to understand his developed MPM analysis method in Reference 1.

Stress, Strain, & Young's modulus:
Prior to his medical research work, he was an engineer in the various fields of structural engineering (aerospace, naval defense, and earthquake engineering), mechanical engineering (nuclear power plant equipments, and computer-aided-design), and electronics engineering (computers, semiconductors, and software robot).

The following excerpts come from the internet public domain, including Google and Wikipedia:

"Strain - ε:
Strain is the "deformation of a solid due to stress" - change in dimension divided by the original value of the dimension - and can be expressed as
ε = dL / L
where
ε = strain (m/m, in/in)
dL = elongation or compression (offset) of object (m, in)
L = length of object (m, in)

Stress - σ:
Stress is force per unit area and can be expressed as
$\sigma = F / A$
where
σ = *stress (N/m2, lb/in2, psi)*
F = applied force (N, lb)
A = stress area of object (m2, in2)

Stress includes tensile stress, compressible stress, shearing stress, etc.

E, Young's modulus:
It can be expressed as:
E = stress / strain
  $= \sigma / \varepsilon$
  $= (F / A) / (dL / L)$
where
E = Young's Modulus of Elasticity (Pa, N/m2, lb/in2, psi) was named after the 18th-century English physicist Thomas Young.

Elasticity:
Elasticity is a property of an object or material indicating how it will restore it to its original shape after distortion. A spring is an example of an elastic object - when stretched, it exerts a restoring force which tends to bring it back to its original length.

Plasticity:
When the force is going beyond the elastic limit of material, it is into a "plastic' zone which means even when force is removed, the material will not return back to its original state (Figure 1).

Based on various experimental results, the following table lists some of Young's modulus associated with different materials:

Nylon: 2.7 GPa
Concrete: 17-30 GPa
Glass fibers: 72 GPa
Copper: 117 GPa
Steel: 190-215 GPa
Diamond: 1220 GPa

Young's modules in the above table are ranked from soft material (low E) to stiff material (higher E)."

Professor James Andrews taught the author strength of materials and linear elasticity at the University of Iowa and Professor Norman Jones taught him nonlinear and dynamic plastic behaviors of structures at Massachusetts Institute of Technology. These two great academic mentors provided him with the foundational knowledge to understand these two important subjects in engineering.

Highlights of linear elastic glucose theory:

Here is the step by step explanation for the predicted PPG equation using linear elastic glucose theory as described in References 9 through 22:

(1) Baseline PPG equals to 97% of FPG value, or 97% * (weight * GH.f-Modulus).
(2) Baseline PPG plus increased amount of PPG due to food, i.e. plus (carbs/sugar intake amount * GH.p-Modulus).
(3) Baseline PPG plus increased PPG due to food, and then subtracts reduction amount of PPG due to exercise, i.e. minus (post-meal walking k-steps * 5).
(4) The Predicted PPG equals to Baseline PPG plus the food influences, and then subtracts the exercise influences.

The linear elastic glucose equation is:

Predicted PPG =
*(0.97 * GH.f-modulus * Weight) +(GH.p-modulus * Carbs&sugar) - (post-meal walking k-steps * 5)*

Where
(1) Incremental PPG = Predicted PPG - Baseline PPG + Exercise impact
(2) GH.f-modulus = FPG / Weight
(3) GH.p-modulus = Incremental PPG / Carbs intake

Therefore,

*GH.p-modulus = (PPG - (0.97 * FPG) + (post-meal walking k-steps * 5)) / (Carbs&Sugar intake)*

By using this linear equation, a diabetes patient only needs the input data of body weight, carbs & sugar intake amount, and post-meal walking steps in order to calculate the predicted PPG value without obtaining any measured glucose data.

In early 2014, the author came up with the analogy between theory of elasticity and plasticity and the severity of his diabetes conditions when he was developing his mathematical model of metabolism using topology concept and finite element method.

On 10/14/2020, by utilizing the concept of Young's modulus with stress and strain, which was taught in engineering schools, he initiated and engaged this linear elastic glucose behaviors research. The following paragraphs describe his research findings at different stages:

1) He discovered that there is a "pseudo-linear" relationship existing between carbs & sugar intake amount and incremental PPG amount. Based on this finding, he defined the first glucose coefficient of GH.p-modulus for PPG.
2) Similar to Young's modulus relating to stiffness of engineering inorganic materials, he found that the GH.p-modulus is dependent upon the patient's severity level of

diabetes, i.e. the patient's glucose sensitivity on carbs/sugar intake amount, which reflects this patient's health state of liver cells and pancreatic beta cells.

3) Comparable to GH.p-modulus for PPG, in 2017, he uncovered a similar pseudo-linear relationship existing between weight and FPG with high correlation coefficient of above 90%. Therefore, he defined the second glucose coefficient of GH.f-modulus as the FPG value divided by the weight value. This GH.f-modulus is related to the severity of combined chronic diseases, including both obesity and diabetes. More than 33 million Americans, about 1 in 10, have diabetes, and approximately **90% to 95%** of them have type 2 diabetes (T2D), where **86%** also have problems with being overweight or obese. In other words, 7.7% to 8.2 % of the US population or 25 to 27 million Americans have issues with both obesity and diabetes.

4) He inserted these two glucose coefficients of GH.p-modulus and GH.f-modulus, into the predicted PPG equation to remove the burden of collecting measured glucoses by patients.

5) By experimenting and calculating many predicted PPG values over a variety of time length from different diabetes patients with different health conditions, he finally revealed that GH.p-modulus seems to be "near-constant" or "pseudo-linearized" over a short period of 3 to 4 months. This short period is compatible with the known lifespan of human red blood cells, which are living organic cells. This is quite different from the engineering inorganic materials, such as steel or concrete which can last for an exceptionally long period of time. The same conclusion was observed using his monthly GH.p-modulus data during the COVID-19 period in 2020 when his lifestyle became routine and stabilized.

6) He used three US clinical cases during the 2020 COVID-19 period to delve into the hidden characteristics of the physical parameters and their biomedical relationships. More importantly, through the comparison study in Part 7, he found explainable biomedical interpretations of his two defined glucose coefficients of GH.p-modulus and GH.f-modulus.

7) He conducted a PPG boundary analysis by discovering a lower bound and an upper bound of predicted PPG values for eight hypothetical standard cases and three US specific clinical cases. The derived numerical values of these two boundaries make sense from a biomedical viewpoint and also matched the situations of the three US clinical cases. He conducted two extreme stress tests, i.e. increasing carbs/sugar intake amount to 50 grams per meal and boosting post-meal walking steps to 5k after each meal, to examine the impacts on the lower bound and upper bound of PPG values.

8) Based on six international clinical cases, he further explored the influences from the combination of obesity and diabetes. Using a "lifestyle medicine" approach, he offered recommendations to reduce their PPG from 130-150 mg/dL down to below 120 mg/dL via reducing carbs/sugar intake and increasing exercise level in walking.

9) Based on his neuroscience research work using both 126 solid eggs and 159 liquid

eggs with a very low carbs/sugar intake amount of ~2.5 grams, producing two totally different sets of PPG data and waveforms based on neurosciences viewpoint. He has also identified a different set of much higher values for GH.p-modulus from the very low carbs/sugar intake of egg meals. Even though this egg neuroscience research results can be served as a special boundary case, it has also further proven that the GH.p-modulus is influenced directly by the human brain and nervous system.

10) He compared the above two egg meals results, including PPG values and glucose coefficients, in particular the GH.p-modulus, against the total results of his 2,843 meals. He discovered the vast differences of GH.p-modulus magnitudes and also learned the tight relationship between GH.p-modulus value and carbs/sugar intake amount. By distinguishing the GH.p-modulus results from the special boundary cases of 12.7 for liquid egg meals and 20.7 for solid egg meals, his general GH.p-modulus values from his 2,843 total meals are 2.1 using finger PPG and 3.4 using sensor PPG.

11) He used his 365 egg meal data from his neurosciences research papers to further calculate detailed variations of their associated GH.p-modulus.

12) He applied the linear elastic glucose theory to formulate certain guidelines as a part of his practical "lifestyle medicine" approach for family medicine branch.

13) He calculates three GH.p-modulus values, 1.8, 2.2, and 1.8, for three different periods, i.e. pre-virus period, COVID-19 period, and total period, respectively. This data range between 1.8 to 2.2 matches with his observed personal lifestyle and acquired biomedical knowledge through his medical research work during the past 9 years.

Results:

Figures 1 and 2 show the 90-days moving average value of FPG, PPG, Carbs/sugar intake amount, and post-meal walking steps for finger glucose case and sensor glucose case, respectively.

Here again is the step by step explanation for the predicted PPG equation:

(1) Baseline PPG equals to 97% of FPG value, or 97% * (weight * GH.f-Modulus).
(2) Baseline PPG plus increased amount of PPG due to food, i.e. plus (carbs/sugar intake amount * GH.p-Modulus).
(3) Baseline PPG plus increased PPG due to food, and then subtracts reduction amount of PPG due to exercise, i.e. minus (post-meal walking k-steps * 5).
(4) The Predicted PPG equals to Baseline PPG plus the food influences, and then subtracts the exercise influences.

The linear elastic glucose equation is:

Predicted PPG =
(0.97 * GH.f-modulus * Weight) +(GH.p-modulus * Carbs&sugar) - (post-meal walking k-steps * 5)

Where
(1) Incremental PPG = Predicted PPG - Baseline PPG + Exercise impact
(2) GH.f-modulus = FPG / Weight
(3) GH.p-modulus = Incremental PPG / Carbs intake

Therefore,

GH.p-modulus = (PPG - (0.97 * FPG) + (post-meal walking k-steps * 5)) / (Carbs&Sugar intake)

The following is the list of his average values in the form of FPG, PPG, Carbs&sugar intake grams, Walking k-steps for both finger and sensor cases.

Finger: (110, 113, 13.64, 4.249)
Sensor: (111, 132, 13.64, 4.249)

During this period from 8/5/2018 to 11/27/2020, the Sensor PPG is 17% higher than the Finger PPG while the Sensor FPG is almost identical to the Finger FPG.

Figure 4 is the combined data tables deploying the GH.p-modulus equation. For better viewing and comparing purposes, the author presents the collected results from both paper No. 369 for three different time periods (Reference 23) and paper No. 370 for finger glucose and sensor glucose cases during the same period of 8/5/2018-11/27/2020.

For the comparison between finger and sensor, the average GH.p-modulus value for finger glucoses is 2.0, while the average GH.p-modulus value for the sensor glucoses is 3.3. This higher GH.p-modulus value for the sensor glucoses is a result finding from the higher sensor PPG values (+19 mg/dL or +17%).

Furthermore, the comparison of the data from three different time periods in Reference 23 (No. 369), the GH.p-modulus value of 2.0 for finger glucoses are within the boundary of 1.8 for both 2017-2019 (pre-virus) period and 2017-2020 total period and 2.2 for the 2020 COVID-19 period (Reference 22). The reason for the +0.2 GH.p difference from the pre-virus period and total period is due to the combination of his lower FPG (-6 mg/dL), lower PPG (-3 mg/dL), and lower carbs/sugar intake amount (-0.7 grams).

However, the GH.p-modulus value of 3.3 for sensor glucoses are +1.3 higher than finger glucose GH.p value, and +1.5 higher than the 2017-2019 pre-virus period and 2017-2020 total period, and +1.1 higher than the 2020 COVID-19 period. The reason for the higher GH.p values from the sensor glucose GH.p is due to its higher PPG values: 19 mg/dL higher than finger, 16 mg/dL higher than pre-virus period, 23 mg/dL higher than virus period, and 18 mg/dL higher than total period. It should be noted that both finger and sensor cases have identical carbs/sugar intake amount and post-meal walking k-steps.

In summary, the GH.p-modulus value coordinates with a patient's weight, FPG, PPG, carbs/sugar intake, and post-meal exercise that fluctuates within a reasonable numerical range. In this study, the GH.p-modulus indeed reflects the general health conditions of the author.

Conclusions:

The study in this article calculates and analyzes the glucose coefficient of GH.p-modulus values over the period from 8/5/2018 through 11/27/2020 using both finger glucoses and sensor glucoses. The calculated GH.p-modulus values are 2.0 for finger glucoses, and 3.3 for sensor glucoses.

This paper investigates the likely situations of the author's health conditions and lifestyle details based on two different glucose measuring methods. These two GH.p-modulus values have a relatively small and insignificant variance of 1.2, which is between 2.0 and 3.2. Actually, any number located between the range of 1.8 to 3.3, even if it skews toward the higher side of this scale, can be used as an application to the GH.p-modulus for PPG prediction.

This study utilizes a step by step illustration, moving from the difference between PPG and FPG, going through the Incremental PPG, and then arriving at the Predicted PPG. In the described steps, the most important variable of the linear elastic glucose behaviors is the coefficient of GH.p-modulus (similar to Young's modules in theory of engineering elasticity). That is why the author has conducted a massive amount of research on linear elastic glucose behaviors theory in order to acquire a good and solid understanding for the GH.p-modulus.

References:

Hsu, Gerald C., eclaireMD Foundation, USA, No. 310: "Biomedical research methodology based on GH-Method: math-physical medicine"

1. Hsu, Gerald C., eclaireMD Foundation, USA, No. 345: "Application of linear equations to predict sensor and finger based postprandial plasma glucoses and daily glucoses for pre-virus, virus, and total periods using GH-Method: math-physical medicine"

2. Hsu, Gerald C., eclaireMD Foundation, USA, No. 97: "A simplified yet accurate linear equation of PPG prediction model for T2D patients (GH-Method: math-physical medicine)"

3. Hsu, Gerald C., eclaireMD Foundation, USA, No. 99: "Application of linear equation-based PPG prediction model for four T2D clinic cases (GH-Method:

math-physical medicine)"

4. Hsu, Gerald C., eclaireMD Foundation, USA, No. 339: "Self-recovery of pancreatic beta cell's insulin secretion based on 10+ years annualized data of food, exercise, weight, and glucose using GH-Method: math-physical medicine)

5. Hsu, Gerald C., eclaireMD Foundation, USA, No. 340: "A neural communication model between brain and internal organs, specifically stomach, liver, and pancreatic beta cells based on PPG waveforms of 131 liquid egg meals and 124 solid egg meals)

6. Hsu, Gerald C., eclaireMD Foundation, USA, No. 349: "Using Math-Physics Medicine to Predict FPG"

7. Hsu, Gerald C., eclaireMD Foundation, USA, No. 264: "Community and Family Medicine via Doctors without distance: Using a simple glucose control card to assist T2D patients in remote rural areas (GH-Method: math-physical medicine)"

8. Hsu, Gerald C., eclaireMD Foundation, USA, No. 346: "Linear relationship between carbohydrates & sugar intake amount and incremental PPG amount via engineering strength of materials using GH-Method: math-physical medicine, Part 1"

9. Hsu, Gerald C., eclaireMD Foundation, USA, No. 349: "Investigation on GH modulus of linear elastic glucose with two diabetes patients data using GH-Method: math-physical medicine, Part 2"

10. Hsu, Gerald C., eclaireMD Foundation, USA, No. 349: "Investigation of GH modulus on the linear elastic glucose behavior based on three diabetes patients' data using the GH-Method: math-physical medicine, Part 3"

11. Hsu, Gerald C., eclaireMD Foundation, USA, No. 356: "Coefficient of GH.f-modulus in the linear elastic fasting plasma glucose behavior study based on health data of three diabetes patients using the GH-Method: math-physical medicine, Part 4 "

12. Hsu, Gerald C., eclaireMD Foundation, USA, No. 357: "High accuracy of predicted postprandial plasma glucose using two coefficients of GH.f-modulus and GH.p-modulus from linear elastic glucose behavior theory based on GH-Method: math-physical medicine, Part 5"

13. Hsu, Gerald C., eclaireMD Foundation, USA, No. 358: "Improvement on the prediction accuracy of postprandial plasma glucose using two biomedical coefficients of GH-modulus from linear elastic glucose theory based on GH-Method: math-physical medicine, Part 6"

14. Hsu, Gerald C., eclaireMD Foundation, USA, No. 359: "High glucose predication accuracy of postprandial plasma glucose and fasting plasma glucose during the COVID-19 period using two glucose coefficients of GH-modulus from linear elastic glucose theory based on GH-Method: math-physical medicine, Part 7"

15. Hsu, Gerald C., eclaireMD Foundation, USA, No. 360: "Investigation of two glucose coefficients of GH.f-modulus and GH.p-modulus based on data of 3 clinical cases during COVID-19 period using linear elastic glucose theory of GH-Method: math-physical medicine, Part 8"

16. Hsu, Gerald C., eclaireMD Foundation, USA, No. 361: "Postprandial plasma glucose lower and upper boundary study using two glucose coefficients of GH-modulus from linear elastic glucose theory based on GH-Method: math-physical medicine, Part 9"

17. Hsu, Gerald C., eclaireMD Foundation, USA, No. 362: "Six international clinical cases demonstrating prediction accuracies of postprandial plasma glucoses and suggested methods for improvements using linear elastic glucose theory of GH-Method: math-physical medicine, Part 10"

18. Hsu, Gerald C., eclaireMD Foundation, USA, No. 363: "A special Neuro-communication influences on GH.p-modulus of linear elastic glucose theory based on data from 159 liquid egg and 126 solid egg meals using GH-Method: math-physical medicine, Part 11"

19. Hsu, Gerald C., eclaireMD Foundation, USA, No. 364: "GH.p-modulus study of linear elastic glucose theory based on data from 159 liquid egg meals, 126 solid egg meals, and 2,843 total meals using GH-Method: math-physical medicine, Part 12"

20. Hsu, Gerald C., eclaireMD Foundation, USA, No. 365: "Detailed GH.p-modulus values at 15-minute time intervals for a synthesized sensor PPG waveform of 159 liquid egg meals, and 126 solid egg meals using linear elastic glucose theory of GH-Method: math-physical medicine, Part 13"

21. Hsu, Gerald C., eclaireMD Foundation, USA, No. 367: "A lifestyle medicine model for family medical practices based on 9-years of clinical data including food, weight, glucose, carbs/sugar, and walking using linear elastic glucose theory and GH-Method: math-physical medicine (Part 14)"

22. Hsu, Gerald C., eclaireMD Foundation, USA, No. 369: "GH.p-modulus study during 3 periods using finger-piercing glucoses and linear elastic glucose theory (Part 15) of GH-Method: math-physical medicine"

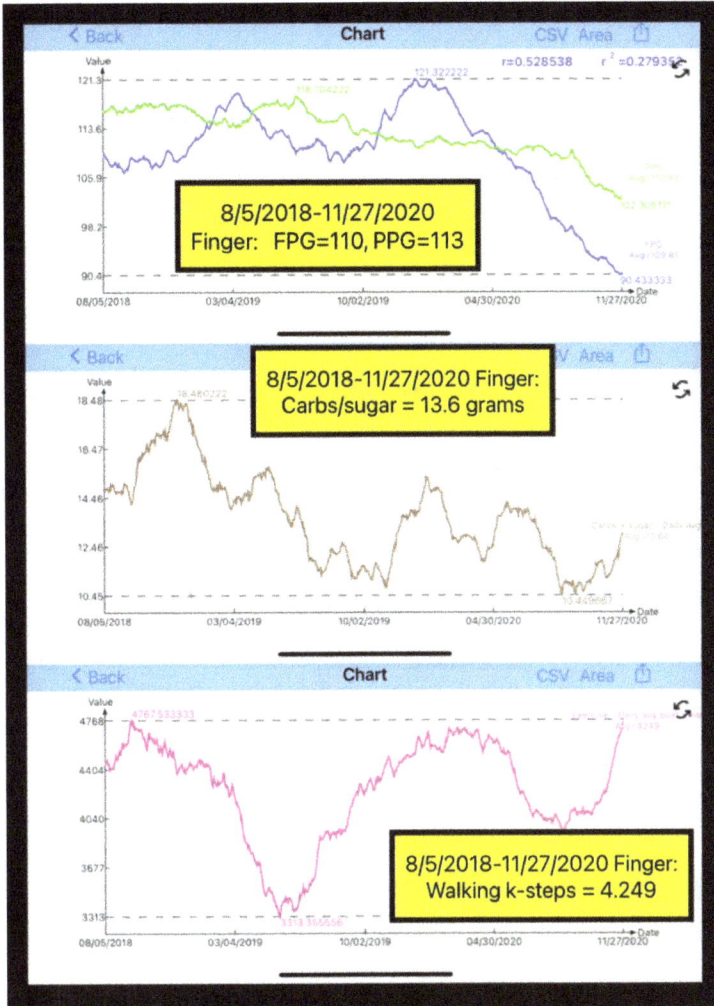

Figure 1: Finger measured FPG, PPG, Carbs, Walking during 8/5/2018 - 11/27/2020

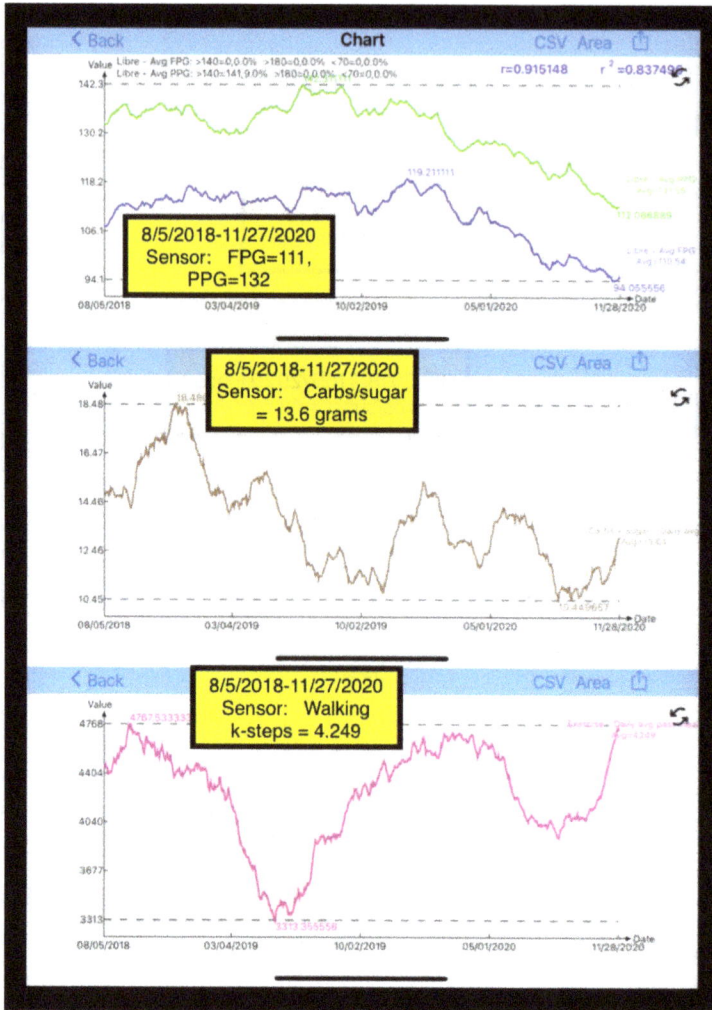

Figure 2: Sensor measured FPG, PPG, Carbs, Walking during 8/5/2018 - 11/27/2020

(8/5/18-11/27/20)	Finger	Sensor
PPG	113	132
FPG	110	111
Carbs gram	13.6	13.6
Walking k-steps	4.25	4.25
(8/5/18-11/27/20)	Finger	Sensor
GH.p (avg. data)	2.0	3.3

Finger	Y2017-2019	Y2020	Y2017-2020
PPG	116	109	114
FPG	116	106	114
Carbs gram	14.3	12.7	13.9
Walking k-steps	4.32	4.37	4.33
Finger	Y2017-2019	Y2020	Y2017-2020
GH.p (avg. data)	1.8	2.2	1.8

Figure 3: GH.p-modulus values for both finger and sensor and 3 different time periods

A summarized investigation report of GH.p-modulus values using linear elastic glucose theory of GH-Method: math-physical medicine, Part 17 (No. 371)

Gerald C. Hsu
eclaireMD Foundation, USA
11/29/2020

Abstract:

This article is Part 17 of the author's linear elastic glucose behavior study. It summarizes key conclusions from the first 16 segments of his research work regarding the data range of GH.p-modulus values (References 9 through 23).

This research report includes the following:

(1) The author's personal data and GH.p-modulus values;
(2) The data and GH.p-modulus values of three US patients and two Myanmar patients;
(3) The low-bound and high-bound analysis from eight hypothetical standard cases of different carbs/sugar intake amounts and post-meal walking steps;
(4) The data with high quite GH.p-modulus values from a special investigation case using 285 egg meals with neuroscience influences.

The following paragraphs describe his key variable definitions and mathematical operations of obtaining the GH.p-modulus:

(1) Baseline PPG equals to 97% of fasting plasma glucose (FPG) value, or 97% * (weight * GH.f-Modulus).
(2) Baseline PPG plus increased amount of PPG due to food, i.e. plus (carbs/sugar intake amount * GH.p-Modulus).
(3) Baseline PPG plus increased PPG due to food, and then subtracts reduction amount of PPG due to exercise, i.e. minus (post-meal walking k-steps * 5).
(4) The Predicted PPG equals to Baseline PPG plus the food influences, and then subtracts the exercise influences.

The linear elastic glucose equation is:

Predicted PPG =
(0.97 * GH.f-modulus * Weight) +(GH.p-modulus * Carbs&sugar) - (post-meal walking k-steps * 5)

Where,

(1) Incremental PPG = Predicted PPG - Baseline PPG + Exercise impact
(2) GH.f-modulus = FPG / Weight
(3) GH.p-modulus = Incremental PPG / Carbs intake

Therefore,

GH.p-modulus = (PPG - (0.97 * FPG) + (post-meal walking k-steps * 5)) / (Carbs&Sugar intake)

This study is a summarized report of the author's previous 16 segments of research articles on linear elastic glucose theory. He focuses on the GH.p-Modulus using four different data groups which cover patients of different nationalities, varying time periods, comparison between pre-virus vs. COVID-19 periods, finger glucoses vs. sensor glucoses, hypothetical boundary analysis (upper bound and lower bound), and a special neuroscience study of egg meals to arrive at the following observed conclusion.

In summary, the author presumes that most patients still having a reasonable normal lifestyles, their GH.p-Modulus value should be located between 1.0 and 6.0. In this study of linear elastic glucose theory, the GH.p-modulus indeed reflects the actual general health conditions and lifestyle details of a patient.

Practical advice of GH.p-Modulus to patients:

(1) If you have a record for some of your glucoses, carbs/sugar intake amount, and post-meal walking steps, then you may use this equation to calculate your GH.p-Modulus:

GH.p-Modulus = ((0.97*FPG) + (post-meal k-steps*5)) / (Carbs&sugar amount)

(2) If you don't have your data stored, then you may apply the following suggestions: *If your diabetes conditions is moderate (HbA1C ~7.0 & glucose ~150 mg/dL), then use 1.8 to 2.2 for your GH.p-Modulus; and if your diabetes conditions is more serious (HbA1C >8.0 & glucose >180 mg/dL), then use 2.5 to 3.3 for your GH.p-Modulus.*

(3) Normally, the GH.p-Modulus should be within 1.5 to 2.5; however, *if you want to be more conservative in predicting your PPG, then you may use the GH.p-Modulus* greater than 3.0 in the following equation:

Predicted PPG = (0.97 * FPG) + (GH.p-Modulus * carbs& sugar) - (post-meal walking k-steps * 5)

Introduction:

This article is Part 17 of the author's linear elastic glucose behavior study. It summarizes key conclusions from the first 16 segments of his research work regarding the data range of GH.p-modulus values (References 9 through 23).

This research report includes the following:

(1) The author's personal data and GH.p-modulus values;
(2) The data and GH.p-modulus values of three US patients and two Myanmar patients;
(3) The low-bound and high-bound analysis from eight hypothetical standard cases of different carbs/sugar intake amounts and post-meal walking steps;
(4) The data with quite high GH.p-modulus values from a special investigation case using 285 egg meals with neuroscience influences.

Methods:

Background:

To learn more about the author's GH-Method: math-physical medicine (MPM) methodology, readers can refer to his article to understand his developed MPM analysis method in Reference 1.

Stress, Strain, & Young's modulus:

Prior to his medical research work, he was an engineer in the various fields of structural engineering (aerospace, naval defense, and earthquake engineering), mechanical engineering (nuclear power plant equipments, and computer-aided-design), and electronics engineering (computers, semiconductors, and software robot).

The following excerpts come from the internet public domain, including Google and Wikipedia:

"Strain - ε:
Strain is the "deformation of a solid due to stress" - change in dimension divided by the original value of the dimension - and can be expressed as
$\varepsilon = dL / L$
where
ε = strain (m/m, in/in)
dL = elongation or compression (offset) of object (m, in)
L = length of object (m, in)

Stress - σ:
Stress is force per unit area and can be expressed as
$\sigma = F / A$
where
σ = stress (N/m2, lb/in2, psi)
F = applied force (N, lb)
A = stress area of object (m2, in2)

Stress includes tensile stress, compressible stress, shearing stress, etc.

E, Young's modulus:
It can be expressed as:
E = stress / strain
  = σ / ε
  = (F / A) / (dL / L)
where
E = Young's Modulus of Elasticity (Pa, N/m2, lb/in2, psi) was named after the 18th-century English physicist Thomas Young.

Elasticity:
Elasticity is a property of an object or material indicating how it will restore it to its original shape after distortion. A spring is an example of an elastic object - when

stretched, it exerts a restoring force which tends to bring it back to its original length.

Plasticity:
When the force is going beyond the elastic limit of material, it is into a "plastic' zone which means even when force is removed, the material will not return back to its original state (Figure 1).

Based on various experimental results, the following table lists some of Young's modulus associated with different materials:

Nylon: 2.7 GPa
Concrete: 17-30 GPa
Glass fibers: 72 GPa
Copper: 117 GPa
Steel: 190-215 GPa
Diamond: 1220 GPa

Young's modules in the above table are ranked from soft material (low E) to stiff material (higher E)."

Professor James Andrews taught the author strength of materials and linear elasticity at the University of Iowa and Professor Norman Jones taught him nonlinear and dynamic plastic behaviors of structures at Massachusetts Institute of Technology. These two great academic mentors provided him with the foundational knowledge to understand these two important subjects in engineering.

Highlights of linear elastic glucose theory:
Here is the step by step explanation for the predicted PPG equation using linear elastic glucose theory as described in References 9 through 24:

(1) Baseline PPG equals to 97% of FPG value, or 97% * (weight * GH.f-Modulus).
(2) Baseline PPG plus increased amount of PPG due to food, i.e. plus (carbs/sugar intake amount * GH.p-Modulus).
(3) Baseline PPG plus increased PPG due to food, and then subtracts reduction amount of PPG due to exercise, i.e. minus (post-meal walking k-steps * 5).
(4) The Predicted PPG equals to Baseline PPG plus the food influences, and then subtracts the exercise influences.

The linear elastic glucose equation is:

Predicted PPG =
(0.97 * GH.f-modulus * Weight) +(GH.p-modulus * Carbs&sugar) - (post-meal walking k-steps * 5)

Where
(1) Incremental PPG = Predicted PPG - Baseline PPG + Exercise impact
(2) GH.f-modulus = FPG / Weight

(3) GH.p-modulus = Incremental PPG / Carbs intake

Therefore,

GH.p-modulus = (PPG - (0.97 * FPG) + (post-meal walking k-steps * 5)) / (Carbs&Sugar intake)

By using this linear equation, a diabetes patient only needs the input data of body weight, carbs & sugar intake amount, and post-meal walking steps in order to calculate the predicted PPG value without obtaining any measured glucose data.

In early 2014, the author came up with the analogy between theory of elasticity and plasticity and the severity of his diabetes conditions when he was developing his mathematical model of metabolism using topology concept and finite element method.

On 10/14/2020, by utilizing the concept of Young's modulus with stress and strain, which was taught in engineering schools, he initiated and engaged this linear elastic glucose behaviors research. The following paragraphs describe his research findings at different stages:

1) He discovered that there is a "pseudo-linear" relationship existing between carbs & sugar intake amount and incremental PPG amount. Based on this finding, he defined the first glucose coefficient of GH.p-modulus for PPG.

2) Similar to Young's modulus relating to stiffness of engineering inorganic materials, he found that the GH.p-modulus is dependent upon the patient's severity level of diabetes, i.e. the patient's glucose sensitivity on carbs/sugar intake amount, which reflects this patient's health state of liver cells and pancreatic beta cells.

3) Comparable to GH.p-modulus for PPG, in 2017, he uncovered a similar pseudo-linear relationship existing between weight and FPG with high correlation coefficient of above 90%. Therefore, he defined the second glucose coefficient of GH.f-modulus as the FPG value divided by the weight value. This GH.f-modulus is related to the severity of combined chronic diseases, including both obesity and diabetes. More than 33 million Americans, about 1 in 10, have diabetes, and approximately 90% to 95% of them have type 2 diabetes (T2D), where 86% also have problems with being overweight or obese. In other words, 7.7% to 8.2 % of the US population or 25 to 27 million Americans have issues with both obesity and diabetes.

4) He inserted these two glucose coefficients of GH.p-modulus and GH.f-modulus, into the predicted PPG equation to remove the burden of collecting measured glucoses by patients.

5) By experimenting and calculating many predicted PPG values over a variety of time length from different diabetes patients with different health conditions, he finally revealed that GH.p-modulus seems to be "near-constant" or "pseudo-linearized" over a short period of 3 to 4 months. This short period is compatible with the known lifespan

of human red blood cells, which are living organic cells. This is quite different from the engineering inorganic materials, such as steel or concrete which can last for an exceptionally long period of time. The same conclusion was observed using his monthly GH.p-modulus data during the COVID-19 period in 2020 when his lifestyle became routine and stabilized.

6) He used three US clinical cases during the 2020 COVID-19 period to delve into the hidden characteristics of the physical parameters and their biomedical relationships. More importantly, through the comparison study in Part 7, he found explainable biomedical interpretations of his two defined glucose coefficients of GH.p-modulus and GH.f-modulus.

7) He conducted a PPG boundary analysis by discovering a lower bound and an upper bound of predicted PPG values for eight hypothetical standard cases and three US specific clinical cases. The derived numerical values of these two boundaries make sense from a biomedical viewpoint and also matched the situations of the three US clinical cases. He conducted two extreme stress tests, i.e. increasing carbs/sugar intake amount to 50 grams per meal and boosting post-meal walking steps to 5k after each meal, to examine the impacts on the lower bound and upper bound of PPG values.

8) Based on six international clinical cases, he further explored the influences from the combination of obesity and diabetes. Using a "lifestyle medicine" approach, he offered recommendations to reduce their PPG from 130-150 mg/dL down to below 120 mg/dL via reducing carbs/sugar intake and increasing exercise level in walking.

9) Based on his neuroscience research work using both 126 solid eggs and 159 liquid eggs with a very low carbs/sugar intake amount of ~2.5 grams, producing two totally different sets of PPG data and waveforms based on neurosciences viewpoint. He has also identified a different set of much higher values for GH.p-modulus from the very low carbs/sugar intake of egg meals. Even though this egg neuroscience research results can be served as a special boundary case, it has also further proven that the GH.p-modulus is influenced directly by the human brain and nervous system.

10) He compared the above two egg meals results, including PPG values and glucose coefficients, in particular the GH.p-modulus, against the total results of his 2,843 meals. He discovered the vast differences of GH.p-modulus magnitudes and also learned the tight relationship between GH.p-modulus value and carbs/sugar intake amount. By distinguishing the GH.p-modulus results from the special boundary cases of 12.7 for liquid egg meals and 20.7 for solid egg meals, his general GH.p-modulus values from his 2,843 total meals are 2.1 using finger PPG and 3.4 using sensor PPG.

11) He used his 365 egg meal data from his neurosciences research papers to further calculate detailed variations of their associated GH.p-modulus.

12) He applied the linear elastic glucose theory to formulate certain guidelines as a part of his practical "lifestyle medicine" approach for the family medicine branch.

13) He calculates three GH.p-modulus values, 1.8, 2.2, and 1.8, for three different periods, i.e. pre-virus period, COVID-19 period, and total period, respectively. This data range of between 1.8 to 2.2 matches with his observed personal lifestyle and acquired biomedical knowledge through his medical research work during the past 9 years.

14) He calculates two GH.p-modulus values, 2.0 and 3.3, for two different measured glucoses, i.e. finger-piercing measured glucoses and CGM sensor collected glucoses, respectively. This GH.p-Modulus difference between 2.0 and 3.3 mainly reflects the average sensor PPG value is 17% higher than the average finger PPG value.

Results:

Figures 1, 2, 3 and 4 show the calculated GH.p-Modulus values based on different input data of FPG, PPG, Carbs/sugar intake amount, and post-meal walking steps for the following four different data groups with a variety of situations:

(1) The author's personal data and GH.p-modulus values;
(2) The data and GH.p-modulus values of three US patients and two Myanmar patients;
(3) The low-bound and high-bound analysis from eight hypothetical standard cases of different carbs/sugar intake amounts and post-meal walking steps;
(4) The data with quite high GH.p-modulus values from a special investigation case using 285 egg meals with neuroscience influences.

Here again is the step by step explanation for the predicted PPG equation:

(1) Baseline PPG equals to 97% of FPG value, or 97% * (weight * GH.f-Modulus).
(2) Baseline PPG plus increased amount of PPG due to food, i.e. plus (carbs/sugar intake amount * GH.p-Modulus).
(3) Baseline PPG plus increased PPG due to food, and then subtracts reduction amount of PPG due to exercise, i.e. minus (post-meal walking k-steps * 5).
(4) The Predicted PPG equals to Baseline PPG plus the food influences, and then subtracts the exercise influences.

The linear elastic glucose equation is:

Predicted PPG =
*(0.97 * GH.f-modulus * Weight) +(GH.p-modulus * Carbs&sugar) - (post-meal walking k-steps * 5)*

Where
(1) Incremental PPG = Predicted PPG - Baseline PPG + Exercise impact
(2) GH.f-modulus = FPG / Weight
(3) GH.p-modulus = Incremental PPG / Carbs intake

Therefore,

GH.p-modulus = (PPG - (0.97 * FPG) + (post-meal walking k-steps * 5)) / (Carbs&Sugar intake)

The following is the list of the GH.p-Modulus values for the four groups in the form of (low-end of GH.p, and high-end of GH.p):

Group 1, the author: (1.8, 3.3)
Group 2, clinical cases: (1.0, 3.6)
Group 3, standard cases: (2.0, 6.0)
Group 4, neuroscience: (13, 21)

Figure 1 depicts the data analysis results from the author himself. Using three different time periods, it shows the GH.p data range of 1.8 to 2.2. However, if using two different glucose measurement devices, it depicts the GH.p data range of 2.0 for finger glucoses and 3.3 for sensor glucoses. Group 1 has a GH.p data range between 1.8 and 3.3.

Figure 2 reflects the data analysis results from three US patients and two Myanmar patients. Group 2 with five different patients have a GH.p data range between 1.0 and 3.6.

Figure 3 illustrates the data analysis results from eight "hypothetical standard cases" with different amounts of carbs/sugar intake and post-meal exercise. Group 3 with the eight hypothetical standard cases have a GH.p data range between 2.0 and 6.0.

Figure 4 represents the data analysis results from 285 "neuroscience investigation meals" having the same food ingredients of one large egg with an extremely low carbs/sugar intake amount of 0.76 gram from egg alone for each meal while always maintaining ~4.3k post-meal walking steps. These 285 experimental results show that solid egg meals (135 mg/dL at peak PPG) is 31 mg/dL higher than liquid egg meals (104 mg/dL at peak PPG). This strange and unique physical phenomenon cannot be explained clearly or satisfactorily using the traditional knowledge of internal medicine and food nutrition. It is a result from the biomedical neural communication model between the brain and internal organs, specifically stomach, intestine, liver, and pancreas. The calculated values of GH.p-Modulus in Group 4 is 12.7 for liquid egg meals and 20.7 for solid egg meals. Therefore, Group 4 of the special neuroscience experiment indeed demonstrates a special case of high-end GH.p-Modulus values.

The GH.p-modulus value coordinates with a patient's weight, FPG, PPG, carbs/sugar intake, and post-meal exercise that fluctuates within a reasonable numerical range. When the author combines the results from Groups 1, 2, and 3, he obtains a data range for GH.p-Modulus values between 1.0 and 6.0.

Conclusions:

This study is a summarized report of the author's previous 16 segments of research articles on linear elastic glucose theory. He focuses on the GH.p-Modulus using four different data groups which cover patients of different nationalities, varying time periods, comparison between pre-virus vs. COVID-19 periods with different lifestyles, finger glucoses vs. sensor glucoses, hypothetical boundary analysis (upper bound and lower bound), and a special neuroscience study of 285 egg meals to arrive at the following observed conclusion.

In summary, the author presumes that most patients having a reasonable normal lifestyles, their GH.p-Modulus value should be located between 1.0 and 6.0. In this study, the GH.p-modulus indeed reflects the actual general health conditions and lifestyle details of a patient.

Practical advice of GH.p-Modulus to patients:

(1) If you have a record for some of your glucoses, carbs/sugar intake amount, and post-meal walking steps, then you may use this equation to calculate your GH.p-Modulus:

GH.p-Modulus = ((0.97*FPG) + (post-meal k-steps*5)) / (Carbs&sugar amount)

(2) If you don't have your data stored, then you may apply the following suggestions: *If your diabetes conditions is moderate (HbA1C ~7.0 & glucose ~150 mg/dL), then use 1.8 to 2.2 for your GH.p-Modulus; and if your diabetes conditions is more serious (HbA1C >8.0 & glucose >180 mg/dL), then use 2.5 to 3.3 for your GH.p-Modulus.*

(3) Normally, the GH.p-Modulus should be within 1.5 to 2.5; however, *if you want to be more conservative in predicting your PPG, then you may use the GH.p-Modulus greater than 3.0 in the following equation:*

Predicted PPG = (0.97 * FPG) + (GH.p-Modulus * carbs& sugar) - (post-meal walking k-steps * 5)

References:

1. Hsu, Gerald C., eclaireMD Foundation, USA, No. 310: "Biomedical research methodology based on GH-Method: math-physical medicine"

2. Hsu, Gerald C., eclaireMD Foundation, USA, No. 345: "Application of linear equations to predict sensor and finger based postprandial plasma glucoses and daily glucoses for pre-virus, virus, and total periods using GH-Method: math-physical medicine"

3. Hsu, Gerald C., eclaireMD Foundation, USA, No. 97: "A simplified yet accurate linear equation of PPG prediction model for T2D patients (GH-Method: math-physical medicine)"

4. Hsu, Gerald C., eclaireMD Foundation, USA, No. 99: "Application of linear equation-based PPG prediction model for four T2D clinic cases (GH-Method: math-physical medicine)"

5. Hsu, Gerald C., eclaireMD Foundation, USA, No. 339: "Self-recovery of pancreatic beta cell's insulin secretion based on 10+ years annualized data of food, exercise, weight, and glucose using GH-Method: math-physical medicine)

6. Hsu, Gerald C., eclaireMD Foundation, USA, No. 340: "A neural communication model between brain and internal organs, specifically stomach, liver, and pancreatic beta cells based on PPG waveforms of 131 liquid egg meals and 124 solid egg meals)

7. Hsu, Gerald C., eclaireMD Foundation, USA, No. 349: "Using Math-Physics Medicine to Predict FPG"

8. Hsu, Gerald C., eclaireMD Foundation, USA, No. 264: "Community and Family Medicine via Doctors without distance: Using a simple glucose control card to assist T2D patients in remote rural areas (GH-Method: math-physical medicine)"

9. Hsu, Gerald C., eclaireMD Foundation, USA, No. 346: "Linear relationship between carbohydrates & sugar intake amount and incremental PPG amount via engineering strength of materials using GH-Method: math-physical medicine, Part 1"

10. Hsu, Gerald C., eclaireMD Foundation, USA, No. 349: "Investigation on GH modulus of linear elastic glucose with two diabetes patients data using GH-Method: math-physical medicine, Part 2"

11. Hsu, Gerald C., eclaireMD Foundation, USA, No. 349: "Investigation of GH modulus on the linear elastic glucose behavior based on three diabetes patients' data using the GH-Method: math-physical medicine, Part 3"

12. Hsu, Gerald C., eclaireMD Foundation, USA, No. 356: "Coefficient of GH.f-modulus in the linear elastic fasting plasma glucose behavior study based on health data of three diabetes patients using the GH-Method: math-physical medicine, Part 4"

13. Hsu, Gerald C., eclaireMD Foundation, USA, No. 357: "High accuracy of predicted postprandial plasma glucose using two coefficients of GH.f-modulus and GH.p-modulus from linear elastic glucose behavior theory based on GH-Method: math-physical medicine, Part 5"

14. Hsu, Gerald C., eclaireMD Foundation, USA, No. 358: "Improvement on the prediction accuracy of postprandial plasma glucose using two biomedical coefficients of GH-modulus from linear elastic glucose theory based on GH-Method: math-physical medicine, Part 6"

15. Hsu, Gerald C., eclaireMD Foundation, USA, No. 359: "High glucose predication accuracy of postprandial plasma glucose and fasting plasma glucose during the COVID-19 period using two glucose coefficients of GH-modulus from linear elastic glucose theory based on GH-Method: math-physical medicine, Part 7"

16. Hsu, Gerald C., eclaireMD Foundation, USA, No. 360: "Investigation of two glucose coefficients of GH.f-modulus and GH.p-modulus based on data of 3 clinical cases during COVID-19 period using linear elastic glucose theory of GH-Method: math-physical medicine, Part 8"

17. Hsu, Gerald C., eclaireMD Foundation, USA, No. 361: "Postprandial plasma glucose lower and upper boundary study using two glucose coefficients of GH-modulus from linear elastic glucose theory based on GH-Method: math-physical medicine, Part 9"

18. Hsu, Gerald C., eclaireMD Foundation, USA, No. 362: "Six international clinical cases demonstrating prediction accuracies of postprandial plasma glucoses and suggested methods for improvements using linear elastic glucose theory of GH-Method: math-physical medicine, Part 10"

19. Hsu, Gerald C., eclaireMD Foundation, USA, No. 363: "A special Neuro-communication influences on GH.p-modulus of linear elastic glucose theory based on data from 159 liquid egg and 126 solid egg meals using GH-Method: math-physical medicine, Part 11"

20. Hsu, Gerald C., eclaireMD Foundation, USA, No. 364: "GH.p-modulus study of linear elastic glucose theory based on data from 159 liquid egg meals, 126 solid egg meals, and 2,843 total meals using GH-Method: math-physical medicine, Part 12"

21. Hsu, Gerald C., eclaireMD Foundation, USA, No. 365: "Detailed GH.p-modulus values at 15-minute time intervals for a synthesized sensor PPG waveform of 159 liquid egg meals, and 126 solid egg meals using linear elastic glucose theory of GH-Method: math-physical medicine, Part 13"

22. Hsu, Gerald C., eclaireMD Foundation, USA, No. 367: "A lifestyle medicine model for family medical practices based on 9-years of clinical data including food, weight, glucose, carbs/sugar, and walking using linear elastic glucose theory and GH-Method: math-physical medicine (Part 14)"

23. Hsu, Gerald C., eclaireMD Foundation, USA, No. 369: "GH.p-modulus study during 3 periods using finger-piercing glucoses and linear elastic glucose theory (Part 15) of GH-Method: math-physical medicine"

24. Hsu, Gerald C., eclaireMD Foundation, USA, No. 370: "GH.p-modulus study using both finger and sensor glucoses and linear elastic glucose theory (Part 16) of GH-Method: math-physical medicine (No. 370)

(8/5/18-11/27/20	Finger	Sensor
PPG	113	132
FPG	110	111
Carbs gram	13.6	13.6
Walking k-steps	4.25	4.25
(8/5/18-11/27/20	Finger	Sensor
GH.p (avg. data)	2.0	3.3

Finger	Y2017-2019	Y2020	Y2017-2020
PPG	116	109	114
FPG	116	106	114
Carbs gram	14.3	12.7	13.9
Walking k-steps	4.32	4.37	4.33
Finger	Y2017-2019	Y2020	Y2017-2020
GH.p (avg. data)	1.8	2.2	1.8

Figure 1: The author's case of 3 different time periods and 2 different glucose measuring devices

	Case A	Case B	Case C
Obesity	Male	Female	Young
Diabetes	T2D	T2D	Obesity
Avg. Height (")	69	64	71
BMI	25	27	41
Weight (lbs)	171	155	292
FPG (mg/dL)	101	103	105
GH.f-modulus	0.59	0.66	0.36
Baseline PPG	98	100	102
GH.p-modulus	3.6	2.6	1.0
Carbs/Sugar (g)	12.34	9.81	12.38
Carbs * GH.p	44	26	12

	Case A	Case B	Case C
Carbs/Sugar (g)	12.34	9.81	12.38
Baseline + Carbs	142	125	114
Walking K-steps	4.35	2.13	1.04
- PPG from Walk	-22	-11	-5
Predicted PPG	121	115	109

T2D Patients	Case M1	Case M2	Case U1	Case U2	Case U3	Improved M1	Improved M2
Weight (pound)	150	237	167	157	273	150	200
FPG (mg/dL)	141	137	101	103	105	120	120
GH.f-modulus	0.94	0.58	0.60	0.66	0.38	0.80	0.60
Baseline PPG 9mg/dL)	137	133	98	100	102	116	116
GH.p-modulus	1.4	1.6	3.6	2.6	1.0	1.4	1.6
Carbs/Sugar (standard gram)	15.42	15.35	12.34	9.81	12.38	13.00	13.00
Carbs *GH.p-modulus	22	25	44	26	12	18	21
Walking (standard k-steps)	1.0	2.5	4.4	2.1	1.0	2.5	2.5
T2D Patients	Case M1	Case M2	Case U1	Case U2	Case U3	Improved M1	Improved M2
Predicted PPG	153.4	145.0	120.6	114.8	109.0	122.1	124.7
Measured PPG	153.0	145.6	120.8	113.9	109.9	121.6	123.5
T2D Patients	Case M1	Case M2	Case U1	Case U2	Case U3	Improved M1	Improved M2
Accuracy of Predicted PPG	100%	100%	100%	101%	99%	100%	101%

Figure 2: Clinic cases of 3 US and 2 Myanmar patients

Results of Boundary Analysis	Lower-Bound	Upper-Bound
BMI	25	35
Height (inch)	64	69
Weight (pound)	146	237
FPG (mg/dL)	100	150
GH.f-modulus	0.42	1.03
Baseline PPG 9mg/dL)	97	146
GH.p-modulus	2.0	6.0
Carbs/Sugar (standard gram)	10	25
Carbs/Sugar (extreme gram)	10	50
Carbs *GH.p (standard gram)	20	150
Carbs *GH.p (extreme gram)	20	300
Walking (standard k-steps)	1	4
Walking (extreme k-steps)	1	5
Predicted PPG (standard case)	97	276
Predicted PPG (extreme case)	92	475

	Case 1	Case 2	Case 3	Case 4	Case 5	Case 6	Case 7	Case 8	Case A	Case B	Case C
Gender	Man	Man	Man	Man	Woman	Woman	Woman	Woman	Male	Female	Young
Obesity	No Obesity	No Obesity	Obesity	Obesity	No Obesity	No Obesity	No Obesity	Obesity	No Obesity	No Obesity	Obesity
Diabetes	No Diabetes	Diabetes	No Diabetes	Diabetes	No Diabetes	Diabetes	No Diabetes	Diabetes	Pre-Diabetes	Pre-Diabetes	Pre-Diabetes
Weight (lbs)	169	169	237	237	146	146	204	204	171	195	292
FPG (mg/dL)	100	150	100	150	100	150	100	150	101	103	105
Carbs/Sugar (g)	10	10	15	15	20	20	25	25	12.34	9.81	52.38

	Case 1	Case 2	Case 3	Case 4	Case 5	Case 6	Case 7	Case 8	Case A	Case B	Case C
Predicted PPG (1K)	112	201	122	231	132	261	142	291	121	115	109
Predicted PPG (2K)	107	196	117	226	127	256	137	286	121	115	109
Predicted PPG (4K)	97	186	107	216	117	246	127	276	121	115	109

	Case 1	Case 2	Case 3	Case 4	Case 5	Case 6	Case 7	Case 8	Case A	Case B	Case C
Predicted PPG (2.3K)	105	194	115	224	125	254	135	284	121	115	109

	Case 1	Case 2	Case 3	Case 4	Case 5	Case 6	Case 7	Case 8	Case A	Case B	Case C
GH.f-modulus	0.6	0.9	0.4	0.6	0.7	1.0	0.5	0.7	0.59	0.66	0.36
GH.p-modulus	2.0	6.0	2.0	6.0	2.0	6.0	3.0	6.0	3.6	3.6	1.0

Figure 3: 8 Hypothetical standard cases to study upper-bound and lower-bound of GH.p-Modulus

Total: 5/5/2018-11/7/2020	Meals:	159	126	2843	2843
	The Author	Liquid Eggs	Solid Eggs	All Meals - Sensor	All Meals -Finger
	GH.f-modulus (%)	59	64	64	64
	Sensor FPG (mg/dL)	100	109	110	110
Formula	Weight (pound)	170	172	171	171
= FPG / Weight	GH.f-modulus	0.59	0.64	0.64	0.64
= 0.97 * Weight * GH.f-modulus	Baseline PPG (mg/dL)	97	106	106	106
	GH.p-modulus	12.7	20.7	3.4	2.1
	Carbs&Sugar (gram)	2.8	2.2	13.8	13.8
	Carbs *GH.p-modulus	35	46	46	28
	Walking (k-steps)	4.2	4.7	4.3	4.3
= Baseline+Carbs*GH.p-Walk*5	Predicted PPG	111.3	128.3	131.0	113.0
	Measured PPG (mg/dL)	111.3	128.3	131.0	113.0
= Predicted PPG / Measured PPG	Accuracy of Predicted PPG	100%	100%	100%	100%
	The Author	Liquid Eggs	Solid Eggs	All Meals - Sensor	All Meals -Finger
	Carbs&Sugar (gram)	2.8	2.2	13.8	13.8
= predcted PPG - Baseline PPG + K-steps*5	Incremental PPG (mg/dL)	35.4	45.6	46.3	28.3
= Incremental PPG / Carbs&Sugar	GH.p-modulus	12.7	20.7	3.4	2.1

Figure 4: Special case of quite high GH.p-Modulus values from 285 egg experimental meals to demonstrate the brain and neuro-scientific influences on GH.p-Modulus

Using Candlestick Charting Techniques to Investigate Glucose Behaviors using GH-Method: Math-Physical Medicine (No.76)

Gerald C. Hsu
eclaireMD Foundation, USA

Introduction:

This paper describes investigation results of glucose behaviors based on both finger and sensor data using candlestick charting techniques.

Method:

A Japanese merchant, who traded in the rice market in Osaka, Japan, started the candlestick charting around 1850. An American, Steve Nison brought the candlestick patterns to the Western world in 1991. These techniques are largely used in today's stock market to predict the price direction or action.

On 4/17/2018, the author had an idea to study glucose behavior by using the candlestick chart (aka "K-Line") and subsequently developed a customized software to analyze his big glucose data. The analogies between fluctuations of stock price and glucose value are as follows:

(1) Stock prices are closely related to the psychology of the buyer/seller, which is similar to the glucoses related to a patient's behavior psychology.
(2) When there are more buyers than sellers, the price goes up, which is similar to the glucose value rising when carbs/sugar intake (buyer) increases.
(3) When there are more sellers than buyers, price goes down, which is similar to the glucose value decreasing when exercise (seller) increases.

During the period of 5/5/2018 through 5/7/2019, the author collected 26,886 glucose data via a sensor placed on his upper left arm (Figure 1: 73.06 measurements/day). He defined (OHLC) open value as his recorded glucose at 7:00, closed value at 23:30, lowest glucose within a day as the minimum value, highest as the maximum value, and average glucose as the daily average value of ~73 recorded data. Based on these 368 candlestick bars, glucose patterns and moving trends can be observed and analyzed through further mathematical and statistical operations. Finally, he interpreted these operational results with his acquired knowledge of biomedical phenomena in order to discover some hidden medical truth and potential health dangers.

Since the stock market is much more lucrative than the medical research field, it attracts more talented mathematicians and engineers to work in the financial industry. As a result, the author decided to import the candlestick techniques and apply them to his medical research activities in order to learn and gain from other intellectuals' knowledge and experiences.

Results:

Here are some of his research findings:

(1) The sensor-monitor data fluctuate between a band of 50 to 250 mg/dL, while the finger-piercing data fluctuate between a band of 96 to 136 mg/dL. The finger data covers a mere 20% range of sensor area (Figure 2: bottom portion of 23% to 43%). This means that the existing finger-piercing glucose testing results cover only the

lower half of the sensor collected data range which will miss many of the glucose spikes.

(2) By using segmentation pattern analysis (Figure 3 & 4), further calculations have revealed that on the high glucose segment, 31.2% of the total glucose data are above 140 mg/dL (with an average glucose of 160 mg/dL, equal to A1C>7.2%, diabetes) and 4.5% of the total glucose data are above 180 mg/dL (with an average glucose of 199 mg/dL, equal to A1C>8.5% severe T2D). These high glucose values are the source of diabetes induced complications such as heart attack, stroke, thyroid and kidney issues, eye and foot problems.

(3) On the low glucose segment, there are 0.2% of the total data below 70 mg/dL with an average glucose of 65 mg/dL. These low glucose values could cause life-threatening conditions from insulin shock. Fortunately, the author has been careful on controlling his low glucose conditions, especially during sleeping hours at night.

(4) Average FPG (average value between open and close values) is lower than the daytime's average glucose (summation of 3 PPG periods and glucose data between meals).

(5) This paper presents partial analysis results based on a candlestick chart over 368 days period. Future detailed glucose analysis of candlestick bars within a day (i.e. "intraday" analysis) would reveal more information regarding the glucose moving trend and detailed patterns within a day.

Conclusion:

This paper has further demonstrated the power of observation of the glucose phenomena, derivation of mathematical equations, application of various computational tools, and finally combined with biomedical interpretations to discover and predict more biomedical findings regarding the human body.

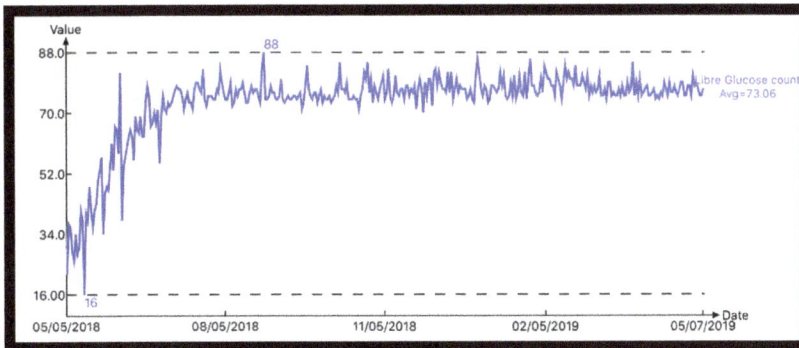

Figure 1: Sensor glucose measurements per day

535

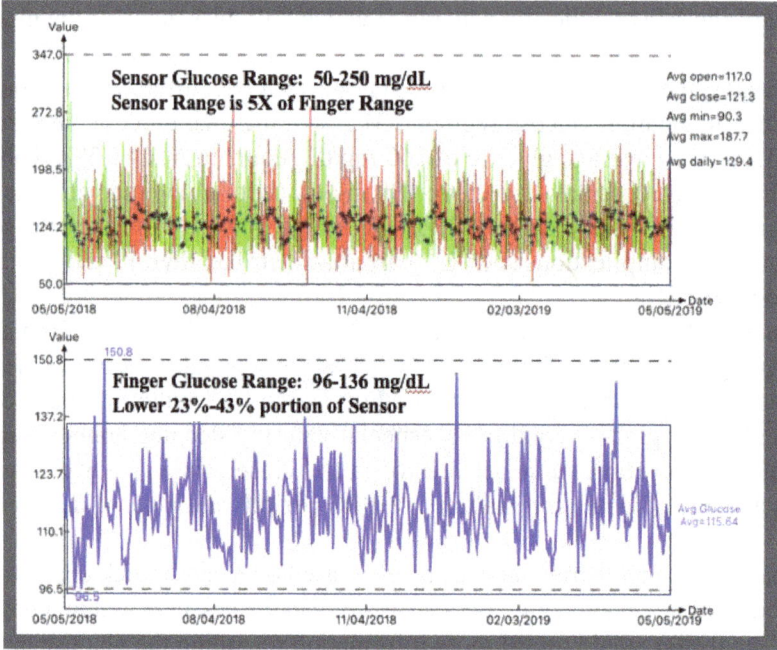

Figure 2: Finger-piercing glucose data are located at lower half of Sensor-based glucose data range

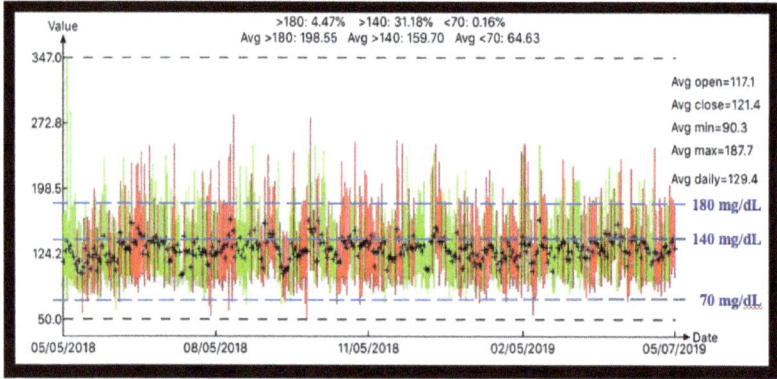

Figure 3: Candlestick chart of daily sensor-based glucose data

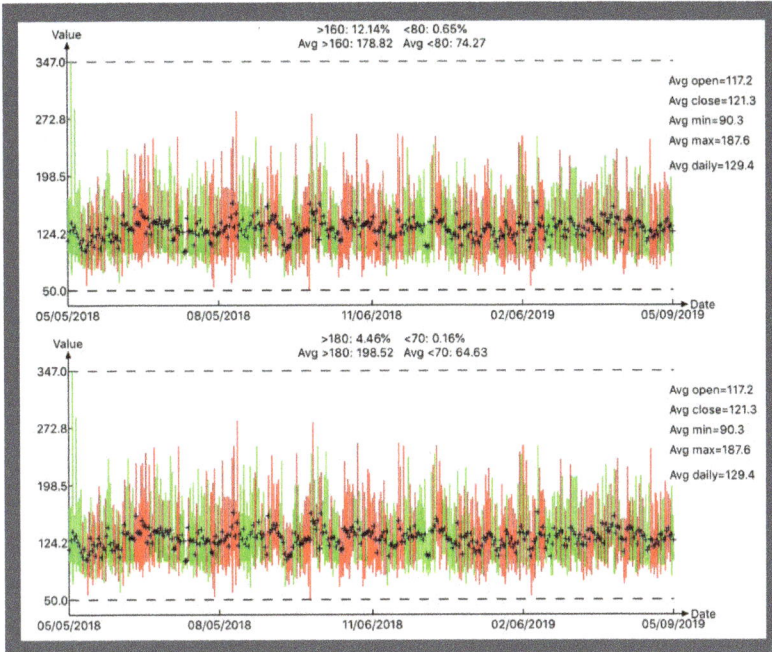

Figure 4: Segmented Sensor Candlestick Glucose

www.ingramcontent.com/pod-product-compliance
Lightning Source LLC
Chambersburg PA
CBHW072006230326
41598CB00082B/6810